COLOR ATLAS AND SYNOPSIS
OF ELECTROPHYSIOLOGY

NOTICE

COLOR ATLAS AND SYNOPSIS OF ELECTROPHYSIOLOGY

EDITORS

Emile G. Daoud, MD, FACC, FHRS

Professor, Internal Medicine

Section Chief, Cardiac Electrophysiology

Ross Heart Hospital

The Ohio State University Wexner Medical Center

Columbus, Ohio

Steven J. Kalbfleisch, MD, FACC, FHRS

Professor, Internal Medicine

Medical Director, Cardiac Electrophysiology Laboratory

Ross Heart Hospital

The Ohio State University Wexner Medical Center

Columbus, Ohio

SERIES EDITOR

William T. Abraham, MD, FACP, FACC, FAHA, FESC

Professor of Medicine, Physiology, and Cell Biology

Chair of Excellence in Cardiovascular Medicine

Director, Division of Cardiovascular Medicine

Deputy Director, Davis Heart and Lung Research Institute

The Ohio State University

Columbus, Ohio

New York   Chicago   San Francisco   Athens   London   Madrid   Mexico City
Milan   New Delhi   Singapore   Sydney   Toronto

Color Atlas and Synopsis of Electrophysiology

1 2 3 4 5 6 7 8 9 0 CTP/CTP 18 17 16 15

ISBN 978-0-07-178626-3
MHID 0-07-178626-0

This book was set in Perpetua by Cenveo Publisher Services.
The editors were Sarah Henry and Christie Naglieri.
The production supervisor was Richard Ruzycka.
Project management was provided by Kritika Kaushik, Cenveo® Publisher Services.
The cover designer was Thomas De Pierro.
CTPS was the printer and binder.

Library of Congress Cataloging-in-Publication Data

Color atlas and synopsis of electrophysiology/[edited by] Emile Daoud, Steven Kalbfleisch.
      p. ; cm.
   Includes bibliographical references and index.
   ISBN 978-0-07-178626-3 (hardcover) -- ISBN 0-07-178626-0 (hardcover)
   I. Daoud, Emile G., editor.   II. Kalbfleisch, Steven Jack, editor.
   [DNLM: 1. Electrophysiologic Techniques, Cardiac—Atlases.
2. Electrophysiologic Techniques, Cardiac—Case Reports.   3. Arrhythmias, Cardiac—diagnosis—Atlases.   4. Arrhythmias, Cardiac—diagnosis—Case Reports.   5. Arrhythmias, Cardiac—therapy—Atlases.   6. Arrhythmias, Cardiac—therapy—Case Reports.   7. Cardiac Resynchronization Therapy Devices—Atlases.   8. Cardiac Resynchronization Therapy Devices—Case Reports.   9. Catheter Ablation—methods—Atlases.   10. Catheter Ablation—methods—Case Reports. WG 17]
  QP341
  612'.01427—dc23
                    2014023699

McGraw-Hill Education books are available at special quantity discounts to use as premiums and sales promotions or for use in corporate training programs. To contact a representative, please visit the Contact Us pages at www.mhprofessional.com.

DEDICATION

We wish to extend our thanks and appreciation to our families for tolerating the hours of training and practice that are required to work in this evolving field. Also, we wish to thank Dr. Fred Morady for his guidance and mentorship during our training and early careers and for still providing insight when needed.

Emile G. Daoud, MD, FACC, FHRS
Steven J. Kalbfleisch, MD, FACC, FHRS

CONTENTS

Nazem Akoum, MD, MS
Comprehensive Arrhythmia Research & Management Center
University of Utah Health Sciences Center
Division of Cardiovascular Medicine
Section of Cardiac Electrophysiology
Salt Lake City, Utah

Sana M. Al-Khatib, MD, MHS
Duke Clinical Research Institute and Department of Medicine
Duke University School of Medicine
Durham, North Carolina

Roi Altit, MD
Fellow, Cardiovascular Diseases
Lankenau Heart Institute
Wynnewood, Pennsylvania

Anish Amin, MD
The Ohio State University
Division of Cardiovascular Medicine
Davis Heart and Lung Research Institute
Columbus, Ohio

Laura Arbour, MD, FRCPC
Department of Medical Genetics
University of British Columbia, Island Medical Program
Victoria, British Columbia, Canada

Khaled Awad, MD
Assistant Professor
Division of Cardiac Electrophysiology,
Birmingham School of Medicine, University of Alabama
Birmingham, Alabama

Yousef Bader, MD
Fellow in Clinical Cardiac Electrophysiology
Tufts Medical Center
Boston, Massachusetts

Nitish Badhwar, MBBS
Cardiac Electrophysiology Section, Division of Cardiology
University of California, San Francisco, School of Medicine
San Francisco, California

Rong Bai, MD
Texas Cardiac Arrhythmia Institute
St. David's Medical Center
Austin, TX

Chirag Barbhaiya, MD
Brigham and Women's Electrophysiology Division of Cardiology
Brigham and Women's Hospital
Boston, Massachusetts

Conor Barrett, MD
Al-Sabah Arrhythmia Institute
St. Luke's Hospital
New York, New York

Richard Bayer II, MD
Medical University of South Carolina
Charleston, South Carolina

Peter H. Belott, MD, FACC, FHRS
Sharp Grossmont Hospital
La Mesa, California

David G. Benditt, MD
Cardiac Arrhythmia and Syncope Center, Cardiovascular Division
Department of Medicine, University of Minnesota Medical School
Minneapolis, Minnesota

Benjamin Berte, MD
Hôpital Cardiologique du Haut-Lévêque
Bordeaux-Pessac, France

Luigi Di Biase MD, PhD, FACC, FHRS
Albert Einstein College of Medicine
Montefiore Hospital
New York, New York

Dan Blendea, MD
Cardiac Arrhythmia Service and Cardiac Unit
Massachusetts General Hospital
Boston, Massachusetts

Frank Bogun, MD
Division of Cardiology
University of Michigan Medical Center
Ann Arbor, Michigan

S. Mark Borganelli, MD
University of Mississippi Medical Center
Jackson, Mississippi

J. Michael Boyd, PharmD, BCPS
Specialty Practice Pharmacist, Cardiology
Richard M. Ross Heart Hospital
The Ohio State University Wexner Medical Center
Columbus, Ohio

Pedro Brugada, MD
Heart Rhythm Management Center, Cardiovascular Division
UZ Brussel, Vrije Universiteit Brussel
Brussels, Belgium

J. David Burkhardt, MD
Albert Einstein College of Medicine
Montefiore Hospital
New York, New York

Alfred E. Buxton, MD
Professor of Medicine
Harvard Medical School
Director of the Clinical Electrophysiology Laboratory
Beth Israel Deaconess Medical Center
Boston, Massachusetts

Hugh Calkins, MD
Division of Cardiology
Johns Hopkins University School of Medicine
Baltimore, Maryland

CONTRIBUTORS

David J. Callans, MD
Professor of Medicine, University of Pennsylvania
Department of Cardiology
Hospital of the University of Pennsylvania
Philadelphia, Pennsylvania

Shawn Campbell, MEM
Medical College of Virginia
Richmond, Virginia

Ruben Casado-Arroyo, MD
Heart Rhythm Management Center, Cardiovascular Division,
UZ Brussel, Vrije Universiteit Brussel
Brussels, Belgium

Aman Chugh, MD, FACC, FHRS
Associate Professor of Medicine
Section of Cardiac Electrophysiology
University of Michigan Ann Arbor, Michigan

Edmond M. Cronin, MB BCh BAO
Interventional Electrophysiology
Henry Low Heart Center Hartford Hospital
Hartford, Connecticut

Stephan Danik, MD
Al-Sabah Arrhythmia Institute
St. Luke's Hospital
New York, New York

Emile G. Daoud, MD, FACC, FHRS
Professor, Internal Medicine
Section Chief, Cardiac Electrophysiology
Ross Heart Hospital
The Ohio State University Wexner Medical Center
Columbus, Ohio

Barry LS Detloff, BS
Cardiac Arrhythmia and Syncope Center, Cardiovascular Division
Department of Medicine, University of Minnesota Medical School
Minneapolis, Minnesota

Oana Dickinson, MD
Cardiac Arrhythmia and Syncope Center, Cardiovascular Division
Department of Medicine, University of Minnesota Medical School
Minneapolis, Minnesota

Kenneth A. Ellenbogen, MD, FHRS
Virginia Commonwealth University Medical Center
Medical College of Virginia
Richmond, Virginia

Andrew E. Epstein, MD, FAHA, FACC, FHRS
Professor of Medicine
Electrophysiology Section, Division of Cardiovascular Medicine
University of Pennsylvania
Chief, Cardiology Section
Philadelphia VA Medical Center
Philadelphia, Pennsylvania

Essa Essa, MD
Ross Heart Hospital
The Ohio State University Wexner Medical Center
Columbus, Ohio

N.A. Mark Estes, MD
Director, New England Cardiac Arrhythmia Center
Professor, Tufts University School of Medicine
Tufts Medical Center
Boston, Massachusetts

Gregory K. Feld, MD
Division of Cardiology, Cardiac Electrophysiology Program
Sulpizio Family Cardiovascular Center
University of California, San Diego
La Jolla, California

Sunita J Ferns MD, MRCPCH
Assistant Professor of Pediatrics
Director, Pediatric Invasive Electrophysiology
The University of North Carolina
Chapel Hill, North Carolina

M. Alaric Franzos, MD
Walter Reed National Military Medical Center
Department of Cardiology, Division of Electrophysiology
The F. Edward Hebert School of Medicine
Uniformed Services University
Bethesda, Maryland

Daniel J. Friedman, MD
Cardiac Arrhythmias Service
Massachusetts General Hospital
Boston, Massachusetts

Paul A. Friedman, MD, FACC, FHRS
Professor of Medicine
Mayo Clinic College of Medicine
Rochester, Minnesota

J. Joseph Gallinghouse, MD
Texas Cardiac Arrhythmia Institute
St. David's Medical Center
Austin, Texas

Michael R. Gold, MD, PhD
Director, Division of Cardiology
Medical University of South Carolina
Charleston, South Carolina

Blair P. Grubb, MD, FACC
Professor of Medicine and Pediatrics
Director, Clinical Cardiac Electrophysiology
School of Medicine
Health and Life Science Campus
The University of Toledo
Toledo, Ohio

Haris M. Haqqani, MBBS (Hons), PhD
Senior Lecturer
School of Medicine, University of Queensland
Department of Cardiology
The Prince Charles Hospital
Queensland, Australia

Mark Haigney, MD
Walter Reed National Military Medical Center
Department of Cardiology, Division of Electrophysiology
The F. Edward Hebert School of Medicine
Uniformed Services University
Bethesda, Maryland

Michel Haïssaguerre, MD
Hôpital Cardiologique du Haut-Lévêque
Bordeaux-Pessac, France

Ismail Hamam, MD
Electrophysiology Section
The Ohio State University Wexner Medical Center
Columbus, Ohio

James H. Hamilton, IV, MD
University of Mississippi Medical Center
Jackson, Mississippi

E. Kevin Heist MD, PhD
Cardiac Arrhythmia Service and Cardiac Unit
Massachusetts General Hospital
Boston, Massachusetts

Paul L. Hess, MD
Duke Clinical Research Institute and Department of Medicine
Duke University School of Medicine
Durham, North Carolina

Rodney Horton, MD
Texas Cardiac Arrhythmia Institute
St. David's Medical Center
Austin, Texas

Mahmoud Houmsse, MD, FACP, FACC, FHRS
The Ohio State University Wexner Medical Center
Columbus, Ohio

Patrick Hranitzky, MD
Texas Cardiac Arrhythmia Institute
St. David's Medical Center
Austin, Texas

John D. Hummel, MD
Electrophysiology Section
The Ohio State University Wexner Medical Center
Columbus, Ohio

Pierre Jaïs, MD
Hôpital Cardiologique du Haut-Lévêque
Bordeaux-Pessac, France

Steven Kalbfleisch, MD,FACC,FHRS
Professor, Internal Medicine
Medical Director, Cardiac Electrophysiology Laboratory
Ross Heart Hospital
The Ohio State University Wexner Medical Center
Columbus, Ohio

Jonathan M. Kalman, MBBS, PhD
Department of Cardiology
Royal Melbourne Hospital
University of Melbourne
Melbourne, Australia

Naomi J. Kertesz, MD
Director of Electrophysiology and Pacing
Nationwide Children's Hospital
Associate Professor of Pediatrics
Ohio State University
Columbus, Ohio

Clarence Khoo MD, FRCPC
Assistant Professor of Medicine
Cardiac Sciences Program
University of Manitoba
Winnipeg, Manitoba, Canada

Bradley P. Knight, MD, FACC, FHRS
Director of Cardiac Electrophysiology
Bluhm Cardiovascular Institute of Northwestern University
Professor of Medicine
Feinberg School of Medicine
Northwestern University
Chicago, Illinois

Matthias Koopmann, MD
Comprehensive Arrhythmia Research & Management Center
University of Utah Health Sciences Center
Division of Cardiovascular Medicine
Section of Cardiac Electrophysiology
Salt Lake City, Utah

Andrew Krahn, MD, FRCPC
Division of Cardiology
University of British Columbia
Vancouver, British Columbia, Canada

Rakesh Latchamsetty, MD
Cardiovascular Center
University of Michigan Hospital
Ann Arbor, Michigan

Byron K. Lee, MD
Associate Professor of Medicine
Director of the Electrophysiology Laboratories and Clinics
Cardiac Electrophysiology Section, Division of Cardiology
University of California, San Francisco, School of Medicine
San Francisco, California

Yehoshua C. Levine, MD
Clinical Fellow in Medicine, Harvard Medical School
Clinical Cardiac Electrophysiology Fellow
Beth Israel Deaconess Medical Center
Boston, Massachusetts

Han S. Lim, MBBS, PhD
Université Victor Segalen Bordeaux II
Bordeaux, France

Zhenguo Liu, MD, PhD
Division of Cardiovascular Medicine
Department of Internal Medicine
The Ohio State University Wexner Medical Center
Columbus, Ohio

Malini Madhavan, MBBS
Assistant Professor of Medicine
Mayo Clinic College of Medicine
Rochester, Minnesota

Moussa Mansour, MD
Cardiac Arrhythmia Service and Cardiac Unit
Massachusetts General Hospital
Boston, Massachusetts

Nassir Marrouche, MD
Director, Comprehensive Arrhythmia Research & Management Center
University of Utah Health Sciences Center
Salt Lake City, Utah

Kelly M.W. McDonnell, DO
Medical College of Virginia
Richmond, Virginia

Thomas McGarry, MD
Division of Cardiology, Cardiac Electrophysiology Program
Sulpizio Family Cardiovascular Center
University of California, San Diego
La Jolla, California

Greg Michaud, MD
Director, Center for Advanced Management of Atrial Fibrillation
Brigham and Women's Electrophysiology Division of Cardiology
Assistant Professor of Medicine, Harvard Medical School
Boston, Massachusetts

Agnieszka Mochon, MD
Fellow, Cardiovascular Diseases
Lankenau Heart Institute
Wynnewood, Pennsylvania

Sanghamitra Mohanty, MD
Texas Cardiac Arrhythmia Institute
St. David's Medical Center
Austin, Texas

Fred Morady, MD
Cardiovascular Center
University of Michigan Hospital
Ann Arbor, Michigan

Talal Moukabary, MD
Fellow, Clinical Cardiac Electrophysiology
Penn State College of Medicine
Hershey, Pennsylvania

Brittney Murray, MS
Division of Cardiology
Johns Hopkins University School of Medicine
Baltimore, Maryland

Gerald V. Naccarelli, MD, FHRS
Bernard Trabin Chair in Cardiology
Professor of Medicine
Chief, Division of Cardiology
Penn State College of Medicine
Hershey, Pennsylvania

Koonlawee Nademanee, MD
Director of Pacific Rim Electrophysiology Research Institute
Los Angeles, California and Bangkok, Thailand

Andrea Natale, MD, FHRS, FESC, FACC
Albert Einstein College of Medicine
Montefiore Hospital
New York, New York

Matthew Needleman, MD
Walter Reed National Military Medical Center
Department of Cardiology, Division of Electrophysiology
The F. Edward Hebert School of Medicine
Uniformed Services University
Bethesda, Maryland

Justin Ng, MD
Brigham and Women's Electrophysiology Division of Cardiology
Brigham and Women's Hospital
Boston, Massachusetts

Jeffrey E. Olgin, MD
Cardiac Electrophysiology Section, Division of Cardiology
University of California, San Francisco, School of Medicine,
San Francisco, California

Hakan Oral, MD
Huetwell Professor of Cardiovascular Medicine
Professor of Internal Medicine
Director, Cardiac Arrhythmia Service
University of Michigan
Ann Arbor, Michigan

Rod Passman, MD, MSCE
Professor of Medicine
Northwestern University Feinberg School of Medicine
Bluhm Cardiovascular Institute
Chicago, Illinois

Alessandro Paoletti Perini, MD
Texas Cardiac Arrhythmia Institute
St. David's Medical Center
Austin, Texas

Sean D. Pokorney, MD, MBA
Duke Clinical Research Institute and Department of Medicine
Duke University School of Medicine
Durham, North Carolina

Venkata Krishna Puppala, MD
Cardiac Arrhythmia and Syncope Center, Cardiovascular Division
Department of Medicine, University of Minnesota Medical School
Minneapolis, Minnesota

Farbod Raiszadeh, MD, PhD
Albert Einstein College of Medicine
Montefiore Hospital
New York, New York

Troy Rhodes, MD, PhD, FHRS, CCDS
Assistant Professor of Medicine
Division of Cardiology, Electrophysiology Section
University of Mississippi Medical Center
Jackson, Mississippi

Jorge Romero, MD
Montefiore Medical Center
Albert Einstein College of Medicine
New York, New York

Steven Rothman, MD
Clinical Associate Professor
Lankenau Institute of Medical Research
Chief, Cardiovascular Division
Lankenau Medical Center
Wynnewood, Pennsylvania

Christopher P. Rowley, MD
Medical University of South Carolina
Charleston, South Carolina

Jeremy N. Ruskin, MD
Cardiac Arrhythmia Service and Cardiac Unit
Massachusetts General Hospital
Boston, Massachusetts

Wajeeha Saeed, MD
Albert Einstein College of Medicine
Bronx, New York

Shubhayan Sanatani, MD, FRCPC
Department of Pediatrics
University of British Columbia
Vancouver, British Columbia, Canada

Javier E. Sanchez, MD
Texas Cardiac Arrhythmia Institute
St. David's Medical Center
Austin, Texas

Pasquale Santangeli, MD
Electrophysiology Section
Cardiovascular Division
University of Pennsylvania

Francesco Santoro, MD
Texas Cardiac Arrhythmia Institute
St. David's Medical Center
Austin, Texas

M. Rizwan Sardar, MD
Lankenau Heart Institute
Wynnewood, Pennsylvania

Sharon Shen, MD
Division of Cardiology, Department of Internal Medicine
Feinberg School of Medicine
Northwestern University
Chicago, Illinois

Jagmeet P. Singh, MD, DPhil
Cardiac Arrhythmias Service
Massachusetts General Hospital
Boston, Massachusetts

Mohamad C.N. Sinno, MD
CoDirector, Atrial fibrillation program St. Elizabeth Healthcare
St. Elizabeth Physicians
Edgewood, Kentucky

Melissa J. Snider, PharmD, BCPS, CLS
Specialty Practice Pharmacist, Ambulatory Care
Clinical Assistant Professor, College of Pharmacy
The Ohio State University Wexner Medical Center
Richard M. Ross Heart Hospital
Columbus, Ohio

Amy C. Sturm, MS, LCGC
Associate Professor, Internal Medicine
Division of Human Genetics, Department of Internal Medicine
Dorothy M. Davis Heart and Lung Research Institute
The Ohio State University Wexner Medical Center
Columbus, Ohio

Kevin Thomas, MD
Fellow, Cardiac Electrophysiology
Loyola University Stritch School of Medicine
Maywood, Illinois

Gery F. Tomassoni, MD, FACC, FHRS
Electrophysiologist
Central Baptist Hospital
Lexington, Kentucky

Jose Tores, MD
Ross Heart Hospital
The Ohio State University Wexner Medical Center
Columbus, Ohio

Niraj Varma, MD, PhD, FRCP
Department of Cardiovascular Medicine
Cleveland Clinic
Cleveland, Ohio

CONTRIBUTORS

Tomos Walters, MBBS, BMedSc
Department of Cardiology
Royal Melbourne Hospital
University of Melbourne
Melbourne, Australia

Kristel Wauters, MD
Heart Rhythm Management Center, Cardiovascular Division,
UZ Brussel, Vrije Universiteit Brussel
Brussels, Belgium

Erich F. Wedam, MD
Walter Reed National Military Medical Center
Department of Cardiology, Division of Electrophysiology
The F. Edward Hebert School of Medicine
Uniformed Services University
Bethesda, Maryland

Raul Weiss, MD
Professor, Internal Medicine
Ross Heart Hospital
The Ohio State University Wexner Medical Center
Columbus, Ohio

David J. Wilber, MD
Director of Cardiology and Professor of Medicine
Loyola University Stritch School of Medicine
Maywood, Illinois

Bruce L. Wilkoff, MD
Director, Cardiac Pacing and Tachyarrhythmia Devices
Department of Cardiovascular Medicine
Professor of Medicine
Cleveland Clinic Lerner College of Medicine of Case Western
Reserve University
Cleveland, Ohio

Jeffrey R. Winterfield, MD
Clinical Electrophysiologist and Assistant Professor of Medicine
Loyola University Medical Center
Maywood, Illinois

Kar-Lai Wong, MD, FACC
Lankenau Heart Institute
Wynnewood, Pennsylvania

Within the field of cardiology the subspecialty of cardiovascular electrophysiology has been one of the most dynamic and rapidly evolving subspecialties over the last few decades. The electrophysiology laboratory has gone from being a place where only diagnostic testing was performed to a place where therapeutic interventions, often curative, are now routinely accomplished. This evolution from a diagnostic to therapeutic laboratory has been driven primarily by parallel advancements in the fields of both implantable devices and ablation therapies.

As an example, advances in device technology have allowed the implantable defibrillator to go from being a large device placed in the abdominal wall and requiring a thoracotomy for placement to being a small device placed prepectorally and performed transvenously. Along with the technological advancements in the defibrillator came a paradigm shift in the use of the device. Defibrillator therapy went from being used exclusively for secondary prevention of sudden death to being a cornerstone for primary prevention of sudden death in high-risk patient groups. This change in the indications for defibrillator implantation led to an explosion in the use of this technology across a wide range of disease subgroups. Advances in pacing therapy along with a better understanding of the role of dyssynchrony in heart failure have led to a synergy between the heart failure specialist and the electrophysiologist in treating heart failure patients with resynchronization pacing therapy. Some of the most significant advancements in the field of electrophysiology for both treatment and a mechanistic understanding of arrhythmias have come from the evolution of ablation therapy. This is now considered first-line therapy for many arrhythmias and is quickly becoming a mainstay of treatment for some of our most challenging arrhythmias such as atrial fibrillation and ventricular tachycardia in structural heart disease. The ablation procedure has gone from a relatively simple fluoroscopy-based procedure to one that now often incorporates three-dimensional electroanatomical mapping and advanced preprocedural cardiac imaging.

With all of these advances it has been challenging, even for the electrophysiologist, to keep up with the latest technologies and the indications for the use of these technologies. The purpose of this book is to use a case-based approach to help the general cardiologist and electrophysiologist better understand the basics of electrophysiology, the clinical approach to managing arrhythmia syndromes, and when and how to use some of the latest technologies for treating the arrhythmia patient.

The editors would like to thank the authors who contributed their time and expertise to make the chapters possible and Ms. Sherri Artis for her assistance in organizing the compilation of these chapters for the book. We both wish to thank our families for tolerating the hours of training and practice that are required to work in this evolving field. We also wish to thank Dr. Fred Morady for his guidance and mentorship during our training and early careers and for still providing insight when needed.

Emile G. Daoud, MD, FACC, FHRS
Steven J. Kalbfleisch, MD, FACC, FHRS

DIAGNOSTIC ELEC-TROPHYSIOLOGY—MAPPING, IMAGING, AND PACING MANEUVERS

1 ABLATION OF VENTRICULAR TACHYCARDIA USING CARTO 3-DIMENSIONAL ELECTROANATOMICAL MAPPING SYSTEM

Kevin Thomas, MD, David J. Wilber, MD,
Jeffrey R. Winterfield, MD

CASE PRESENTATION

An 83-year-old woman with a history of coronary artery disease, ischemic cardiomyopathy, atrial fibrillation, diabetes mellitus, and hypertension presented to clinic for evaluation of recurrent ventricular tachycardia (VT). The patient has a biventricular pacing defibrillator (ICD), initially placed for primary prevention 6 years earlier, and there were no detected ventricular arrhythmias until approximately 6 months prior to presenting when she had a first episode of sustained VT, postoperatively after hip surgery. She has since had multiple episodes of VT requiring ICD therapies (both antitachycardia pacing as well as shock) despite treatment with dual antiarrhythmic medications (sotalol and mexiletine). Her past surgical history includes two coronary artery bypass surgeries as well as a bioprosthetic mitral valve replacement. Her echocardiogram revealed an ejection fraction of 20% with basal inferior aneurysm and akinetic inferior and infero-lateral walls.

The patient was admitted to the hospital for antiarrhythmic drug washout in preparation for VT ablation. On the evening prior to the scheduled procedure, she had a spontaneous episode of her clinical VT, which was of right bundle morphology with a superior axis and positive concordance across the precordium at a cycle length of 370 ms, which was successfully terminated with internal defibrillation from her ICD.

The following day the patient was brought to the electrophysiology lab. Programmed stimulation was performed to assess electrophysiologic properties of the ventricles and for arrhythmia induction.

Using the CARTO 3-dimensional electroanatomical mapping system (Biosense Webster, Diamond Bar, CA), mapping was performed in the left ventricle both in sinus rhythm and after induction of tachycardia.

BACKGROUND

The mechanism of VT in the presence of coronary artery disease and prior myocardial infarction is reentry within the scar and the border between infarcted and normal tissue (border zone). The surface QRS morphology of the VT is generated by the reentrant wavefront exiting the scar at a distinct site or sites along the border zone and can be used to localize the site of origin.[1] Areas within the scar that are critical to the reentrant circuit are marked by channels of slow conduction that are protected by areas of functional or anatomic conduction block.[2–4] Isolated and late potentials seen in areas of scar during sinus rhythm indicate the presence of surviving myocyte fiber bundles

that are a necessary component of these critical isthmuses.[5] Targets for ablation include these critical isthmuses within the scar as well as identified exit sites along the scar border. Identification of these targets rely upon the ability to accurately map (1) areas of scar, dense scar, and border zone, (2) sites within the scar and scar border that have abnormal local electrical activity, and (3) the channels of slow conduction within scar that are participating in the reentrant circuit. This can be performed with a combination of substrate, entrainment, and pace-mapping.

Electroanatomical Mapping

Three-dimensional anatomical mapping has been utilized for over a decade to aid in mapping and ablation of a wide variety of arrhythmias, including VT.[6–8] In addition to constructing accurate chamber anatomy and allowing the operator to view real-time catheter position and movement, the ability to display visual representations of myocardial substrate and arrhythmia propagation has revolutionized the way substrate, activation, and entrainment mapping are performed and interpreted. Newer features include the ability to automatically compare and evaluate paced morphologies to a stored template for more accurate pace-mapping.

The CARTO 3-D electroanatomical mapping system utilizes ultra-low intensity magnetic fields emitted from nine coils placed beneath the table. A sensor in the catheter tip senses the strength each of the magnetic fields, which decay as a function of distance from the emitting coil. Using this information, the position of the tip of catheter in space can be triangulated and then visually represented on a computer screen in real time. The ability to know the precise spatial location of the catheter(s) with the CARTO 3-D system has been shown to be associated with reductions in procedure time, fluoroscopy time, and radiofrequency energy delivery time when compared to non–3-dimensional mapping systems as well as other commercially available 3-dimensional mapping systems that utilize a current-based, rather than magnetic-based, localization system.[9]

DIAGNOSIS

In our patient, programmed stimulation resulted in two distinct hemodynamically stable monomorphic VT (Figure 1-1A and B).

- VT1: Induced with triple extrastimuli from right ventricular catheter, had a right bundle, right superior morphology with abrupt loss precordial pattern between V_2–V_3 and a CL = 430 ms.
- VT2: Right bundle, right inferior with late (V_6) precordial transition and a CL = 460 ms. Initially seen after pace termination of VT1 but later was able to be induced with double extrastimuli.

MANAGEMENT

Substrate Mapping

Substrate mapping was then performed during sinus rhythm (Figure 1-2) using a 2-mm tip mapping catheter (NOGA). Standard bipolar voltage criteria for identification of scar were used based on clinically accepted norms[10]: >1.5mV represented normal tissue, 0.5mV to 1.5mV represented scar border zone, and <0.5mV represented dense scar. However, recent in vivo imaging data suggest scar distribution identified by gadolinium delayed enhancement, while generally in agreement with clinical criteria, may be more variable.[11]

ABLATION OF VENTRICULAR TACHYCARDIA USING
CARTO 3-DIMENSIONAL ELECTROANATOMICAL
MAPPING SYSTEM

SECTION I
DIAGNOSTIC ELECTROPHYSIOLOGY—
MAPPING, IMAGING, AND
PACING MANEUVERS

3

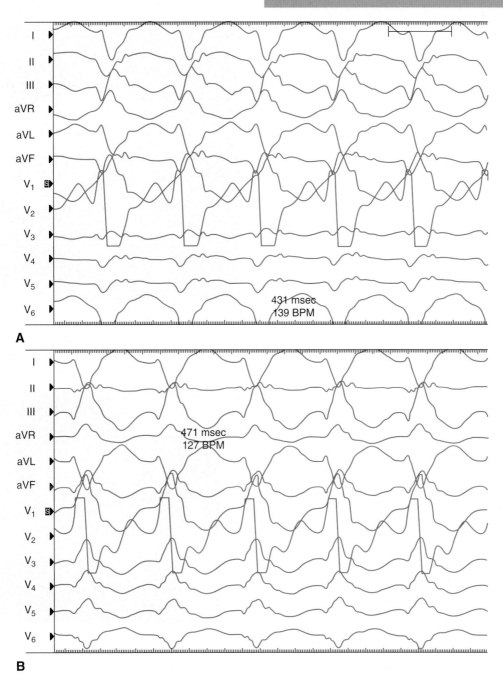

FIGURE 1-1 Monomoprhic VTs induced with programmed stimulation. VT1 (A) and VT2 (B).

A total of 440 endocardial sites were sampled with a total LV chamber volume of 226 cc. A large, dense inferior wall scar representing 41.1% of the total myocardium was seen with a basal inferior wall aneurysm. Areas of late potentials were identified and tagged both at the scar border as well as in the scar itself (Figure 1-3).

Pace-Mapping

Pace-mapping using CARTO-3 Paso Module for automated comparison of paced morphology to stored template was then performed at previously identified sites of late potentials within the scar and along the scar border. Sites of excellent pace-maps (correlation >90%) were tagged (Figure 1-5A). Each of our encountered VT had excellent pace-map matches at various sites in and around the previously defined scar.

- VT1: Pace-mapped to a site of previously identified late potentials at the scar border zone on the lateral side of the midinferior wall (Figures 1-4A and 1-4B).

- VT2: Pace-mapped to a site of late potentials along the scar border on the inferolateral free wall as well as to a site of late potentials within the dense scar (Figure 1-6A) where there was a long (109 ms) pacing stimulus to QRS duration.

Entrainment Mapping and Ablation

Entrainment mapping is used to characterize the reentrant circuit[4,12] and identify a protected isthmus critical to the maintenance of the tachycardia that can be targeted for ablation.

Characteristics of entrainment at a particular site that are predictive of success of ablation include:

1. Concealed fusion: entrained QRS identical to tachycardia QRS

2. Postpacing interval minus tachycardia cycle length difference (PPI-TCL) ± 30 msec

3. When pacing from the site, the stimulus to QRS duration of >60 msec

4. Ratio of stimulus-to-QRS duration to TCL of <0.7

5. Stimulus-to-QRS to the local electrogram recorded from the catheter during VT-to-QRS difference ± 10 msec.[5,13]

Tachycardia was reinduced in our patient via programmed stimulation, and entrainment mapping was performed. Entrainment of VT1 near the previously identified site of best pace-map match was concealed with a short postpacing interval minus tachycardia cycle length difference (PPI-TCL). Radiofrequency ablation at this site terminated the tachycardia (Figures 1-6A and 1-6B).

Following ablation of VT1, programmed stimulation was again performed and resulted in induction of clinical VT2. Pace-mapping at sites with previously identified late potentials revealed a site in dense scar with an excellent match to the VT2 QRS morphology, and long S-QRS interval (Figure 1-5A). Of interest, a similar match was identified at a site on the lateral scar border, with a short S-QRS interval, indicating the exit of the circuit from scar to normal myocardium (Figure 1-5B). These findings are compatible with an anatomically fixed pathway. Entrainment from the site within dense scar was consistent with a critical isthmus site. Ablation at this site terminated the VT (Figures 1-7A and 1-7B).

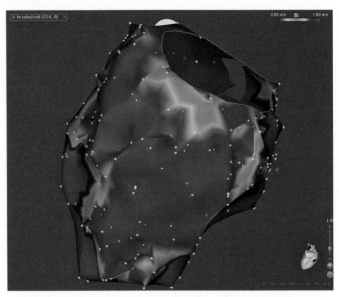

FIGURE 1-2 Substrate map of LV (PA projection) created using CARTO 3-D electroanatomical mapping system (Biosense Webster, Diamond Bar, CA) showing large inferior scar.

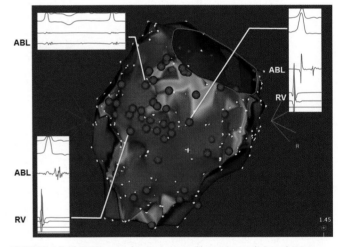

FIGURE 1-3 CARTO map showing tagged late potentials (purple). Inset: Intracardiac electrograms showing three distinct late potential appearances from three separate areas of the scar/scar border. Ablation catheter recording marked with ABL; RV catheter recording marked with RV.

ABLATION OF VENTRICULAR TACHYCARDIA USING
CARTO 3-DIMENSIONAL ELECTROANATOMICAL
MAPPING SYSTEM

SECTION I
DIAGNOSTIC ELECTROPHYSIOLOGY—
MAPPING, IMAGING, AND
PACING MANEUVERS

5

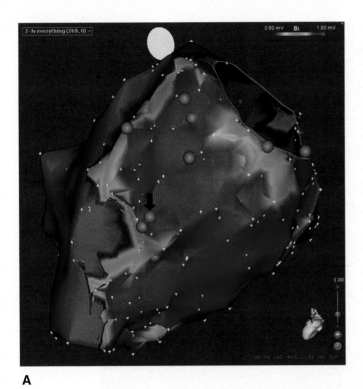

A

FIGURE 1-4A Sites of good pace-maps. Arrow: site of best pace-map match for VT1.

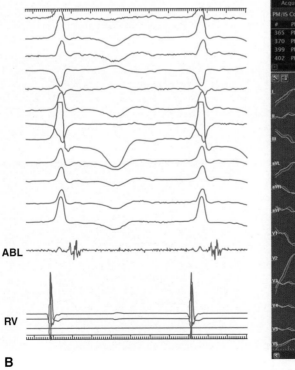

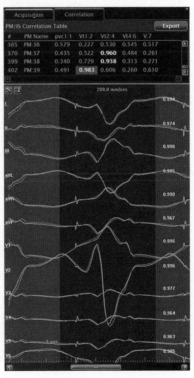

B

FIGURE 1-4B Intracardiac electrogram showing late potential at site near perfect pace-map match for VT1. (Right) PASO comparison of pace-map morphology at this site with stored VT1 template showing >98% match. Green: paced QRS. Yellow: stored VT1 template. Ablation catheter recording marked with ABL; RV catheter recording marked with RV.

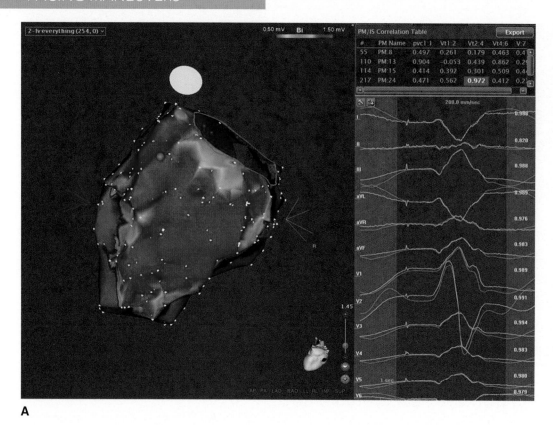

A

FIGURE 1-5A (Left) CARTO map showing site of best pace-map match for VT2, located in dense scar. (Right) PASO comparison of pace-map morphology at this site with stored VT2 template showing >97% match. Note the long S-QRS interval from a site deep within scar. Green: paced QRS. Yellow: stored VT2 template.

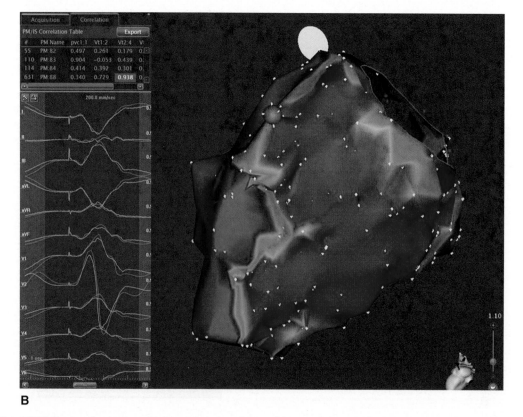

B

FIGURE 1-5B (Right) CARTO map showing excellent pace-map match for VT2, located at the lateral scar border. (Left) PASO comparison of pace-map morphology at site (orange) on lateral scar border to stored VT2 template showing >93% match. Note the shorter S-QRS interval from a site on the scar border compared with the deeper scar site in Figure 1-6A. Green: paced QRS. Yellow: stored VT2 template.

ABLATION OF VENTRICULAR TACHYCARDIA USING
CARTO 3-DIMENSIONAL ELECTROANATOMICAL
MAPPING SYSTEM

SECTION I
DIAGNOSTIC ELECTROPHYSIOLOGY—
MAPPING, IMAGING, AND
PACING MANEUVERS

7

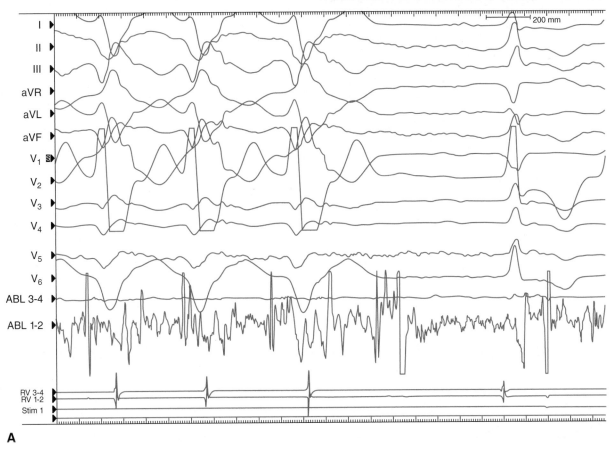

A

FIGURE 1-6A Termination of VT1 during ablation at site that demonstrates late potential in sinus rhythm and near perfect pace-map. Entrainment from this site in VT appeared concealed with a short PPI-TCL.

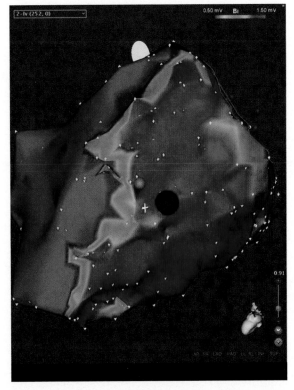

FIGURE 1-6B CARTO map showing relationship of best pace-map site (orange) to site of termination during ablation (green).

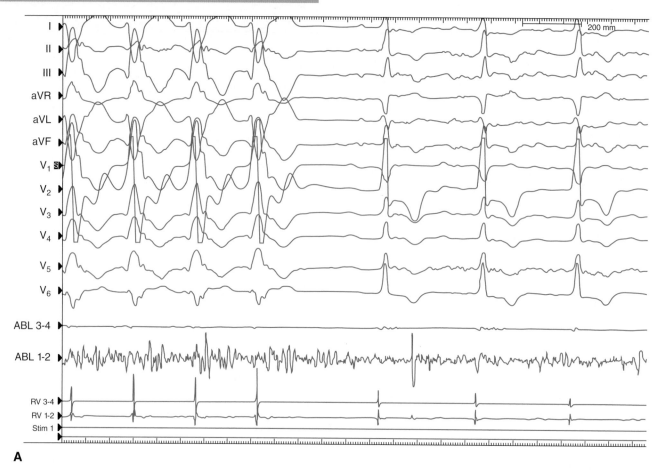

A

FIGURE 1-7A Termination of VT2 with ablation from site of entrainment in dense scar.

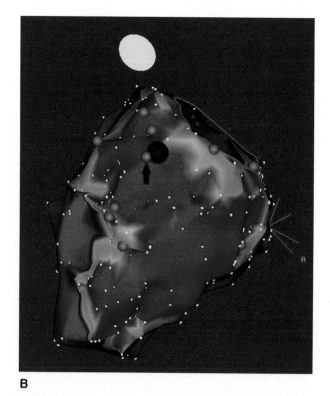

B

FIGURE 1-7B CARTO map showing relationship of site of best pace-map match for VT2 (orange, arrow) within scar to site of termination (green) for VT2.

ABLATION OF VENTRICULAR TACHYCARDIA USING
CARTO 3-DIMENSIONAL ELECTROANATOMICAL
MAPPING SYSTEM

SECTION I
DIAGNOSTIC ELECTROPHYSIOLOGY—
MAPPING, IMAGING, AND
PACING MANEUVERS

9

FOLLOW-UP

Further programmed stimulation failed to induce any sustained VT. Ablation was then performed at previously marked sites of good pace-maps as well as at sites of late potentials along the scar border (Figure 1-8). An approach to eliminate sites where local abnormal ventricular activity is present during sinus or paced rhythm has been shown to improve outcomes in substrate-based ablations when compared to the endpoint of noninducibility alone.[14] Since the initial ablation, the patient has been free of VT for 3 months without the aid of antiarrhythmic drug therapy.

CONCLUSION

Ventricular tachycardia as a result of prior myocardial infarction is associated with significant morbidity and can have profound effects on quality of life. Healed scar and the border zone between scar and normal tissue presents the necessary substrate for reentrant VT in this group of patients. Ablation targets include protected critical isthmuses of slow conduction within the scar as well as the exit sites near the scar border. Target sites can be identified by a variety of techniques, including identification and tagging of late and/or isolated potentials, entrainment mapping, and pace-mapping. Depending on the specific clinical presentation and tachycardia characteristics, a combination of these techniques, as illustrated by this case, may best facilitate optimal outcomes.

Three-dimensional electroanatomical mapping has become an essential tool in VT ablation because of its ability to (1) accurately construct chamber geometry, (2) delineate scar topography, (3) provide a spatial anatomic template on which relevant physiologic features of electrical activation during sinus rhythm and multiple tachycardias can displayed, analyzed, and compared, and (4) track the location of ablation lesions relative to critical anatomy and physiology previously identified. By providing real-time catheter position and navigation, these systems help minimize radiation exposure to both patient and operator. Newer advancements, including multi-electrode mapping and qualitative ablation lesion evaluation, promise to further enhance the mapping and ablation of a wide variety of cardiac arrhythmias, including VT.

In our case, the CARTO 3-dimensional electroanatomical mapping system aided us in accurately defining the location and extent of myocardial scar, identifying and tagging areas of abnormal electrical activity, and quantitatively comparing paced morphologies to our clinical VTs. Each of these features contributed to the performance of an efficient, safe, and ultimately successful ablation.

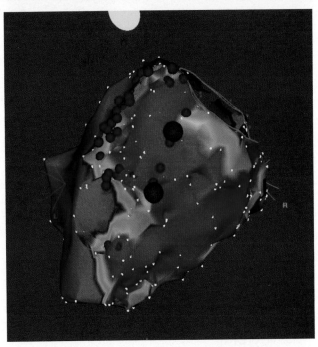

FIGURE 1-8 CARTO map showing full set of ablation lesions (red) as well as sites of termination during ablation (green).

REFERENCES

1. Josephson ME, Callans DJ. Using the twelve-lead electrocardiogram to localize the site of origin of ventricular tachycardia. *Heart Rhythm.* 2005;2(4):443-446.

2. De Chillou C, Lacroix D, Klug D, et al. Isthmus characteristics of ventricular tachycardia after myocardial infarction. *Circulation.* 2002;105(6):726-731.

3. Brunckhorst CB, Stevenson WG, Soejima K, et al. Relationship of slow conduction detected by pace-mapping to ventricular tachycardia re-entry circuit sites after infarction. *J Am Coll Cardiol.* 2003;41:802-809.

4. Stevenson WG, Khan H, Sager P, et al. Identification of reentry circuit sites during catheter mapping and radiofrequency ablation of ventricular tachycardia late after myocardial infarction. *Circulation.* 1993;88:1647-1670.

5. Bogun F, Bahu M, Knight BP, et al. Comparison of effective and ineffective target sites that demonstrate concealed entrainment in patients with coronary artery disease undergoing radiofrequency ablation of ventricular tachycardia. *Circulation.* 1997;95:183-190.

6. Kottkamp H, Hindricks G, Breithardt G, Borggrefe M. Three-dimensional electromagnetic catheter technology: electroanatomical mapping of the right atrium and ablation of ectopic atrial tachycardia. *J Cardiovasc Electrophysiol.* 1997;8(12):1332-1337.

7. Nakagawa H, Jackman WM. Use of a three-dimensional, non-fluoroscopic mapping system for catheter ablation of typical atrial flutter. *Pacing Clin Electrophysiol.* 1998;21(6):1279-1286.

8. Stevenson, et al. Identification and ablation of macroreentrant ventricular tachycardia with the CARTO electroanatomical mapping system. *Pacing Clin Electrophysiol.* 1998;21(7):1448-1456.

9. Khaykin Y, Oosthuizen R, et al. CARTO-guided vs. NavX-guided pulmonary vein antrum isolation and pulmonary vein antrum isolation performed without 3-D mapping: effect of the 3-D mapping system on procedure duration and fluoroscopy time. *J Interv Card Electrophysiol.* 2011;30(3):233-240.

10. Wilber DJ. Post infarction ventricular tachycardia: substrate approaches. In: Wilber DJ, Packer DL, Stevenson WG, eds. *Radiofrequency Catheter Ablation of Cardiac Arrhythmias: Basic Concepts and Clinical Applications.* 3rd ed. Blackwell Oxford UK; 2008:326-341.

11. Wijnmaalen AP, et al. Head-to-head comparison of contrast-enhanced magnetic resonance imaging and electroanatomical voltage mapping to assess post-infarct scar characteristics in patients with ventricular tachycardias: real-time image integration and reversed registration. *Eur Heart J.* 2011;32:104-114.

12. Stevenson WG, Friedman PL, Sager PT, et al. Exploring postinfarction reentrant ventricular tachycardia with entrainment mapping. *J Am Coll Cardiol.* 1997;29:1180-1189.

13. El-Shalakany A, Hadjis T, Papageorgiou P, et al. Entrainment/mapping criteria for the prediction of termination of ventricular tachycardia by single radiofrequency lesion in patients with coronary artery disease. *Circulation.* 1999;99:2283-2289.

14. Jais P, Maury P, Khairy P, et al. Elimination of local abnormal ventricular activities: a new end point for substrate modification in patients with scar-related ventricular tachycardia. *Circulation.* 2012;125(18):2184-2196.

THREE-DIMENSIONAL ELECTROANATOMIC
MAPPING FOR ABLATION OF CARDIAC ARRHYTHMIAS:
ENSITE NAVX AND ENSITE ARRAY

SECTION I
DIAGNOSTIC ELECTROPHYSIOLOGY—
MAPPING, IMAGING, AND
PACING MANEUVERS

11

2 THREE-DIMENSIONAL ELECTROANATOMIC MAPPING FOR ABLATION OF CARDIAC ARRHYTHMIAS: ENSITE NAVX AND ENSITE ARRAY

Rod Passman, MD, MSCE

CASE PRESENTATION 1: RADIOFREQUENCY ABLATION OF POST-MAZE ATRIAL FLUTTER

PATIENT STORY

A 63-year-old man status post-mitral and tricuspid valve repair and biatrial maze procedure 4 years ago presents with palpitations. The patient denied any chest pain, presyncope, or syncope with these palpitations. An ECG (Figure 2-1) demonstrated atypical atrial flutter.

PATHOPHYSIOLOGY

- Post-maze atrial tachycardias occur more frequently in the right atrium.

- Most common mechanism is the persistence of electrical conduction through regions that were targeted for prior surgical ablation or the creation of a central anatomic barrier to conduction. In each of these mechanisms, a macroreentrant circuit is created that was maintained by protected anatomic boundaries.

- In some cases, the reentrant circuit involves a region of incompletely ablated tissue such as the musculature of the coronary sinus

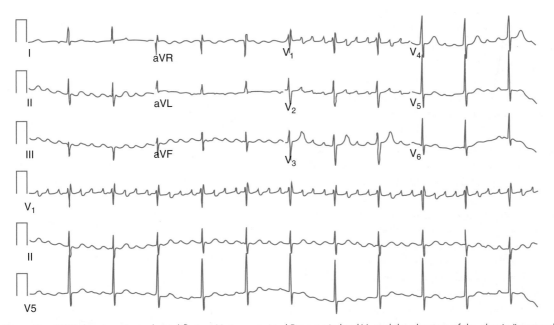

FIGURE 2-1 Presenting ECG showing atypical atrial flutter. Note organized P waves in lead V_1 and the absence of the classic "sawtooth" pattern in the inferior leads.

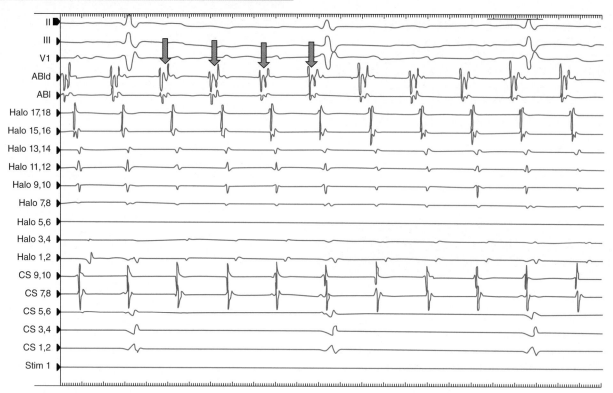

FIGURE 2-2 Intracardiac electrograms showing a right atrial flutter with narrow split potentials in the posterior right atrium near the superior aspect of the intercaval incision.

or the junction of the intercaval right atrial incision and the superior vena cava (Figure 2-2).

• The creation of surgical barriers may have allowed reentry to occur around a central obstacle that was functional (either the crista terminalis in the right atrium or Bachmann's bundle in the left atrium).

MANAGEMENT

• Cardioversion alone is unlikely to offer a long-term cure for atrial tachycardias that arise remote from the time of surgery.

• Antiarrhythmic therapy is a treatment option, though the long-term efficacy in this situation is unknown.

• Ablation has a high success rate for these arrhythmias; however, the identification of the critical sites for ablation often requires the use of an electroanatomic mapping system.

  ○ An electroanatomic map was created to define the reentrant circuit (Figure 2-3). The entire cycle length of the tachycardia was present in the right atrium. Entrainment mapping was used to localize the critical isthmus of tissue that was targeted for catheter ablation.

  ○ Optimal ablation sites were those with a postpacing interval within 20 ms of the tachycardia cycle length at which fractionated or narrowly split electrograms were recorded.

  ○ Once a suitable ablation site was recorded, high-output pacing was performed to assess for phrenic nerve capture (yellow circles show sites of phrenic nerve capture).

  ○ If phrenic nerve capture was absent, radiofrequency current was applied using a 4-millimeter irrigated catheter at a maximum power of 35 watts. The arrhythmia terminated at the

THREE-DIMENSIONAL ELECTROANATOMIC
MAPPING FOR ABLATION OF CARDIAC ARRHYTHMIAS:
ENSITE NAVX AND ENSITE ARRAY

SECTION I
DIAGNOSTIC ELECTROPHYSIOLOGY—
MAPPING, IMAGING, AND
PACING MANEUVERS

13

site of radiofrequency ablation between the superior margin of the posterior intercaval incision (blue circles represent site of termination; brown circles represent additional ablation sites).

° The use of an electroanatomic mapping system was essential to create a virtual recreation of the atrial anatomy, mark anatomic sites of importance, and to guide catheter ablation lesions.

ELECTROANATOMIC MAPPING SYSTEM: ST. JUDE MEDICAL ENSITE NAVX

The St. Jude Medical EnSite NavX system is a 3-dimensional impedance-based mapping system that allows the user to nonfluoroscopically locate electrodes in the human body. The NavX system uses constant current over a set of six patches (anterior-posterior, side-to-side, cranial-caudal) (Figure 2-4) and Ohm's law to create an impedance gradient across the thorax. When an electrode is placed inside this established impedance gradient, NavX measures the local impedance and calculates the position along that plane. This location is calculated along multiple axes to create a 3-dimensional navigation field. The NavX system can locate up to 132 electrodes simultaneously and updates electrode location approximately 204 times per second creating near real-time 3-D catheter visualization. The system can also save the coordinates of each electrode relative to a positional reference; as the electrodes move, additional data is stored, allowing the user to create a 3-D model of the endocardial surface. This model aids in reproducibly maneuvering to desired locations in the heart, to denote the locations of critical anatomic structures, and to mark sites of ablation or other sites of interest. The system is also capable of saving local bipolar and unipolar electrograms; this data can be used to create a variety of voltage and activation timing maps that can also assist in locating the optimal ablation location for various arrhythmias. Types of maps that can be created with EnSite NavX include:

• Geometry

• Ablation points

• Voltage

• Propagation

• Activation

• Complex fractionated electrogram

• Dominant frequency

The St. Jude Medical EnSite Array offers a viable solution for complex or nonsustained arrhythmias. The Array is a balloon catheter constructed of a handmade wire mesh consisting of 64 individual electrodes and is the only noncontact mapping tool on the market (Figure 2-5). The balloon is filled with a heparinized saline and contrast mixture. Unlike traditional contact mapping techniques, noncontact mapping can display mapping data of an entire atrium from a single heartbeat without moving a roving catheter. The software processes unipolar electrograms to create both local activation time and voltage maps. These maps are displayed on a color-coded scale and can be viewed as either static or dynamic maps. Catheter movement is displayed in real time, and traditional contact data may also be collected with the Array.

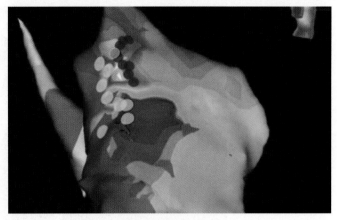

FIGURE 2-3 A high-density geometry and activation map of the right atrium was created primarily using a duodeca catheter looped around the right atrium. This catheter was rotated around the chamber allowing for rapid mapping, collecting 10 activation points at a time. Internal/external interpolation controls how near to the geometry each timing point was collected to help ensure good contact. Reentry (versus standard) map display helps determine what percentage of the atrial flutter cycle length is present in the specific chamber and colors are evenly distributed along the cycle length. Low voltage identification (grey areas) help locate areas of scar/electrical barriers. Varying lesion colors displayed here help distinguish good ablation sites in very close proximity to sites associated with phrenic nerve capture.

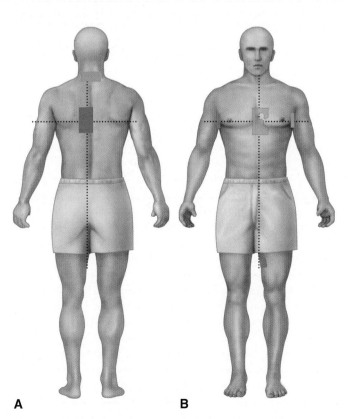

A   B

FIGURE 2-4 Position of body surface patches used with the NavX system. The six-patch configuration is used to create electroanatomic gradients used to localize multiple electrodes in a 3-D space.

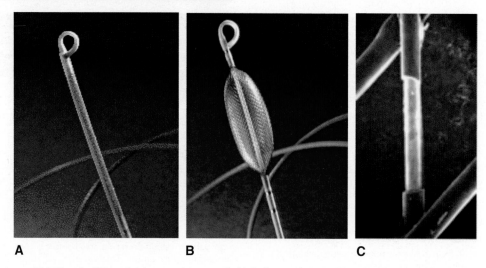

A **B** **C**

FIGURE 2-5 EnSite Array. (A) 9-French, 110-cm body, open lumen with the balloon in low profile. (B) A 7.5-ml balloon inflated, stainless steel mesh. (C) Microscopic view of single microelectrodes on the balloon mesh.

USES OF 3-D MAPPING

- Define anatomy
- Tag location of critical anatomic landmarks
- Localize arrhythmia circuit with activation map
- Track ablation lesions
- Limit fluoroscopy

CASE PRESENTATION 2: RADIOFREQUENCY ABLATION OF ATRIOVENTRICULAR NODAL REENTRANT TACHYCARDIA

PATIENT STORY

A 22-year-old woman with no significant past medical history presents to the emergency department (ED) with palpitations. The patient reports that the episodes began around age 18, occur 4 to 5 times per year, usually last several minutes, and have an abrupt onset and offset. In the ED, her ECG showed a narrow complex, short RP tachycardia at a rate of 180 beats per minute (Figure 2-6A and B). Adenosine terminated the tachycardia. The patient underwent an electrophysiologic study where she was found to have typical atrioventricular nodal reentry tachycardia (AVNRT) (Figure 2-6C). Since the target for ablation in AVNRT is the slow pathway, there is a risk for inadvertent heart block if lesions are delivered close to the compact AV node. A 3-D mapping system is helpful to provide a high-resolution detailed map of the cardiac anatomy including the location the coronary sinus os, which is a marker for location of the slow pathway and the atrioventricular node. Utilization of the "shadow" feature allowed for the display of the exact positioning of the catheter location where His potentials could be reliably recorded. With these important structures defined, coupled with electrogram information recorded at the site of catheter ablation, radiofrequency lesion can be safely delivered while minimizing the risk of injury to the AV node or coronary sinus (Figure 2-7). In addition, use of 3-D mapping allowed for a successful ablation while reducing fluoroscopy exposure in this young patient.

THREE-DIMENSIONAL ELECTROANATOMIC
MAPPING FOR ABLATION OF CARDIAC ARRHYTHMIAS:
ENSITE NAVX AND ENSITE ARRAY

SECTION I
DIAGNOSTIC ELECTROPHYSIOLOGY—
MAPPING, IMAGING, AND
PACING MANEUVERS

15

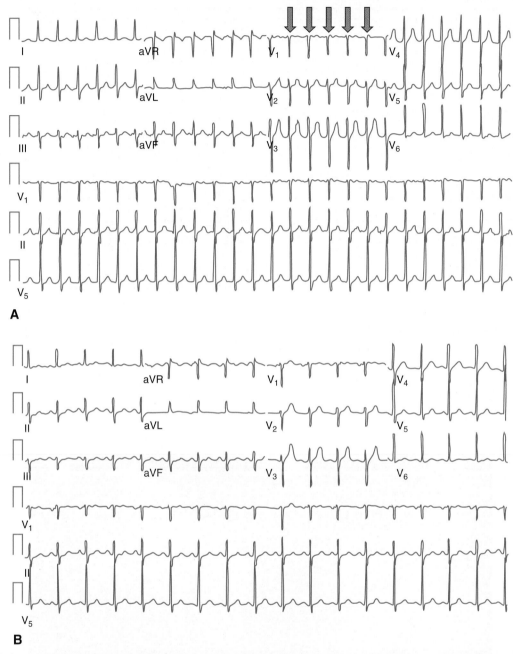

FIGURE 2-6 (A) ECG of AVNRT shows a narrow complex short RP tachycardia with P waves buried in the terminal portion of the QRS interval in (most easily seen in lead V_1 (arrows). (B) ECG in sinus rhythm; note absence of P waves in the terminal portion of lead V_1. (C) Intracardiac electrograms demonstrate long AH times and short (<70 msec) septal VA times consistent with typical AVNRT.

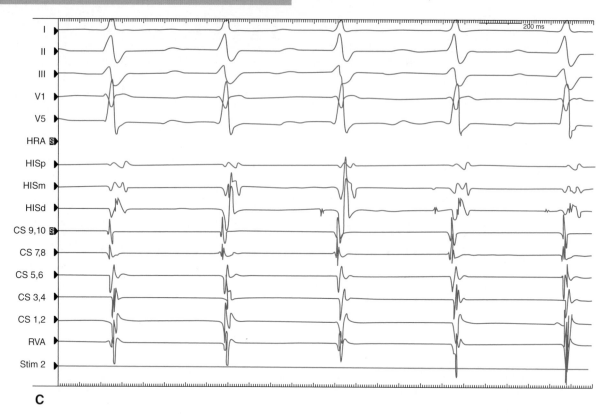

C

FIGURE 2-6 (*Continued*)

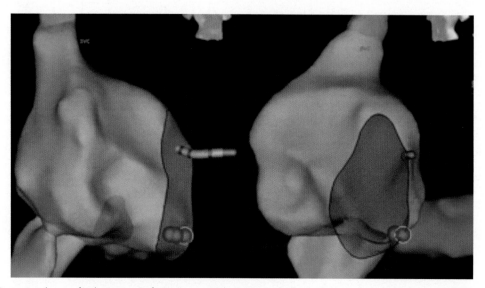

FIGURE 2-7 Three-dimensional map of right atrium. (Left: RAO view; Right: LAO view). The coronary sinus can be seen extending posterior and leftward (green), and the area of the His bundle is marked by the shadow of a catheter crossing the anteroseptal region of the tricuspid valve. Radiofrequency modification of the slow pathway was performed. The red circles represent sites of successful lesions with junction ectopic beats.

THREE-DIMENSIONAL ELECTROANATOMIC
MAPPING FOR ABLATION OF CARDIAC ARRHYTHMIAS:
ENSITE NAVX AND ENSITE ARRAY

SECTION I
DIAGNOSTIC ELECTROPHYSIOLOGY—
MAPPING, IMAGING, AND
PACING MANEUVERS

17

CASE 3: RADIOFREQUENCY ABLATION OF RIGHT VENTRICULAR OUTFLOW TRACT PREMATURE VENTRICULAR DEPOLARIZATIONS

PATIENT STORY

A 47-year-old woman with no significant past medical history complained of palpitations. She denied presyncope, syncope, chest pain, or dyspnea on exertion. Her ECG (Figure 2-8) showed frequent monomorphic PVCs, both isolated and in pairs, in a left bundle/inferior axis morphology. Her echo shows normal contractile function, and a Holter showed NSR with 43% monomorphic isolated PVCs and couplets and no NSVT. A stress test showed no ischemia. Her PVCs failed to decrease on β-adrenergic blockers, and the patient underwent EP study and ablation.

MANAGEMENT

- For asymptomatic individuals with normal ejection fraction and a PVC burden of <20%, no specific therapy is required.

- Treatment is necessary for symptomatic individuals or with those who have a reduced ejection fraction that is possibly tachycardia-mediated.

- β-Adrenergic blockers and verapamil may be used to suppress RVOT PVCs and are frequently used as first-line therapy.

- Antiarrhythmic drugs can also be considered.

- Radiofrequency ablation has a high success rate, low complication rate, and can avoid the need for long-term medical therapy in this often young and otherwise healthy patient population.

  ○ Figure 2-9: Using EnSite NavX, a spiral catheter ("lasso" catheter) was used to map the PVCs in the RVOT. The earliest site was localized to the superior septal region just under the pulmonic valve (white region).

  ○ Figure 2-10: Pace-mapping confirmed a 12/12 match with activation demonstrating local EGMs 31 msec prior to the onset of the PVC. Successful ablation was performed at that site.

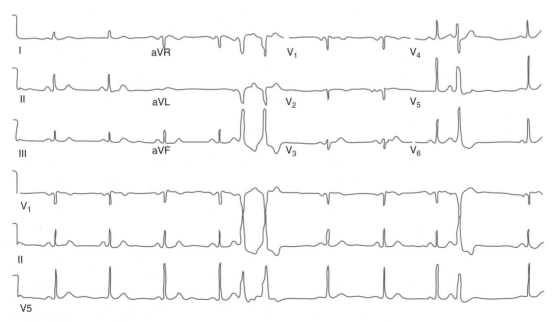

FIGURE 2-8 Baseline ECG showing PVCs.

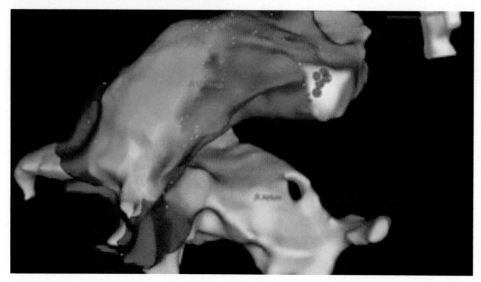

FIGURE 2-9 The EnSite system was used to collect 113 points from the 10 electrodes of a spiral catheter to simultaneously display local activation timing data and geometry. The use of multipolar catheters decreases the time spent collecting arrhythmia data. Any mapping catheter can be used to collect this data with the EnSite system. The use of standard activation timing map (versus reentrant) was used to display the earliest ventricular signal as white (then red through purple as signals get later). This area was then more closely evaluated as a potential ablation site, and successful ablation was performed in this region (brown lesions).

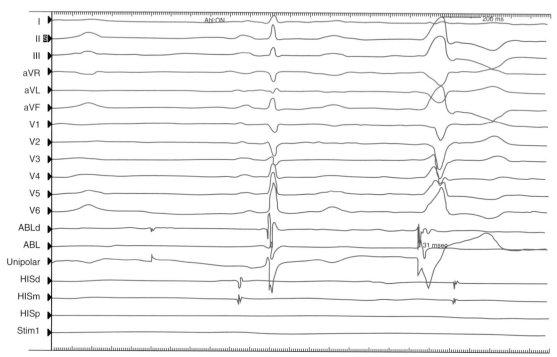

FIGURE 2-10 Intracardiac EGM demonstrating onset of RVOT PVC 31 msec prior to surface QRS onset. Unipolar tracing demonstrates characteristic QS pattern.

THREE-DIMENSIONAL ELECTROANATOMIC
MAPPING FOR ABLATION OF CARDIAC ARRHYTHMIAS:
ENSITE NAVX AND ENSITE ARRAY

SECTION I
DIAGNOSTIC ELECTROPHYSIOLOGY—
MAPPING, IMAGING, AND
PACING MANEUVERS

19

CASE 4: RADIOFREQUENCY ABLATION OF LEFT ATRIAL FLUTTER FOLLOWING AN ABLATION FOR ATRIAL FIBRILLATION

PATIENT STORY

The patient is a 64-year-old man with a history of hypertension, a permanent pacemaker for atrioventricular nodal dysfunction, and symptomatic paroxysmal atrial fibrillation who underwent wide area circumferential ablation 2 years ago. He presents with dyspnea on exertion and was found to be in atrial flutter (Figure 2-11).

PATHOPHYSIOLOGY

- The development of left atrial tachycardias or atrial flutters occurs in 1% to 50% of patients.

- New onset left atrial flutters are more common following wide area circumfrential ablation using radiofrequency energy as opposed to pulmonary vein isolation alone or cryoballoon ablation.

- The risk of postablation left atrial flutters increases in patients with persistent AF, enlarged atria, or when linear lesions have been used.

- Left atrial flutters following ablation of AF are often due to macroreentrant circuits around the prior roof or mitral annular linear lesions.

- Nonreentrant focal arrhythmias can also occur around lesion edges.

MANAGEMENT

- Left atrial flutters occurring within the 3-month blanking period following the index ablation may respond to cardioversion alone.

- Rate control is often problematic given the rapid ventricular rates associated with atrial flutter in general and the paradoxically faster rates seen with the slower atrial flutters often seen with diseased atrium.

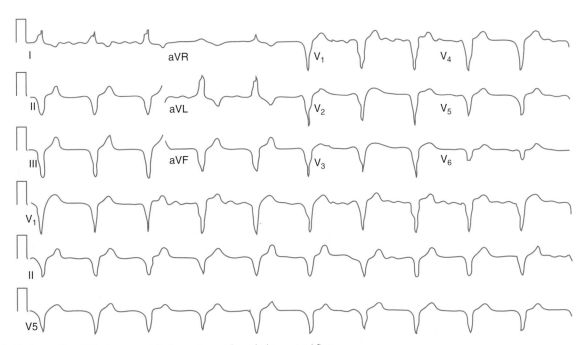

FIGURE 2-11 Presenting ECG shows ventricular pacing with underlying atrial flutter.

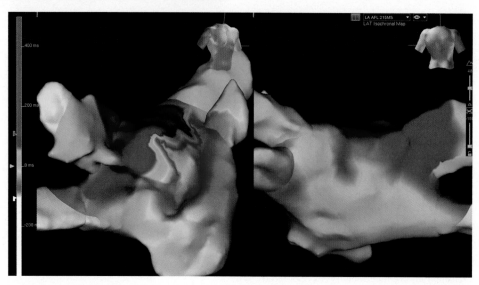

FIGURE 2-12 A 10-pole circular mapping catheter was used to create the left atrial geometry and activation map simultaneously. The use of a multipolar catheter allowed for the creation of maps with several hundrend data points in just a few minutes. Electrograms from a catheter in the coronoary sinus were used as a timing reference for the activation map. The propagation map shows the entire cycle length of the atrial flutter with "early" activation (white area) over the roof region closest to the right superior pulmonary vein. Analysis of the data shows where "early" activation (white area) penetrates "late" activation (purple) near the right superior pulmonary vein.

- Response rates to antiarrhythmic therapy are thought to be low.

- Ablation remains a highly effective approach to these arrhythmias.

  ○ EnSite NavX was used to create an activation map of the atrial flutter. Figure 2-12 shows an activation map of a left atrial flutter propagating over the left atrial roof. This map shows the full range of color from white to purple indicating that the full cycle length of the tachycardia (240 msec) is present in the left atrium. Entrainment mapping was used to confirm the location as part of the flutter circuit.

  ○ Intracardiac electrograms from the anterior roof portion near the right superior pulmonary vein shows fractionated electrograms. Ablation at this site successfully terminated the tachycardia (Figure 2-13A and B).

CASE 5: RADIOFREQUENCY ABLATION OF A NONSUSTAINED ATRIAL TACHYCARDIA USING THE ENSITE ARRAY

PATIENT STORY

A 56-year-old woman with hypertension and asthma developed intermittent palpitations. They generally occurred on a daily basis, and she describes episodes of waking up at night with her heart beating really fast. These episodes lasted about 10 minutes and occurred once per month. Her workup included an echocardiogram that showed normal left ventricular function and no evidence of structural heart disease. An event monitor documented paroxysms of supraventricular tachycardia (Figure 2-14).

PATHOPHYSIOLOGY

- ATs can be caused by automaticity, triggered activity, and microreentry.

- Three-quarters of ATs arise from the right atrium, the majority near the crista terminalis.

- Of those originating in the left atrium, the pulmonary veins are the most common site.

THREE-DIMENSIONAL ELECTROANATOMIC
MAPPING FOR ABLATION OF CARDIAC ARRHYTHMIAS:
ENSITE NAVX AND ENSITE ARRAY

SECTION I
DIAGNOSTIC ELECTROPHYSIOLOGY—
MAPPING, IMAGING, AND
PACING MANEUVERS

21

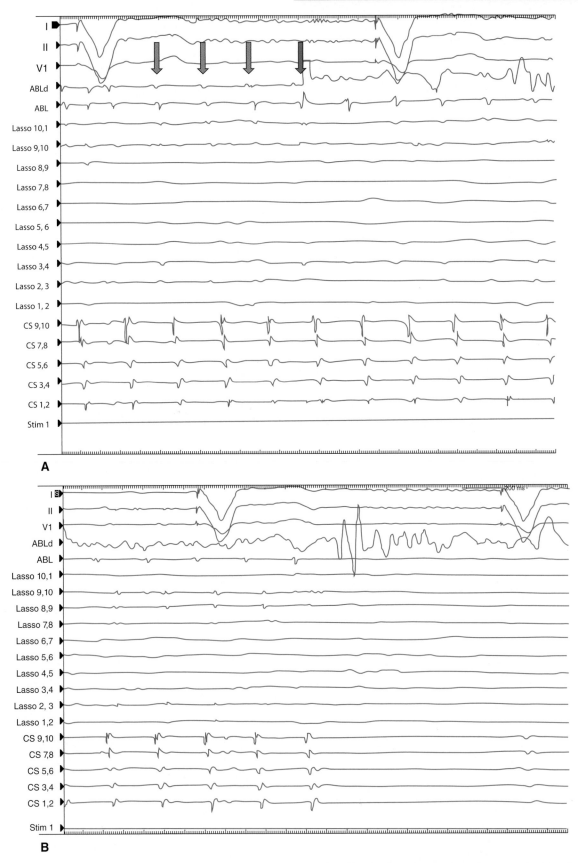

FIGURE 2-13 (A) IEGMs of left atrial flutter. Ablation catheter at anterior aspect of roof line by the right superior pulmonary vein shows fractionated electrograms (blue arrows). Onset of radiofrequency energy also pictured (red arrow). (B) Termination of atrial flutter at sight of breakthrough at prior ablation roof line.

MANAGEMENT

- Atrial tachycardia may be responsive to β-blockers and calcium channel blockers.

- Antiarrhythmic drugs may be used as second-line agents.

- Ablation of AT has a high success rate, but the inability to sustain the tachycardia may make ablation challenging. When the AT cannot be sustained, noncontact mapping with EnSite Array offers a viable treatment option.

  - Figure 2-15: EnSite Array shows the sinus node and the earliest activation site (EA) along the superior aspect of the crista terminalis.
  - Figure 2-16 shows an isochronal activation of the atrial tachycardia.
  - Figure 2-17 shows ablation catheter at the site of EA, which is 35 ms pre–p-wave. Ablation at this site rendered the AT noninducible.

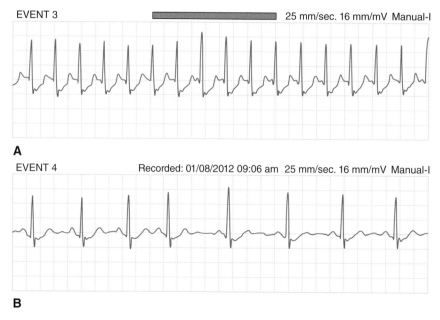

FIGURE 2-14 Event monitor shows a long RP tachycardia at 160 beats per minute. Sinus rhythm with sinus arrhythmia is also pictured.

THREE-DIMENSIONAL ELECTROANATOMIC
MAPPING FOR ABLATION OF CARDIAC ARRHYTHMIAS:
ENSITE NAVX AND ENSITE ARRAY

SECTION I
DIAGNOSTIC ELECTROPHYSIOLOGY—
MAPPING, IMAGING, AND
PACING MANEUVERS

23

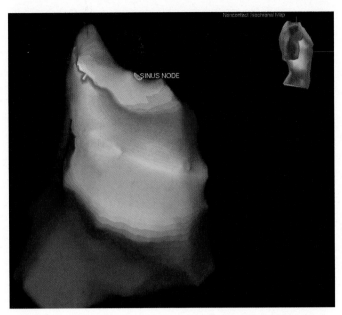

FIGURE 2-15 EnSite Array has the ability to produce a noncontact isochronal map based on the extrapolated unipolar data of a single beat. The isochronal map shows the timing activation for a sinus beat in the right atrium. Earliest activation (white) is shown high lateral in the region of the sinus node with activation spreading in a cranial-to-caudal direction.

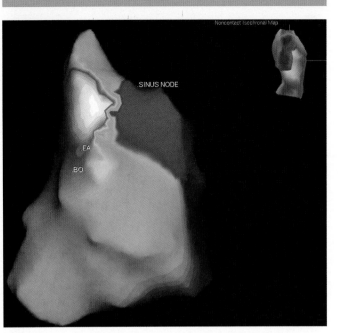

FIGURE 2-16 The image shows an isochronal activation of the atrial tachycardia. This isochronal map shows earliest activation (white) in the high posterior lateral region of the right atrium with the activation continuing posterior and medial with the latest activation being anterior. This activation pattern is likely due to the crista terminalis blocking conduction in the anterior direction. Successful ablation was performed at the site of early activation.

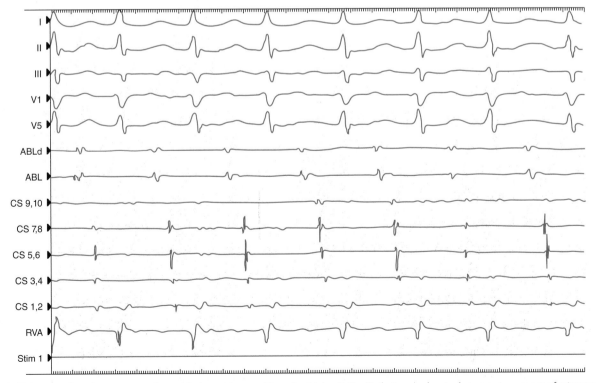

FIGURE 2-17 Intracardiac electrograms show ablation catheter with early atrial activity. Catheter was located at superior aspect of crista terminalis at the site of the EA seen on EnSite Array.

REFERENCES

1. Ventura R, Rostock T, Klemm HU, et al. Catheter ablation of common-type atrial flutter guided by three-dimensional right atrial geometry reconstruction and catheter rracking using cutaneous patches. *J Cardiovasc Electrophysiol.* 2004;15(10):1157-1161.

2. Krum D, Goel A, Hauck J, et al. Catheter location, tracking, cardiac chamber geometry creation, and ablation using cutaneous patches. *J Interv Card Electrophysiol.* 2005;12:17-22.

3. Chinitz LA, Sethi JS. How to perform noncontact mapping. *Heart Rhythm.* 2006;3:120.

4. Earley M, Showkathali R, Alzetani M, et al. Radiofrequency ablation of arrhythmias guided by non-fluoroscopic catheter location: a prospective randomized trial. *Eur Heart J.* 2006;27:1223-1229.

5. Reddy VY, Morales G, Ahmed H, et al. Catheter ablation of atrial fibrillation without the use of fluoroscopy. *Heart Rhythm.* 2010;7:1644-1653.

6. Razminia M, Manankil MF, Eryazici PL, et al. Nonfluoroscopic catheter ablation of cardiac arrhythmias in adults: feasibility, safety, and efficacy. *J Cardiovasc Electrophysiol.* 2012;23(10):1078-1086.

3 INTRACARDIAC ECHOCARDIOGRAPHY FOR TRANSSEPTAL ACCESS

Gery F. Tomassoni MD, FACC, FHRS

CASE PRESENTATION

A 66-year-old woman with a past medical history of hypertension, diabetes, and symptomatic paroxysmal atrial fibrillation (AF) was transferred for radiofrequency catheter ablation (RFCA) of the pulmonary veins. The patient had failed multiple antiarrhythmic medications and was extremely symptomatic during the AF episodes, which were increasing in frequency and duration. A previous attempt at RFCA failed due to difficulty in gaining transseptal access to the left atrium. Intracardiac echocardiography (ICE) was not used during the procedure. Laboratory evaluation was unremarkable including thyroid function tests. A 12-lead ECG confirmed AF during her symptoms. Baseline 12-lead ECG in normal sinus rhythm and an echocardiogram were normal.

EVOLUTION AND UTILITY OF ICE

- The use of ICE in the electrophysiology (EP) laboratory has increased dramatically in the past 15 years as more and more patients are undergoing left-sided procedures.

- As procedures are becoming increasingly more complex, several limitations have become apparent when using fluoroscopy as the primary imaging tool, including poor visualization of soft tissue structures and significant radiation exposure to both the patient and physician.

- As a result, ultrasound imaging techniques that are characterized by real-time high quality soft tissue imaging are now readily available.

- ICE in the EP lab allows:
  - direct visualization of all relevant anatomical structures and their relationship to catheters during the procedure.
  - assessment of unusual anatomical septal and left (LA) variations.
  - guiding site-specific transseptal puncture (TSP) along the septum.
  - functional analysis such as flow measurements and early monitoring for complications.

ICE CATHETERS AND GUIDANCE FOR TRANSSEPTAL ACCESS IN EP LAB

- ICE uses high-frequency ultrasound for cardiac imaging. Most commercially available ICE catheters provide sector-based imaging using a phased-array transducer.[1]

- Phased-array ICE:
  - allows for a greater frequency range and a greater depth of field resulting in higher imaging resolution.[2]
  - has the ability to acquire Doppler and color flow imaging.[2]
  - uses a catheter with a deflectable tip that is easy to steer and maneuver.

- TSP was first described in 1960, predominantly for the diagnostic evaluation of valvular heart disease.[3] With the emergence of therapeutic procedures for structural heart disease and RFCA, there has been a revival in the use of transseptal catheterization. Despite high success rates and overall low complication rates, complications of fluoroscopic-guided transseptal catheterization still exist and include the following:
  - pericardial effusion with or without cardiac tamponade
  - cardiac and aortic perforation
  - myocardial infarction
  - air embolization
  - thrombus formation on the transseptal sheath
  - CVA/TIA (4)

- Since the fossa ovalis (FO) is easily recognizable on ICE, this imaging modality is well established at facilitating safe TSP.

- In addition, ICE allows for direct imaging of the structures important for assuring an optimal puncture site including the FO, the posterior left atrial wall, and the aorta.[5]

- Finally, ICE has been shown to be extremely useful in many cardiac interventional procedures that require transseptal access, including RFCA (AF, SVT, and VT), percutaneous LAA occlusion, ASD device closure, and mitral valvuloplasty.[6]

MANAGEMENT AND PATHOPHYSIOLOGY

Procedure

- After the patient arrived to the EP lab, typical venous access was obtained from both the femoral and internal jugular veins.

- A phased-array ICE transducer was advanced from the left femoral vein to the level of the right atrium (RA). The FO was visualized demonstrating a double layered or membrane interatrial septum (Figure 3-1).

- Prior to transseptal access, intravenous heparin was initiated to maintain an ACT >350 seconds.

- After the dilator, 8 Fr transseptal sheath, and Brockenbrough needle (BRK-1) was advanced into the SVC, the assembly was retracted until the tip was engaged in the FO. The angle of the sheath and dilator was directed in a posterior manner for easier access to the posteriorly directed pulmonary veins. Mechanical pressure applied at the FO was performed causing "tenting" (Figure 3-2).

- The needle tip was then advanced across both septum, and the location was confirmed with pressure monitoring and bubbles seen in the LA by ICE. A second TSP was performed in a similar fashion.

- RFCA and isolation of the pulmonary veins was done successfully without complications.

INTERATRIAL SEPTAL VARIATIONS

- Many different interatrial septal variations exist that can have a significant impact on TSP.[7] In addition to the double septum (see Figure 3-1), the variations include:
  - an FO with a thickened septum
  - an FO with a thickened, enlarged superior limbus

- ◦ patent FO with a tunnel
- ◦ a large intra-atrial aneurysm
- ◦ a fenestrated septum with multiple defects (Figure 3-3)

- Each septal variation has its own unique set of challenges making TSP extremely difficult. The use of ICE is invaluable in these circumstances. Not only does it confirm the appropriate location and angle of the TSP, but it also allows for recognition of immediate complications (Figure 3-4).

- This case demonstrated the utility of ICE allowing visualization of a double membrane and ultimately safe passageway to the LA so that PV isolation could be successfully performed.

ADDITIONAL BENEFITS OF ICE

- While performing RFCA of AF, the goal of TSP is to cross the FO at lower end of the septum and posteriorly for easier access to pulmonary veins, especially the right inferior vein.

- An anterior TSP higher along the septum can be helpful for procedures such as insertion of LAA occlusive devices and ablation of left ventricle VT.

- ICE can guide the location of TSP in patients with structural heart disease and previous cardiac procedures such as ASD closure devices (Figure 3-5).

- Repeat left-sided procedures after previous TSP and patients with valvular surgery can have excessive interatrial scarring, making TSP nearly impossible. New tools such as radiofrequency-assisted TSP and needle-tipped guidewires have been specially designed for such an issue.[8,9]

- ICE-guided ablation can monitor thrombus formation on sheaths, endocardial lesion sites, and coagulum formation on ablation electrodes.[5]

- ICE has been used effectively to guide antral isolation for atrial fibrillation as opposed to ostial isolation.[5]

- ICE can also identify the location of the esophagus during the ablative procedure in an attempt to avoid esophageal ulceration or fistula formation[10] (see Figure 3-4).

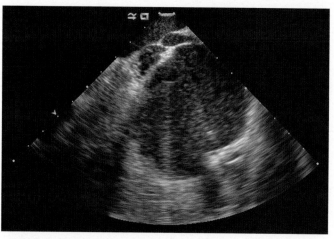

FIGURE 3-1 ICE image from RA demonstrating the variation of a double layered or membrane interatrial septum.

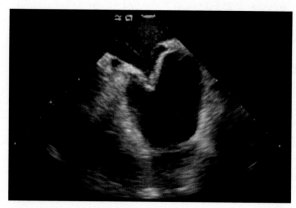

FIGURE 3-2 RA ICE image showing "tenting" of both interatrial septums. During TSP, ICE imaging allows direct visualization of the transseptal sheath and dilator apparatus as it enters the interatrial septum during retraction from the SVC. When the dilator tip engages the FO, "tenting" of the FO is seen.

INTRACARDIAC ECHOCARDIOGRAPHY FOR
TRANSSEPTAL ACCESS

SECTION I
DIAGNOSTIC ELECTROPHYSIOLOGY—
MAPPING, IMAGING, AND
PACING MANEUVERS

27

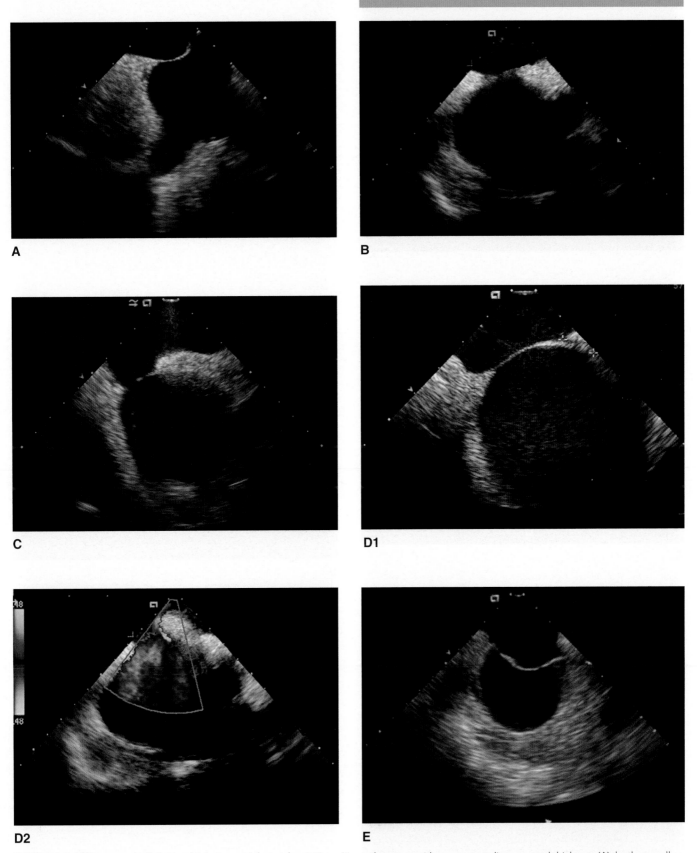

FIGURE 3-3 ICE images depicting multiple interatrial septal variations. Normal septum with an average diameter and thickness (A), both a small diameter and thickened FO (B), a small diameter normal thickness FO with a thickened, enlarged superior limbus (C), patent FO with tunnel (D1, D2), a large intra-atrial aneurysm (E), and a fenestrated septum with multiple defects demonstrated with Doppler color flow (F). The patent FO with tunnel is depicted with asterisks (D1) and doppler color flow (D2).

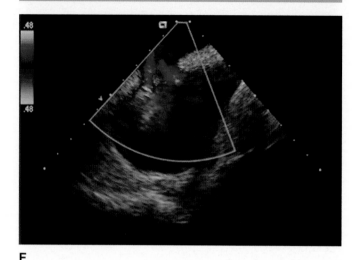

F

FIGURE 3-3 (*Continued*)

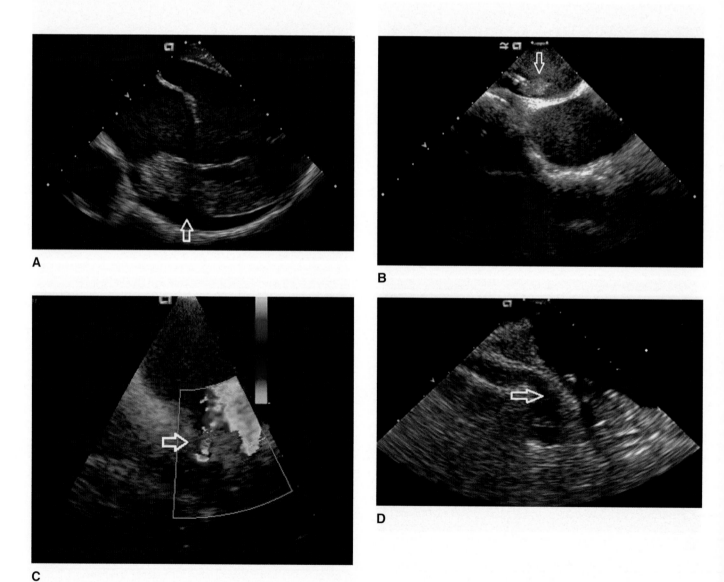

A

B

C

D

FIGURE 3-4 ICE images of potential complications from transseptal catheterization and RFCA. Early detection of a pericardial effusion (arrow) (A), thrombus formation (arrow) on transseptal sheath (B), and LIPV (arrow) stenosis (C). In addition, ICE can help prevent esophageal damage by identifying its location (arrow) behind the LA prior to RFCA (D).

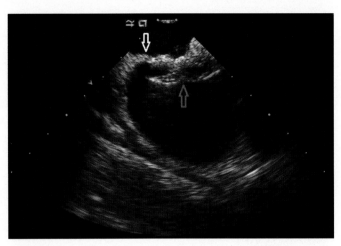

FIGURE 3-5 An ICE image showing the presence of an ASD device (red arrow). The white arrow depicts a safe location for TSP below or inferior to the ASD.

REFERENCES

1. Kim SS, Hijazi ZM, Lang RM, et al. The use of intracardiac echocardiography and other intracardiac imaging tools to guide noncoronary cardiac interventions. *J Am Coll Cardiol*. 2009;53(23):2117-2128.

2. Packer DL, Stevens CL, Curley MG, et al. Intracardiac phase-array imaging. *J Am Coll Cardiol*. 2002;39(3):509-516.

3. Brockenbrough E, Braunwald E. A new technique for left ventricular angiography and transseptal left heart catheterization. *Am J Cardiol*. 1960;6:219-231.

4. De Ponti R, Cappato R, Olsson SB, et al. Trans-septal catheterization in the electrophysiology laboratory: Data from a multicenter survey spanning 12 years. *J Am Coll Cardiol*. 2006;47:1037-1042.

5. Saliba W, Thomas J. Intracardiac echocardiography during catheter ablation of atrial fibrillation. *Europace*. 2008;10:iii42-iii47.

6. Hijazi ZM, Shiykumar K, Sahn D. Intracardiac echocardiography (ICE) during interventional and electrophysiological cardiac catheterization. *Circulation*. 2009;119(4):587-596.

7. Schernthaner C, Danmayr F, Daburger A, et al. High incidence of echocardiographic abnormalities of the interatrial septum in patients undergoing ablation for atrial fibrillation. *Echocardiography*. 2013;30(4):402-406.

8. Shah DP, Knight BP. Transseptal catheterization using a powered radiofrequency transseptal needle. *J Interv Card Electrophysiol*. 2010;27(1):15-16.

9. Wieczorek WM, Hoeltgen R, Akin E, et al. Use of a novel needle wire in patients undergoing transseptal puncture associated with severe septal tenting. *J Interv Card Electrophysiol*. 2010;27(1):9-13.

10. Cummings JE, Schweikert RA, Saliba WI, et al. Assessment of temperature, proximity, and course of the esophagus during radiofrequency ablation within the left atrium. *Circulation*. 2005;112:459-464.

4 DIAGNOSTIC MANEUVERS FOR SUPRAVENTRICULAR TACHYCARDIA: VAV, VAAV, PPI, AND VA LINKING

Sharon Shen, MD, and Bradley P. Knight, MD

CASE PRESENTATION

A 55-year-old man without significant past medical history presents to clinic for consultation regarding the management of paroxysmal supraventricular tachycardia (PSVT). He states that he first noted rapid palpitations approximately 6 months ago shortly after hip surgery. Palpitations were rapid and regular with abrupt onset and offset. Several episodes lasted 3 to 6 hours. He endorsed about 8 to 10 episodes over the past few months. LV function by echocardiogram was normal. He had previously seen another physician a few months prior who inserted an implantable loop recorder. Interrogation of his ILR showed a regular tachycardia at 120 bpm.

CASE EXPLANATION

This is an example of a typical patient who will undergo catheter ablation for symptomatic SVT. To choose a target for ablation, however, the mechanism of tachycardia must first be determined. This chapter will focus on the diagnostic pacing maneuvers of ventricular and atrial overdrive pacing. For the purposes of this chapter, the term "entrainment" refers to acceleration of the atrial or ventricular electrograms to the pacing cycle length (CL) during overdrive pacing from the ventricle or atrium, respectively, with resumption of the original tachycardia upon cessation of pacing.

VENTRICULAR OVERDRIVE PACING

A useful first pacing maneuver during PSVT induced in the electrophysiology laboratory is to entrain the tachycardia from the ventricle. In this patient, a regular tachycardia with a 1:1 AV relationship, CL of 580 ms, and a septal VA time of 130 ms is induced in the EP lab. The differential diagnosis includes atypical atrioventricular nodal reentry tachycardia (AVNRT), orthodromic atrioventricular reentry tachycardia (AVRT), and atrial tachycardia (AT). Ventricular overdrive pacing at a CL 10 ms shorter than the tachycardia CL produces the response shown in Figure 4-1A.

VAV OR VAAV

- Assessment of the electrogram sequence following the last paced ventricular complex can be used to differentiate between AT and an AV node-dependent arrhythmia (AVNRT or AVRT).[1,2]

- *The principle*: Overdrive ventricular pacing in tachycardia often results in 1:1 retrograde conduction whereby the atrial rate accelerates to the ventricular pacing rate. With either AVNRT or AVRT, the last entrained beat conducts via the retrograde limb of the circuit (AV nodal pathway or accessory pathway [AP]) and then anterograde down the AV node displaying an "atrial-ventricular" response (VAV) as is the case in this patient (see Figures 4-1A and 4-1B).

- Conversely, during entrainment in AT, both retrograde and anterograde conduction occurs via the AV node. Therefore, upon cessation of pacing, the last entrained atrial beat finds the AV node refractory displaying an "atrial-atrial-ventricular" response described as VAAV (Figures 4-2A and 4-2B).

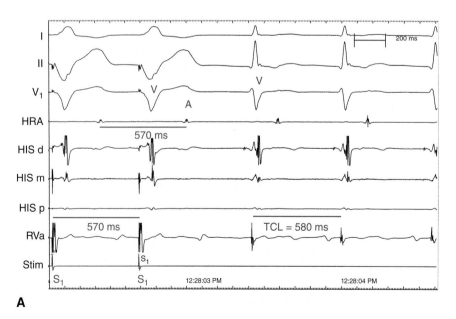

A

FIGURE 4-1A An example of ventricular overdrive pacing during PSVT is shown. During tachycardia, ventricular overdrive pacing was performed at 10 ms shorter than the tachycardia CL. After confirming acceleration of the atrial CL to the pacing CL, ventricular pacing was stopped, and the response to cessation of pacing was observed to be VAV.

DIAGNOSTIC MANEUVERS FOR SUPRAVENTRICULAR
TACHYCARDIA: VAV, VAAV, PPI, AND VA LINKING

SECTION I
DIAGNOSTIC ELECTROPHYSIOLOGY—
MAPPING, IMAGING, AND
PACING MANEUVERS

31

- Assessment of the retrograde atrial activation sequence (RAAS) during entrainment is useful; if the RAAS of the entrained complex is different from that in tachycardia, a diagnosis of AT or bystander AP is suggested (see Figure 4-2A).

- *Pseudo VAAV*: Caution should be exercised in identifying the last entrained atrial beat as prolonged retrograde conduction can give the false appearance of a VAAV response (Figure 4-3).

THE POSTPACING INTERVAL

- Useful for differentiating atypical AVNRT from AVRT using a septal AP.[3]

- Postpacing interval minus tachycardia CL (PPI-TCL) >115 ms suggests atypical AVNRT (Figure 4-4).

- PPI-TCL <115 ms suggests a septal AP-mediated AVRT (Figure 4-5).

- *The Principle:* As the ventricle is an obligate member of the AVRT circuit, namely the RV pacing site is near the circuit, entrainment from the ventricle results in a shorter PPI compared to that in AVNRT.

- *Pitfall:* This calculation includes anterograde AV conduction. If the first AH interval after pacing is stopped is longer than the AH during SVT, it can falsely prolong the PPI.

- Alternatively, a second calculation that only measures the difference in VA conduction is the stimulus to A interval minus VA interval during tachycardia (SA-VA) where >85 ms suggests atypical AVNRT (see Figure 4-4) and <85 ms suggests a septal AP-mediated AVRT (see Figure 4-5).

- Exception to both calculations exists in very slowly conducting accessory pathways whereby marked cycle length-dependent conduction delay can increase the PPI and SA values.[4]

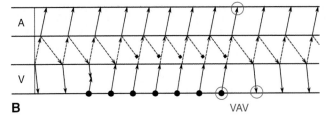

FIGURE 4-1B Ladder diagram for VAV response.

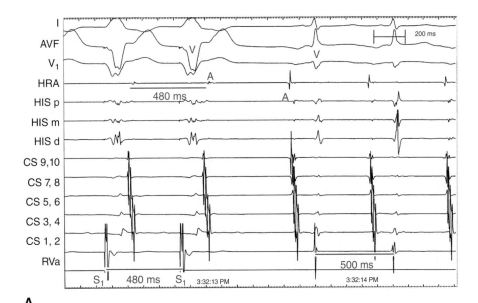

A

FIGURE 4-2A An example of a "VAAV response" to entrainment pacing from the ventricle during a long RP tachycardia. After cessation of overdrive pacing, the electrogram response is VAAV consistent with the patient's diagnosis of AT. Note also the change in the atrial activation sequence during ventricular pacing consistent with AT.

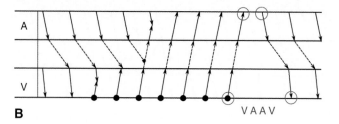

B

FIGURE 4-2B Ladder diagram of VAAV response.

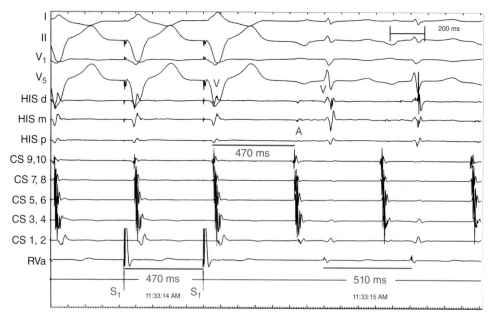

FIGURE 4-3 "Pseudo VAAV" in a patient with atypical AVNRT.

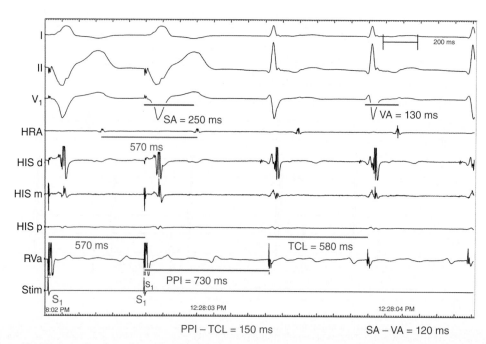

FIGURE 4-4 PPI-TCL and SA-VA example of a patient with AVNRT. PPI-TCL >115 ms and SA-VA >85 ms are both consistent with a diagnosis of AVNRT.

DIAGNOSTIC MANEUVERS FOR SUPRAVENTRICULAR
TACHYCARDIA: VAV, VAAV, PPI, AND VA LINKING

SECTION I
DIAGNOSTIC ELECTROPHYSIOLOGY—
MAPPING, IMAGING, AND
PACING MANEUVERS

33

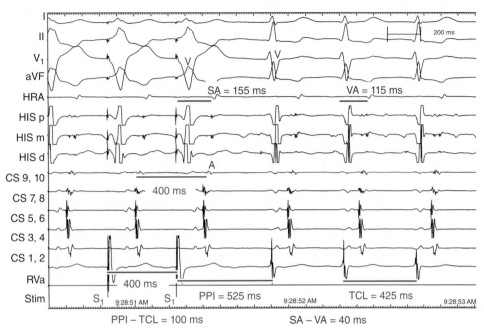

FIGURE 4-5 PPI-TCL and SA-VA example of a patient with a septal AP-mediated AVRT. As the ventricle is a part of the AVRT circuit, RV pacing as a result is near the circuit lending to a shorter PPI and shorter SA interval. PPI-TCL <115 ms and SA-VA <85 ms are consistent with this patient's diagnosis of a septal AP-mediated AVRT.

Keys to Performing This Maneuver

- Pace the ventricle at a CL 10 to 40 ms shorter than the tachycardia CL.
- Confirm ventricular capture.
- Confirm that the atrial CL equals the pacing CL.
- Identify the last entrained atrial depolarization.
- Identify the next ventricular depolarization.
- Characterize the response as VAV or VAAV.
- If the mechanism is now between atypical AVNRT and AVRT, calculate PPI-TCL or SA-VA.

ATRIAL OVERDRIVE PACING

Another useful pacing maneuver in tachycardia is to entrain from the atrium. This pacing maneuver can be used to assess for VA linking and effectively exclude AT.

VA Linking

- Pace the atrium 10 to 40 ms shorter than the tachycardia CL to entrain the ventricle.
- Compare the VA interval of the first return beat after cessation of pacing to the VA interval during tachycardia.
- If the VA interval is unchanged, this suggests that atrial activation is linked to ventricular activation (Figure 4-6) thus excluding AT as the mechanism.
- VA linking is not 100% predictive as coincident events can rarely result in apparent VA linking and 3% of AVNRT do not show VA linking.[2]

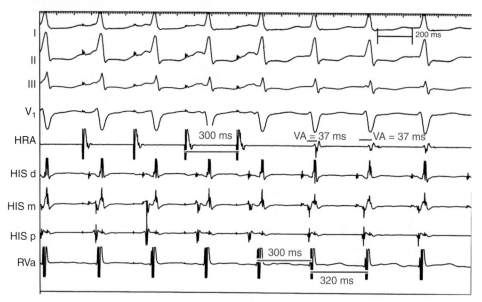

FIGURE 4-6 VA linking in a patient with AVNRT. Upon cessation of atrial overdrive pacing, the last entrained ventricular beat has the same VA time as that in tachycardia, suggesting that the timing of atrial activation is linked to the timing of ventricular activation.

REFERENCES

1. Knight BP, Zivin A, Souza J, et al. A technique for the rapid diagnosis of atrial tachycardia in the electrophysiology laboratory. *J Am Coll Cardiol*. 1999;33(3):775-781.

2. Knight BP, Ebinger M, Oral H, et al. Diagnostic value of tachycardia features and pacing maneuvers during paroxysmal supraventricular tachycardia. *J Am Coll Cardiol*. 2000;36:574-582.

3. Michaud GF, Tada H, Chough S, et al. Differentiation of atypical atrioventricular node reentrant tachycardia from orthodromic reciprocating tachycardia using a septal accessory pathway by the response to ventricular pacing. *J Am Coll Cardiol*. 2001;38:1163-1167.

4. Bennett MT, Leong-Sit P, Gula LJ, et al. Entrainment for distinguishing atypical atrioventricular node reentrant tachycardia from atrioventricular reentrant tachycardia over septal accessory pathways with long-rp [corrected] tachycardia. *Circ Arrhythm Electrophysiol*. 2011;4:506-509.

DIAGNOSTIC MANEUVERS FOR SUPRAVENTRICULAR
TACHYCARDIA: PVC ON HIS AND PARA-HISIAN PACING

SECTION I
DIAGNOSTIC ELECTROPHYSIOLOGY—
MAPPING, IMAGING, AND
PACING MANEUVERS

35

5 DIAGNOSTIC MANEUVERS FOR SUPRAVENTRICULAR TACHYCARDIA: PVC ON HIS AND PARA-HISIAN PACING

Sharon Shen, MD, and Bradley P. Knight, MD

CASE PRESENTATION

A 24-year-old man without significant past medical history presents to clinic for management of paroxysmal supraventricular tachycardia (PSVT). He recalls palpitations since he was a teenager, but the episodes were generally infrequent and not bothersome. Over the past few months, however, episodes have become more frequent, occurring once per week, with the last episode prompting a visit to the emergency department. At that time, a regular, narrow QRS tachycardia at 145 bpm was noted and terminated with adenosine. Baseline ECG shows normal sinus rhythm with normal intervals and absence of preexcitation. The patient elected to undergo catheter ablation.

CASE EXPLANATION

This clinical scenario, in particular the patient's young age, raises suspicion for a concealed accessory pathway (AP) participating in atrioventricular reentrant tachycardia (AVRT). This chapter will focus on the diagnostic maneuvers of His-refractory ventricular extrastimulus testing, otherwise known as delivering a "PVC on His" and

para-Hisian pacing, two maneuvers frequently used to determine the presence of a concealed or retrogradely conducting AP.

PVC ON HIS

In this patient with a suspected AP participating in tachycardia, a useful maneuver to consider during tachycardia is to deliver a ventricular extrastimulus when the His bundle is refractory and assess its effect on the atrium (Figure 5-1).[1]

- Advancement of atrial activation with a PVC delivered during PSVT when the His bundle should be refractory as seen in this patient indicates that a retrogradely conducting AP is present, but it may not necessarily participate in tachycardia. Although unlikely, an atrial tachycardia with a concealed bystander AP cannot be excluded.

- A His-synchronous PVC that *terminates* the tachycardia without preexcitation of the atrium is diagnostic of AVRT (Figure 5-2). An atrial tachycardia would not terminate under those conditions. Note that in this example there was an attempt to entrain the atrium with ventricular pacing, but pacing terminated tachycardia. Careful examination showed that the first beat of the pacing train occurred during the His bundle refractory period and ultimately provided the diagnosis of AVRT.

- *The Principle:* A PVC that preexcites the atrium must do so via an AP because when the His-Purkinje system (HPS) is refractory during PSVT, a PVC cannot conduct to the atrium through the HPS. Similarly, a PVC that terminates tachycardia without preexciting the atrium must have occurred as a result of causing block in the AP. When atrial activation is *delayed* with a PVC delivered during His refractoriness, the maneuver is also diagnostic for AVRT because an AP must be participating in the tachycardia.

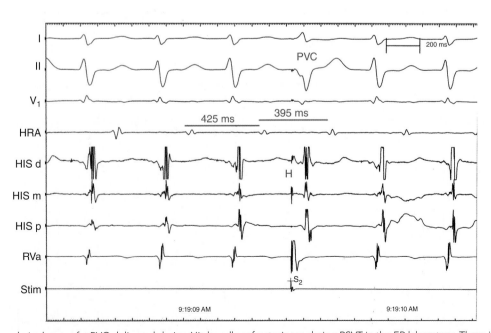

FIGURE 5-1 An example is shown of a PVC delivered during His bundle refractoriness during PSVT in the EP laboratory. There is preexcitation of the atrium with a His-synchronous PVC, which is evidence of an accessory pathway but is not diagnostic of AVRT. Although unlikely, an atrial tachycardia with a concealed bystander accessory pathway cannot be excluded. The His bundle is refractory as seen by the coincident antegrade His potential. Thus, retrograde conduction of the PVC must have occurred over an accessory pathway.

- *Pitfall:* Preexcitation of the atrium may not occur despite the presence of an AP if the pacing site is far from the ventricular insertion of the AP; the ability of the ventricular extrastimulus to enter the reentrant circuit before ventricular activation over the normal pathway is affected by (1) the conduction time from the ventricular stimulation site to the AP, (2) the local ventricular refractory period, and (3) the tachycardia cycle length.

Keys to Performing This Maneuver

- Scan diastole with PVCs at progressively shorter coupling intervals (decrease by 10 ms).

- Confirm ventricular capture.

- Look for shortening of the A-A interval with the longest coupled PVC.

- Confirm that the PVC is delivered when the His bundle is refractory either by a manifest His potential (see Figure 5-1) or that the stimulus is less than 35 to 55 ms before the next expected His potential (see Figure 5-2).

- An alternative method is to examine the atrial response during overdrive ventricular pacing when the ventricular complexes appear fused. Fusion confirms anterograde activation of the His bundle during the initiation of overdrive pacing. Preexcitation of the atrium with a fused ventricular complex therefore indicates the presence of an AP (Figure 5-3).

PARA-HISIAN PACING

- Useful maneuver performed during sinus rhythm to evaluate for the presence of a septal AP.[2]

- Incremental high-output pacing during sinus rhythm is performed at the site of the largest His bundle recording with various stimulation intensities to achieve (1) simultaneous ventricular and His bundle (and/or right bundle branch) capture and (2) ventricular capture alone.

- Simultaneous ventricular and His bundle capture results in both anterograde and retrograde conduction via the HPS with the anterograde conduction resulting in a relatively narrow QRS morphology.

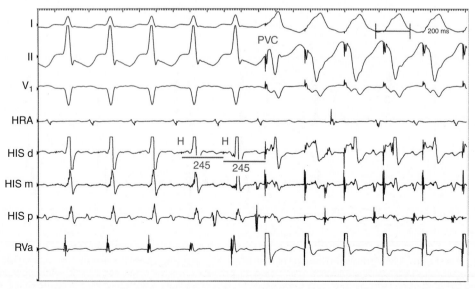

FIGURE 5-2 Termination of tachycardia with a His-synchronous PVC without preexcitation of the atrium is shown. This is diagnostic of AVRT.

DIAGNOSTIC MANEUVERS FOR SUPRAVENTRICULAR
TACHYCARDIA: PVC ON HIS AND PARA-HISIAN PACING

SECTION I
DIAGNOSTIC ELECTROPHYSIOLOGY—
MAPPING, IMAGING, AND
PACING MANEUVERS

37

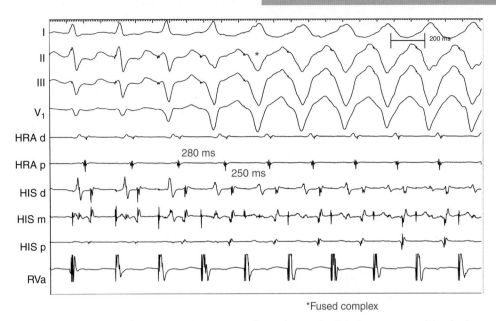

*Fused complex

FIGURE 5-3 Preexcitation of the atrium with a fused ventricular extrastimulus is shown. The fused appearance of the third ventricular extrastimulus confirms that the His bundle was activated anterogradely. Preexcitation of the atrium in this situation offers the same evidence as when a PVC is delivered when the His is refractory and confirms the presence of an accessory pathway.

- *Nodal Response:* In the absence of an AP, retrograde conduction occurs over the His bundle with a stimulus to His (SH) interval of 0, followed by atrial activation where the stimulus to atrium (SA) interval equals the His to atrium (HA) interval. With a decrease in the pacing output, His bundle capture is lost (confirmed by a widening in the QRS) and anterograde conduction occurs over ventricular myocardium. His activation is delayed (SH increases) as it now follows retrograde activation of the right bundle leading to an increase in the SA interval (Figure 5-4A).

- *Extranodal Response:* As retrograde conduction occurs over the AP instead of the AV node, the SA interval remains unchanged (Figure 5-4B).

- Carefully examine that the retrograde atrial activation sequence is unchanged; a change suggests that retrograde conduction could be occurring over multiple pathways, either over multiple APs, fast and slow AV node pathways, or simultaneously over the AV node and AP.

- *Pitfalls:* Although an extranodal response has a positive predictive value of 83% for AVRT, the sensitivity is only 47% when assessed for all forms of APs.[1] Ability to elicit an extranodal response is limited by the how far the AP is located from the pacing site and how slowly it conducts.

Keys to Performing This Maneuver

- Identify (1) simultaneous His bundle and ventricular capture and (2) ventricular capture only with varying the pacing stimulus output.

- Confirm the absence of atrial capture.

- Confirm that the retrograde atrial activation sequence is unchanged.

- Compare the SA intervals at the earliest atrial activation.

  ○ SA increases with loss of His bundle capture → nodal response (Figure 5-5A).

  ○ SA unchanged → extranodal response (Figure 5-5B).

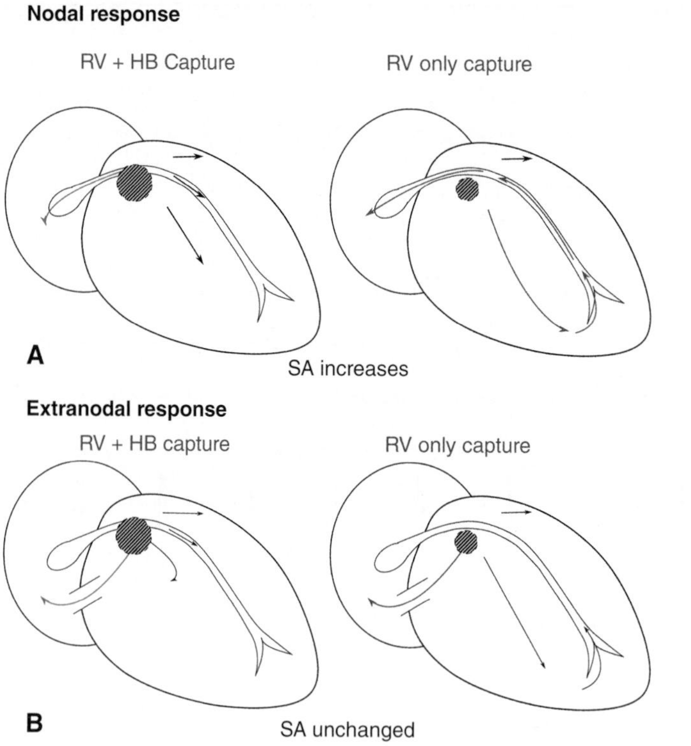

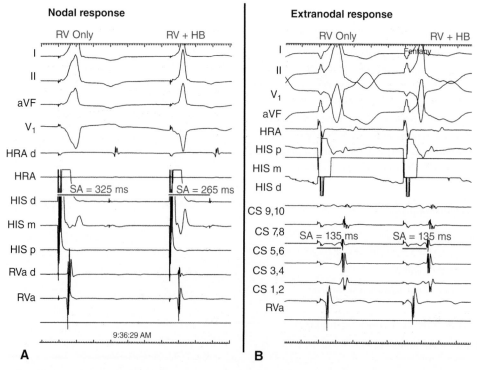

FIGURE 5-4 Para-Hisian pacing. (A) *Nodal response:* High-output pacing at the His bundle (HB) captures both the HB and right ventricle (RV), whereby anterograde and retrograde activation occurs over the His-Purkinje system leading to a short stimulus to atrium (SA) interval. At a lower pacing output, only the ventricle is paced, and retrograde atrial activation is delayed (SA increases) as it now follows retrograde right bundle activation. (B) *Extranodal response:* As retrograde conduction occurs over the accessory pathway and not the AV node, the SA interval is unchanged upon loss of HB capture.

FIGURE 5-5 Examples of nodal (A) and extranodal (B) responses to para-Hisian pacing.

DIAGNOSTIC MANEUVERS FOR SUPRAVENTRICULAR
TACHYCARDIA: PVC ON HIS AND PARA-HISIAN PACING

SECTION I
DIAGNOSTIC ELECTROPHYSIOLOGY—
MAPPING, IMAGING, AND
PACING MANEUVERS

39

REFERENCES

1. Knight BP, Ebinger M, Oral H, et al. Diagnostic value of tachycardia features and pacing maneuvers during paroxysmal supraventricular tachycardia. *J Am Coll Cardiol*. 2000;36(2):574-582.

2. Hirao K, Otomo K, Wang X, et al. Para-Hisian pacing. A new method for differentiating retrograde conduction over an accessory AV pathway from conduction over the AV node. *Circulation*. 1996;94(5):1027-1035.

6 ATRIAL TACHYCARDIA AND CARDIAC ANATOMY: CRISTA TERMINALIS

Tomos Walters, MBBS, BMedSc, Jonathan M. Kalman, MBBS, PhD

CASE PRESENTATION

A 55-year-old previously well woman presented with fatigue and progressively increasing exertional dyspnea. She appeared unwell, with clinical features of decompensated left ventricular (LV) failure. An ECG revealed long runs of a narrow complex long R-P tachycardia with a P-wave morphology similar to that of the occasional sinus beats observed (Figure 6-1). A transthoracic echocardiogram (TTE) revealed a dilated cardiomyopathy with an LV ejection fraction LVEF of 32%. Cardiac MRI demonstrated minimal myocardial fibrosis and coronary arteries were free of disease. Assessment in the electrophysiology laboratory confirmed a sustained tachycardia with a TCL of 460 msec, a VAAHV response to entrainment from the ventricular apex, and an earliest site of atrial activation in the region of the high crista terminalis (CT). Mapping identified the earliest atrial activation at this location, 20 msec ahead of the P wave. Ablation at this location resulted in speeding and termination of the tachycardia, which could subsequently not be induced with either atrial pacing or isoprenaline. Over 6 months there was no evidence of recurrent tachycardia. All clinical evidence of heart failure resolved, and repeat TTE demonstrated normalization of LV structure and function.

EPIDEMIOLOGY

Focal atrial tachycardia (FAT) is a relatively uncommon form of supraventricular tachycardia (SVT) encountered in the electrophysiology laboratory in adults, accounting for no more than 15% of studies performed for management of SVT.[1] While reports differ, FAT appears to be equally present in men and women and to be overrepresented in younger patients.[2,3] The single most common location for FAT is the crista terminalis. Tachycardias arising from the CT show a particular preponderance in women and are relatively more likely to arise in older patients.

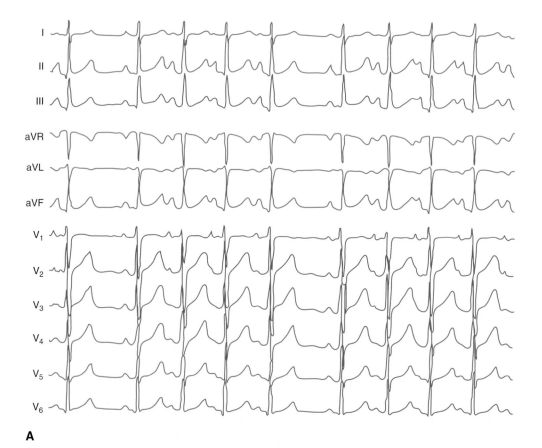

A

FIGURE 6-1 Patient TM. (A) Twelve-lead ECG showing recurrent bursts of FAT. Tachycardia P-wave morphology is similar to the sinus P-wave morphology. Biphasic (+/−) in V1, positive in lead I and negative in aVL indicates a CT origin. Positive morphology in the inferior leads indicates a position high on the CT. (B) Intracardiac electrograms EGMs. The earliest atrial signal is from the distal bipole of a catheter laid along the CT. (C) The upper left panel shows a coronal view of an anatomic specimen of the RA, with the CT running anterior to the SVC os and down the posterolateral right atrial wall before terminating anterior to the IVC. The lower left panel shows the electroanatomic map localizing the earliest site of activation during tachycardia to the superior CT, anteromedial to the SVC-RA junction. The panels on the right show LAO and RAO images of the catheter laid along the CT and of the ablation catheter at the time of successful termination of the tachycardia. (CT = crista terminalis; SVC = superior vena cava; IVC = inferior vena cava; FO = foramen ovale; CS os = coronary sinus os; RA = right atrium.) (D) The mapping catheter records an EGM 20 ms ahead of the P wave. Ablation at this location successfully terminated the tachycardia.

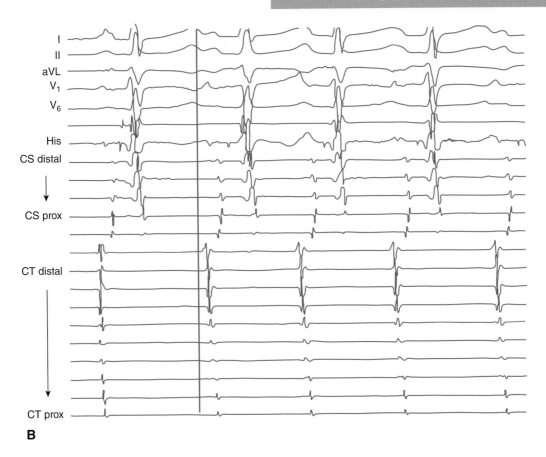

B

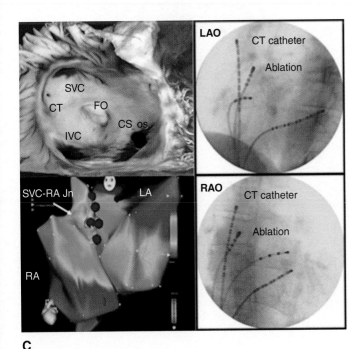

C

FIGURE 6-1 (*Continued*)

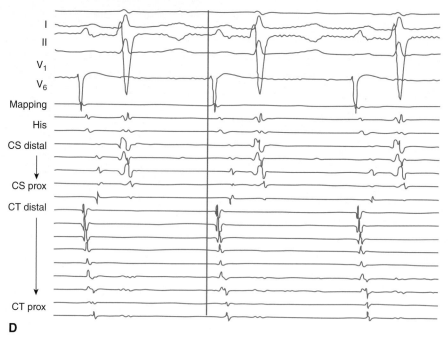

D

FIGURE 6-1 (*Continued*)

Patients may present with specific symptoms of variable severity that include palpitations, chest discomfort, dyspnea, fatigue, dizziness and syncope, with a first symptomatic event between the ages of 10 and 39 years in the majority.[1] In a subset, the mode of presentation relates to the development of a tachycardia-mediated cardiomyopathy (TCM), reported in 10% in a single-center series of 345 patients with no preexisting structural heart disease.[4]

PATHOPHYSIOLOGY

FAT is characterized by an identifiable focal origin with subsequent centrifugal atrial activation, with a mechanism based in any of abnormal automaticity, triggered activity, or microreentry.[2,5] Precise definition of the electrophysiological mechanism of a given FAT may be difficult because of overlapping features and is of less relevance in the ablation era.

FAT has been thought to arise in structurally normal atria. There is, however, evidence from surgical specimens of myocardial inflammation, infiltration, or fibrosis in almost 50% of cases,[6] which may be reflected in areas of low voltage and electrogram fractionation on electroanatomic maps.

FAT in the absence of significant structural heart disease is recognized to cluster in particular anatomic locations (Figure 6-2). Characteristic locations in the right atrium include the tricuspid annulus, the right perinodal region, the ostium of the coronary sinus, and the trabeculated right atrial appendage, with the most common site of origin along the long axis of the CT.[7,8] In the largest published series, 73% were found to have their origin in the right atrium, with 43% clustered along the CT. Of these 47% were located in the superior portion, 47% in the mid portion, and 6% in the inferior portion.

DIAGNOSIS

In the absence of significant structural heart disease, the surface ECG P-wave morphology provides a noninvasive guide to the location of the tachycardia focus (Figures 6-2 and 6-3). Leads V_1 and aVL are most useful

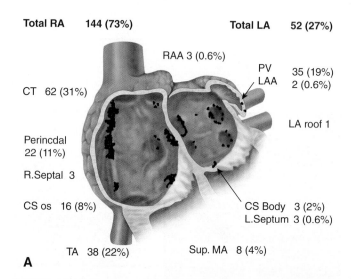

A

FIGURE 6-2 (A) Clustering of 196 FATs in 186 consecutive patients undergoing catheter ablation. A coronal section through the heart at the atrioventricular junction, with the atrioventricular valves removed. (CS = coronary sinus; CT = crista terminalis; LA = left atrium; LAA = left atrial appendage; MA = mitral annulus; PV = pulmonary vein; RA = right atrium; RAA = right atrial appendage; TA = tricuspid annulus.). (B) A P-wave algorithm using the anterior precordial leads, lead aVL, the inferior leads, and any change in the V_1 P wave between tachycardia and sinus rhythm. When tested prospectively, this algorithm correctly located the focus in 93% of cases.

ATRIAL TACHYCARDIA AND CARDIAC ANATOMY:
CRISTA TERMINALIS

SECTION I
DIAGNOSTIC ELECTROPHYSIOLOGY—
MAPPING, IMAGING, AND
PACING MANEUVERS

43

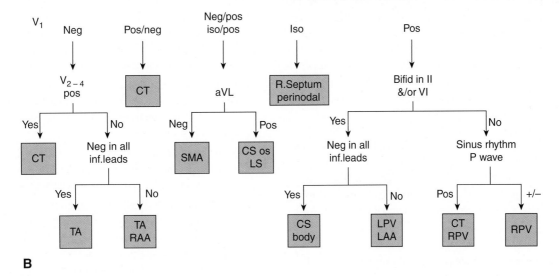

B

FIGURE 6-2 (*Continued*)

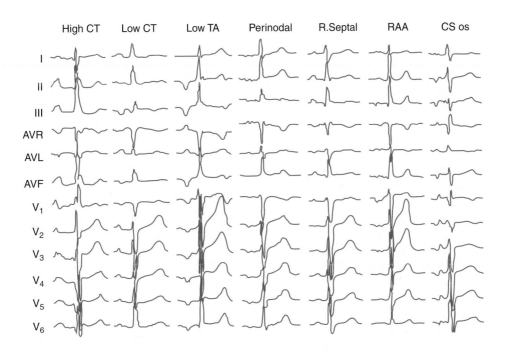

FIGURE 6-3 Representative example of tachycardia P waves from common right atrial locations.

- Foci around the tricuspid annulus (TA) are identified by a negative P wave in V_1, which may be bifid, and a positive or isoelectric P wave in aVL. As with foci on the CT, the morphology in the inferior leads depends on the relative superior-inferior positioning of the focus around the TA.

- The superior TA and the right atrial appendage (RAA) are anatomically very close and often have very similar P-wave morphologies.

- P waves arising from the perinodal region or interatrial septum are relatively narrow, with lead V_1 being isoelectric or biphasic (–/+). The greatest diagnostic imprecision in interpretation of P-wave morphology is for midline tachycardias.

- For FAT arising from the coronary sinus (CS) ostium, lead V_1 has an initial component that is either isoelectric or slightly inverted followed by a positive component (iso /+ or –/+). Moving across the precordium, the initial component becomes more negative, and the second component becomes isoelectric. Lead aVL is positive and the P waves are deeply negative in the inferior leads.

in identifying a left or right atrial origin.[8,9] A positive or biphasic (−/+) morphology in V_1 is highly suggestive of a left atrial location, and either a negative or biphasic (+/−) morphology is strongly associated with a right atrial focus. A positive or biphasic P wave in aVL is associated with a right atrial location, with a positive predictive value of 83.3% and a negative predictive value of 84.6%. Predictive accuracy is most limited for foci in the midline, including those arising from the high CT.

Kistler et al reported 62 FATs arising specifically from the CT.[8] Lead V_1 manifests a positive P wave in 25%, a biphasic (+/−) P wave in 67%, and a negative P wave in 7%. All had a negative morphology in lead aVR and a positive P wave in lead I, and 89% manifest a negative or isoelectric P wave in lead aVL. Tachycardias from the high and midportions of the CT typically manifest an upright inferior P wave.

MANAGEMENT

There is a paucity of robust studies assessing the relative efficacy of the various pharmacologic management strategies. Class Ia, class Ic, and class III antiarrhythmic agents have been used to attempt chronic suppression of a tachycardia focus, but the reported success rates are disappointing. Quinidine and procainamide have demonstrated success in only 20% of cases, while flecainide and encainide have been reported successful in over 50%.[10] Several small studies have demonstrated higher success rates with sotalol[11] and with amiodarone, but the toxicity of these agents, in particular amiodarone, limits their applicability.

Over the past 20 years catheter ablation has evolved to become the cornerstone management technique, offering the potential for definitive cure with a low risk of major complications. Activation mapping with multipolar catheters, or more usually a 3-dimensional mapping system, is employed to localise the focus. The onset of the bipolar electrogram recorded at the site of successful ablation typically precedes the P-wave onset by >20 msec. Atrioventricular block or ventricular pacing may be required to fully reveal the P wave, the onset of which can then be defined in relation to activation at a stable endocardial reference such as a coronary sinus bipole. Recording a QS unipolar electrogram[12] may aid in localizing a successful ablation site. Some studies have suggested that the signal at the successful site may be fractionated or multicomponent, but this has not been a consistent finding.[7] Mapping of infrequent ectopy may be aided by the use of a non-contact mapping system, which can provide over 3000 virtual electrograms from a single beat.[13]

Catheter ablation of FAT in contemporary practice is highly successful. Although radiofrequency ablation is the standard approach, cryoablation is an alternative in the perinodal area. Series including both right and left atrial foci have reported success rates between 69% and 100%, with very low rates of major complications that may, depending on the site of ablation, include pericardial effusion and tamponade, phrenic nerve injury, sinoatrial and atrioventricular node injury, and pulmonary vein stenosis.[3,14] Long-term recurrence rates are low, varying between 0% and 33%,[15] with predictors of recurrence being a left atrial focus, older age, coexistent cardiac disease, and multiple foci.[16] In patients with TCM, catheter ablation has been associated with a long-term drug-free success rate of 87%, and LV function typically returns to normal within 3 months.[4]

REFERENCES

1. Rodriguez LM, de Chillou C, Schläpfer J, et al. Age at onset and gender of patients with different types of supraventricular tachycardias. *Am J Cardiol.* 1992;70(13):1213-1215.

2. Chen SA, Chiang CE, Yang CJ, et al. Sustained atrial tachycardia in adult patients. Electrophysiological characteristics, pharmacological response, possible mechanisms, and effects of radiofrequency ablation. *Circulation.* 1994;90(3):1262-1278.

3. Kammeraad JAE, Balaji S, Oliver RP, et al. Nonautomatic focal atrial tachycardia: characterization and ablation of a poorly understood arrhythmia in 38 patients. *Pacing Clin Electrophysiol.* 2003;26(3):736-742.

4. Medi C, Kalman JM, Haqqani H, et al. Tachycardia-mediated cardiomyopathy secondary to focal atrial tachycardia: long-term outcome after catheter ablation. *J Am Coll Cardiol.* 2009;53(19):1791-1797.

5. Saoudi N, Cosío F, Waldo A, et al. A classification of atrial flutter and regular atrial tachycardia according to electrophysiological mechanisms and anatomical bases; a Statement from a Joint Expert Group from The Working Group of Arrhythmias of the European Society of Cardiology and the North American Society of Pacing and Electrophysiology. *Eur Heart J.* 2001;22:1162-1182.

6. McGuire MA, Johnson DC, Nunn GR, Yung T, Uther JB and Ross DL. Surgical therapy for atrial tachycardia in adults. *J Am Coll Cardiol.* 1989;14(7):1777-1782.

7. Kalman JM, Olgin JE, Karch MR, Hamdan M, Lee RJ and Lesh MD. "Cristal Tachycardias": origin of right atrial tachycardias from the crista terminalis identified by intracardiac echocardiography. *J Am Coll Cardiol.* 1998;31(2):451-459.

8. Kistler PM, Roberts-Thomson KC, Haqqani HM, et al. P-wave morphology in focal atrial tachycardia: development of an algorithm to predict the anatomic site of origin. *J Am Coll Cardiol.* 2006;48(5):1010-1017.

9. Tang CW, Scheinman MM, Van Hare GF, et al. Use of P wave configuration during atrial tachycardia to predict site of origin. *J Am Coll Cardiol.* 1995;26(5):1315-1324.

10. Kuck KH, Kunze KP, Schlüter M, Duckeck W. Encainide versus flecainide for chronic atrial and junctional ectopic tachycardia. *Am J Cardiol.* 1988;62(19):37L-44L.

11. Colloridi V, Perri C, Ventriglia F, Critelli G. Oral sotalol in pediatric atrial ectopic tachycardia. *Am Heart J.* 1992;123(1):254-256.

12. Tang K, Ma J, Zhang S, et al. Unipolar electrogram in identification of successful targets for radiofrequency catheter ablation of focal atrial tachycardia. *Chin Med J.* 2003;116(10):1455-1458.

13. Wieczorek M, Salili AR, Kaubisch S, Hoeltgen R. Catheter ablation of non-sustained focal right atrial tachycardia guided by virtual noncontact electrograms. *Europace.* 2011;13(6):876-882.

14. Anguera I, Brugada J, Roba M, et al. Outcomes after radio frequency catheter ablation of atrial tachycardia. *Am J Cardiol.* 2001;87(7):886-890.

15. Roberts-Thomson KC, Kistler PM, Kalman JM. Focal atrial tachycardia II: management. *Pacing Clin Electrophysiol.* 2006;29(7):769-778.

16. Chen SA, Tai CT, Chiang CE, Ding YA, Chang MS. Focal atrial tachycardia: reanalysis of the clinical and electrophysiologic characteristics and prediction of successful radiofrequency ablation. *J Cardiovasc Electrophysiol.* 1998;9(4):355-365.

CASE STUDIES IN SUPRAVENTRICULAR TACHYCARDIA

7 TYPICAL ATRIOVENTRICULAR NODAL REENTRANT TACHYCARDIA

Mahmoud Houmsse, MD, and Anish Amin, MD

CASE PRESENTATION

A 31-year-old woman with a 10-year history of palpitations is referred for an electrophysiologic (EP) study and consideration for radiofrequency ablation (RFA) for recurrent symptomatic paroxysmal supraventricular tachycardia (PSVT). Her symptoms start suddenly and are associated with chest pain and shortness of breath. The index episode terminated suddenly before she arrived at the emergency department (ED). Her initial evaluation, including 12-lead electrocardiogram (ECG), thyroid function testing, and echocardiogram was not revealing. Empiric medical therapy with atenolol initially suppressed her PSVT; however, breakthrough episodes have occurred over the past few months. Her most recent episode was recorded on an ECG as a narrow QRS complex tachycardia without an obvious P wave compared to baseline ECG (Figure 7-1A and B). Valsalva maneuver did not affect the tachycardia, and intravenous adenosine was administered, which successfully terminated her arrhythmia. Therapeutic options, including changing medical therapy versus EP

study and RFA of her PSVT, were discussed with her. She requested the latter option since her symptoms were not controlled on medical therapy. Her EP study demonstrated dual AV node physiology and easily inducible typical atrioventricular nodal reentrant tachycardia (AVNRT). Slow pathway mapping and ablation was performed successfully, and postablation she had no inducible tachycardia or evidence of slow pathway function. Her atenolol was discontinued, and she has had no further episodes of tachycardia after long-term follow-up.

EPIDEMIOLOGY

AVNRT is the most common type of regular narrow QRS complex SVT and accounts for approximately 60% to 70% of cases. There is a higher incidence in women and younger individuals, with the mean age of symptom onset at 30 years.[1,2] The slow-fast variant of AVNRT accounts for nearly 90% of all AVNRT and is therefore referred to as typical AVNRT.

CLINICAL PRESENTATION

The onset of symptoms with AVNRT are usually paroxysmal in nature occurring suddenly without warning, but in some patients episodes can be brought on during high adrenergic states such as exercise. Symptoms that occur during AVNRT, like other forms of PSVT, are nonspecific and include palpitations, shortness of breath, chest pain, and dizziness. Frank syncope occurs rarely and appears to be rate-related since it is uncommon at rates less than 170 bpm.[3]

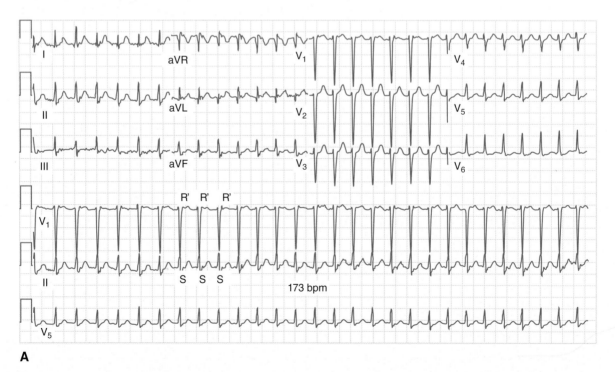

FIGURES 7-1A AND 7-1B Twelve-lead ECG during typical AVNRT and normal sinus rhythm. During typical AVNRT, the QRS complex is usually narrow, and the P wave is often absent due to simultaneous activation of the atrium and ventricle. If, however, the atrial depolarization is slightly delayed, a portion of the P wave may be seen at the end of the QRS complex and be manifest as a pseudo R' wave in lead V1 or a pseudo S wave in the inferior leads. Figure 7-1A was taken during tachycardia at a rate of 173 bpm. No clear P wave was discernible, but terminal deflections were seen in leads V1 and II consistent with pseudo R' and pseudo S waves (labeled R' and S, respectively). A comparison to the baseline ECG (shown in Figure 7-1B) is required to confirm this, and as can be seen there were no R' or S waves in leads V1 or II during normal sinus rhythm.

Comments:

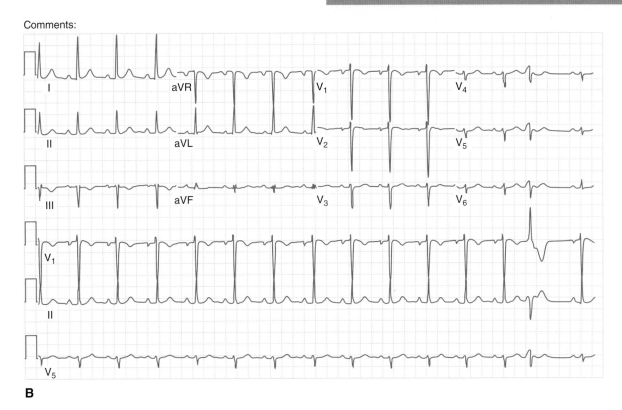

B

FIGURES 7-1A AND 7-1B (*Continued*)

ANATOMY

AVNRT utilizes both AV nodal and peri-AV nodal tissue as substrate for the reentrant circuit.[2] This circuit is located within the triangle of Koch, which is boarded by the tricuspid annulus anteriorly, the tendon of Todoro posteriorly, and the coronary sinus inferiorly (Figure 7-2A and B). The triangle of Koch is divided into three zones: anterior, middle, and posterior. The anterior zone is located at the apex of the triangle and contains the compact AV node and initial portion of the His bundle. The middle zone is located just inferior to the anterior zone, and the posterior zone is located at the base of the triangle and contains the ostium of the coronary sinus. The fast and slow pathways that make up the reentrant circuit for typical AVNRT are also located within the triangle of Koch. The fast pathway is located in the anterior portion of the triangle in close proximity to the compact AV node. The slow pathway is found in the middle or posterior portions of the triangle often around the coronary sinus ostium. The fast and slow pathways join at the lower and upper common pathways. The latter is located within the AV node proximal to the bundle of His.[4] Understanding this anatomy is especially important when ablative therapy is contemplated. Energy delivery in the anterior zone targeting the fast pathway carries a significant risk of creating AV block since this is where the compact AV node and proximal His bundle are located.

ELECTROPHYSIOLOGY

The basic components of a typical AVNRT circuit are a slow pathway that conducts in the antegrade direction, a fast pathway that conducts in the retrograde direction, and upper and lower common pathways which link the fast and slow pathways. Antegrade conduction over

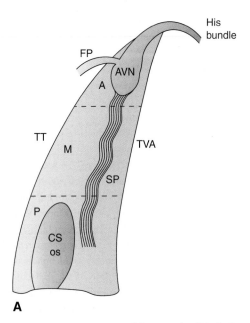

A

FIGURES 7-2A AND 7-2B Anatomy of the triangle of Koch. Figure 7-2A depicts the anatomy in the right anterior oblique (RAO) view, and Figure 7-2B depicts the anatomy in the left anterior oblique (LAO) view. The triangle of Koch is bordered anteriorly by the tricuspid valve annulus (TVA), posteriorly by the Tendon of Todaro (TT), and inferiorly by the coronary sinus ostium (CS os). The anterior (A) zone contains the compact atrioventricular node (AVN) and the fast pathway (FP). The middle (M) and posterior zones contain the slow pathway (SP), and the posterior zone also includes the coronary sinus ostium (CS os).

both a fast and slow AV nodal pathway ("dual AV nodal physiology") can usually be demonstrated in patients with typical AVNRT. The fast pathway has more rapid conduction but usually has a longer refractory period compared to the slow pathway. When an appropriately timed premature atrial contraction occurs, it will block in the fast pathway and conduct over the slow pathway to the His bundle and ventricle resulting in significant prolongation of the AH and PR intervals compared to the normal sinus beat. This electrophysiologic (EP) phenomenon of changing conduction from the fast to the slow pathway is known as an "AV nodal Jump."[5] During an EP study, an AV nodal jump is defined as a 50 ms increase in the AH interval corresponding to a 10 ms decrease in the A1-A2coupling interval during atrial extrastimulus testing (Figure 7-3A and B).

The finding of antegrade dual AV nodal physiology only defines the presence of antegrade fast and slow pathways, but it does not demonstrate the existence of a retrograde fast pathway, which is a necessary component of the AVNRT circuit. The presence of a retrograde fast pathway is suggested when there is rapid ventriculo-atrial (VA) conduction during ventricular pacing. Some patients with typical AVNRT may have very poor VA conduction or VA dissociation during baseline EP testing and may require the addition of an isoproterenol infusion to elicit fast pathway conduction.[5] The presence of a retrograde fast pathway is confirmed if an AV nodal echo can be demonstrated during atrial pacing maneuvers (Figure 7-4). An AV nodal echo is the result of antegrade conduction down the slow pathway to the lower common pathway and then simultaneous conduction retrograde over the fast pathway to the atrium and antegrade over the His-Purkinje system to the ventricle. It is this simultaneous or "in parallel" conduction along with very rapid retrograde fast pathway conduction that results in the short VA times (≤70 ms recorded on the His bundle catheters) that are characteristic of typical AVNRT. In some cases the VA time during tachycardia may be zero or even negative. This can occur if the conduction time from the lower common pathway retrograde to the atrium is equal to or faster than the antegrade conduction time to the ventricle. If after an AV node echo the slow pathway is not refractory, then antegrade conduction can occur over the slow pathway, and typical AVNRT can be induced (Figure 7-5A and B).

The AV relationship during sustained typical AVNRT is almost always 1:1; however, the atrium and ventricle are not obligatory components of the tachycardia circuit, and therefore AV or VA block can occur without termination of the arrhythmia.[6] Infra-Hisian block below the lower common pathway is relatively common at the onset of AVNRT but usually extinguishes quickly as the bundle of His refractory period accommodates overtime. Block above the upper common pathway during AVNRT resulting in VA conduction block is far less common than AV block but has been reported.[7]

DIAGNOSIS

The clinical presentation and ECG findings of typical AVNRT, although suggestive of the diagnosis, are not specific for it, and therefore EP testing is needed to confirm the tachycardia mechanism.

Diagnostic Criteria for Typical AVNRT during EP Testing

- Induction
  - Induction is dependent upon developing a critical degree of AH prolongation (Figure 7-5A and B).[8]

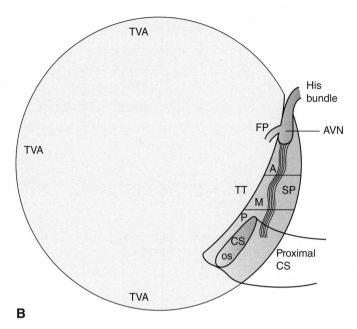

B

FIGURES 7-2A AND 7-2B (Continued)

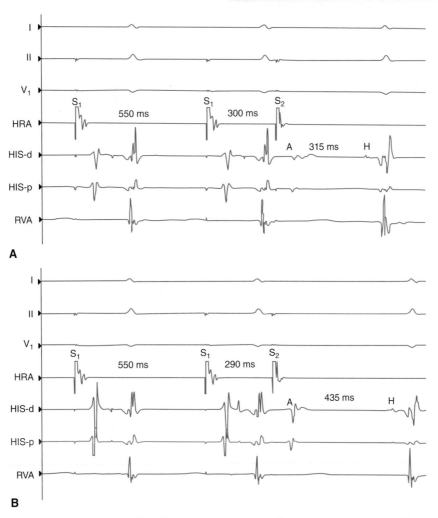

FIGURES 7-3A AND 7-3B Dual AV nodal physiology. These figures demonstrate atrial extrastimulus pacing at a drive train of 550 ms. Shown are surface leads I, II, and V_1 and intracardiac recordings from the high right atrium (HRA), His bundle distal (His-d), His bundle proximal (His-p), and right ventricle apex (RVA). In Figure 7-3A, with an S_2 coupling interval of 300 ms the corresponding atrial to His (AH) interval is 315 ms. In Figure 7-3B the S_1S_2 coupling interval is 290 ms with a corresponding AH interval of 435 ms, an increase of 120 ms. An AH interval increase of >50 ms for a decrement in the S_1S_2 coupling of 10 ms defines an AV nodal jump and indicates the presence of antegrade dual AV nodal physiology.

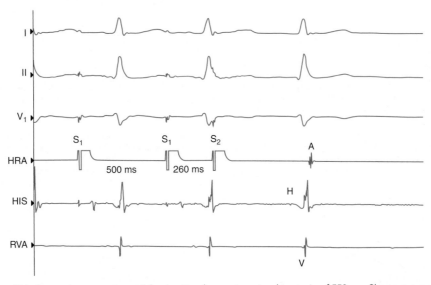

FIGURE 7-4 AV nodal echo. This figure demonstrates atrial extrastimulus pacing at a drive train of 550 ms. Shown are surface leads I, II, and V_1 and intracardiac recordings from the high right atrium (HRA), His bundle (His), and right ventricle apex (RVA). An S_1S_2 coupling interval of 260 ms results in conduction down the slow pathway and a prolonged AH interval. At this degree of AH prolongation an atrial event (A) with a short VA conduction time occurs. This is an AV nodal echo and confirms the presence of retrograde fast pathway conduction.

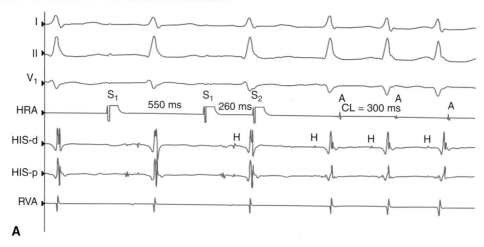

A

FIGURE 7-5A Initiation of AVNRT. Figure 7-5A demonstrates atrial extrastimulus pacing at a drive train of 550 ms. Shown are surface leads I, II, and V_1 and intracardiac recordings from the high right atrial (HRA), His bundle distal (His-d), His bundle proximal (His-p), and right ventricular apex (RVA). An S_1S_2 coupling interval of 260 ms results in antegrade conduction down the slow pathway and initiation of typical AVNRT at a cycle length of 300 ms. The atrial, His, and ventricular electrograms are labeled A, H, and V, respectively, on the intracardiac recordings.

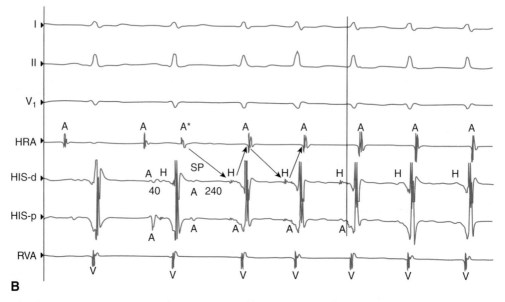

B

FIGURE 7-5B This figure demonstrates a spontaneous premature atrial contraction (PAC) initiating typical AVNRT. Shown are surface leads I, II, and V_1 and intracardiac recordings from the high right atrium (HRA), His bundle distal (His-d), His bundle proximal (His-p), and right ventricle apex (RVA). The atrial, ventricular, and His bundle electrograms are labeled A, V, and H, respectively, on the intracardiac recordings. The first two beats conduct over the fast pathway with an AH interval of 40 ms. The third atrial beat (A*) is a spontaneous premature atrial contraction, which blocks in the fast pathway and conducts over the slow pathway (SP = down arrows, AH = 240 ms). Subsequent retrograde conduction occurs over the fast pathway (up arrows), and tachycardia is initiated. The onset of the QRS is denoted as a solid line, and the earliest A is seen on the proximal His bundle recording. The VA time during tachycardia measured at proximal His bundle is 0 ms (solid line). The very short VA time during AVNRT is the result of simultaneous conduction from the lower common pathway retrograde to the atrium via the fast pathway and antegrade to ventricle via the His bundle ("conduction in parallel") as well as rapid retrograde fast pathway conduction.

○ Induction is usually achieved by atrial burst or extrastimulus pacing but can occasionally be seen after ventricular overdrive pacing.

- Timing
  ○ Septal VA interval ≤70 ms.
  ○ The earliest retrograde atrial activation is usually recorded near the compact AV node at the apex of the triangle of Koch on the His bundle recording catheter. In a small percentage (<10%) the earliest retrograde atrial activation may be recorded at the coronary sinus ostium or along the left side of the atrial septum.[9]

- Entrainment
  ○ Atrial overdrive pacing at a rate slightly faster than the tachycardia should result in acceleration of the ventricular rate to the pacing rate with a long antegrade conduction time consistent with continued conduction down the slow pathway.
    ▪ Upon termination of atrial pacing, if the tachycardia continues, the VA relationship on the first return tachycardia beat should be roughly the same as during stable tachycardia ("VA linking").[8]
    ▪ Antegrade block in the slow pathway terminates tachycardia.
  ○ Ventricular overdrive pacing from the right ventricle: Ventricular pacing entrainment is said to be present if pacing at a cycle length slightly shorter than the tachycardia cycle length (20 to 30 ms shorter) results in acceleration of the atrial rate to the pacing rate and upon termination the tachycardia continues.
    ▪ Features of ventricular pacing entrainment of AVNRT (Figure 7-6)[8]
    ▪ An atrial-ventricular response postpacing

    ▪ Postpacing interval (PPI)–Tachycardia cycle length (TCL) difference >115 ms
    ▪ Stimulus to A interval (SA)–tachycardia VA interval >85 ms

Note: For ventricular pacing impulses to reach the AVNRT circuit they have to conduct retrograde through the His bundle to the AV node. Therefore, there must be complete capture of the ventricle without fusion prior to entrainment of AVNRT. Also, since the ventricle is not part of the reentrant circuit of typical AVNRT, VA dissociation during pacing does not rule out AVNRT as a possible mechanism.

DIFFERENTIAL DIAGNOSIS

The differential diagnosis for a very short septal VA time (<70 ms) tachycardia includes typical AVNRT, atrial tachycardia, and non-reentrant junctional tachycardia. An atrial tachycardia can usually be excluded by demonstrating an atrial-ventricular response after ventricular pacing entrainment. If ventricular pacing entrainment can't be achieved, then atrial pacing maneuvers which demonstrate VA linking are useful to rule out atrial tachycardia as the mechanism. Although nonreentrant junctional tachycardia is a much less common arrhythmia, it can be quite difficult to differentiate from typical AVNRT since the VA timing relationships and response to ventricular overdrive pacing can be identical. A useful technique to help differentiate these arrhythmias has been described using PACs introduced during tachycardia. If a PAC introduced late into the tachycardia cycle length results in a short AV time (indicative of fast pathway conduction) and the tachycardia does not terminate, this rules out

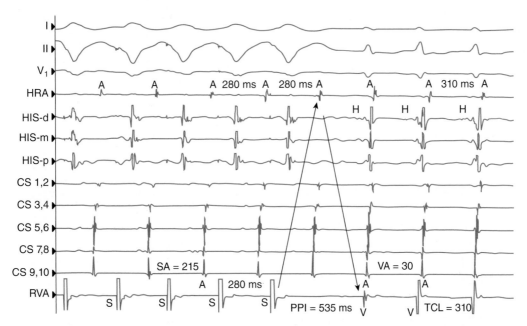

FIGURE 7-6 Entrainment of AVNRT during ventricular pacing. Shown are surface leads I, II, and V₁ and intracardiac recordings from the high right atrium (HRA), His bundle distal (His-d), His bundle mid (His-m), His bundle proximal (His-p), coronary sinus (CS) distal (1,2) to proximal (9,10), and right ventricle apex (RVA). The atrial, ventricular, and his bundle electrograms are labeled A, V, and H respectively on the intracardiac recordings. right ventricular pacing (S₁) at a cycle length of 280 ms was performed during AVNRT, which had a cycle length of 310 ms. Ventricular pacing advanced the atrial electrogram to the ventricular pacing rate of 280 ms (1st arrow), and upon termination of pacing the tachycardia continued indicating that the tachycardia was entrained by pacing. The postpacing response was an AV response (2nd arrow), which rules out an atrial tachycardia as the mechanism. AV reentrant tachycardia was ruled out by the very short VA time (30 ms) measured at the CS ostium (CS 9,10), making typical AVNRT the correct diagnosis. The long postpacing interval (PPI)–tachycardia cycle length (TCL) difference of more than 115 ms (535 − 310 = 225 ms) and long stimulus to A interval (SA)–tachycardia VA interval difference of more than 85 ms (215 − 30 = 185 ms) after RV pacing entrainment are characteristic of AVNRT.[8]

AVNRT as the mechanism. If a PAC introduced early in the tachycardia cycle length affects the subsequent ventricular timing with a long AV interval (suggestive of slow pathway conduction), this is highly suggestive of AVNRT as the mechanism.[10]

MANAGEMENT

The aggressiveness of treatment for termination or prevention of AVNRT depends on the clinical scenario. The American College of Cardiology (ACC) and the American Heart Association (AHA) guidelines give an in-depth discussion of the management of patients with supraventricular arrhythmias, and the reader is directed there for a more comprehensive review.[11]

- Termination strategy
  - Hemodynamically unstable: Most patients with typical AVNRT are stable, but some patients may present with severe symptoms or hypotension, which require urgent restoration of sinus rhythm. This can be achieved by either an intravenous (IV) push of adenosine or direct current (DC) cardioversion.
  - Hemodynamically stable
    - Vagal maneuvers such as the Valsalva maneuver can be tried first.[12]
    - Adenosine is the next step if vagal maneuvers fail. Adenosine is >80% effective in terminating AVNRT.[13] It should be used with caution or avoided in patients with severe bronchospastic lung disease.
    - IV nondihydropyridine calcium channel blockers (verapamil or diltiazem) or IV β-blockers are the second-line drug therapy. Potential side effects of these agents include hypotension and bradycardia.[14]

- Preventive strategy: Symptomatic and frequent AVNRT is usually treated with either long-term pharmacologic therapy or catheter-based ablative therapy. Patient preference as well as drug tolerance are the main factors in selecting either therapy.

  - Nondihydropyridine calcium channel blockers and β-blockers are first-line agents.
  - Class I and III antiarrhythmics can be effective but are usually avoided because of the increased risk of serious side effects (ie, proarrhythmia). These agents can be considered if calcium or β-blockers are not effective and ablation is not an option.
    - Catheter ablation is the therapy of choice for:
      - Patients who fail or do not desire long-term medical therapy.
      - Patients with highly symptomatic or poorly tolerated AVNRT.

Ablation Strategies

The overall success rate for AVNRT ablation is high (>95%), and the recurrence rate after successful ablation is low (<5%). Ablation techniques targeting both the fast pathway and slow pathway have been described, but because of the much lower incidence of heart block (<1%) with the slow pathway approach, this has become the preferred technique. The slow pathway is targeted by positioning the tip of the ablation catheter in the middle or posterior zones of the triangle of Koch, often around the coronary sinus ostium. These regions are searched for locations with a fractionated atrial electrogram and A:V electrogram ratio of <1 (typically on the order of 1:3) (Figure 7-7). After an acceptable site is found, radiofrequency (RF) energy can be delivered in a titrated fashion, starting at a low power of 10 to 15 watts and progressively increasing the wattage to a target of 25 to 35 watts. During energy delivery, continuous monitoring of the rhythm for the emergence of a junctional rhythm and for any sign of AV block is of critical importance. The development of a relatively slow stable junctional rhythm with 1:1 VA conduction during RF delivery is the desired response (Figure 7-8). The occurrence of a junctional rhythm indicates that the ablation lesion is affecting tissue with a connection to the AV node. The presence of 1:1 VA conduction during the junctional rhythm is an indicator that fast pathway function is intact and that the patient will not have AV block after the ablation is terminated. If at any time during the ablation there is evidence of disruption

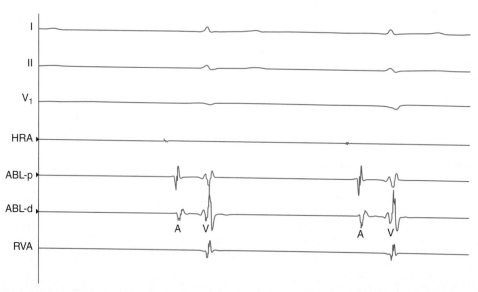

FIGURE 7-7 Slow pathway ablation target site. Shown are surface leads I, II, and V₁ and intracardiac recordings from the high right atrium (HRA), ablation proximal (ABL-p), ablation distal (ABL-d), and right ventricle apex (RVA). The atrial, ventricular, and electrograms are labeled A and V, respectively, on the intracardiac recordings. The ideal slow pathway site should have an A/V ratio <1 along with a fractionated atrial electrogram as seen on the ablation distal recording.

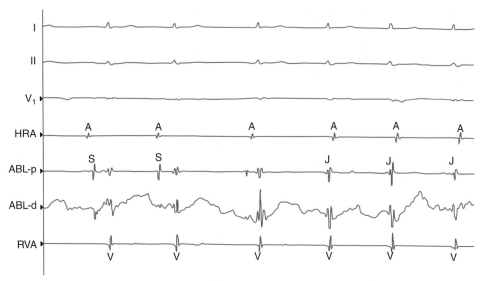

FIGURE 7-8 Junctional beats during slow pathway catheter ablation. Shown are surface leads I, II, and V₁ and intracardiac recordings from the high right atrium (HRA), ablation proximal (ABL-p), ablation distal (ABL-d), and right ventricular apex (RVA). The atrial and ventricular electrograms are labeled A and V, respectively, on the intracardiac recordings. The first two beats are sinus beats (S), and on the third beat there is a change in the atrial activation sequence with the atrial electrogram on the AB p occurring before the atrial electrogram on the HRA, indicating the emergence of a junctional rhythm and the last three beats are clearly junctional (J). It should be noted that during the junctional rhythm there is consistent 1:1 conduction to the atrium with a short VA time indicating that fast pathway conduction is intact.

of rapid VA conduction (VA block or a significant change in VA time), the application should be terminated immediately to minimize the risk of high grade AV block. The primary endpoint for ablation is to render the patient noninducible. In patients where reproducibility of tachycardia induction was not reliable, secondary endpoints such as elimination or modification of slow pathway function can be used. It is important to understand that it is not necessary to completely eliminate all slow pathway function and that the presence of a single AV node echo is an acceptable endpoint in most patients.

REFERENCES

1. Liuba I, Jönsson A, Säfström K, Walfridsson H. Gender-related differences in patients with atrioventricular nodal reentry tachycardia. *Am J Cardiol*. 2006;97(3):384-388.

2. Goyal R, Zivin A, Souza J, et al. Comparison of the ages of tachycardia onset in patients with atrioventricular nodal reentrant tachycardia and accessory pathway-mediated tachycardia. *Am Heart J*. 1996;132:765-767.

3. Wood KA, Drew BJ, Scheinman MM. Frequency of disabling symptoms in supraventricular tachycardia. *Am J Cardiol*. 1997;79:145-149.

4. McGuire MA, Janse MJ, Ross DL. "AV nodal" reentry: Part II: AV nodal, AV junctional, or atrio-nodal reentry? *J Cardiovasc Electrophysiol*. 1993;4:573-586.

5. Moe GK, Preston JB, Burlington H. Physiologic evidence for a dual A-V transmission system. *Circ Res*. 1956;4:357-375.

6. Man KC, Brinkman K, Bogun F, et al. 2:1 atrioventricular block during atrioventricular node reentrant tachycardia. *J Am Coll Cardiol*. 1996;28:1770-1774.

7. Otomo K, Okamura H, Noda T, et al. Unique electrophysiologic characteristics of atrioventricular nodal reentrant tachycardia with different ventriculoatrial block patterns: effects of slow pathway ablation and insights into the location of the reentrant circuit. *Heart Rhythm*. 2006;3:544-554.

8. Knight BP, Ebinger M, Oral H, et al. Diagnostic value of tachycardia features and pacing maneuvers during paroxysmal supraventricular tachycardia. *J Am Coll Cardiol*. 2000;36:574-582.

9. Anselme F, Papageorgiou P, Monahan K, et al. Presence and significance of the left atrionodal connection during atrioventricular nodal reentrant tachycardia. *Am J Cardiol*. 1999;83:1530-1536.

10. Padanilam BJ, Manfredi JA, Steinberg LA, Olson JA, Fogel RI, Prystowsky EN. Differentiating junctional tachycardia and atrioventricular node re-entry tachycardia based on response to atrial extrastimulus pacing. *J Am Coll Cardiol*. 2008;52:1711-1717.

11. Blomström-Lundqvist C, Scheinman MM, Aliot EM, et al. ACC/AHA/ESC guidelines for the management of patients with supraventricular arrhythmias—executive summary: a report of the American College of Cardiology/American Heart Association Task Force on Practice Guidelines and the European Society of Cardiology Committee for Practice Guidelines (Writing Committee to Develop Guidelines for the Management of Patients With Supraventricular Arrhythmias). *Circulation*. 2003;108:1871-1909.

12. Belz MK, Stambler BS, Wood MA, Pherson C, Ellenbogen KA. Effects of enhanced parasympathetic tone on atrioventricular nodal conduction during atrioventricular nodal reentrant tachycardia. *Am J Cardiol*. 1997;80:878-882.

13. Glatter KA, Cheng J, Dorostkar P, et al. Electrophysiologic effects of adenosine in patients with supraventricular tachycardia. *Circulation*. 1999;99:1034-1040.

14. Dougherty AH, Jackman WM, Naccarelli GV, Friday KJ, Dias VC. Acute conversion of paroxysmal supraventricular tachycardia with intravenous diltiazem. IV Diltiazem Study Group. *Am J Cardiol*. 1992;70:587-592.

8 AV NODAL REENTRANT TACHYCARDIA: ATYPICAL

Patrick Hranitzky, MD, Luigi Di Biase, MD, PhD,
Rodney Horton, MD, J. David Burkhardt, MD,
Andrea Natale, MD

CASE PRESENTATION

A 37-year-old woman presented with a long-standing history of intermittent palpitations that initially occurred 1 to 2 times per month but which have now progressed to 8 times per month. She was originally diagnosed with anxiety disorder after a 24-hour Holter monitor revealed sinus rhythm and sinus tachycardia, and she was placed on a β-blocker. She had minimal improvement in her symptoms and was intolerant of the β-blocker due to fatigue. One month prior to her initial clinic visit, she had an emergency department (ED) visit where her heart rate was documented at 180 bpm, but was interpreted as sinus tachycardia despite abrupt termination in the ED prior to obtaining a 12-lead ECG. She denied any history of syncope and stated that her palpitations would initially only last seconds, but now last anywhere from 10 to 45 minutes. She cannot identify any specific triggers other than when she assumes an upright posture after leaning over to pick something up. Her past medical history is otherwise unremarkable. An echocardiogram revealed normal left ventricular systolic function and no structural abnormalities. Laboratory values were all within normal limits. A 12-lead ECG was obtained at the initial clinic visit (Figure 8-1) and revealed sinus rhythm without preexcitation. She was scheduled for electrophysiologic testing where she was discovered to have both typical and atypical atrioventricular nodal reentrant tachycardia (AVNRT). A successful radiofrequency ablation was performed of the slow pathway. At follow-up there has been no recurrent arrhythmia or palpitations.

SIGNS/SYMPTOMS

The history and symptoms are quite consistent with AVNRT, which is typically characterized by an abrupt onset and termination. Episodes may last from seconds to hours. Many patients will report that they will often experience the episodes after they lean over to pick something up. The heart rate is usually rapid, ranging from 150 to 250 beats per minute (bpm). It is usually 180 to 200 bpm in adults; in children, the rate may exceed 250 bpm. In the absence of structural heart disease, it is usually well tolerated.

Common symptoms include the following:

- Palpitations
- Dizziness
- Anxiety/nervousness
- Lightheadedness
- Chest discomfort/fullness
- Neck pulsations (often due to near simultaneous contraction of the atria and ventricles)
- Presyncope

Syncope is rare, but may occur in patients with a rapid ventricular rate or prolonged tachycardia due to poor ventricular filling, decreased cardiac output, hypotension, and reduced cerebral perfusion.

The lack of ECG documentation is not unusual as these episodes are often quite brief. In the atypical form of AVNRT the ECG often reveals a long RP interval and can be misinterpreted as sinus tachycardia;

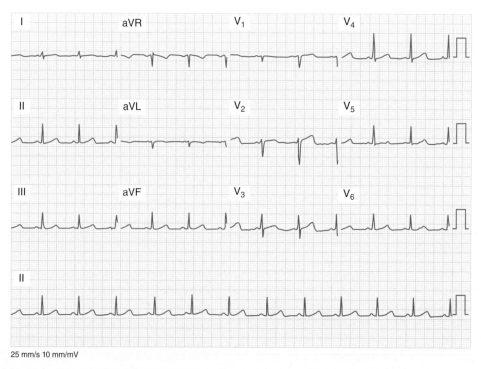

25 mm/s 10 mm/mV

FIGURE 8-1 Initial ECG revealing sinus rhythm with a normal axis and intervals and no evidence of preexcitation.

however, the P waves (if discernable) are usually inverted in the inferior leads (II, III, and AVF).

EPIDEMIOLOGY

Paroxysmal supraventricular tachycardia (PSVT) has a prevalence of 2.25 per 1000 population and an incidence of 35 per 100,000 person-years. AVNRT is the most common cause of PSVT and is the underlying arrhythmia in 60% of these patients.[1-3] Of the patients presenting with AVNRT, 11% to 15% will present with the atypical form.[4-7] There is a 3:1 predominance of AVNRT in women.[8-10] AVNRT may occur in persons of any age. It is common in young adults, but some patients do not present until their seventh or eighth decade or later. AVNRT is considered less common in newborns and increases in prevalence throughout childhood. However, some reports suggest that AVNRT may be underrecognized in infancy.[11]

ETIOLOGY AND PATHOPHYSIOLOGY

AVNRT (typical and atypical) occurs due to reentry within two (or more) anatomically and functionally distinct pathways located within the region of the AV node; they are known as the fast and the slow pathways and have different electrophysiologic characteristics. The fast pathway is characterized by its more anterior and superior location within the right atrial septum and its relatively shorter conduction time and longer effective refractory period (ERP), whereas the slow pathway is typically located inferiorly and posteriorly and has a relatively longer conduction time and an ERP that typically is short when compared to fast pathway ERP (Figure 8-2). There may be multiple slow pathways in as many as 5% of patients with AVNRT.[12] As previously mentioned, these separate pathways are usually anatomically discrete, but dual AV nodal physiology is a common finding during EP studies and is not synonymous with AVNRT. There are two forms of AVNRT that are usually described and include the typical form (ie, slow-fast) and the atypical form

(ie, fast-slow or slow-slow), referring to the anterograde-retrograde conduction over the pathways during tachycardia. In the typical form the conduction moves in the anterograde direction through the slow pathway and in the retrograde direction through the fast pathway. In the atypical form, the conduction moves either anterograde in the fast pathway and retrograde in the slow pathway, or anterograde and retrograde through two slow pathways. Either of these scenarios can result in a long RP interval during tachycardia.[6,7,13-18] Typically, retrograde CS activation is concentric (Figures 8-3A and B and 8-4) as the inputs of the fast and slow pathways usually reside at the anterior/superior right atrial septum and the inferior/posterior right atrial septum, respectively. However, eccentric CS activation is seen in approximately 5% of all AVNRT and 32% to 80% of atypical AVNRT due to leftward inferior nodal extensions which are densely populated with transitional cells.[7,15,18] In most patients with AVNRT, the tachycardia is initiated when a premature complex (atrial or ventricular) is blocked in the one pathway (usually the fast pathway with a longer refractory period) and conducts in the other pathway (usually the slow pathway with a shorter refractory period). While the impulse conducts in one pathway, the other pathway recovers so that the impulse can conduct in the opposite direction thus completing the loop of reentry.

DIAGNOSIS

The definitive diagnosis of AVNRT (typical or atypical) can only be made with electrophysiologic testing. The hallmark of AVNRT is the presence of dual AV node physiology which is defined as a >50 ms "jump" in the atrial-His interval (AH) between a 10 ms S_1S_2 decrement during atrial-programmed stimulation. This is evident in this patient (see Figures 8-3A and B and 8-4). An HA jump during ventricular pacing or programmed stimulation is frequently seen in patients with atypical AVNRT and was present in this patient (Figure 8-5).

Approximately 85% of patients presenting with atypical AVNRT will also have inducible typical AVNRT.[7] AVNRT can be initiated by ectopic atrial or ventricular beats. The typical form is usually initiated

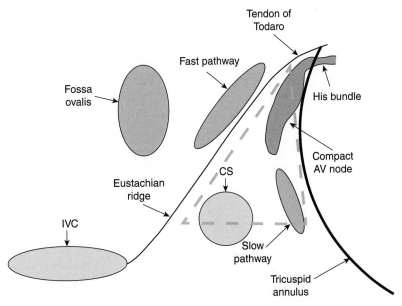

FIGURE 8-2 Schematic reprenating an RAO projection of the right atrial septum. The fast and slow pathways are depicted in red and yellow, respectively. The dotted red line represents the borders of the triangle of Koch.

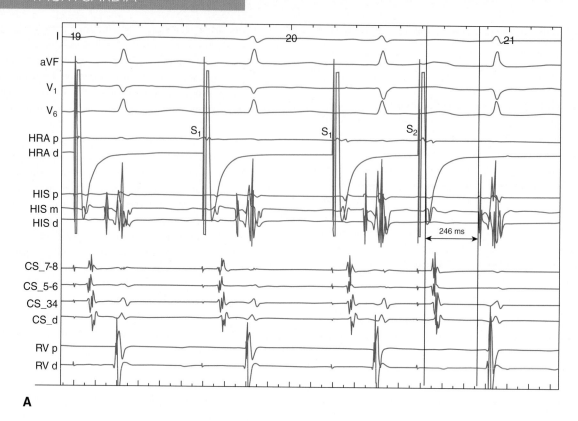

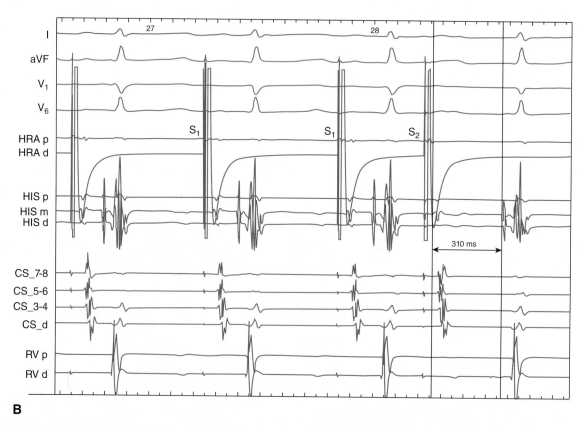

FIGURE 8-3 Programmed electrical stimulation is performed from the high right atrial catheter. Simultaneous recordings are taken from the proximal and distal high right atrium (HRA p, HRA d), the proximal, mid, and distal His bundle (HIS p, HIS m, HIS d), the proximal to distal coronary sinus (CS_7,8 to CS_d), and the proximal and distal right ventricular apex (RVA p, RVA d). (A): Decremental conduction has occurred down the fast pathway, and the AH interval measures 246 ms. (B) After a 10-ms decrement in the S$_2$, there is a 64 ms "jump" in the AH interval consistent with dual AV nodal physiology.

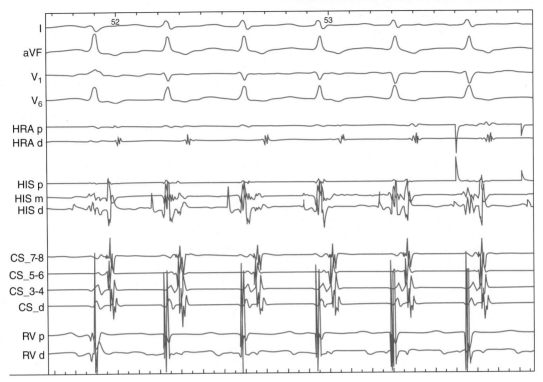

FIGURE 8-4 Typical AVNRT in this patient as evidenced by a long AH interval and short VA interval during tachycardia.

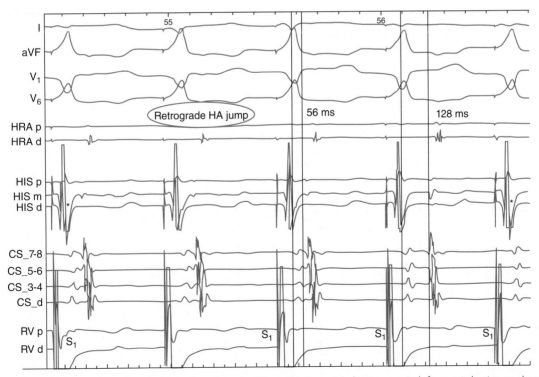

FIGURE 8-5 During a ventricular pacing drive in this patient there is a 72-ms HA "jump" indicating a switch from conduction up the retrograde fast pathway to the retrograde slow pathway. Note that the earliest atrial activation switches from the proximal His (HIS p) to the proximal CS (CS_7,8). The asterisks on the first and last beat indicate the retrograde His deflection.

by atrial ectopic beats that block in the fast pathway and travel anterograde via the slow pathway. The resulting arrhythmia results in near simultaneous activation of the atria and ventricles (see Figure 8-4). The atypical form can be induced with atrial or ventricular extrastimuli or may occur during an atrial or ventricular pacing drive (Figure 8-6). Some of the distinguishing features of the various forms of AVNRT are as follows[7,17]:

- Typical
  - Slow-fast → VA <60 ms and AH > HA during tachycardia, earliest retrograde atrial activation at the His bundle
- Atypical
  - Fast-slow → often no jump seen, VA >60 ms and HA > AH during tachycardia, earliest retrograde atrial activation near CS os
  - Slow-slow → AH jump often seen, VA >60 and AH > HA during tachycardia, earliest retrograde atrial activation near CS os

There is frequently quite a bit of cycle length variability during atypical AVNRT, which may be due to multiple slow pathways or presence of an upper or lower common pathway[6,12,15,16] and is seen in this patient (Figures 8-7 and 8-8).

AVNRT must be differentiated from other forms of supraventricular tachycardia (SVT) including:

- Atrial tachycardia
- Orthodromic reciprocating tachycardia
- Sinus tachycardia
- Sinus node reentry

Differentiation of these forms of SVT is done during electrophysiologic testing. Sinus mechanisms as well as nonseptal atrial tachycardias demonstrate the earliest atrial activation away from

the septum and thus can usually be excluded by looking at atrial activation.

A septal atrial tachycardia with 1:1 conduction to the ventricle can mimic AVNRT and can usually be excluded with ventricular entrainment. A VAV response to ventricular entrainment will typically exclude atrial tachycardia as the mechanism.

Orthodromic reciprocating tachycardia using a septal accessory pathway is a bit more challenging and can be differentiated using one or more of the following criteria[19-22]:

- SA-VA (if >110 ms → AVNRT, if <100 ms → ORT via septal AP)
  - Where SA is the interval between the stimulus artifact and the atrial signal on the HRA catheter during RV pacing and VA is the interval between the ventricular signal on the RV catheter and the atrial signal on the HRA catheter during tachycardia.
- PPI-TCL (if >115 ms → AVNRT)
  - Where PPI is the postpacing interval measured on the RV catheter between the last entrained beat and the first return beat and the TCL is the tachycardia cycle length.
- Introduction of a ventricular extrastimulus during His bundle refractoriness → if no atrial preexcitation this is consistent with AVNRT
- Preexcitation index (if >100 → AVNRT)
  - Preexcitation index (PI) is the V_1V_1 interval during tachycardia minus the longest V_1V_2 at which atrial preexcitation occurs
  - PI = V_1V_1 - V_1V_2
- Para-Hisian pacing (if nodal response → AVNRT)

Demonstrations of these maneuvers in this patient are seen in Figures 8-9 to 8-11.

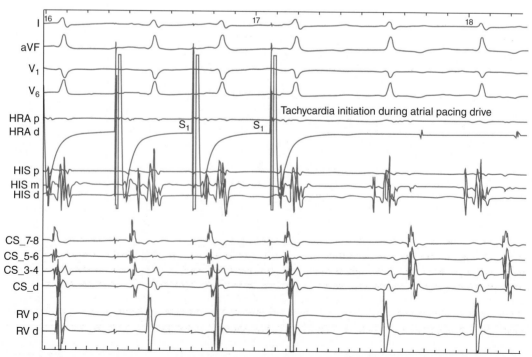

FIGURE 8-6 Initiation of atypical AVNRT during an atrial pacing drive. Notice the long AH interval on the HIS catheter and the longer VA time when compared to the typical form in Figure 8-4.

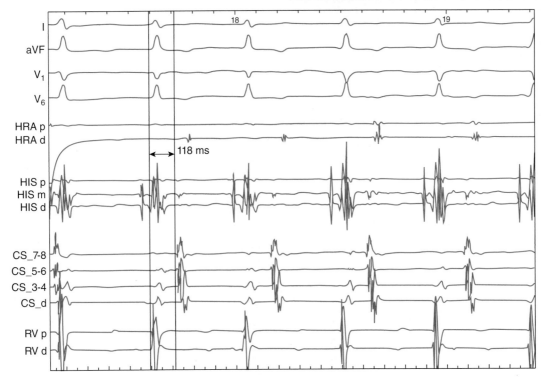

FIGURE 8-7 Beat-to-beat variations in the VA time during atypical AVNRT in this patient. Note the long VA time (>100 ms).

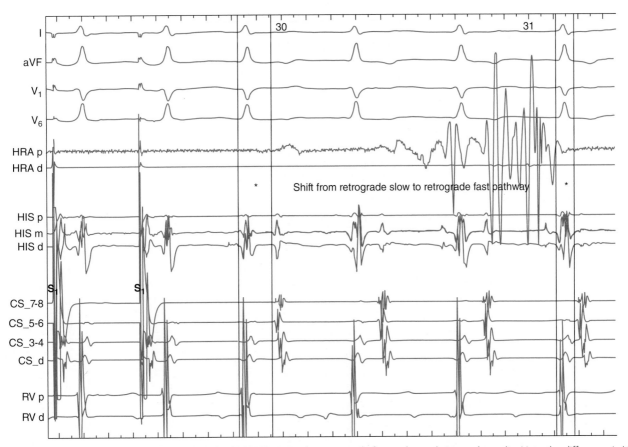

FIGURE 8-8 Example of a switch from the retrograde slow pathway to the retrograde fast pathway during tachycardia. Note the difference in VA times between the beats annotated with asterisks.

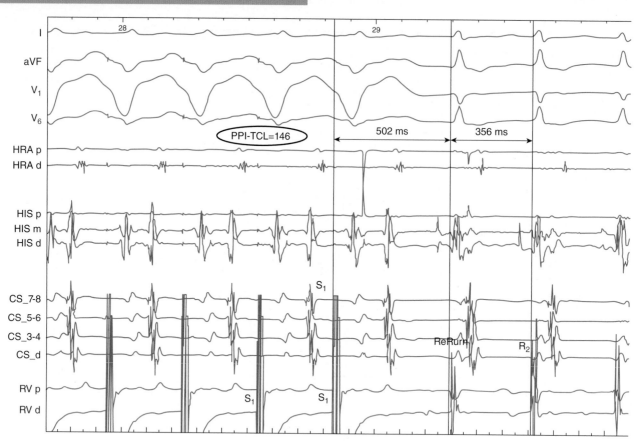

FIGURE 8-9 Entrainment from the RV catheter reveals a V-A-H-V response excluding an atrial tachycardia. The postpacing interval minus the tachycardia cycle length is 146 ms, which is consistent with AVNRT.

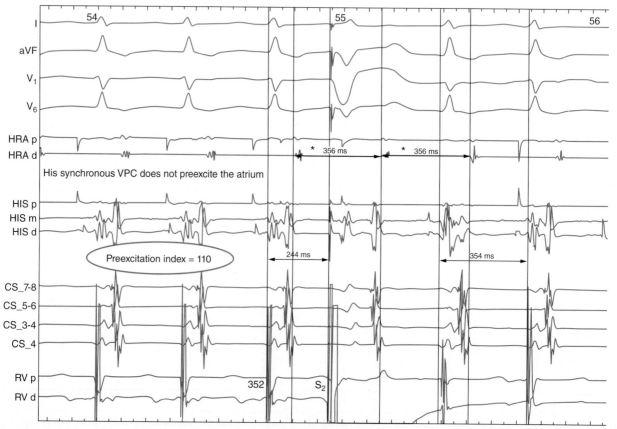

FIGURE 8-10 This figure demonstrates a His-synchronous ventricular extrastimulus during tachycardia. There is no change in the atrial cycle length as annotated with the asterisks. In addition, the preexcitation index is calculated and is 110. Both findings are consistent with AVNRT.

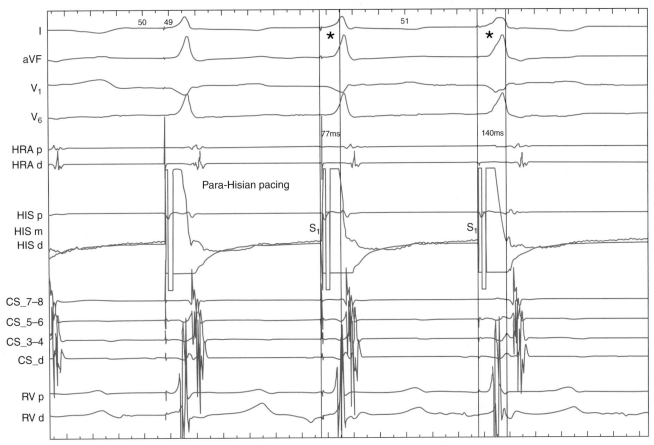

FIGURE 8-11 Para-Hisian pacing is performed on the patient. There is a nodal response as the SA interval varies by greater than 60 ms between His capture (left asterisk) and RV capture (right asterisk).

MANAGEMENT (ACUTE)

Relaxation or vagal maneuvers alone may terminate an episode of AVNRT. The successful management of an acute episode, however, depends on the symptoms, the presence of underlying heart disease, and the natural history of previous episodes.

- Vagal maneuvers
  - Valsalva maneuver
  - Carotid sinus massage (avoid if known cerebrovascular disease)
  - Dive reflex → submerge face in cold water
    - These maneuvers can also be tried after each pharmacologic approach
- Pharmacologic intervention
  - Intravenous adenosine 6-12 mg
  - Intravenous β-blocker
    - eg, metoprolol 5 mg (may be repeated if necessary)
  - Intravenous calcium channel blocker
    - eg, erapamil 5 mg
    - eg, diltiazem 10 mg
- Synchronized direct current cardioversion
  - Used when the patient has hemodynamic compromise or if drug conversion fails and the patient continues to be symptomatic
  - 100 joules usually adequate
    - Rarely necessary for AVNRT

MANAGEMENT (LONG-TERM)

Prevention can be obtained in part by avoidance of exacerbating factors or triggers. Some of these include:

- Caffeine
- Foods high in theobromine (eg, coffee, tea, chocolate)
- Alcohol
- Pharmacologic stimulants (eg, pseudoephedrine, theophylline)

Long-term management is usually accomplished with pharmacologic or catheter-based therapy.

- Pharmacologic (given orally)
  - β-Blockers (eg, metoprolol, atenolol)
  - Calcium channel blockers (eg, verapamil, diltiazem)
  - Digitalis (rarely used)
  - (The previous three agents must be given with caution in patients with prolonged PR intervals to avoid high degree AV block. However, the fast pathway inserts into the central fibrous body distal to the AV node and is less subject to beta-blockers and calcium channel blockers)
  - Antiarrhythmic drugs (rarely used)
    - Sodium channel blockers (eg, flecainide, propafenone)
      - Flecainide depresses conduction in the fast pathway
    - Potassium channel blockers (eg, sotalol)
      - More drug intolerance
      - Considered drug of choice for refractory AVNRT in pregnant women not undergoing catheter ablation

***The fast pathway inserts into the central fibrous body distal to the AV node, is less subject to β-blockers and calcium channel blockers, and has less decremental conduction.

- Catheter-based therapy
  - The cornerstone of therapy for patients with symptomatic AVNRT is catheter ablation. This procedure is highly effective (91%-99% acute success for all forms of AVNRT), safe (<2% serious complication risk), and provides a durable, long-term cure.
    - AV block in <1%.
    - Typically involves ablation of the slow pathway.
      - Successful slow pathway site usually results in accelerated junctional rhythm when radiofrequency energy is applied (Figure 8-12).
    - Fast pathway ablation is done superior to the Tendon of Todaro.
      - Less frequently performed due to higher recurrence rates and greater risk of AV block.
    - Single echos following catheter ablation are not associated with higher recurrence rate and occur in ~25% following catheter ablation.
    - Ablation may be required inside the CS at the site of earliest retrograde atrial activation.[15,16,18]
      - More frequent in atypical form.
      - Ablation at these sites may not produce junctional rhythm.

- In rare cases, ablation on the left side of the septum maybe required (Figure 8-13).
  - Usually junctional rhythm is seen at this site.
    - Recurrence rate is higher for atypical versus typical AVNRT (3%-8.3% versus 0.5%),[8-10,17,23-25]
    - Safe and effective in patients with prolonged PR interval.[26-29]
    - Cryothermal ablation may be advantageous in patients with a smaller triangle of Koch.[30]
      - Less destruction of tissue architecture, thus should AV block occur it is likely reversible.
      - Cryoablation results in adherence of catheter to heart tissue providing greater stability.
      - No junctional rhythm is seen during cryoablation.
      - Similar efficacy as radiofrequency.
- Inappropriate sinus tachycardia is seen in ~10% following catheter ablation of the slow pathway.
  - Usually persists for 1 to 6 weeks, up to 6 months.

PROGNOSIS

The prognosis for patients with AVNRT is usually good in the absence of structural heart disease. Most patients respond to medications to prevent recurrence or to catheter ablation, which is approximately 95% curative and has a low risk of complications. Catheter ablation is the preferred method of treatment for most patients.

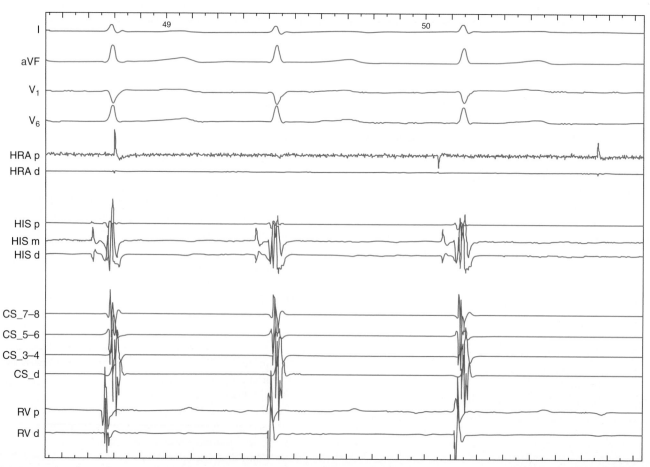

FIGURE 8-12 Accelerated junctionals during radiofrequency application at the slow pathway.

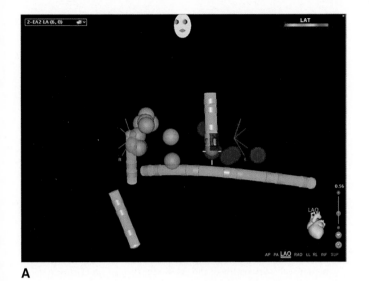

A

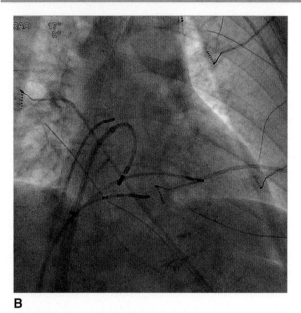

B

C

FIGURE 8-13 Example of a rare case where ablation on the left side of the septum was required to achieve slow pathway ablation and AVNRT noninducibility. Top left shows a 3-D map cloud of the His bundle (yellow dots) and the left-sided lesions (red dots) where the slow pathway was ablated. Top right image shows a fluoroscopy image of the ablation catheter in the left side of the septum at the successful site. The bottom image shows junctional rhythm during ablation.

REFERENCES

1. Belhassen B, Fish R, Glikson M, et al. Noninvasive diagnosis of dual AV node physiology in patients with AV nodal reentrant tachycardia by administration of adenosine-5′-triphosphate during sinus rhythm. *Circulation.* 1998;98(1):47-53.

2. Elvas L, Gursoy S, Brugada J, Andries E, Brugada P. Atrioventricular nodal reentrant tachycardia: a review. *Can J Cardiol.* 1994;10(3):342-348.

3. Kreiner G, Frey B, Gossinger HD. Atrioventricular nodal reentry tachycardia in patients with sinus node dysfunction: electrophysiologic characteristics, clinical presentation, and results of slow pathway ablation. *J Cardiovasc Electrophysiol.* 1998;9(5):470-478.

4. Crawford TC, Mukergi S, Good E, et al. Utility of atrial and ventricular cycle length variability in determining the mechanism of paroxysmal supraventricular tachycardia. *J Cardiovasc Electrophysiol.* 2007;18(7):698-703.

5. Fujiki A, Sakamoto T, Sakabe M, et al. Junctional rhythm associated with ventriculoatrial block during slow pathway ablation in atypical atrioventricular nodal reentrant tachycardia. *Europace.* 2008;10(8):982-987.

6. Heinroth KM, Kattenbeck K, Stabenow I, Trappe HJ, Weismuller P. Multiple AV nodal pathways in patients with AV nodal reentrant tachycardia—more common than expected? *Europace.* 2002;4(4):375-382.

7. Hwang C, Martin DJ, Goodman JS, et al. Atypical atrioventricular nodal reciprocating tachycardia masquerading as tachycardia using a left-sided accessory pathway. *J Am Coll Cardiol.* 1997;30(1):218-225.

8. Jackman WM, Beckman KJ, McClelland JH, et al. Treatment of supraventricular tachycardia due to atrioventricular nodal reentry by radiofrequency catheter ablation of slow-pathway conduction. *N Engl J Med.* 1992;327(5):313-318.

9. Chen SA, Chiang CE, Tsang WP, et al. Selective radiofrequency catheter ablation of fast and slow pathway in 100 patients with atrioventricular nodal reentrant tachycardia. *Am Heart J.* 1993;125(1):1-10.

10. Lee MA, Morady F, Kadish A, et al. Catheter modification of the atrioventricular junction with radiofrequency energy for control of atrioventricular nodal reentry tachycardia. *Circulation.* 1991;83(3):827-835.

11. Blaufox AD, Warsy I, D'Souza M, Kanter R. Transesophageal electrophysiological evaluation of children with a history of supraventricular tachycardia in infancy. *Pediatr Cardiol.* 2011;32(8):1110-1114.

12. Tai CT, Chen SA, Chiang CE, et al. Multiple anterograde atrioventricular node pathways in patients with atrioventricular node reentrant tachycardia. *J Am Coll Cardiol.* 1996;28(3):725-731.

13. Langberg JJ, Kim YN, Goyal R, et al. Conversion of typical to "atypical" atrioventricular nodal reentrant tachycardia after radiofrequency catheter modification of the atrioventricular junction. *Am J Cardiol.* 1992;69(5):503-508.

14. Strickberger SA, Kalbfleisch SJ, Williamson B, et al. Radiofrequency catheter ablation of atypical atrioventricular nodal reentrant tachycardia. *J Cardiovasc Electrophysiol.* 1993;4(5):526-532.

15. Otomo K, Nagata Y, Uno K, et al. Atypical atrioventricular nodal reentrant tachycardia with eccentric coronary sinus activation: electrophysiological characteristics and essential effects of left-sided ablation inside the coronary sinus. *Heart Rhythm.* 2007;4(4):421-432.

16. Otomo K, Nagata Y, Uno K, et al. Irregular atypical atrioventricular nodal reentrant tachycardia: incidence, electrophysiological characteristics, and effects of slow pathway ablation. *Heart Rhythm.* 2007;4(12):1507-1522.

17. Goldberger J, Brooks R, Kadish A. Physiology of "atypical" atrioventricular junctional reentrant tachycardia occurring following radiofrequency catheter modification of the atrioventricular node. *Pacing Clin Electrophysiol.* 1992;15(12):2270-2282.

18. Nam GB, Rhee KS, Kim J, et al. Left atrionodal connections in typical and atypical atrioventricular nodal reentrant tachycardias: activation sequence in the coronary sinus and results of radiofrequency catheter ablation. *J Cardiovasc Electrophysiol.* 2006;17(2):171-177.

19. Gonzalez-Torrecilla E, Almendral J, Garcia-Fernandez FJ, et al. Differences in ventriculoatrial intervals during entrainment and tachycardia: a simpler method for distinguishing paroxysmal supraventricular tachycardia with long ventriculoatrial intervals. *J Cardiovasc Electrophysiol.* 2011;22(8):915-921.

20. Michaud GF, Tada H, Chough S, et al. Differentiation of atypical atrioventricular node re-entrant tachycardia from orthodromic reciprocating tachycardia using a septal accessory pathway by the response to ventricular pacing. *J Am Coll Cardiol.* 2001;38(4):1163-1167.

21. Miles WM, Yee R, Klein GJ, et al. The preexcitation index: an aid in determining the mechanism of supraventricular tachycardia and localizing accessory pathways. *Circulation.* 1986;74(3):493-500.

22. Jackman WM, Beckman KJ, McClelland J, et al. Para-Hisian RV pacing site for differentiating retrograde conduction over septal accessory pathway and AV node. *Pacing Clin Electrophysiol.* 1991;14:670.

23. Haisaguerre M, Gaita F, Fischer B, et al. Elimination of atrioventricular nodal reentrant tachycardia using discrete slow potentials to guide application of radiofrequency energy. *Circulation.* 1992;85(6):2162-2175.

24. Mitrani RD, Klein LS, Hackett K, et al. Radiofrequency ablation for atrioventricular nodal reentrant tachycardia: comparison between fast (anterior) and slow (posterior) pathway ablation. *J Am Coll Cardiol.* 1993;21(2):432-441.

25. Jazayeri MR, Hempe SL, Sra JS, et al. Selective transcatheter ablation of the fast and slow pathways using radiofrequency energy in patients with atrioventricular nodal reentrant tachycardia. *Circulation.* 1992;85(4):1318-1328.

26. Sra JS, Jazayeri MR, Blanck Z, et al. Slow pathway ablation in patients with atrioventricular node reentrant tachycardia and a prolonged PR interval. *J Am Coll Cardiol.* 1994;24(4):1064-1068.

27. Basta MN, Krahn AD, Klein GJ, et al. Safety of slow pathway ablation in patients with atrioventricular node reentrant tachycardia and a long fast pathway effective refractory period. *Am J Cardiol.* 1997;80(2):155-159.

28. Natale A, Greenfield RA, Geiger MJ, et al. Safety of slow pathway ablation in patients with long PR interval: further evidence of fast and slowpathway interaction. *Pacing Clin Electrophysiol.* 1997;20(6):1698-703.

29. Dhala A, Bremner S, Deshpande S, et al. Efficacy and safety of atrioventricular nodal modification for atrioventricular nodal reentrant tachycardia in the pediatric population. *Am Heart J.* 1994;128(5):903-907.

30. Skanes AC, Dubuc M, Klein GJ, et al. Cryothermal ablation of the slow pathway for the elimination of atrioventricular nodal reentrant tachycardia. *Circulation.* 2000;102(23):2856-2860.

ATRIOVENTRICULAR
RECIPROCATING
TACHYCARDIA: RIGHT-SIDED

SECTION II
CASE STUDIES IN SUPRAVENTRICULAR
TACHYCARDIA

65

9 ATRIOVENTRICULAR RECIPROCATING TACHYCARDIA: RIGHT-SIDED

Aman Chugh, MD

CASE PRESENTATION

A 55-year-old man was referred to for electrophysiologic evaluation for Wolff-Parkinson-White (WPW) syndrome. Although he had noted palpitations for many years, they were initially brief and responded to vagal maneuvers. He had previously undergone an attempt at catheter ablation of a right-sided accessory pathway (AP) at another institution. The procedure was unsuccessful and was terminated secondary to transient atrioventricular (AV) nodal conduction block. An event monitor after the ablation procedure revealed supraventricular tachycardia (SVT) at a heart rate of 190 bpm with a right bundle branch block pattern. There was no history of syncope or a family history of unexplained sudden death. There is a remote history of cardiomyopathy, which was attributed to viral etiology, and has since resolved.

The 12-lead electrocardiogram (ECG) showed sinus rhythm with ventricular preexcitation. The pattern of preexcitation was a bit unusual but was compatible with a right anterior free wall accessory pathway (AP), likely inserting superiorly on the tricuspid annulus (Figure 9-1). The electrophysiology procedure was performed under conscious sedation. In the baseline state, no supraventricular tachycardia could be induced.

With isoproterenol infusion, SVT at a cycle length of 340 ms could be easily induced (Figure 9-2). Diagnostic maneuvers confirmed the presence of orthodromic atrioventricular reciprocating tachycardia (AVRT) (see Figures 9-2 to 9-4). The earliest atrial activation during AVRT was at the anterior tricuspid annulus (Figure 9-5). Mapping during sinus rhythm also revealed that the earliest ventricular activation occurred at the anterior tricuspid annulus (approximately 12 o'clock in the left anterior oblique view) (Figure 9-6). Catheter stability at the target site was suboptimal, as the catheter would frequently dislodge into the right atrial appendage or into the right ventricle. Radiofrequency energy was applied during sinus rhythm with an irrigated-tip ablation catheter (Surround Flow, Biosense-Webster, Diamond Bar, CA) at 35 watts, which only had a transient effect on the AP. Increasing the power to 45 watts finally eliminated preexcitation (Figures 9-7 to 9-9), and also rendered the tachycardia noninducible despite isoproterenol infusion. The patient has been free of palpitations for 2 years in the absence of rate- or rhythm-controlling medications.

EPIDEMIOLOGY

AVRT is the most common sustained arrhythmia in patients with WPW syndrome. It is the second most common arrhythmia mechanism in patients presenting for catheter ablation of paroxysmal SVT. In patients undergoing catheter ablation of AVRT/WPW syndrome, right free wall APs account for about 15% of cases. Left free wall and septal accessory pathways are found in about 60% and 25% of patients, respectively. The prevalence of the WPW pattern, that is, evidence of ventricular preexcitation without arrhythmic symptoms, is estimated to be about 2 to 4 per 1000 individuals.[1]

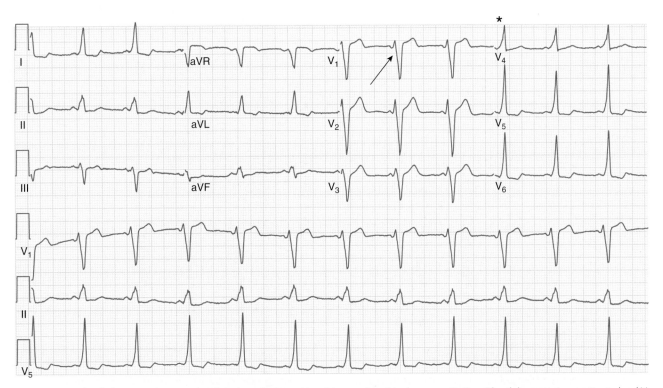

FIGURE 9-1 A 12-lead electrocardiogram showing sinus rhythm with evidence of ventricular preexcitation. The delta wave is negative in lead V_1 (arrow) and the transition (asterisk) in the precordial leads occurs between leads V_3 and V_4, compatible with a right free wall accessory pathway.

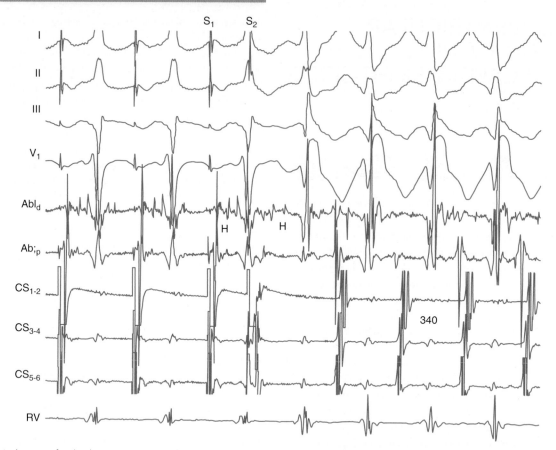

FIGURE 9-2 Induction of orthodromic atrioventricular reciprocating tachycardia (ORT) with programmed atrial stimulation. After a drive train at 400 ms (S_1), a single atrial extrastimulus (S_2) is introduced at 210 ms. The extrastimulus blocks in the accessory pathway and conducts over the specialized conduction system, yielding supraventricular tachycardia. The mechanism of a tachycardia whose induction depends upon conduction block in the accessory pathway is very likely to be ORT. Abl = ablation; CS = coronary sinus; H His; RV = right ventricle.

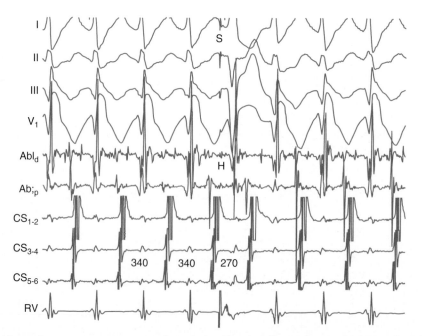

FIGURE 9-3 Response to a His-synchronous premature ventricular complex ("S") during supraventricular tachycardia. The premature ventricular complex (PVC) results in advancement of the subsequent atrial electrogram (from 340 to 270 ms), which confirms the presence of an accessory pathway.

ATRIOVENTRICULAR
RECIPROCATING
TACHYCARDIA: RIGHT-SIDED

SECTION II
CASE STUDIES IN SUPRAVENTRICULAR
TACHYCARDIA

67

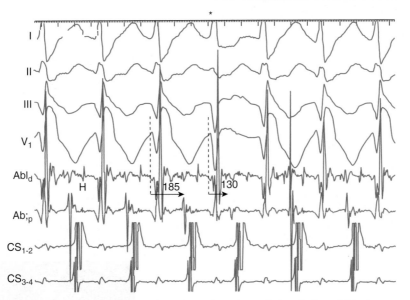

FIGURE 9-4 The ventriculoatrial (VA) time during supraventricular tachycardia with a right bundle branch block pattern is 185 ms, as compared with 130 ms during the narrow QRS complex (asterisk). This observation proves that the mechanism of the tachycardia is orthodromic reciprocating tachycardia (ORT) utilizing a right free wall accessory pathway. (Although the QRS morphology during tachycardia was that of a right bundle branch block pattern, there were several instances in which a narrow QRS complex appeared spontaneously. The narrow QRS complex was *always* followed by a shorter VA time.)

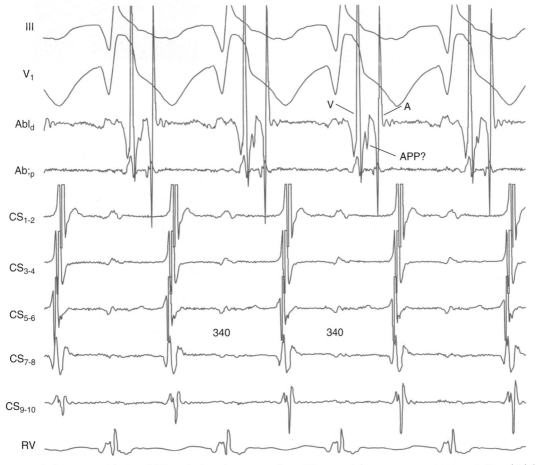

FIGURE 9-5 Prior to radiofrequency ablation, ORT was induced to ensure that a His potential was not present at target site, which had afforded the earliest ventricular activation during sinus rhythm. Note the possible accessory pathway potential (APP) between the ventricular and atrial electrograms.

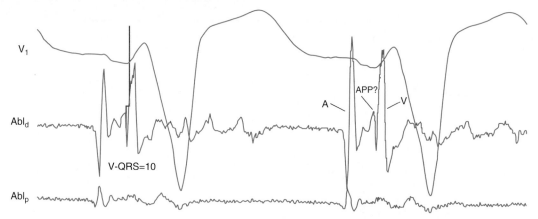

FIGURE 9-6 Bipolar electrogram during sinus rhythm, recorded by the ablation (Abl) catheter at the site where radiofrequency energy eliminated conduction over the accessory pathway. The activation time (V-QRS) is relatively modest, but there may also be an accessory pathway potential (APP) present.

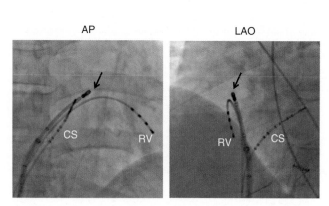

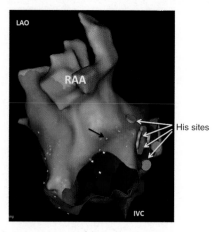

FIGURE 9-7 Fluoroscopic view showing the position of the ablation catheter (arrow) at the site on the tricuspid annulus where radiofrequency ablation eliminated preexcitation. AP = posterior; LAO = left anterior oblique.

FIGURE 9-8 Activation map of the right atrium (RA) showing that the earliest ventricular activation (arrow) was found at the anterior tricuspid annulus (12 o'clock). A His potential could be recorded relatively diffusely over the septal region. IVC inferior vena cava; RAA = right atrial appendage.

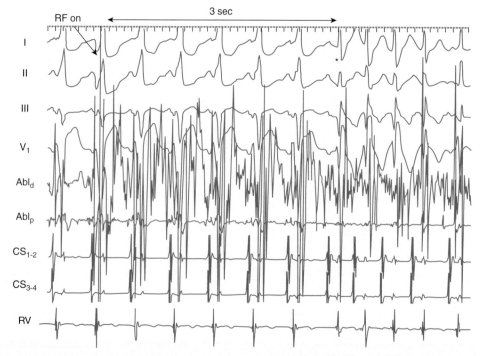

FIGURE 9-9 Initiation of radiofrequency (RF) energy at the anterior tricuspid annulus readily eliminates preexcitation (asterisk). There was no longer evidence of retrograde activation over the pathway or tachycardia.

ATRIOVENTRICULAR
RECIPROCATING
TACHYCARDIA: RIGHT-SIDED

SECTION II
CASE STUDIES IN SUPRAVENTRICULAR
TACHYCARDIA

69

ETIOLOGY AND PATHOPHYSIOLOGY

Ventricular preexcitation is mediated by anomalous muscular tracts that connect the atrium and ventricle along the mitral or tricuspid annulus. Patients with WPW syndrome are usually otherwise healthy, and no significant abnormalities are found on cardiovascular testing. Occasionally, AVRT may occur in the context of overt heart disease, such as Ebstein anomaly or hypertrophic cardiomyopathy.

Orthodromic AVRT (or ORT) is due to a macroreentrant circuit that involves anterograde activation of the specialized conduction system and retrograde activation over the AP. During ORT, typically a narrow complex tachycardia is inscribed on the 12-lead ECG, with retrograde P waves obscured by the ST segment. In cases of a slowly conducting AP, retrograde conduction may be delayed such that the P wave is found after the T wave, resulting in a long RP tachycardia. Classically, such pathways insert near the posteroseptal area, resulting in negative P waves in the inferior leads. These slowly conducting pathways may result in frequent or nearly incessant bouts of tachycardia, ie, permanent junctional reciprocating tachycardia (PJRT). Frequent tachycardia may be associated with left ventricular dysfunction, which resolves after elimination of the AP.

Much less commonly, one may encounter antidromic AVRT or ART during which the circus movement involves anterograde conduction along the AP and retrograde conduction over the normal conduction system or another AP. The ECG in this case shows a wide QRS-complex tachycardia, the morphology of which does not resemble a typical bundle branch block pattern. The QRS complex during ART is maximally preexcited and may be mistaken for ventricular tachycardia.

One may encounter less common forms of AVRT mediated by APs that do not insert along the AV ring. These include atriofascicular, nodofascicular, and nodoventricular pathways. Conduction along these pathways is decremental and may not be apparent on the resting ECG. Atriofascicular pathways connect the atrium to the right bundle branch and are incapable of retrograde conduction. Nodofascicular or nodoventricular pathways connect the AV node and proximal right bundle or the right ventricular myocardium, respectively. Fasciculoventricular APs connect the distal right bundle branch to the ventricular myocardium. As such, the ECG shows only subtle preexcitation in patients with a fasciculoventricular pathway. These pathways are thought not to participate in AVRT but may act as bystanders during supraventricular tachycardia.

DIAGNOSIS AND DIFFERENTIAL DIAGNOSIS

In a patient with a history of paroxysmal supraventricular tachycardia, the presence of preexcitation on the 12-lead ECG during sinus rhythm increases the odds that the mechanism of the tachycardia is ORT as opposed to atrioventricular nodal reentrant tachycardia (AVNRT) or atrial tachycardia (AT). Often, the 12-lead ECG during SVT does not contain clues that may be diagnostic of ORT. If a narrow complex tachycardia is initiated after anterograde conduction block over the AP, the mechanism is very likely to be ORT. Prolongation of the RP interval during bundle branch block is diagnostic of ORT utilizing an AP located ipsilateral to the blocked bundle branch.

Diagnosis of ORT is usually made in the electrophysiology laboratory. Development of a bundle branch block during ORT provides important diagnostic information. Prolongation of the ventriculoatrial (VA) interval by >30 ms during SVT with a bundle branch block is diagnostic of ORT utilizing an AP that is located ipsilateral to the blocked bundle branch (see Figure 9-4). There is less of an increment in the VA interval with development of a bundle branch block during ORT mediated by a septal accessory pathway. Insertion of a His-synchronous premature ventricular complex (PVC) during supraventricular tachycardia may provide mechanistic insights. Advancement or delay of the subsequent atrial electrogram confirms the presence of an AP. Termination of the tachycardia without affecting the atrial electrogram proves that the mechanism is ORT (Figure 9-10). Differentiation between typical AVNRT and ORT is straightforward. However, differentiation between atypical AVNRT and ORT using a septal AP usually requires a few diagnostic maneuvers. After ruling out the possibility of atrial tachycardia (by observing an A-V response after cessation of ventricular overdrive pacing that entrains the tachycardia), the difference between the postpacing interval and the tachycardia cycle length helps discern between the two possibilities. If the difference is less than 115 ms, the diagnosis is very likely to be ORT.[2] Even if the tachycardia terminates during the entrainment attempt, the maneuver can still be helpful. The number of fully paced ventricular complexes (as compared to fused complexes) required to advance the atrial electrogram to the paced rate can be helpful in differentiating between AVNRT and ORT. A prior study showed that ORT could be reset with one fully paced complex as compared with a mean of 3.7 beats for AVNRT.[3] The delta-AH (ie, the difference between the atrio-His (AH) interval during pacing from the high right atrium at the tachycardia cycle length and that during tachycardia) can be quite helpful in differentiating between atypical AVNRT and ORT using a septal AP. During ORT (and atrial tachycardia), the delta-AH is minimal. However, the AH interval during pacing is longer than that during AVNRT owing to *sequential* activation of the atrium and specialized conduction system during atrial pacing. During atypical AVNRT, after retrograde activation over the slow pathway, there is nearly *simultaneous* activation of the atrium and His bundle, leading to a pseudo-AH interval. A prior study showed that the delta-AH interval was >40 ms in 80% of patients with atypical AVNRT whereas it was never >10 to 20 ms in patients with ORT (or AT).[4]

Para-Hisian pacing is a useful maneuver to determine whether retrograde activation is occurring over the AV node or septal accessory pathway. High-output pacing is performed from the His bundle catheter, and the output is then gradually decreased. With high output pacing, both the ventricular myocardium and the His bundle (V+H) are captured resulting in a relatively narrow QRS. As the output is lowered, only the ventricular myocardium (V) is captured resulting a wider QRS. Then the stimulus-to-atrial electrogram interval (SA) during the narrow and wide QRS is compared. If the SA interval is the same, then retrograde conduction is occurring over a septal AP since pathway activation depends only upon ventricular activation. If the SA interval with a narrow QRS paced complex is shorter, then retrograde activation is occurring over the AV node. The reason that the SA is shorter with the narrow QRS paced complex (ie, during V + H capture) is that retrograde conduction needs only to commence from the proximal aspect of the specialized conduction system to the atrium. With the wide QRS paced complex (ie, during ventricular capture only), the SA interval is longer because

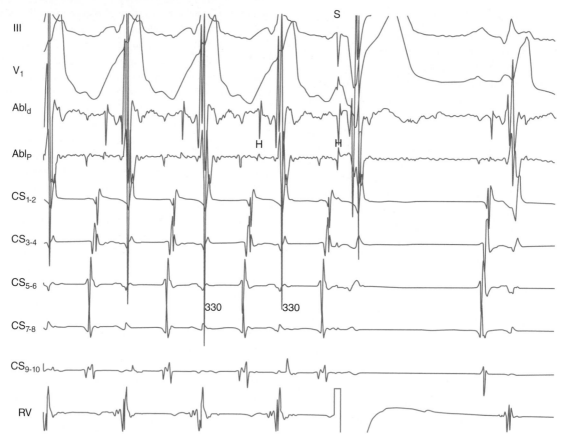

FIGURE 9-10 In another patient with multiple right free wall accessory pathways, a His-synchronous PVC ("S") terminates supraventricular tachycardia, proving that the mechanism of the tachycardia is ORT.

atrial activation depends upon a series of steps: ventricular activation, followed by engagement of the Purkinje network, His bundle, and then the AV node. Para-Hisian pacing is also helpful in determining whether a septal AP has been successfully ablated.

MANAGEMENT

Asymptomatic Individuals with Preexcitation

An Italian study from a few years ago revealed that the prognosis for most asymptomatic persons with incidentally discovered preexcitation is good.[5] Specifically, 293 patients with a WPW pattern underwent a diagnostic electrophysiologic evaluation. Over a median follow-up of 67 months, 262 individuals (89%) remained asymptomatic. AVRT was noted in 14 persons (5%) during follow-up. Potentially life-threatening arrhythmias were noted in 17 patients (6%). Although one of the latter individuals suffered an aborted cardiac arrest, there were no deaths. The investigators identified young age, inducibility, and a short AP anterograde effective refractory period ($\leq$250 ms) as predictors of potentially life threatening events. Importantly, spontaneous disappearance of the delta wave on the ECG was noted in 30% of the study population. Since the event rate of individuals with incidental preexcitation is low, a conservative approach is reasonable in most situations. The care of pilots, bus drivers, athletes, or others in whom ventricular preexcitation is discovered on routine testing (ie, in the absence of symptoms) should be individualized.

Medical Management

The acute management of a patient with AVRT is similar to that of a patient with paroxysmal supraventricular tachycardia in general. In the hemodynamically stable patient, intravenous adenosine is indicated to terminate the tachycardia. In the acute setting (eg, a patient presenting to the emergency department with SVT) it may not be known whether the patient has manifest preexcitation during sinus rhythm. Since adenosine administration may result in atrial fibrillation (AF) in about 10% of patients, in the patient with underlying preexcitation, AF may result in rapid conduction over the accessory pathway. The ECG may show an irregular, wide complex tachycardia (owing to varying fusion between activation over the AP and the AV node) with heart rates >200 bpm. This may be met with hemodynamic collapse and/or ventricular fibrillation requiring immediate transthoracic cardioversion/defibrillation. Although the emergency department is well prepared to deal with such a situation, other medical facilities (eg, student health services) may be less prepared should adenosine administration result in preexcited AF.

Patients with hemodynamically stable antidromic AVRT may be treated with intravenous ibutilide or procainamide. Patients presenting with tachycardia and hemodynamic instability or serious symptoms such as angina or heart failure should undergo prompt cardioversion.

ATRIOVENTRICULAR
RECIPROCATING
TACHYCARDIA: RIGHT-SIDED

SECTION II
CASE STUDIES IN SUPRAVENTRICULAR
TACHYCARDIA

71

MAPPING AND ABLATION OF RIGHT-SIDED AVRT

Patients with recurrent SVT that is thought to be due to AVRT or AF in the setting of ventricular preexcitation should undergo catheter ablation given the favorable risk/benefit ratio. The pathway responsible for AVRT can be eliminated in >95% of patients with a low risk of complications, such as serious bleeding, thromboembolism, and stroke (all <1%). Patients with a septal AP need to be counseled that the risk of AV block requiring a pacemaker is obviously higher than with free wall APs, but the risk is still small (about 1%). In a case of a para-Hisian accessory pathway (Figure 9-11), AV block may be avoided by targeting the noncoronary cusp of the aortic valve (Figure 9-12). In patients with a midseptal accessory pathway, cryomapping may be helpful in determining whether the pathway can be safely ablated. In some cases where the AP cannot be ablated without injury to the conduction system, patients are best treated with a combination of rhythm- and rate-controlling medications. Posteroseptal APs may be ablated outside the ostium of the coronary sinus, from the inferoseptal mitral annulus or from within the coronary sinus or one of its ventricular branches.[6] Varying VA times may also reveal the presence of multiple accessory pathways responsible for ORT (Figure 9-13).

Troubleshooting

Some studies have suggested that the recurrence rate following catheter ablation of right free wall APs may be greater than that of left free wall accessory pathways. In most cases, this is probably related to suboptimal contact/stability during ablation of APs located at the lateral, anterolateral, and anterior aspects of the tricuspid annulus. Utilization of a long sheath is helpful in order to improve contact at these locations. Deflectable sheaths (eg, Agilis, St. Jude Medical) may also be useful in difficult cases. To approach the free wall aspect of the tricuspid annulus, the operator carefully advances the catheter and sheath assembly from the 6 o'clock position superiorly in the left anterior oblique view. The tension on the handle is released, and the assembly is rotated toward the target site on the annulus, while seeking an atrial and ventricular electrogram on the distal bipole of the ablation catheter. Some have also advocated a superior mapping approach from the right internal jugular vein in order to improve stability in this region. Tachycardia termination during radiofrequency ablation leads to a sudden change in the heart rate, and may lead to catheter dislodgement and suboptimal lesion delivery. Ventricular pacing at a rate approximating that of the tachycardia may help prevent the sudden change in rate and abrupt catheter dislodgement from the target site. It should also be noted that right free wall APs may insert at some distance away from the annulus, even as high as the base of the right atrial appendage. Three-dimensional mapping may be helpful in mapping challenging right free wall APs.[7]

PATIENT EDUCATION

Patients who are diagnosed with paroxysmal SVT and whose ECG during sinus rhythm reveals evidence of ventricular preexcitation

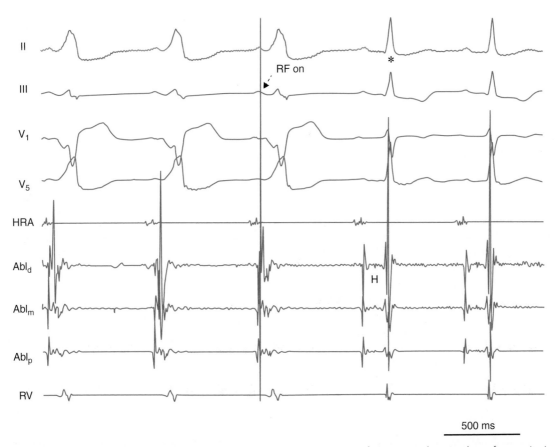

FIGURE 9-11 Catheter ablation of a para-Hisian accessory pathway. Shortly after initiation of RF current, there is a loss of preexcitation (*). A small His electrogram is apparent on the electrogram recorded by the distal bipole of the ablation catheter. Note that there is no RF-induced junctional ectopy, which would prompt the immediate discontinuation of RF energy.

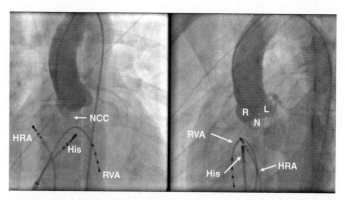

FIGURE 9-12 An aortogram showing the location of the noncoronary cusp (NCC), where radiofrequency ablation was applied to eliminate a para-Hisian accessory pathway. "L" and "R" refer to left and right coronary cusp.

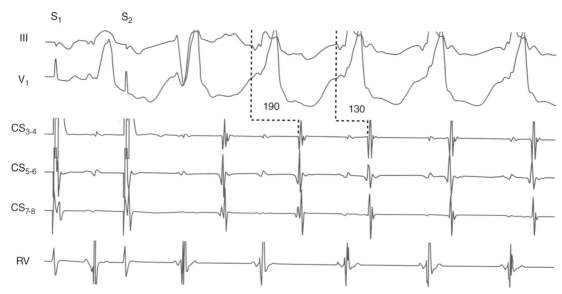

FIGURE 9-13 Example of multiple pathways responsible for ORT. Programmed atrial stimulation induced a tachycardia with varying ventriculoatrial (VA) times. The varying VA intervals were due to two different tachycardias, and the mechanisms of both were due to ORT. The longer VA interval corresponded to retrograde activation over a right lateral accessory pathway, and the shorter over a right anterior accessory pathway.

(ie, WPW syndrome) should be advised about vagal maneuvers that may help abort long episodes of tachycardia. They should also be told about the risk of syncope and sudden death, although the risk is small. Patients with paroxysmal SVT that is thought to be mediated by an accessory pathway should be referred to an electrophysiologist to discuss the risks and benefits of catheter ablation. Patients should be told that catheter ablation successfully eliminates that AP responsible for ORT with a low risk of complication. The risk of AV conduction block should be discussed with patients with septal APs. Patients in whom ventricular preexcitation is discovered incidentally should be advised that a conservative approach is reasonable since of risk of syncope and sudden death is low.

REFERENCES

1. Klein GJ, Gula LJ, Krahn AD, Skanes AC, Yee R. WPW pattern in the asymptomatic individual: has anything changed? *Circ Arrhythm Electrophysiol.* 2009;2(2):97-99.

2. Michaud GF, Tada H, Chough S, et al. Differentiation of atypical atrioventricular node re-entrant tachycardia from orthodromic reciprocating tachycardia using a septal accessory pathway by the response to ventricular pacing. *J Am Coll Cardiol.* 2001;38: 1163-1167.

3. Dandamudi G, Mokabberi R, Assal C, et al. A novel approach to differentiating orthodromic reciprocating tachycardia from atrioventricular nodal reentrant tachycardia. *Heart Rhythm.* 2010;7:1326-1329.

4. Man KC, Niebauer M, Daoud E, et al. Comparison of atrial-His intervals during tachycardia and atrial pacing in patients with long RP tachycardia. *J Cardiovasc Electrophysiol.* 1995;6: 700-710.

5. Santinelli V, Radinovic A, Manguso F, et al. Asymptomatic ventricular preexcitation: a long-term prospective follow-up study of 293 adult patients. *Circ Arrhythm Electrophysiol.* 2009;2:102-107.

ATRIOVENTRICULAR
RECIPROCATING
TACHYCARDIA: RIGHT-SIDED

SECTION II
CASE STUDIES IN SUPRAVENTRICULAR
TACHYCARDIA

73

6. Stavrakis S, Jackman WM, Nakagawa H, et al. Risk of coronary artery injury with radiofrequency ablation and cryoablation of epicardial posteroseptal accessory pathways within the coronary venous system. *Circ Arrhythm Electrophysiol*. 2014;7:113-119.

7. Long DY, Dong JZ, Liu XP, et al. Ablation of right-sided accessory pathways with atrial insertion far from the tricuspid annulus using an electroanatomical mapping system. *J Cardiovasc Electrophysiol*. 2011;22:499-505.

10 AV RECIPROCATING TACHYCARDIA: LEFT-SIDED

Dan Blendea MD, PhD, E. Kevin Heist MD, PhD,
Jeremy N. Ruskin, MD, Moussa Mansour, MD

CASE PRESENTATION

An 84-year-old woman with history of hypertension presented with palpitations, dizziness, and dyspnea. Upon arrival in the emergency department (ED) the ECG showed a wide-complex tachycardia at a rate of 155 bpm. This was a short RP tachycardia with left bundle branch block (LBBB) QRS morphology similar to that in sinus rhythm (Figure 10-1). The patient received 6 mg of adenosine IV and converted to sinus rhythm. The ECG in sinus rhythm revealed LBBB. There was no evidence of ventricular preexcitation.

In the ED the patient recalled having episodes of palpitations for the past 3 years. Initially she described intermittent "blips" in her chest without associated chest pain or dyspnea. Later, episodes of palpitations became more frequent and more protracted, prompting two prior visits to the ED. Each time tachycardia, thought to be supraventricular tachycardia, resolved with adenosine. The patient received diltiazem, with limited improvement in the frequency and duration of the episodes of palpitations. Three years prior to the current presentation she was diagnosed with LBBB. At that time the workup included

an echocardiogram that revealed left atrial enlargement and normal left ventricular systolic function, and an exercise myocardial perfusion imaging stress test without evidence of ischemia or infarction.

Given the recurrent episodes of symptomatic supraventricular tachycardia, the patient underwent an electrophysiology (EP) study. With ventricular pacing, the atrial activation was eccentric—earliest at the distal dipole of the coronary sinus catheter situated in a lateral position (CS 1-2; Figure 10-2) suggesting retrograde conduction via a lateral accessory pathway (AP). With atrial pacing, conduction was decremental, via the AV node. The retrograde effective refractory period of the AP was 330 ms at a 600 ms driving train. At baseline, single echos were seen (Figure 10-3). Supraventricular tachycardia with a cycle length of 400 ms (heart rate 150 bpm) was induced with atrial extrastimuli (Figure 10-4). The surface ECG was similar to the ECG on presentation in the ED. The earliest atrial activation was again at the CS 1-2 electrode. Ventricular entrainment revealed a VAV response. His-synchronous PVCs advanced the subsequent A as well as the tachycardia (Figure 10-5). These maneuvers were consistent with orthodromic atrioventricular reentrant tachycardia (AVRT), using a concealed left lateral AP. A transseptal puncture was performed, and radiofrequency applications were delivered to the area of the earliest activation at the left lateral region during ventricular pacing. Pathway conduction was abolished at the successful site after 3 seconds of RF application (Figure 10-6). Postablation there was midline and decremental AV conduction with no evidence for dual AV nodal physiology. There was no retrograde VA conduction. The patient tolerated the procedure well. At follow-up there has been no recurrence of arrhythmia symptoms, and the ECG remained unchanged.

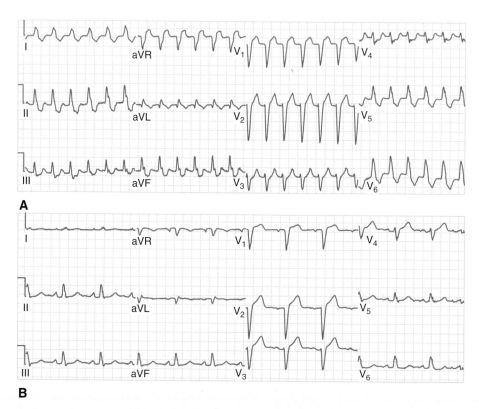

FIGURE 10-1 Twelve-lead ECG during tachycardia (A) with LBBB QRS morphology similar to that in sinus rhythm (B).

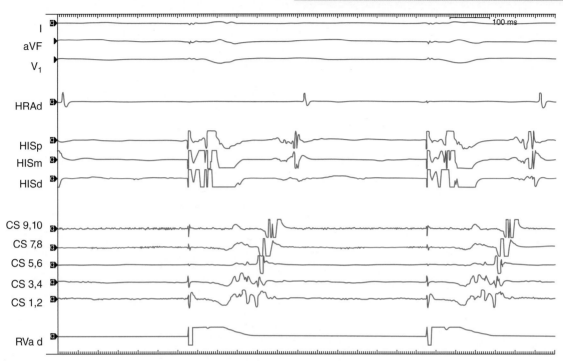

FIGURE 10-2 With ventricular pacing the atrial activation was eccentric—earliest at the distal dipole of the coronary sinus catheter (CS 1-2) suggesting retrograde conduction via a left lateral accessory pathway. Tracings are shown from surface leads I, aVF, and V₁ as well as HRA, His proximal (HISp), mid (HISm), and distal (HISd), coronary sinus (CS) proximal (9,10) to distal (1,2), and right ventricular apex (RVa).

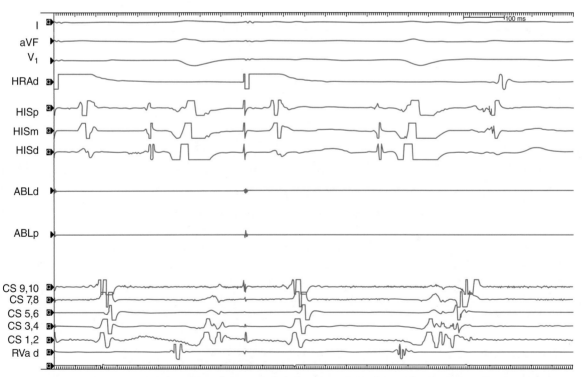

FIGURE 10-3 Single atrial echo beats were seen with atrial extrastimuli. Tracings are shown from surface leads I, aVF, and V₁ as well as HRA, His proximal (HISp), mid (HISm), and distal (HISd), ablation catheter distal (ABLd) and proximal (ABLp), coronary sinus (CS) proximal (9,10) to distal (1,2), and right ventricular apex (RVa).

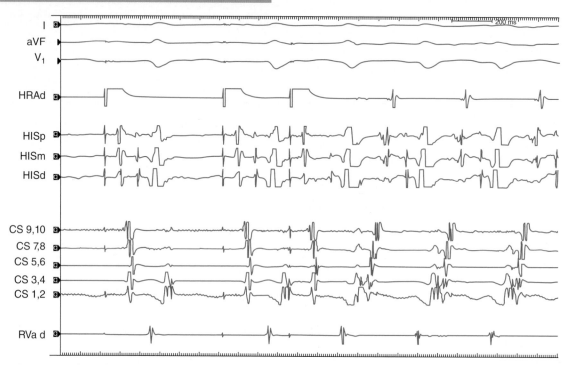

FIGURE 10-4 Supraventricular tachycardia with cycle length of 400 ms (heart rate 150 bpm) was induced with an atrial extrastimulus. Tracings are shown from surface leads I, aVF, and V₁ as well as HRA, His proximal (HISp), mid (HISm), and distal (HISd), coronary sinus (CS) proximal (9,10) to distal (1,2), and right ventricular apex (RVa).

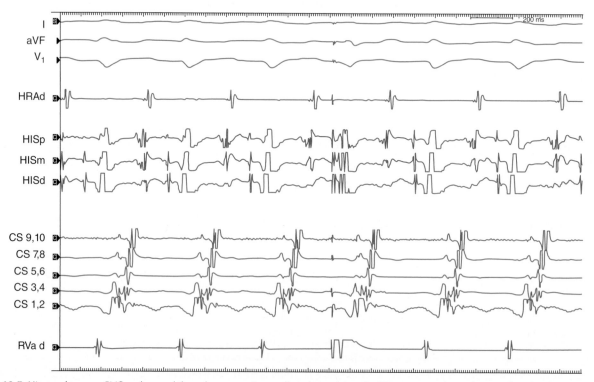

FIGURE 10-5 His-synchronous PVCs advanced the subsequent A as well as the tachycardia. Tracings are shown from surface leads I, aVF, and V₁ as well as HRA, His proximal (HISp), mid (HISm), and distal (HISd), coronary sinus (CS) proximal (9,10) to distal (1,2), and right ventricular apex (RVa).

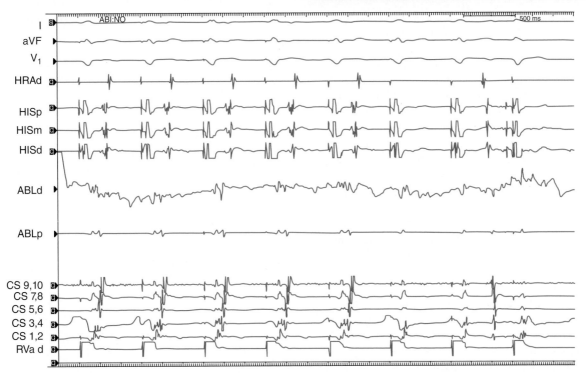

FIGURE 10-6 Pathway conduction was abolished at the successful site after 3 seconds of radiofrequency ablation. Tracings are shown from surface leads I, aVF, and V$_1$ as well as HRA, His proximal (HISp), mid (HISm), and distal (HISd), ablation catheter distal (ABLd) and proximal (ABLp), coronary sinus (CS) proximal (9,10) to distal (1,2), and right ventricular apex (RVa).

EPIDEMIOLOGY, ETIOLOGY, AND PATHOGENESIS

AVRT is the second most common cause of paroxysmal supraventricular tachycardia, but the etiology of AP formation remains largely unknown.[1,2] It is not clear whether the development of atrioventricular connections is genetically determined,[3] due to some environmental exposure, or due to other factors.[1]

The APs are located in the left free wall in approximately 60% of patients undergoing RF ablation, in or adjacent to the interventricular septum in 20% to 30% of patients, and in the right free wall in about 10% of patients.[4,5]

There are gender differences in the clinical characteristics of the APs. Women seem have more concealed accessory pathways (59%) than men (50%).[5] Orthodromic AVRT is more frequent than antidromic AVRT in both men and women.[5] The left free wall locations are similarly encountered in men and in women.[4]

With advancing age, there is a higher prevalence of left-sided APs and a longer duration of the arrhythmia compared to young patients.[6] The incidence of concealed APs and orthodromic AVRT increases with age. The tachycardia cycle length, antegrade and retrograde AP effective refractory periods, antegrade AV node effective refractory periods, and atrial and ventricular effective refractory periods lengthen as the age increases.[6]

Importance of the LBBB

In the present case, it was only after the onset of LBBB at age 81 that the patient started to have palpitations. It is likely that the electrical delay in ventricular conduction caused by LBBB allowed recovery of the retrograde conduction in the left-sided AP and thus initiation and perpetuation of orthodromic AV reentry.

There are reports in the literature of othodromic AVRT using concealed APs facilitated by the onset of ipsilateral bundle branch block. Calo et al described an onset incessant orthodromic AVRT, using a concealed right-sided accessory pathway, after iatrogenic right bundle branch block during an EP study.[7] Another report by Stanke and colleagues described the association between LBBB and development of orthodromic AVRT using a concealed left-sided accessory pathway.[8]

DIAGNOSIS

Preexcitation of the ventricles in patients with Wolff-Parkinson-White (WPW) syndrome results in distinctive changes of the 12-lead ECG configuration with characteristic polarity of the delta wave, QRS polarity, and R/S ratio, respectively, depending on the AP location. Based on these characteristics, several algorithms have been developed to predict AP location from the surface ECG in patients with WPW syndrome. Unfortunately, there are only limited possibilities to predict the localization of concealed atrioventricular APs from a 12-lead surface ECG by analyzing retrograde P-wave polarity during AVRT.[9-11] The analysis of retrograde P-wave polarity during AVRT is often difficult due to the superimposing repolarization. Typically a negative P wave in lead I is indicative of a left free wall location with a 95% positive predictive value.[9] The presence of negative P waves in inferior leads suggests an inferior/posterior location, while positive P waves in all inferior leads indicate a superior/anterior location. Isoelectric or biphasic P waves in any of the inferior leads suggest a left lateral location. A combination of negative P waves in lead I, positive P waves in aVR and V$_1$, and isoelectric P waves in aVL indicate a left lateral location of the AP with 100% positive predictive value.[10] In the present case, the P waves during tachycardia were negative in lead I, positive in lead II, and biphasic in lead III (Figure 10-7), morphology consistent with atrial activation via a left lateral AP.

During EP study, the hallmark of orthodromic AVRT is the requirement of a 1:1 atrial and ventricular activation for maintaining tachycardia. The diagnosis of orthodromic AVRT using a left free wall AP requires demonstration of an eccentric atrial activation sequence earliest along the left atrial free wall. In addition, in orthodromic AVRT there is a constant ventricle-to-atrium conduction time despite changes in the tachycardia cycle length, and typically one can advance the atrial activation by a premature ventricular stimulus delivered during His bundle refractoriness. A left lateral AP is typically associated with a preexcitation index greater than 70 ms.[12] The preexcitation index is defined as the difference between the tachycardia cycle length and the longest coupling interval of a right ventricular apical premature stimulus that advances the atrium.[12,13] A diagnostic feature suggestive of a left free wall pathway is the prolongation of the QRS-to-atrium time during orthodromic AVRT by 35 to 40 ms or longer with the onset of LBBB.[14] Another diagnostic criterion for orthodromic AVRT is the ability to reproducibly terminate the tachycardia with a premature ventricular stimulus delivered during His bundle refractoriness.

Orthodromic AVRTs using left free wall APs must be differentiated from atrial tachycardias originating from areas close to the mitral annulus, which is best accomplished by dissociating the ventricles from the tachycardia.[13] For example, a VAAV response after termination of ventricular pacing that entrains the atrium excludes orthodromic AVRT and confirms atrial tachycardia.[13] About 6% of AV nodal reentrant tachycardias are associated with an eccentric atrial activation sequence earliest in the distal or posterior CS with the shortest VA time with an atrial activation pattern that can be confused with a left-sided concealed AP. The diagnostic criteria that suggest AV nodal reentrant tachycardia rather than AVRT are demonstration of dual AV nodal physiology, inability to advance the atrium with ventricular extrastimuli during His refractoriness, decremental VA conduction, and ability to dissociate the atria and the ventricles from the tachycardia.[13,15]

MAPPING AND ABLATION

Mapping and ablation of left free wall APs may be performed via a transseptal or transaortic approach, the latter facilitating access to the ventricular insertion sites of the APs, but being usually avoided in patients with peripheral vascular disease, aortic stenosis, or small left ventricular dimensions. The transseptal approach allows mapping of the atrial side of the mitral annulus or the annulus itself.[13] Several electrogram characteristics predict successful ablation of a left free wall AP, when mapping is performed during orthodromic AVRT or during ventricular pacing: presence of presumed AP potential, continuous electrical activity, and local VA interval of 25 to 50 ms.[13,16]

Before delivering radiofrequency energy it is important to obtain a stable catheter position. Catheter stability during ablation of left-sided APs is enhanced by use of preformed sheaths. With ventricular pacing to entrain the orthodromic AVRT, the risk of catheter dislodgement with termination of the arrhythmia is diminished. Loss of AP conduction should occur in 1 to 6 seconds after radiofrequency energy delivery, longer times to successful ablation being associated with higher recurrence rates.[13,16,17] In the case of resistant Aps,

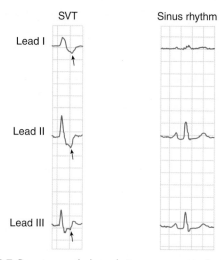

FIGURE 10-7 P-wave morphology during supraventricular tachycardia (SVT) and during sinus rhythm.

irrigated catheters can help delivering higher energies.[18] Epicardial left-sided APs can be approached from within the CS or using direct epicardial mapping and ablation.[19,20]

REFERENCES

1. Hsu JC, Tanel RE, Lee BK, et al. Differences in accessory pathway location by sex and race. *Heart Rhythm*. 2010;7(1):52-66.

2. Ganz LI, Friedman PL. Supraventricular tachycardia. *N Eng J Med*. 1995;332:162-173.

3. Vidaillet HJ, Jr, Pressley JC, Henke E, Harrell FE, Jr, German LD. Familial occurrence of accessory atrioventricular pathways (pre-excitation syndrome). *N Eng J Med*. 1987;317:65-69.

4. Birati EY, Eldar M, Belhassen B. Gender differences in accessory connections location: an Israeli study. *J Interv Card Electrophysiol*. 2012;34:227-229.

5. Huang SY, Hu YF, Chang SL, et al. Gender differences of electrophysiologic characteristics in patients with accessory atrioventricular pathways. *Heart Rhythm*. 2011;8:571-574.

6. Li CH, Hu YF, Lin YJ, et al. The impact of age on the electrophysiological characteristics and different arrhythmia patterns in patients with Wolff-Parkinson-White syndrome. *J Cardiovasc Electrophysiol*. 2011;22:274-279.

7. Calo L, Lamberti F, Golia P, et al. Facilitation of atrioventricular reentrant tachycardia by iatrogenic right bundle branch block. *Ital Heart J*. 2001;2:468-471.

8. Stanke A, Storti C, De Ponti R, Salerno-Uriarte JA. Spontaneous incessant AV reentrant tachycardia related to left bundle branch block and concealed left-sided accessory AV pathway. *J Cardiovasc Electrophysiol*. 1994;5:777-781.

9. Fitzgerald DM, Hawthorne HR, Crossley GH, Simmons TW, Haisty WK, Jr. P wave morphology during atrial pacing along the atrioventricular ring. ECG localization of the site of origin of retrograde atrial activation. *J Electrocardiol*. 1996;29:1-10.

10. Rostock T, Sydow K, Steven D, et al. A new algorithm for concealed accessory pathway localization using T-wave-subtracted retrograde P-wave polarity during orthodromic atrioventricular reentrant tachycardia. *J Interv Card Electrophysiol*. 2008;22:55-63.

11. Tai CT, Chen SA, Chiang CE, et al. A new electrocardiographic algorithm using retrograde P waves for differentiating atrioventricular node reentrant tachycardia from atrioventricular reciprocating tachycardia mediated by concealed accessory pathway. *J Am Coll Cardiol*. 1997;29:394-402.

12. Miles WM, Yee R, Klein GJ, Zipes DP, Prystowsky EN. The preexcitation index: an aid in determining the mechanism of supraventricular tachycardia and localizing accessory pathways. *Circulation*. 1986;74:493-500.

13. Huang SK, Wood MA. *Catheter Ablation of Cardiac Arrhythmias*. Philadelphia, PA: W.B. Saunders; 2006.

14. Yang Y, Cheng J, Glatter K, Dorostkar P, Modin GW, Scheinman MM. Quantitative effects of functional bundle branch block in patients with atrioventricular reentrant tachycardia. *Am J Cardiol*. 2000;85:826-831.

15. Hwang C, Martin DJ, Goodman JS, et al. Atypical atrioventricular node reciprocating tachycardia masquerading as tachycardia using a left-sided accessory pathway. *J Am Coll Cardiol*. 1997;30:218-225.

16. Chen X, Borggrefe M, Shenasa M, Haverkamp W, Hindricks G, Breithardt G. Characteristics of local electrogram predicting successful transcatheter radiofrequency ablation of left-sided accessory pathways. *J Am Coll Cardiol*. 1992;20:656-665.

17. Twidale N, Wang XZ, Beckman KJ, et al. Factors associated with recurrence of accessory pathway conduction after radiofrequency catheter ablation. *Pacing Clin Electrophysiol*. 1991;14:2042-2048.

18. Yamane T, Jais P, Shah DC, et al. Efficacy and safety of an irrigated-tip catheter for the ablation of accessory pathways resistant to conventional radiofrequency ablation. *Circulation*. 2000;102:2565-2568.

19. Ho I, d'Avila A, Ruskin J, Mansour M. Images in cardiovascular medicine. Percutaneous epicardial mapping and ablation of a posteroseptal accessory pathway. *Circulation*. 2007;115:e418-e421.

20. Haissaguerre M, Gaita F, Fischer B, Egloff P, Lemetayer P, Warin JF. Radiofrequency catheter ablation of left lateral accessory pathways via the coronary sinus. *Circulation*. 1992;86:1464-1468.

11 AV RECIPROCATING TACHYCARDIA: EPICARDIAL

E. Kevin Heist, MD, PhD, Dan Blendea, MD,
Jeremy N. Ruskin, MD, Moussa Mansour, MD

CASE PRESENTATION

A 20-year-old man without previous medical history suffered a witnessed cardiac arrest in a locker room shortly after refereeing a wrestling match. He received bystander CPR; when paramedics arrived, he was found to be in preexcited atrial fibrillation with a rapid rate (290 bpm) and was externally shocked to sinus rhythm. His ECG in sinus rhythm demonstrated manifest preexcitation, with deeply negative delta waves in the inferior leads, suggestive of a posteroseptal accessory pathway (AP) (Figure 11-1). He was taken to EP study, which demonstrated the presence of a posteroseptal AP, with antegrade effective refractory period 400/210 ms, and 1:1 A:V conduction via the AP with rapid atrial pacing down to 220 ms, as well as inducible, nonsustained orthodromic AV reciprocating tachycardia (AVRT). Mapping of ventricular activation during sinus rhythm (preexcited) utilizing endocardial access localized the earliest ventricular potentials to the proximal coronary sinus (CS) os, where a small CS diverticulum was identified by contrast venography. Extensive radiofrequency ablation at this region resulted in only transient loss of preexcitation, and cryoablation at this site was also ineffective. The patient then returned for a second procedure with preprocedural CT imaging and percutaneous subxyphoid epicardial access. The earliest preexcited ventricular electrogram using both endocardial and epicardial mapping was identified in the epicardial posteroseptal region (Figures 11-2 and 11-3). After coronary angiography was performed to demonstrate that this site was not adjacent to a coronary artery,

radiofrequency ablation at this site successfully and durably ablated AP conduction (Figure 11-4), and the patient has had no further arrhythmic symptoms.[1]

EPIDEMIOLOGY AND PATHOPHYSIOLOGY

Manifest preexcitation is evident in approximately 0.1% to 0.3% of ECGs,[2] although this underestimates the true prevalence of AP conduction, as many APs are concealed, either due to AV nodal conduction preceding AP conduction or due to lack of anterograde AP conduction. Classic APs result from electrically excitable fibers (bundles of Kent) which pass through the fibrous AV ring, although other types of APs (ie, atriofascicular pathways) have also been extensively described in the literature.[3]

The initial interventional approaches to patients with symptomatic Wolff-Parkinson-White (WPW) syndrome involved cardiac surgical incisions in the region of the AP.[4] Because these incisions were transmural, the exact intramural location of the AP (endocardial, midmyocardial, or epicardial) was generally not relevant for clinical success in most cases. This changed with the advent of catheter ablation,[5] however, as current ablation catheters may not always create transmural lesions, particularly in regions of thick myocardium, such as the AV ring (particularly relevant to AP ablation) and the ventricular septum and left ventricle (relevant to ventricular tachycardia ablation).

If microscopic studies could be performed on all APs, it would be possible to anatomically define the course of each AP, and endocardial/epicardial location could be precisely determined. Because this is obviously not possible in patients, the location of a given AP is typically defined based on activation mapping of the region of earliest atrial and/or ventricular preexcitation and AP potentials, and particularly by success (or lack of success) of ablation at a given site. Epicardial APs are typically defined as those which require epicardial access for successful ablation, as well as APs which map to and/or are successfully ablated from the coronary sinus (CS) and its tributaries, which is an epicardial structure. This is thus a functional rather than a true anatomic classification of endocardial/epicardial location of APs,

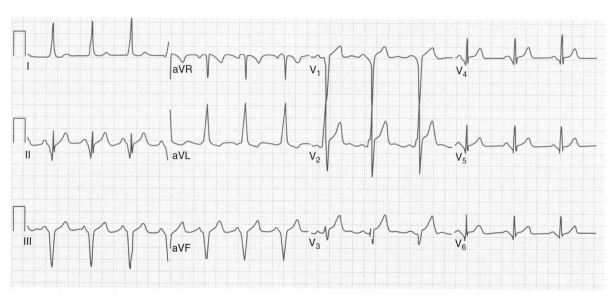

FIGURE 11-1 Twelve-lead ECG after cardioversion, demonstrating manifest preexcitation with deeply negative delta waves in leads II, III, and aVF.

and it should be noted that pericardial mapping (other than mapping within the CS) is rarely performed for a given AP unless ablation from an endocardial approach is unsuccessful. APs requiring pericardial access for successful ablation have generally been reported as single cases or small case series, and so it is currently difficult to estimate their true incidence.[1,6-9] In comparison, APs which have been successfully ablated from within the CS or its tributaries have been described with much greater frequency.[10]

It should be noted that in many cases it is possible to create electrically transmural lesions at the AV ring utilizing only endocardial catheter ablation. Examples of this include cavo-tricuspid isthmus ablation for typical right atrial flutter (which is virtually always successful using endocardial ablation with current techniques and requires transmural electrical block) and mitral isthmus ablation at the AV ring adjacent to the left inferior pulmonary vein (which is successful in some cases using only endocardial ablation, while other cases require combined endocardial and intra-CS ablation[11]). Based on this evidence, it would be reasonable to hypothesize that an AP in the vicinity of the cavo-tricuspid isthmus could be successfully ablated using an endocardial approach in almost all cases regardless of endocardial/epicardial course, while an epicardial or intra-CS AP in the vicinity of the mitral isthmus could be ablated using an endocardial approach in some but not all cases.

The large majority of APs which are thus functionally classified as epicardial are posteroseptal, as is true for the case presented here. It should be noted that the thickness of the myocardium at the AV ring is typically greatest in the posteroseptal region. It is therefore not clear whether anatomically epicardial APs are truly more common in the posteroseptal region compared to other regions, or whether the greater myocardial thickness in the posteroseptal region results in greater difficulty in creating transmural ablation lesions, more often

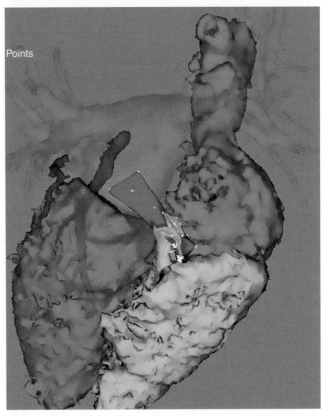

FIGURE 11-2 Site of successful epicardial mapping and ablation. This shows a fusion of electroanatomic mapping from the epicardial space (with colors indicating timing of earliest preexcited ventricular electrogram) with a previously acquired CT scan of the heart. The left and right atria and ventricles can be seen in the CT image, as well as the relevant portions of the right and left circumflex coronary arteries, which are adjacent to the ablation site.

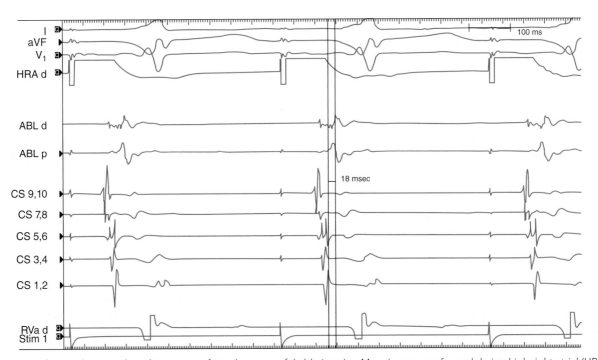

FIGURE 11-3 Surface and intracardiac electrograms from the successful ablation site. Mapping was performed during high right atrial (HRA) pacing. Tracings are shown from surface leads I, V_1, and aVF, as well as HRA, ablation (ABL) proximal and distal electrograms, coronary sinus (CS) proximal (9,10) to distal (1,2), and right ventricular apex (RVa). The earliest accessory pathway (AP) electrograms are noted 18 ms before the onset of the delta wave visualized on the surface leads.

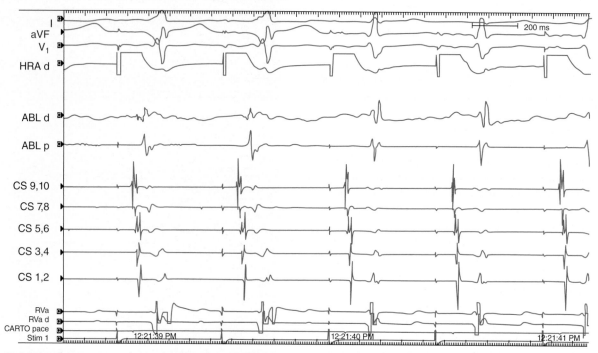

FIGURE 11-4 Loss of preexcitation during ablation. These electrograms (same annotation as Figure 11-3) were obtained during ablation at the same site as Figure 11-3. The first 2 beats show preexcitation on the surface leads, which is no longer evident on the 3rd and subsequent beats. In addition, the short delay between the local atrial and ventricular electrograms in the preexcited beats noted on the ablation catheter lengthens with loss of preexcitation. Loss of preexcitation was noted after 6.5 seconds of ablation at this site and was durable after completion of ablation and administration of IV adenosine.

necessitating an epicardial approach for posteroseptal APs. It should be noted that the proximal CS (and its tributaries such as the takeoff of the middle cardiac vein) contains a muscular coat capable of electrical conduction and contraction,[10] and this may also contribute to the presence of epicardial APs in the posteroseptal location. Other unusual epicardial AP connections such as from the left or right atrial appendage to the ventricle (which in some cases may require a surgical approach for successful interruption of the AP), have also been reported.[12]

APPROACH TO EP STUDY AND ABLATION

Although ECG criteria have been devised to estimate the likelihood that a particular VT will require pericardial access for successful ablation,[13] APs requiring pericardial access are much less common, and no definitive criteria for such APs has been devised. Given that the majority of these APs are posteroseptal, however, preexcitation suggestive of a posteroseptal AP[14] (typically negative delta waves in the inferior leads) suggests a greater likelihood of the requirement for epicardial ablation. It should be noted, however, that only a small minority of posteroseptal APs require pericardial access for successful ablation; most can be ablated from endocardial sites, or from the proximal CS or its tributaries.[10] Given the greater risk of complications from pericardial access[15] compared to traditional endocardial access, it is our opinion that mapping should be attempted from an endocardial/intra-CS approach for virtually all patients requiring AP ablation prior to obtaining pericardial access. For operators skilled in pericardial access and with the proper equipment available, it is certainly reasonable to obtain pericardial access during the same procedure if endocardial and intra-CS mapping/ablation is not successful

and there is reason to believe that this may be due to an epicardial AP (this will generally require reversal of any IV anticoagulation used for the endocardial procedure). Suggestive findings of the need for epicardial access may include a low frequency "far field" electrogram with endocardial mapping at the earliest preexcited site with lack of a sharp AP potential and unsuccessful ablation at that site, particularly for posteroseptal APs (and after extensive CS mapping has been performed). It should also be kept in mind that midseptal sites do not have a corresponding epicardial site, and unsuccessful ablation at a midseptal site should prompt mapping of the septum of the alternate atrium, rather than pericardial access.

Percutaneous pericardial access for AP ablation is essentially identical to the approach described by Sosa and colleagues for ablation of ventricular tachycardia.[16,17] This has been described in great detail in the published literature, but generally involves careful subxyphoid introduction of a round tipped spinal needle using small amounts of contrast to identify the pericardial space, and then advancement of a guidewire and sheath into this space. Fortunately, most AP ablation procedures are performed on patients who have not previously undergone cardiac surgical procedures, and so the pericardial adhesions which may challenge attempts at percutaneous epicardial VT ablation procedures[18] are much less commonly encountered with AP ablation. Once pericardial access has been obtained, epicardial mapping of the AP can be performed in the same manner as endocardial mapping. In almost all cases, endocardial mapping should also be performed, and epicardial ablation only performed if an epicardial site is more favorable (based on typical criteria for AP ablation such as earliest site of preexcitation, presence of AP potentials, etc.) than the best endocardial site.

As is true for other types of epicardial ablation, there is the risk of damage to nearby structures.[15] Proximity to coronary arteries should always be assessed by coronary angiography prior to ablation in most AP locations, and high output pacing prior to ablation to determine proximity to the phrenic nerve may also be important, although typical posteroseptal AP locations are usually distant from either phrenic nerve. The esophagus is also in proximity to the posterior AV groove in many patients, and the strategies currently in use for esophageal protection during AF ablation[19] may also be relevant during ablation of posterior APs from an epicardial approach.

REFERENCES

1. Ho I, d'Avila A, Ruskin J, Mansour M. Images in cardiovascular medicine. Percutaneous epicardial mapping and ablation of a posteroseptal accessory pathway. *Circulation.* 2007;115(16):e418-421.

2. Wellens HJ, Rodriguez LM, Timmermans C, Smeets JP. The asymptomatic patient with the Wolff-Parkinson-White electrocardiogram. *Pacing Clin Electrophysiol.* 1997;20(8):2082-2086.

3. Gandhavadi M, Sternick EB, Jackman WM, Wellens HJ, Josephson ME. Characterization of the distal insertion of atriofascicular accessory pathways and mechanisms of QRS patterns in atriofascicular antidromic tachycardia. *Heart Rhythm.* 2013;10(9):1385-1392.

4. Misaki T, Watanabe G, Iwa T, et al. Surgical treatment of patients with Wolff-Parkinson-White syndrome and associated Ebstein's anomaly. *J Thorac Cardiovasc Surg.* 1995;110(6):1702-1707.

5. Jackman WM, Wang XZ, Friday KJ, et al. Catheter ablation of accessory atrioventricular pathways (Wolff-Parkinson-White syndrome) by radiofrequency current. *N Engl J Med.* 1991;324(23):1605-1611.

6. Schweikert RA, Saliba WI, Tomassoni G, et al. Percutaneous pericardial instrumentation for endo-epicardial mapping of previously failed ablations. *Circulation.* 2003;108(11):1329-1335.

7. Valderrabano M, Cesario DA, Ji S, et al. Percutaneous epicardial mapping during ablation of difficult accessory pathways as an alternative to cardiac surgery. *Heart Rhythm.* 2004;1(3):311-316.

8. de Paola AA, Leite LR, Mesas CE. Nonsurgical transthoracic epicardial ablation for the treatment of a resistant posteroseptal accessory pathway. *Pacing Clin Electrophysiol.* 2004;27(2):259-261.

9. Sapp J, Soejima K, Couper GS, Stevenson WG. Electrophysiology and anatomic characterization of an epicardial accessory pathway. *J Cardiovasc Electrophysiol.* 2001;12(12):1411-1414.

10. Sun Y, Arruda M, Otomo K, et al. Coronary sinus-ventricular accessory connections producing posteroseptal and left posterior accessory pathways: Incidence and electrophysiological identification. *Circulation.* 2002;106(11):1362-1367.

11. Shah AJ, Pascale P, Miyazaki S, et al. Prevalence and types of pitfall in the assessment of mitral isthmus linear conduction block. *Circ Arrhythm Electrophysiol.* 2012;5(5):957-967.

12. Mah D, Miyake C, Clegg R, et al. Epicardial left atrial appendage and biatrial appendage accessory pathways. *Heart Rhythm.* 2010;7(12):1740-1745.

13. Valles E, Bazan V, Marchlinski FE. ECG criteria to identify epicardial ventricular tachycardia in nonischemic cardiomyopathy. *Circ Arrhythm Electrophysiol.* 2010;3(1):63-71.

14. d'Avila A, Brugada J, Skeberis V, Andries E, Sosa E, Brugada P. A fast and reliable algorithm to localize accessory pathways based on the polarity of the QRS complex on the surface ECG during sinus rhythm. *Pacing Clin Electrophysiol.* 1995;18(9):1615-1627.

15. Koruth JS, Aryana A, Dukkipati SR, et al. Unusual complications of percutaneous epicardial access and epicardial mapping and ablation of cardiac arrhythmias. *Circ Arrhythm Electrophysiol.* 2011;4(6):882-888.

16. d'Avila A, Koruth JS, Dukkipati S, Reddy VY. Epicardial access for the treatment of cardiac arrhythmias. *Europace.* 2012;14: Suppl 2:ii13-ii18.

17. Sosa E, Scanavacca M, D'Avila A, et al. Endocardial and epicardial ablation guided by nonsurgical transthoracic epicardial mapping to treat recurrent ventricular tachycardia. *J Cardiovasc Electrophysiol.* 1998;9(3):229-239.

18. Tschabrunn CM, Haqqani HM, Cooper JM, et al. Percutaneous epicardial ventricular tachycardia ablation after noncoronary cardiac surgery or pericarditis. *Heart Rhythm.* 2013;10(2):165-169.

19. Contreras-Valdes FM, Heist EK, Danik SB, et al. Severity of esophageal injury predicts time to healing after radiofrequency catheter ablation for atrial fibrillation. *Heart Rhythm.* 2011;8(12):1862-1868.

12 ATYPICAL ACCESSORY PATHWAYS

Steven J. Kalbfleisch, MD

CASE PRESENTATION

A 29-year-old man presented to the emergency department with complaints of progressive shortness of breath and occasional palpitations. The presenting ECG is shown in Figure 12-1. The patient was admitted to the hospital for further cardiac workup. An echocardiogram demonstrated a reduced left ventricular ejection fraction of 35% with no other significant abnormalities. While on telemetry, the patient was noted to have intermittent termination of his arrhythmia with brief periods of normal sinus rhythm and prompt recurrence of tachycardia. During the periods of sinus rhythm, a 12-lead ECG was obtained and was normal without evidence of pre-excitation. The patient reported that his symptoms of palpitations dated back a few years, but they had become more persistent over the past 6 months.

He was referred to the electrophysiology service for evaluation of possible catheter ablation of his arrhythmia. An electrophysiology study was performed which demonstrated an incessant atrioventricular (AV) reentrant tachycardia utilizing a decremental posteroseptal accessory pathway (AP) with a long conduction time. Mapping during tachycardia revealed a broad atrial insertion of the pathway spanning across the posteroseptal space from the mouth of the coronary sinus ostium to the left posteroseptal region of the mitral annulus. Ablation at the coronary sinus ostium and posteroseptal mitral annulus via a transeptal approach terminated the tachycardia and eliminated pathway conduction (Figure 12-2). The patient was seen at follow-up 2 months after the ablation procedure. His symptoms had abated, no further tachycardia was noted on Holter

monitoring, and there was normalization of the ejection fraction by echocardiography.

EPIDEMIOLOGY

This patient had a classic case of permanent junctional reciprocating tachycardia (PJRT). PJRT is a long RP tachycardia that is associated with deeply negative P waves in the inferior leads and is caused by an "atypical" AP.

A "typical" AP is one that has a rapid and fixed conduction time and is located along the AV groove anywhere except at the anteromedial mitral annulus where the aortic valve sits.[1,2] Both the atrial and ventricular insertions of a typical AP are close to the mitral or tricuspid valve annulus.

A simple definition of an "atypical" accessory pathway is any AP that has either unusual conduction characteristics (long conduction time or decremental conduction) or an unexpected location.

Pathways with unusual locations such as those coursing through the fibrous region of the aortomitral continuity, traveling around the aortic valve through the left anteroseptal region or connecting directly between the right or left atrial appendage and the ventricles, are very rare and have been reported only in small series or isolated case reports.[3-6]

During electrophysiologic testing in patients with an AP, the probability of finding decremental pathway conduction is not rare and in one series was reported to be on the order of 10%.[7] In the majority of cases from this series, the pathways had relatively short conduction times with decremental conduction in the retrograde direction. The most common location for a decremental pathway was in the posteroseptal region (47%).[7]

Two specific variants of atypical APs occur frequently enough and have consistent enough characteristics to form distinct clinical subgroups. These are pathways associated with PJRT and Mahaim fibers. Both of these pathways types are fairly rare, and each type accounts for less than 2.5% of pathways in large ablation series of adult patients.[7-9]

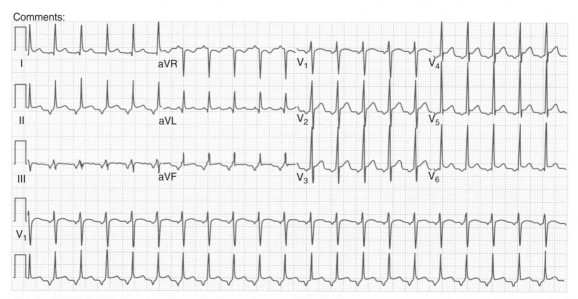

Comments:

FIGURE 12-1 Twelve-lead ECG demonstrating a long RP supraventricular tachycardia at a rate of 130 bpm. Note the deeply inverted P waves in the inferior leads (II, III, aVF), which clearly distinguish this from sinus tachycardia.

Electroanatomic Map

LAO Fluoroscopic View

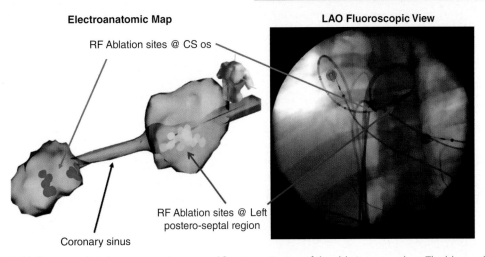

RF Ablation sites @ CS os

RF Ablation sites @ Left
postero-septal region

Coronary sinus

FIGURE 12-2 Shown in this figure are the electroanatomic map and fluoroscopic view of the ablation procedure. The blue and red arrows point to the ablation sites at the coronary sinus ostium (CS os) and left posteroseptal region, respectively. The pathway had a broad atrial insertion requiring ablation on both sides of the posteroseptal space for elimination.

The locations of the most common sites for atypical APs are shown in Figure 12-3.

ETIOLOGY AND PATHOPHYSIOLOGY

APs of the PJRT type have very long conduction times with decremental conduction properties. These pathways essentially only conduct in the retrograde direction and are therefore concealed on the baseline ECG. They are usually located in the posteroseptal region close to the coronary sinus ostium (75% of patients), but pathways with these conduction characteristics can also be found in other locations.[10]

The characteristic tachycardia associated with this type of pathway is a long RP tachycardia with deeply inverted P waves in the inferior leads. The P wave timing is due to the long VA conduction time of the pathway and the morphology of the P wave is the result of earliest activation of the atrium being near the coronary sinus ostium. These tachycardias can be paroxysmal in nature, but in a high percentage of patients they can be nearly incessant. In one large ablation series of 49 patients with PJRT type pathways, the tachycardia was incessant in 47% and led to a tachycardia-induced cardiomyopathy in 16% of cases.[10]

Mahaim fibers, on the other hand, are APs with long conduction times and decremental conduction properties that conduct in the antegrade direction only. These pathways are typically very long in their course, usually originating in the anterolateral right atrium and inserting in the distal right ventricle near the right bundle branch.[11] They behave like a duplicate AV node and His-Purkinje system and are referred to as atriofascicular pathways. The tachycardias associated with these pathways are wide complex preexcited tachycardias with a left bundle branch block configuration (Figure 12-4).

DIAGNOSIS

Diagnosing an AP-mediated tachycardia usually relies on invasive electrophysiologic testing. Determining that the AP has atypical decremental conduction properties is dependent on demonstrating an

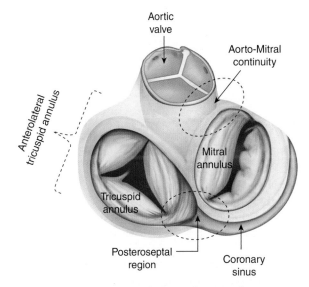

Aortic
valve

Aorto-Mitral
continuity

Anterolateral
tricuspid annulus

Mitral
annulus

Tricuspid
annulus

Posteroseptal
region

Coronary
sinus

FIGURE 12-3 The most common locations for atypical accessory pathways are shown in the areas outlined with a dashed line. The most common variant of Mahaim fibers, atriofascicular pathways, are located along the anterolateral tricuspid annulus. The posteroseptal region is the usual location for pathways responsible for PJRT and is the most common location for any pathway with decremental conduction properties. Pathways located in the aortomitral continuity are atypical by virtue of their location; very rarely pathways can traverse this area, which is a region of dense fibrous tissue that separates the left atrium and ventricle.

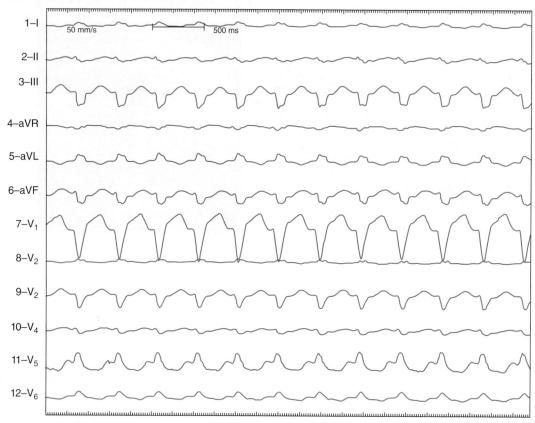

FIGURE 12-4 This 12-lead ECG was recorded during an episode of antidromic tachycardia in a patient with a Mahaim fiber. Because these pathways insert distally into the right ventricle close to the location of the right bundle branch, they have a left bundle superior axis morphology that can closely mimic left bundle branch aberration. The recording was performed at 50 mm/sec, twice the normal sweep speed.

increase in conduction time across the AP of at least 30 msec in the antegrade or retrograde direction with pacing maneuvers.[7] Unlike typical APs, pathways with decremental properties are often sensitive to adenosine, and pathway conduction can be blocked or slowed after its administration.[7]

The diagnosis of a PJRT-type tachycardia should be considered whenever a long RP (RP interval > PR interval) tachycardia is demonstrated on the ECG. Many variants of the initially described tachycardia have been reported, and the term PJRT is now often loosely used to describe any orthodromic reciprocating tachycardia caused by an AP with a very long conduction time.

The pacing maneuver most commonly performed during tachycardia to prove the existence of an extranodal pathway and determine if the pathway participates in the tachycardia is delivery of a PVC when the His bundle is refractory (Figure 12-5). If a PVC is delivered when the His bundle is refractory and the atrial timing is advanced, then an extranodal AP has to be present. If the tachycardia is reset by advancing the atrial activation, then the pathway participates in the tachycardia and is not just a bystander. Other possible responses to a His refractory PVC include delaying the next atrial activation or terminating the tachycardia without affecting atrial activation. Either of these responses also proves both the existence and participation of an AP in the tachycardia.

A Mahaim tachycardia should be considered in otherwise healthy patients who have a wide complex tachycardia of left bundle morphology. During a Mahaim tachycardia the left bundle morphology

is usually relatively narrow (≤0.15 seconds), has a late precordial transition (>V_4), and left axis deviation.[12] These patients often do not manifest preexcitation on their baseline ECG; however, antegrade preexcitation can easily be demonstrated by pacing along the lateral right atrium in close proximity to the atrial insertion of the AP.

DIFFERENTIAL DIAGNOSIS

For any supraventricular arrhythmia with a 1:1 AV relationship, an AP-mediated tachycardia needs to be considered. The only ECG feature that effectively rules out the participation of an AP is the presence of AV block during the tachycardia. This is true because the ventricle is an obligatory part of any tachycardia, which is dependent on AP conduction.

For patients who have a long RP tachycardia with deeply inverted P waves in the inferior leads, the differential diagnosis includes PJRT, atypical AV node reentrant tachycardia, and a septal atrial tachycardia. Differentiating these can usually be accomplished by performing ventricular pacing maneuvers during the tachycardia. For patients with PJRT, the tachycardia should be able to be entrained with ventricular pacing with a postpacing atrial-ventricular response and a tachycardia cycle length postpacing interval difference of less than 115 ms (Figure 12-6).

The differential diagnosis for patients presenting with a left bundle morphology tachycardia includes ventricular tachycardia, supraventricular tachycardia with aberration, and a preexcited tachycardia using an AP for antegrade activation of the ventricle. A short HV

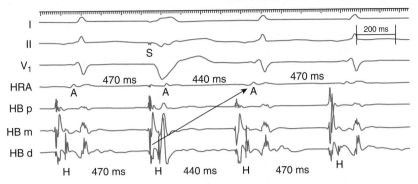

FIGURE 12-5 These are the intracardiac recordings during an episode of PJRT at the time of delivery of a His refractory PVC. Shown are surface leads I, II, and V$_1$ and intracardiac recordings from the high right atrium (HRA) and His bundle proximal, mid, and distal locations (HB p, HB m, and HB d, respectively). The tachycardia cycle length was 470 ms. A ventricular extrastimulus (S) was delivered and captured in the RV apex. The His bundle timing was not affected by the extrastimulus, but the subsequent atrial electrogram was advanced and occurred earlier than expected at an interval of 440 ms, proving the existence of an extranodal accessory pathway. After advancement of the atrial electrogram, the tachycardia was reset (ie, the next His and QRS complex were also advanced), this indicates that the accessory pathway was not just a bystander pathway but also participated in the tachycardia.

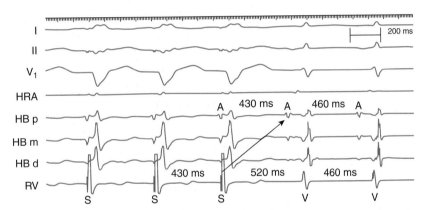

FIGURE 12-6 This tracing is the same as Figure 12-5 with the edition of the right ventricular (RV) recording. The patient was in tachycardia with a tachycardia cycle length (TCL) of 460 ms. Ventricular overdrive pacing at a cycle length of 430 ms was performed. The tachycardia was entrained with acceleration of the atrium to the pacing cycle length. Upon termination of pacing there was an atrial-ventricular response and a postpacing interval (PPI) of 520 ms. The atrial-ventricular response rules out an atrial tachycardia, and the PPI-TCL difference of 60 ms rules out atypical AV node reentrant tachycardia, making AV reentry utilizing long conducting accessory pathway the correct diagnosis.

interval during tachycardia excludes supraventricular tachycardia with aberration from the differential. For patients with antegrade conduction over a Mahaim fiber during tachycardia, atrial stimulation during the tachycardia when the atrial septum is refractory will often preexcite the ventricle without changing the morphology of the ventricular complex thus proving the presence of an AP.

MANAGEMENT

For patients with symptomatic or recurrent AP-mediated tachycardia, ablation of the AP has a class I indication based on current AHA and ACC guidelines.[14]

Ablation of atypical APs can be somewhat more challenging than typical APs since the conduction time across the pathway can be variable, the pathway course can be long and tortuous across the AV groove, and the insertion into the atrium or ventricle can be distant from the AV groove.

Patients with PJRT can be quite difficult to control with antiarrhythmic therapy, especially when the arrhythmia is incessant, and

are usually best treated with ablation therapy.[10] For patients with a tachycardia-mediated cardiomyopathy, the majority of improvement in cardiac function can be expected within the first 2 to 3 months after arrhythmia control.[15] In these patients, close follow-up is required to ensure arrhythmia control. If the arrhythmia is recurrent, further decline in cardiac function can occur quickly and in some cases may be irreversible.

The most common variety of Mahaim fibers, atriofascicular pathways, by their very definition insert distally into the right ventricle near the right bundle branch and almost never conduct in the retrograde direction. The approach to ablating these pathways is to find and target the AP potential along the anterolateral tricuspid annulus (Figure 12-7).[16] These pathways can be associated with Ebstein's anomaly, the presence of multiple APs, and other supraventricular arrhythmias such as AV node reentrant tachycardia, so it is important to do a complete evaluation rather than to assume that the Mahaim fiber is the sole tachyarrhythmia.[17]

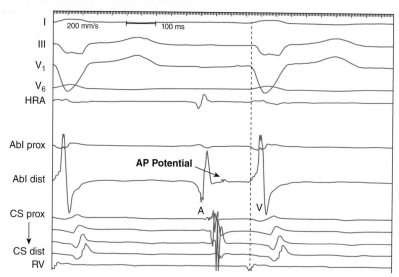

FIGURE 12-7 This tracing shows surface ECG recordings from leads I, III, V₁ and V₆, intracardiac recordings from the high right atrium (HRA), ablation proximal and distal electrode pairs (Abl prox and dist), coronary sinus (CS) proximal (prox) to distal (dist) electrode pairs, and right ventricular (RV) apex. The ablation catheter was placed on the lateral aspect of the tricuspid annulus. Notice the sharp deflection consistent with an accessory pathway (AP) potential between the atrial (A) and ventricular (V) electrograms on the ablation distal recordings. It should also be noted that the RV apical electrogram was early relative to the onset of the QRS complex (dotted line) and ventricular electrogram on the mapping catheter. This indicates that the ventricular insertion of the accessory pathway was distal in the right ventricle near the location of the RV apical catheter.

REFERENCES

1. Anderson RH, Path FRC, Ho SY. Structure and location of accessory muscular atrioventricular connections. *J Cardiovasc Electrophysiol.* 1999;10(8):1119-1123.

2. Nakagawa H, Jackman WM. Catheter ablation of paroxysmal supraventricular tachycardia. *Circulation.* 2007;116(21):2465-2478.

3. Goya M, Takahashi A, Nakagawa H, Iesaka Y. A case of catheter ablation of accessory atrioventricular connection between the right atrial appendage and right ventricle guided by three-dimensional electroanatomic mapping system. *J Cardiovasc Electrophysiol.* 1999;10(8):1112-1118.

4. Tada H, Naito S, Nogami A, Taniguchi K. Successful catheter ablation of an anteroseptal accessory pathway from the noncoronary sinus of valsalva. *J Cardiovasc Electrophysiol.* 2003;14(5):544-546.

5. Tada H, Naito S, Taniguchi K, Nogami A. Concealed left anterior accessory pathways: two approaches for successful ablation. *J Cardiovasc Electrophysiol.* 2003;14(2):204-208.

6. Miyauchi Y, Kobayashi Y, Morita N, et al. Successful radiofrequency catheter ablation of an anteroseptal (superoparaseptal) atrioventricular accessory pathway from the left ventricular outflow tract. *Pacing Clin Electrophysiol.* 2004;27(5):668-670.

7. Chen S, Tai C, Chiang C, et al. Electrophysiologic characteristics, electropharmacologic responses and radiofrequency ablation in patients with decremental accessory pathway. *J Am Coll Cardiol.* 1996;28(3):732-737.

8. Jackman W, Wang X, Friday K, et al. Catheter ablation of accessory atrioventricular pathways (Wolff-Parkinson-White syndrome) by radiofrequency current. *N Engl J Med.* 1991;324(23):1605-1611.

9. Dagres N, Clague J, Kottkamp H, Hindricks G, Breithardt G, Borggrefe M. Radiofrequency catheter ablation of accessory pathways. *Eur Heart J.* 1999;20(24):1826-1832.

10. Meiltz, A, Weber R, Halimi F, et al. Permanent form of junctional reciprocating tachycardia in adults: peculiar features and results of radiofrequency catheter ablation. *Europace.* 2006;8(1):21-28.

11. Haissaguerre M, Cauchemez B, Marcus F, et al. Characteristics of the ventricular insertion sites of accessory pathways with anterograde decremental conduction properties. *Circulation.* 1995;91(4):1077-1085.

12. Sternick EB, Cruz F, Timmermans C, et al. Electrocardiogram during tachycardia in patients with anterograde conduction over a Mahaim fiber: old criteria revisited. *Heart Rhythm.* 2004;4(4):406-413.

13. Michaud G, Tada H, Chough S, et al. Differentiation of atypical atrioventricular node re-entrant tachycardia from orthodromic reciprocating tachycardia using a septal accessory pathway by the response to ventricular pacing. *J Am Coll Cardiol.* 2001;38(4):1163-1167.

14. ACC/AHA/ESC Guidelines for the management of patients with supraventricular arrhythmias—executive summary: a report of the American College of Cardiology/American Heart Association Task Force on Practice Guidelines and the European Society of Cardiology Committee for Practice Guidelines (Writing Committee to Develop Guidelines for the Management of Patients With Supraventricular Arrhythmias). *Circulation.* 2003;108(15):1871-1909.

15. Houmsee M, Tyler J, Kalbfleisch S. Supraventricular tachycardia causing heart failure. *Curr Opin Cardiol.* 2011;26(3):261-269.

16. McClelland JH, Wang X, Beckman KJ, et al. Radiofrequency catheter ablation of right atriofasicular (Mahaim) accessory pathway guided by accessory pathway activation potentials. *Circulation.* 1994, 89(6):2655-2666.

17. Sternick, Lokhandwala Y, Timmermans C, et al. The atrioventricular interval during pre-excited tachycardia: a simple way to distinguish between decrementally or rapidly conducting accessory pathways. *Heart Rhythm.* 2009;6(9):1351-1358.

13 WOLFF-PARKINSON-WHITE SYNDROME AND SUDDEN CARDIAC DEATH

Steven J. Kalbfleisch, MD

CASE PRESENTATION

A 31-year-old man with no prior medical history was brought to the emergency department (ED) after suffering an out-of-hospital cardiac arrest. He reported the onset of a rapid heart rate to a friend after completing a 10-mile run. He began to feel progressively worse and suddenly collapsed. Bystander CPR was initiated, and the EMS was called. Upon arrival, the EMS personal found the patient to be in ventricular fibrillation (Figure 13-1), and he was converted to sinus rhythm with an external shock. The 12-lead ECG obtained upon arrival in the ED (Figure 13-2) demonstrated evidence of ventricular preexcitation with a probable left lateral accessory pathway. A cardiac catheterization and echocardiogram were performed and revealed no evidence of structural heart disease. An electrophysiology study confirmed the presence of a single left lateral accessory pathway. The accessory pathway had an antegrade block cycle length and refractory period of 280 ms and 260 ms, respectively, in the baseline state. Orthodromic reciprocating tachycardia with a cycle length of 400 ms (heart rate of 150 bpm) was easily induced and was hemodynamically stable. After the addition of intravenous isoproterenol at 8 μg/min, the accessory pathway block cycle length and refractory period decreased to <200 ms and

<210 ms, respectively (Figure 13-3). The patient had successful radiofrequency ablation of the accessory pathway performed. At follow-up there was no further arrhythmia symptoms or recurrence of preexcitation on the ECG.

EPIDEMIOLOGY

The prevalence of the Wolff-Parkinson-White (WPW) ECG pattern, which indicates the presence of an accessory pathway causing ventricular preexcitation, is estimated to be on the order of 0.1% to 0.3%.[1,2]

Although there is a clear association between the presence of ventricular preexcitation and sudden cardiac death (SCD), the overall risk of sudden death in this patient population is relatively small.

The incidence of SCD in asymptomatic patients with a WPW ECG pattern is low and estimated to be <0.5% per patient-year.[3]

However, the prevalence of aborted SCD in large series of patients with WPW syndrome referred to an electrophysiology center for treatment of symptomatic arrhythmias is on the order of 1% to 2%, and in approximately 50% of these patients the aborted SCD event was their first arrhythmia symptom.[4,5]

ETIOLOGY AND PATHOPHYSIOLOGY

The mechanism of SCD in WPW patients is most often due to the presence of atrial fibrillation, which conducts rapidly across an accessory pathway and triggers ventricular fibrillation (Figure 13-4).

In the majority of patients with an accessory pathway, the occurrence of atrial fibrillation is triggered by an episode of paroxysmal supraventricular tachycardia (PSVT) due to AV reentrant tachycardia.

Like patients without WPW, patients with WPW can have atrial fibrillation triggered for reasons other than an episode of PSVT. Regardless of the cause of atrial fibrillation, as long as there is rapid conduction across the accessory pathway, the arrhythmia can degenerate into ventricular fibrillation and result in a cardiac arrest.

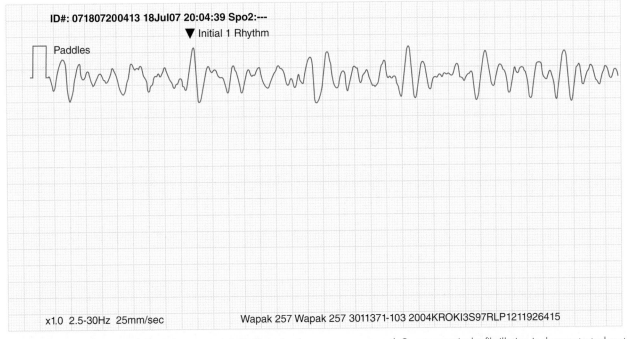

ID#: 071807200413 18Jul07 20:04:39 Spo2:---
▼ Initial 1 Rhythm
Paddles

x1.0 2.5-30Hz 25mm/sec   Wapak 257 Wapak 257 3011371-103 2004KROKI3S97RLP1211926415

FIGURE 13-1 Initial rhythm recorded on the external defibrillator by the emergency squad. Coarse ventricular fibrillation is demonstrated on the ECG strip, which was converted to sinus rhythm by an external 200J shock.

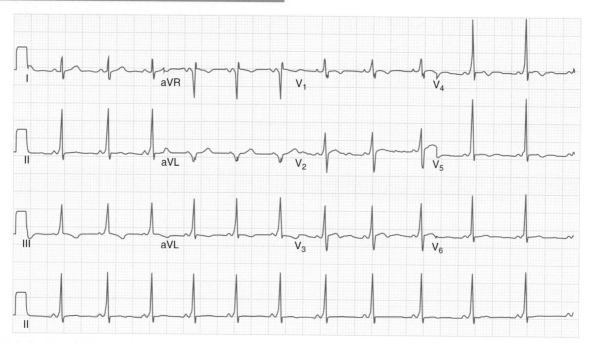

FIGURE 13-2 The12-lead ECG recorded in the emergency department. The WPW pattern is clearly seen on the ECG. The positive delta wave in lead V_1 and negative delta wave in lead aVL are indicative of a left lateral accessory pathway location.

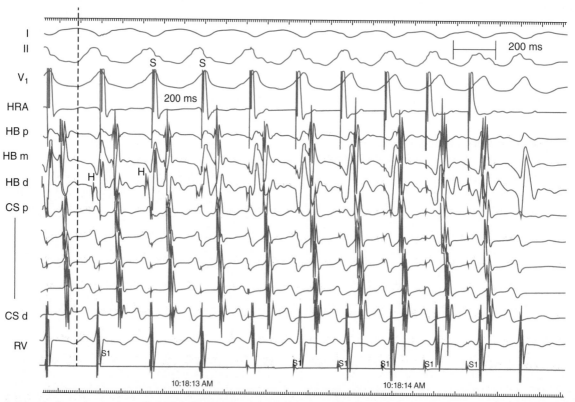

FIGURE 13-3 Tracings from the electrophysiologic study during atrial pacing with an infusion of isoproterenol at 8 μg/min. Shown are recordings from surface leads I, II, and V_1 and intracardiac recordings from the high right atrium (HRA), His bundle proximal, mid, and distal locations (HB p, HB m, and HB d), coronary sinus proximal to distal locations (CS p to CS d), and right ventricular apex (RV). Atrial pacing stimuli (S) are delivered throughout the tracing at a cycle length of 200 ms (300 bpm). A His bundle recording (H) is detected at the beginning of the tracing indicating that initially there was conduction down both the normal AV conduction system and accessory pathway. The HV interval measured from the onset of the first complete QRS complex (dotted line) is –70 ms. There is 1:1 conduction from the atrium to the ventricle across the accessory pathway at 300 bpm during the isoproterenol infusion. This confirms that this is a high-risk accessory pathway and can account for the episode of aborted sudden death.

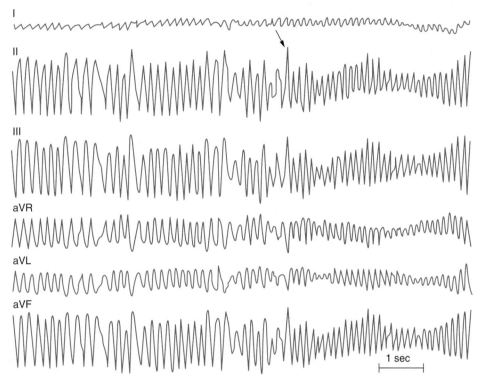

FIGURE 13-4 Atrial fibrillation degenerating to ventricular fibrillation. The initial portion of the image shows atrial fibrillation conducting across and accessory pathway at rates of over 300 bpm. The arrow points to where the rhythm degenerates to ventricular fibrillation.

A number of clinical predictors for the occurrence of SCD in patients with WPW have been described and include male gender, young age, older age, septal accessory pathway location, left lateral accessory pathway location, presence of multiple accessory pathways, history of syncope, and the presence of symptomatic tachycardia. These clinical predictors are very weak and nonspecific, and due to the small numbers of patients in most series the studies often have conflicting data.[4,5]

Patients with baseline intermittent preexcitation on their ECG or telemetry monitors are felt to be at low risk for SCD since this generally indicates that their accessory pathway cannot conduct at rapid rates.

The use of noninvasive testing with stress testing and pharmacologic agents has been advocated for risk stratification of patients with persistent WPW pattern on their ECG. Patients with *abrupt* loss of preexcitation during stress testing or intravenous procainamide are considered at low risk for sudden death since this indicates the presence of a pathway with relatively poor antegrade conduction characteristics.[6]

DIAGNOSIS

The diagnosis of WPW after an episode of aborted SCD is reliant on seeing ventricular preexcitation on the ECG or detecting an antegrade accessory pathway during invasive electrophysiologic testing. It is important to realize that the WPW pattern on the ECG may be subtle and difficult to detect especially if the pathway is located far from the AV node (ie, left lateral accessory pathways) or if AV node conduction is rapid. It is also important to understand that the degree of preexcitation on the baseline ECG is not predicative of whether the pathway is a high risk pathway or not.

Although there are a number of clinical and noninvasive predicators for risk stratifying patients with WPW, the most consistent data for determining whether a pathway is of high risk is with invasive electrophysiologic testing.[4,5,7,8]

If a patient suffers a cardiac arrest and is found to have preexcitation on an ECG, the next step is to determine if the pathway is capable of rapid conduction to cause hemodynamic collapse during atrial fibrillation or trigger ventricular fibrillation. Electrophysiologic testing of patients with WPW who have suffered an aborted cardiac arrest have consistently shown that these patients have very rapid conduction across the pathway as measured by the shortest RR interval during induced atrial fibrillation (<250 ms), atrial effective refractory period (<240 ms), and maximal rate of conduction across the accessory pathway (>250 bpm).[5]

If the pathway does not have very rapid conduction in the baseline state, it is important to retest the patient on isoproterenol. Many pathways will have marked enhancement of conduction during adrenergic stimulation, and it has been noted that a significant percentage of patients with WPW suffer a cardiac arrest during exercise or other periods of high adrenergic tone.[5,9]

DIFFERENTIAL DIAGNOSIS

If a patient survives an episode of aborted sudden death and is found to have a WPW pattern on an ECG, it should not be assumed that the accessory pathway is the etiology, although this is highly likely especially in younger patients without a prior history of cardiac disease.

The WPW ECG pattern can be associated with other forms of organic heart disease, such as Ebstein anomaly and hypertrophic cardiomyopathy, so an evaluation for structural heart disease with some form of cardiac imaging needs to be done prior to electrophysiologic testing.

If the patient does not have structural heart disease and at electrophysiologic testing the patient's accessory pathway is not found to be a high-risk, rapidly conducting pathway, then consideration of other arrhythmic causes of cardiac arrest such as long QT syndrome, Brugada syndrome, catecholaminergic polymorphic ventricular tachycardia, or primary ventricular fibrillation needs to be considered.

MANAGEMENT

For patients presenting with atrial fibrillation and rapid conduction across an accessory pathway, either external cardioversion or intravenous procainamide should be considered, depending upon their hemodynamic status (Figure 13-5). Procainamide slows conduction across the accessory pathway and may convert atrial fibrillation.

Agents that slow AV nodal conduction such as verapamil, diltiazem, or β-blockers should be avoided during the acute episode of atrial fibrillation since they may increase conduction over the accessory pathway and hasten cardiovascular collapse. By blocking AV nodal conduction, these agents decrease the number of impulses that conduct across the AV node, penetrate the accessory pathway in the retrograde direction, and modulate antegrade conduction.

The cornerstone of therapy for patients with symptomatic WPW is radiofrequency catheter ablation. This procedure is highly effective (>95% acute success) and safe (<2% serious complication risk), and it provides a durable long-term cure in high-risk WPW patients with a prior history of cardiovascular collapse.[10]

In patients who are not able to be ablated using percutaneous techniques, consideration for either surgical ablation or long-term medical therapy should be entertained. If antiarrhythmic therapy is chosen,

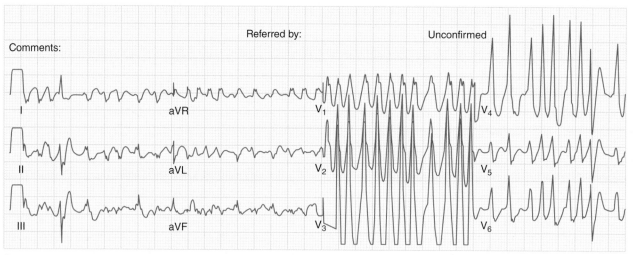

A

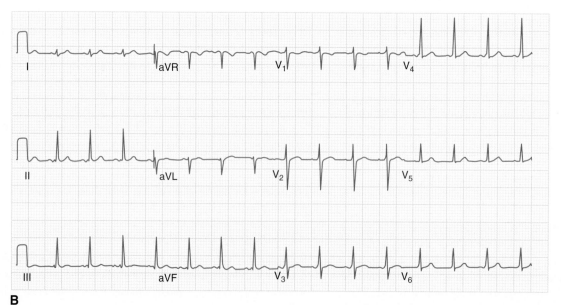

B

FIGURE 13-5 (A) The presenting 12-lead ECG demonstrates atrial fibrillation with rapid conduction across a left-sided accessory pathway. The shortest RR intervals during atrial fibrillation were <200 ms. (B) The patient was converted to sinus rhythm after an external shock, and the 12-lead ECG in sinus rhythm is also shown. Ventricular preexcitation is best seen in leads V₃ and V₄ but is fairly subtle in many of the ECG leads. This case helps demonstrate that the degree of preexcitation on the 12-lead ECG is not a reliable indicator if an accessory pathway is a high-risk pathway.

a drug that slows or blocks antegrade accessory pathway conduction needs to be included to minimize the risk of rapid conduction during atrial fibrillation.

PATIENT EDUCATION

Patients with a history of aborted sudden cardiac death or hemodynamic compromise and WPW need to understand that if their condition is left untreated the recurrence rate is high and that the efficacy and cost-effectiveness of catheter ablation is superior to other treatment strategies.[11]

Patients with an asymptomatic WPW ECG pattern should be counseled that the risk of SCD is low, but not zero, and that if arrhythmia symptoms begin to occur, further evaluation with either telemetry monitoring or invasive electrophysiologic testing is generally recommended.

In asymptomatic patients who have high-risk professions or are competitive athletes, consideration can be given to perform electrophysiologic testing for risk stratification with a goal of ablating a high-risk pathway, if one is present. Because of the risk of triggering life-threatening arrhythmias during competitive athletics, the European Society of Cardiology mandates that all athletes with WPW undergo risk stratification with electrophysiologic testing. The Bethesda Conference on sports eligibility requires electrophysiologic testing in symptomatic WPW patients and considers it advisable for asymptomatic athletes with WPW who are engaged in moderate or high-level competitive sports. Both of these bodies recommend radiofrequency ablation of the WPW if a high-risk pathway is found at electrophysiologic testing to retain athletic eligibility.[12]

REFERENCES

1. Averill KH, Fosmoe RJ, Lamb LE. Electrocardiographic findings in 67,375 asymptomatic subjects, IV: Wolff-Parkinson-White syndrome. *Am J Cardiol.* 1960;6:108-129.

2. Sears GA, Manning GW. The Wolff-Parkinson-White pattern in routine electrocardiography. *Can Med Assoc J.* 1962;87:1213-1217.

3. Munger TM, Packer DL, Hammill SC, et al. A population study of the natural history of Wolff-Parkinson-White syndrome in Olmsted County, Minnesota, 1953-1989. *Circulation.* 1993;87:866-873.

4. Timmermans C, Smeets J, Rodriguez LM, Vrouchos G, Dool V, Wellens HJ. Aborted sudden death in the Wolff-Parkinson-White syndrome. *Am J Cardiol.* 1995;76:492-494.

5. Brembilla-Perrot B, Tatar C, Suty-Selton C. Risk factors of adverse presentation as the first arrhythmia in Wolff-Parkinson-White syndrome. *Pacing Clin Electrophysiol.* 2010;33:1074-1081.

6. Gaita F, Giustetto C, Riccardi R, Mangiardi L, Brusca A. Stress and pharmacologic tests as methods to identify patients with Wolff-Parkinson-White syndrome at risk for sudden death. *Am J Cardiol.* 1989;64:487-490.

7. Pappone C, Santinelli V, Rosanio S, et al. Usefulness of invasive electrophysiologic testing to stratify the risk of arrhythmic events in asymptomatic patients with Wolff-Parkinson-White pattern. *J Am Coll Cardiol.* 2003;41:239-244.

8. Santinelli V, Radinovic A, Manguso F, et al. The natural history of asymptomatic ventricular pre-excitation. *J Am Coll Cardiol.* 2009;53:275-280.

9. Szabo TS, Klein GJ, Sharma AD, Yee R, Milstein S. Usefulness of isoproterenol during atrial fibrillation in evaluation of asymptomatic Wolff-Parkinson-White pattern. *Am J Cardiol.* 1989;63:187-192.

10. Antz M, Weib C, Volkmer M, et al. Risk of sudden death after successful accessory atrioventricular pathway ablation in resuscitated patients with Wolff-Parkinson-White syndrome. *J Cardiovasc Electrophysiol.* 2002;13:231-236.

11. Hogenhuis W, Stevens SK, Wang P, et al. Cost-effectiveness of radiofrequency ablation compared with other strategies in Wolff-Parkinson-White syndrome. *Circulation.* 1993;88:II 437-446.

12. Pelliccia A, Zipes DP, Maron BJ. Bethesda conference #36 and the European Society of Cardiology consensus recommendations revisited. *J Am Coll Cardiol.* 2008;52:1990-1996.

14 ANALYSIS OF CHALLENGING INTRACARDIAC ELECTROGRAMS: CASE I—ORTHODROMIC RECIPROCATING TACHYCARDIA UTILIZING A SEPTAL ACCESSORY PATHWAY VERSUS ATRIAL TACHYCARDIA OR ATRIOVENTRICULAR NODAL REENTRANT TACHYCARDIA

Rakesh Latchamsetty, MD, and Fred Morady, MD

CASE PRESENTATION

A 60-year-old woman with previous history of supraventricular tachycardia (SVT) and who had undergone two prior ablation procedures for SVT presents with recurrent episodes of palpitations and fatigue. The patient's most recent ablation procedure had been performed 1 week earlier. She had presented with nearly incessant tachycardia, and the electrophysiology study had revealed orthodromic reciprocating tachycardia (ORT) utilizing two separate left lateral pathways. The two left-sided accessory pathways were successfully ablated, and the patient remained arrhythmia-free for several days. She now presents to the emergency department in a narrow QRS complex tachycardia with a cycle length of 370 to 430 ms that spontaneously terminates and reinitiates with atrial premature depolarizations (APDs).

The patient arrived in the electrophysiology laboratory in narrow QRS complex tachycardia (Figure 14-1). The tachycardia demonstrates frequent cycle length variability with the septal atrial electrogram at times simultaneous with the QRS complex. During the study, the tachycardia occasionally terminated with spontaneous APDs. Spontaneous reinduction would occur soon thereafter with APDs that did not display atrial-His interval (AH) prolongation.

Cycle length variability as great as 60 ms, as seen in Figure 14-1, is most commonly observed during atrial tachycardia. The occasionally simultaneous activation of the atria and ventricle ruled out orthodromic reciprocating tachycardia (ORT) as a sole diagnosis. Atrioventricular nodal reentrant tachycardia (AVNRT) with multiple slow pathways or multiple coexisting tachycardias could not be ruled out.

Ventricular pacing during the tachycardia revealed a V-A-V response (Figure 14-2). This response eliminates atrial tachycardia as the only mechanism of the tachycardia.[1] The postpacing interval (PPI)

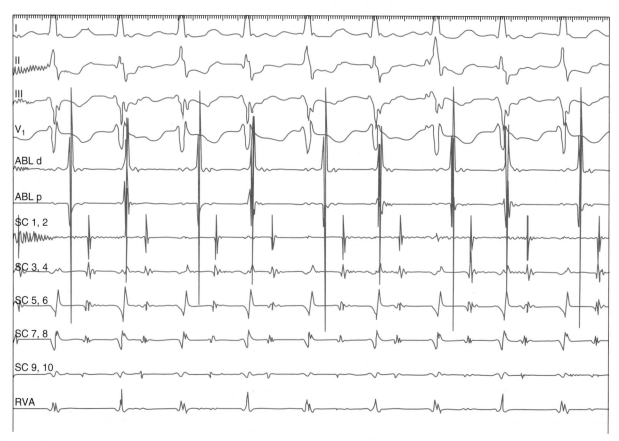

FIGURE 14-1 Patient's presenting rhythm. The ablation catheter is positioned in the low right atrial septum, and a decapolar catheter is positioned in the coronary sinus (SC). Note the significant cycle length variability of the tachycardia with the septal atrial electrogram at times within the QRS complex. ABL = Ablation; d = distal; p = proximal; RVA = right ventricular apex; SC = coronary sinus.

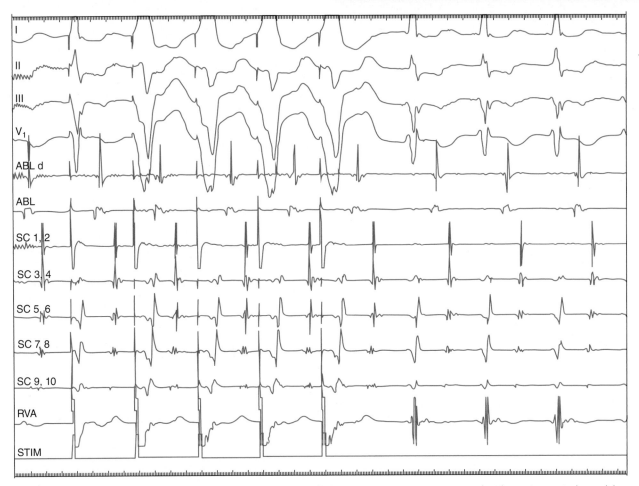

FIGURE 14-2 Entrainment of the tachycardia by ventricular pacing revealed a V-A-V response, consistent with either atrioventricular nodal reentrant tachycardia (AVNRT) or orthodromic reciprocating tachycardia. The postpacing interval minus the tachycardia cycle length was 100 ms, which is inconsistent with AVNRT. ABL = Ablation; d = distal; p = proximal; RVA = right ventricular apex; SC = coronary sinus.

in this tracing exceeded the tachycardia cycle length (TCL) by 100 msec, which is inconsistent with a diagnosis of AVNRT.[2]

Induction by atrial pacing (or spontaneous APDs) was not dependent on critical AH prolongation. Figure 14-3 shows an example of initiation with a single ventricular premature depolarization (VPD) with a V-A-A-V response. As is the case upon cessation of ventricular pacing that entrains a tachycardia, induction with a V-A-A-V response is indicative of an atrial tachycardia.

A single tachycardia mechanism fails to adequately explain all of the findings previously described. The PPI <115 ms following ventricular entrainment made AVNRT unlikely. Initiation of the tachycardia with ventricular pacing followed by a V-A-A-V response as well as the significant tachycardia cycle length variability with lack of stability in the V-A interval confirms the presence of an atrial tachycardia. Entrainment with a V-A-V response with a relatively short PPI-TCL also suggests the presence of an accessory pathway and probable ORT.

Atrial activation mapping during the tachycardia demonstrated earliest atrial activation at the low right atrial septum. Ablation here terminated the tachycardia and rendered it noninducible. Following ablation, ventricular pacing demonstrated VA dissociation, indicating

that both the atrial tachycardia and a posteroseptal accessory pathway were ablated at the same target site. The site of origin of the atrial tachycardia had been at or very close to the atrial insertion of the accessory pathway.

DIAGNOSING CONCEALED SEPTAL ACCESSORY PATHWAYS

Diagnosis of ORT utilizing a concealed septal accessory pathway is made based on tachycardia characteristics and pacing maneuvers during SVT. Differentiation of ORT from atypical AVNRT or in some cases focal atrial tachycardia can be challenging. Here, we describe techniques to differentiate these tachycardia mechanisms.

Para-Hisian pacing can be a valuable tool to confirm the presence of retrograde septal accessory pathway conduction as well as to verify successful septal accessory pathway ablation. The goal of para-Hisian pacing is to pace near the His bundle at high output and to gradually decrease the pacing output to produce complexes with right ventricular plus His capture and complexes with only right ventricular capture. When rapid retrograde conduction proceeds through an accessory pathway, similar conduction times

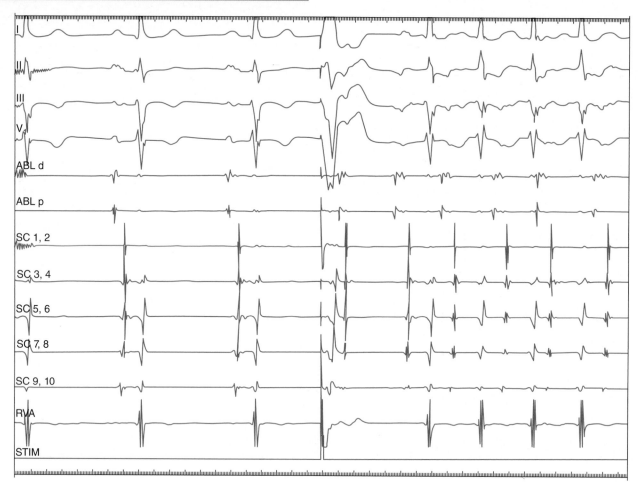

FIGURE 14-3 Tachycardia is initiated with a single ventricular premature depolarization. The method of induction is a V-A-A-V response, strongly indicating atrial tachycardia as the mechanism of the tachycardia. ABL = Ablation; d = distal; p = proximal; RVA = right ventricular apex; SC = coronary sinus.

from the pacing stimulus to the atrial electrogram are expected regardless of His capture. When no retrograde accessory pathway conduction is present, conduction proceeds through the atrioventricular node, and conduction time will be abbreviated with His capture. Caution should be used when interpreting results of this maneuver to ascertain that only the right ventricle and His bundle were captured during pacing (Figure 14-4). Furthermore, slowly conducting and nonseptal accessory pathways can also result in a "nodal" response to this maneuver. Following successful accessory pathway ablation, this maneuver can be repeated to demonstrate a nodal response.

DISTINGUISHING ORTHODROMIC RECIPROCATING TACHYCARDIA UTILIZING A SEPTAL ACCESSORY PATHWAY FROM ATRIAL TACHYCARDIA

With spontaneous tachycardia cycle length variability, changes in atrial electrogram intervals (A-A) will precede and predict changes in the His electrogram intervals (H-H) during atrial tachycardia. Changes in the H-H interval predicting changes in the A-A interval rules out atrial tachycardia as a mechanism and strongly favors ORT or typical AVNRT. Repeated spontaneous termination of the

SVT with an atrial electrogram also eliminates atrial tachycardia from the diagnosis, as maintenance of an atrial tachycardia is independent of atrioventricular nodal conduction. When atrioventricular block is observed during tachycardia, ORT is eliminated as a diagnosis.

Ventricular pacing during SVT that entrains the SVT with resumption of the tachycardia upon pacing termination is a valuable maneuver for differentiating ORT from atrial tachycardia. When a V-A-V response upon pacing termination is elicited, atrial tachycardia can be eliminated as a diagnosis. During this maneuver, a diagnosis of AVNRT can also be excluded when the corrected postpacing interval (PPI) exceeds the tachycardia cycle length (TCL) by <115 msec,[2] or if upright P waves in the inferior surface ECG leads are revealed. Even when ventricular pacing fails to entrain the tachycardia, the results may still be helpful. AV dissociation without interruption of the tachycardia during ventricular pacing eliminates ORT as a tachycardia mechanism (Figure 14-5) and strongly favors an atrial tachycardia or AVNRT with retrograde lower common pathway block. Termination of the tachycardia during ventricular pacing can also be useful to differentiate mechanisms of the tachycardia. When termination occurs with a paced ventricular stimulus at

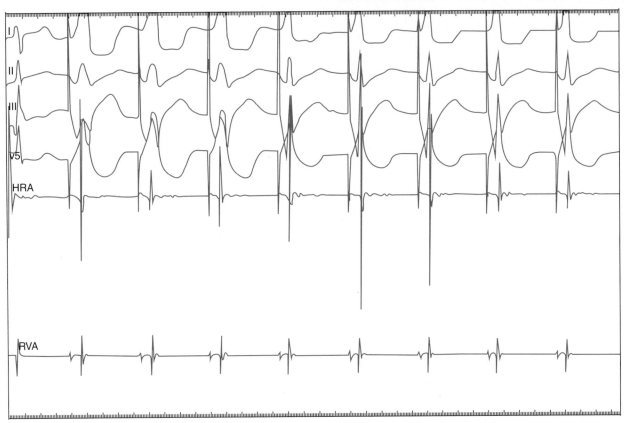

FIGURE 14-4 Pacing is performed at the His level with varying outputs. Similar VA conduction times are seen with both right ventricular capture (first three paced complexes) and His + right ventricular capture (remaining paced complexes). However, the VA conduction time <70 ms is highly suggestive of atrial capture,[5] and therefore this maneuver does not confirm the presence of a septal accessory pathway. HRA = high right atrium; RVA = right ventricular apex.

a time when the His-Purkinje system is refractory, the presence of an accessory pathway is verified. If termination occurs in this setting without advancement of the next atrial electrogram, a diagnosis of ORT is established (Figure 14-6).

If ventricular pacing during the tachycardia fails to establish a diagnosis, atrial pacing during the tachycardia at a slightly faster cycle length than the TCL can also be useful. Consistent resumption of the tachycardia with a constant VA conduction time ("VA linking") supports a diagnosis of ORT (or AVNRT), whereas a variable VA relationship strongly favors an atrial tachycardia (Figure 14-7).

In the majority of cases, the previously described techniques will definitively differentiate ORT from atrial tachycardia. If these pacing maneuvers or tachycardia characteristics fail to establish a clear-cut diagnosis, mapping for the earliest atrial electrogram during the tachycardia can be performed to identify a successful ablation target for either arrhythmia.

DISTINGUISHING ORTHODROMIC RECIPROCATING TACHYCARDIA UTILIZING A SEPTAL ACCESSORY PATHWAY FROM ATRIOVENTRICULAR NODAL REENTRANT TACHYCARDIA

In an SVT with concentric retrograde atrial activation, ORT utilizing a septal accessory pathway can often be distinguished from typical AVNRT using retrograde VA conduction times. Simultaneous atrial and ventricular activation eliminates the possibility of ORT. If atrial activation follows ventricular activation but the interval between the onset of the QRS complex and the septal atrial electrogram is <70 ms, ORT is very unlikely. A longer retrograde VA conduction time can be seen with ORT, typical AVNRT with slower retrograde fast pathway conduction, or atypical AVNRT.

The postpacing interval upon cessation of ventricular pacing that entrains the SVT is a valuable tool for distinguishing AVNRT from ORT. When there is a V-A-V response, a corrected PPI-TCL interval <115 ms essentially rules out AVNRT (Figure 14-8). The PPI is corrected by subtracting any increment in AH interval in the first beat following ventricular pacing compared to the AH intervals during tachycardia.[3] A corrected PPI-TCL >115 ms strongly favors AVNRT as the mechanism, but ORT utilizing a very decremental or nonseptal accessory pathway is not ruled out.

Two other observations during ventricular pacing that entrains the SVT are also helpful in making a diagnosis. A recent study[4] demonstrated that during entrainment, a highly sensitive and specific criteria for ORT is advancement of the atrial electrograms with the first nonfused ventricular paced beat. Also, if fusion between the paced ventricular beat and the tachycardia QRS complex is observed during entrainment, this proves the presence of an extra-nodal pathway.

As in the case highlighted above, multiple mechanisms may be at play and can lead to seemingly contradictory findings. In these cases, one must consider a combination of SVT mechanisms that can explain all the observations noted during tachycardia and with pacing maneuvers.

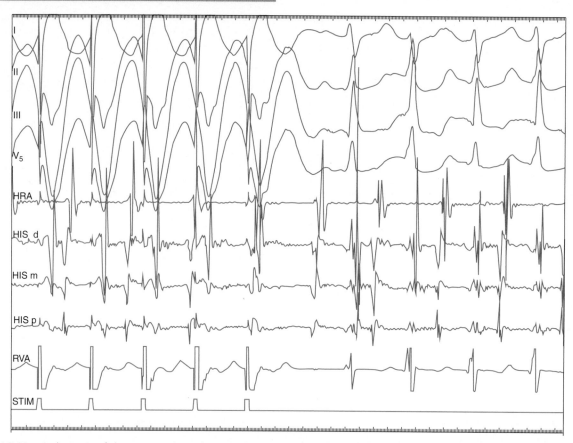

FIGURE 14-5 Ventricular pacing fails to entrain the tachycardia; however, this produces atrioventricular dissociation with continuation of the tachycardia. This is incompatible with a diagnosis of orthodromic reciprocating tachycardia. In this example, the upright P waves in the inferior leads also rules out a diagnosis of atrioventricular nodal reentrant tachycardia and establishes atrial tachycardia as the tachycardia mechanism. d = distal; HRA = high right atrium; m = middle; p = proximal; RVA = right ventricular apex.

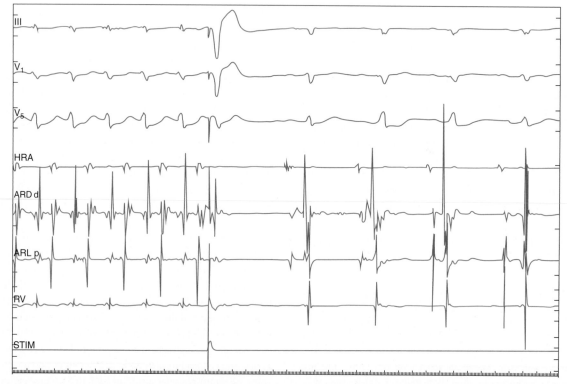

FIGURE 14-6 A premature ventricular stimulus is delivered at a time when the His bundle is refractory. Termination of the tachycardia without advancement of the next atrial electrogram establishes orthodromic reciprocating tachycardia as the mechanism of this tachycardia. ABL = ablation; d = distal; HRA = high right atrium; p = proximal; RV = right ventricle.

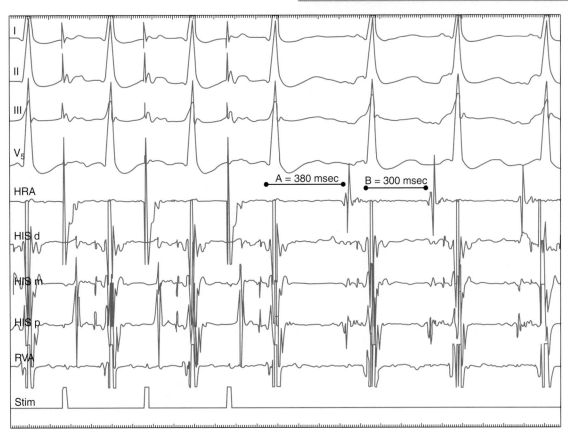

FIGURE 14-7 Following cessation of atrial pacing during tachycardia, the interval between the last entrained ventricular complex and the next atrial electrogram (A) is compared with the interval between the first ventricular complex of the tachycardia to the following atrial electrogram (B). The difference in these measurements here (or lack of "VA linking") supports a diagnosis of atrial tachycardia. d = distal; HRA = high right atrium; m = middle; p = proximal; RVA = right ventricular apex.

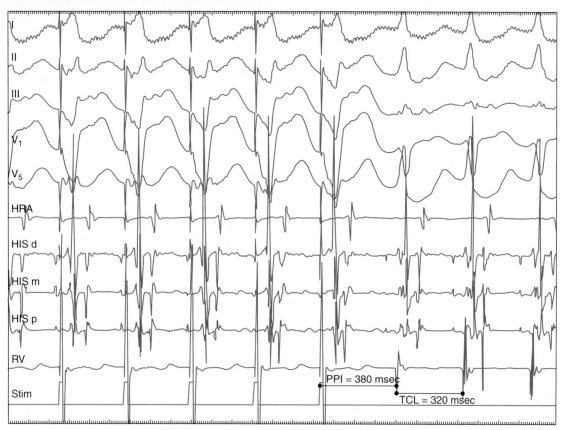

FIGURE 14-8 Following entrainment of the SVT by ventricular pacing, the SVT resumes with a V-A-V response. This coupled with a short post-pacing interval (PPI) minus tachycardia cycle length (TCL) of 60 ms establishes a diagnosis of ORT. d = distal; HRA = high right atrium; m = middle; p = proximal; RV = right ventricle.

REFERENCES

1. Knight BP, Zivin A, Souza J, et al. A technique for the rapid diagnosis of atrial tachycardia in the electrophysiology laboratory. *J Am Coll Cardiol.* 1999;33(3):775-781.

2. Michaud GF, Tada H, Chough S, et al. Differentiation of atypical atrioventricular node re-entrant tachycardia from orthodromic reciprocating tachycardia using a septal accessory pathway by the response to ventricular pacing. *J Am Coll Cardiol.* 2001;38(4):1163-1167.

3. González-Torrecilla E, Arenal A, et al. First postpacing interval after tachycardia entrainment with correction for atrioventricular node delay: a simple maneuver for differential diagnosis of atrioventricular nodal reentrant tachycardias versus orthodromic reciprocating tachycardias. *Heart Rhythm.* 2006;3(6):674-679.

4. Dandamudi G, Mokabberi R, Assal C, et al. A novel approach to differentiating orthodromic reciprocating tachycardia from atrioventricular nodal reentrant tachycardia. *Heart Rhythm.* 2010;7(9):1326-1329.

5. Obeyesekere M, Leong-Sit P, Skanes A, et al. Determination of inadvertent atrial capture during para-Hisian pacing. *Circ Arrhythm Electrophysiol.* 2011;(4)4:510-514.

ANALYSIS OF CHALLENGING INTRACARDIAC
ELECTROGRAMS: CASE II—FOCAL VERSUS
MACROREENTRANT ATRIAL TACHYCARDIA

SECTION II
CASE STUDIES IN SUPRAVENTRICULAR
TACHYCARDIA

101

15 ANALYSIS OF CHALLENGING INTRACARDIAC ELECTROGRAMS: CASE II—FOCAL VERSUS MACROREENTRANT ATRIAL TACHYCARDIA

Rakesh Latchamsetty, MD, and Fred Morady, MD

CASE PRESENTATION

A 62-year-old man with a history of atrial fibrillation and atrial flutter had undergone one previous catheter ablation procedure consisting of pulmonary vein isolation and ablation of the cavotricuspid isthmus. Following this procedure, he had no further episodes of atrial fibrillation but presented several months later with persistent atrial tachycardia. He was taken to the electrophysiology lab for catheter ablation.

The patient presented to the laboratory in atrial tachycardia with 2:1 atrioventricular conduction (Figure 15-1). Upright P waves in V_1 and earliest coronary sinus (CS) atrial activity in the distal CS indicated a left atrial source. Evaluation of the P waves during a period of extended atrioventricular block showed no isoelectric segment in several leads (Figure 15-2). This suggested a macroreentrant mechanism for the tachycardia. Detailed activation mapping was performed in the left atrium and confirmed a macroreentrant circuit revolving around the left pulmonary veins (Figure 15-3).

Rapid atrial pacing at a slightly faster cycle length than the tachycardia cycle length (TCL) was performed at sites believed to be within the macroreentrant circuit. Pacing at the crux of the left superior pulmonary vein (LSPV) and left inferior pulmonary vein demonstrated a postpacing interval (PPI) minus TCL of 20 ms (Figure 15-4). At the junction of the left atrial roof and the LSPV, a multicomponent atrial electrogram was identified that displayed both near-field and far-field components. Rapid atrial pacing at this location revealed a PPI-TCL of zeroms for the near-field component and a PPI-TCL of −20 ms for the far-field component (Figure 15-5). Ablation at this site resulted in termination of the tachycardia (Figure 15-6) and rendered it noninducible.

FOCAL VERSUS MACROREENTRANT ATRIAL TACHYCARDIA

Classification of atrial tachycardia has evolved as diagnostic and therapeutic options for their management have evolved. Original classifications were based on mechanism (enhanced automaticity, triggered activity, and reentry) or appearance on surface ECG. More recently, atrial tachycardias have been classified as either focal or macroreentrant.[1] A macroreentrant tachycardia naturally invokes reentry as a mechanism, whereas a focal atrial tachycardia can utilize any of the three primary tachycardia mechanisms: abnormal automaticity, triggered activity, or reentry.

The commonly accepted gold standard for distinguishing a focal versus macroreentrant tachycardia is the atrial activation pattern. As seen in our case study (Figure 15-3), activation mapping

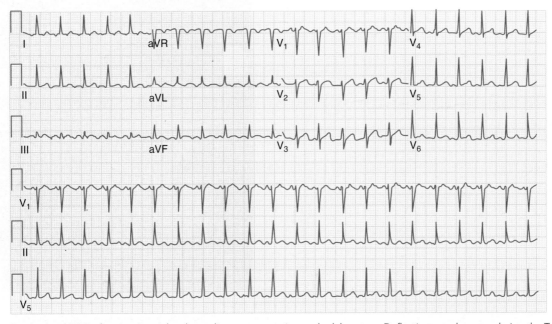

FIGURE 15-1 Twelve-lead ECG of patient's atrial tachycardia on presentation to the laboratory. Deflections can be seen during the T waves in V_1 suggesting 2:1 atrioventricular conduction.

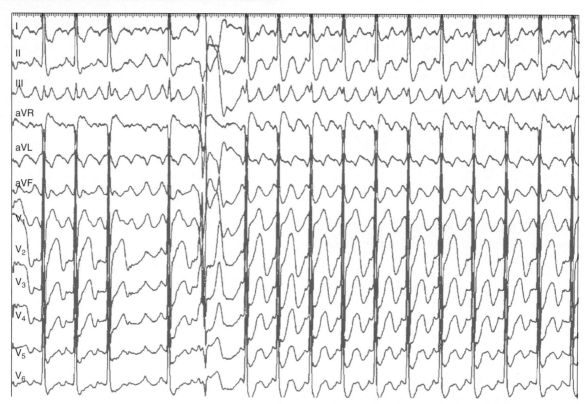

FIGURE 15-2 Surface lead electrocardiogram capturing a period of extended atrioventricular block during the tachycardia. The lack of an isoelectric component in several leads suggests a macroreentrant mechanism for this atrial tachycardia.

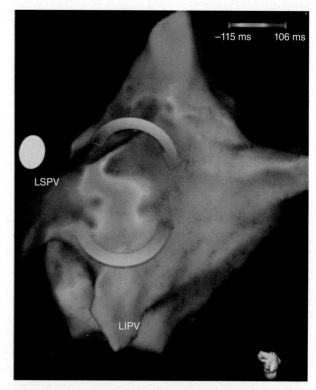

FIGURE 15-3 Activation map in the left atrium revealed a macroreentrant tachycardia through the previously ablated left pulmonary vein antra. Two conduction gaps around the left pulmonary vein antra, one near the roof and the other at the crux, facilitated the reentrant circuit. Note the "early meets late" activation point where the purple and red colors abut. LIPV = left inferior pulmonary vein; LSPV = left superior pulmonary vein.

ANALYSIS OF CHALLENGING INTRACARDIAC
ELECTROGRAMS: CASE II—FOCAL VERSUS
MACROREENTRANT ATRIAL TACHYCARDIA

SECTION II
CASE STUDIES IN SUPRAVENTRICULAR
TACHYCARDIA

103

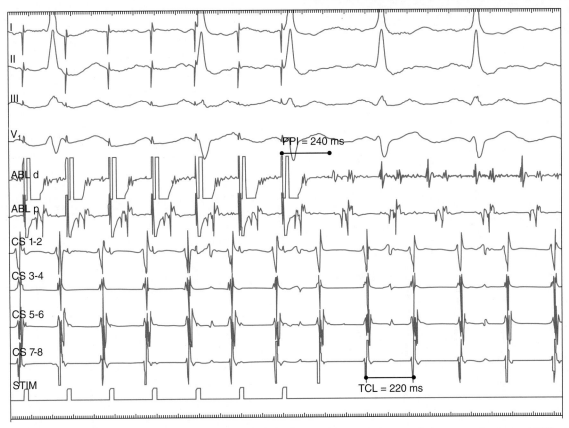

FIGURE 15-4 Rapid atrial pacing at the crux of the left superior and left inferior pulmonary veins revealed a postpacing interval (PPI) minus tachycardia cycle length (TCL) time of just 20 ms, indicating this location was at or very close to the tachycardia circuit. ABL = ablation; CS = coronary sinus; d = distal; p = proximal.

during a macroreentrant atrial tachycardia reveals a circuit with continuous atrial activity that encompasses at least 90% of the TCL and demonstrates an "early meets late" pattern at some point along the circuit.[2] One should note that during mapping of a reentrant circuit, the terms "early" and "late" are arbitrary and depend on the fiducial point used as a reference for atrial timing. In contrast, electroanatomic mapping of a focal atrial tachycardia (Figure 15-7) shows centrifugal activation from a point source usually less than 2 cm in area.

For either mechanism, a detailed map during the tachycardia can identify targets for ablation. For a focal mechanism, the site of earliest atrial activity is targeted. For a macroreentrant circuit, electrical mapping is performed along the circuit to locate areas of slow conduction with a longer duration of fractionated electrograms, ideally at a narrow isthmus bounded by an anatomic obstacle or scar tissue (Figure 15-5). Successful sites for termination of the tachycardia frequently demonstrate an atrial electrogram duration that is >30% of the TCL.[2] Ablation is typically performed across the slow area of conduction and extended linearly to an anatomic obstacle to provide a line of conduction block. Care must be taken to avoid any gaps in this line, as this can facilitate tachycardia recurrence.

Prior to electroanatomic mapping, several observations during tachycardia can provide clues to differentiate a focal versus

macroreentrant mechanism. Cycle length variation >20 ms during the tachycardia is more often seen with a focal tachycardia than with reentrant circuits. A progressive reduction in cycle length at the onset of a tachycardia is suggestive of an automatic mechanism, as is a progressive lengthening of cycle length just before termination.[3] Tachycardia entrainment with rapid atrial pacing is used to identify a reentrant circuit, which can be a mechanism for either a microreentrant (focal) or macroreentrant tachycardia. Variability of the PPI when pacing at different cycle lengths at the same atrial location has been proposed as a sensitive and specific maneuver to differentiate between a focal and macroreentrant source, with a focal source showing greater PPI variability.[4] Automatic sources are prone to overdrive suppression with increasing pacing rates, and microreentrant circuits are believed to be more subject to areas of decremental conduction—both resulting in longer PPIs with more rapid pacing. Decremental conduction may also explain why microreentrant circuits show more cycle length variation than macroreentrant circuits.[5]

P-wave morphology on ECG during a focal atrial tachycardia often displays an isoelectric component in all leads, whereas a macroreentrant tachycardia is expected to reveal continuous atrial activity. However, this finding is not always reliable.[6] With very rapid tachycardia rates or in atria with significant conduction abnormalities

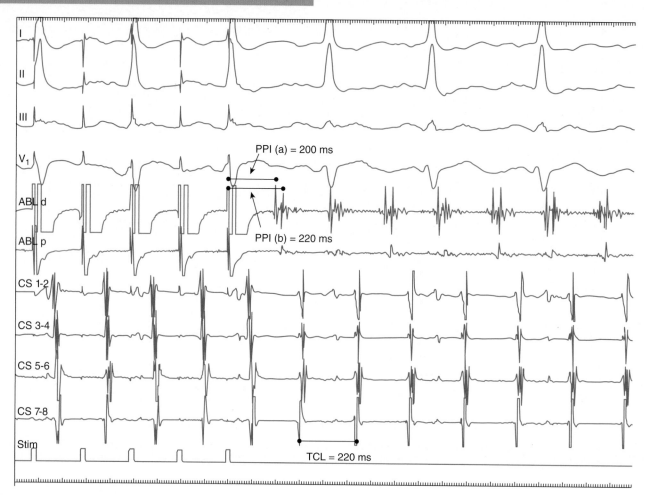

FIGURE 15-5 Rapid atrial pacing from the left atrial roof was performed during tachycardia. Note the multicomponent atrial electrogram at the distal ablation (ABL) catheter. The postpacing interval (PPI) to the initial component representing far-field atrial activity is actually 20 ms less than the tachycardia cycle length (TCL). The PPI to the second, or near-field component of the electrogram matches the TCL. CS = coronary sinus; d = distal; p = proximal.

(commonly seen in patients with prior ablation procedures), an isoelectric component may not be observed with a focal tachycardia. If distinct P waves are difficult to discern because of interference by the QRS complexes on ECG, ventricular pacing or administration of adenosine can often unveil several consecutive P waves for analysis.[1] P wave duration >140 ms has also been shown to be a fairly sensitive and specific marker for a macroreentrant mechanism.[7]

The mechanism of tachycardia initiation and termination can help differentiate tachycardia mechanisms, although these are not entirely sensitive and specific findings. A focal automatic mechanism is more likely to be dependent on isoproterenol for induction and less likely to be induced by pacing.[8] Automatic tachycardias are also more vulnerable to overdrive suppression by rapid atrial pacing. Triggered

and reentrant atrial tachycardias are more likely to be induced with pacing. Triggered activity, in particular, maybe sensitive to specific pacing cycle lengths. Triggered activity is also more likely to be terminated with adenosine, propranolol, verapamil, and the Valsalva maneuver.[8]

Catheter ablation has become common for patients with atrial tachycardias resistant to medical therapy. Technological advances in electroanatomic mapping systems and ablation catheters have improved the ability to diagnose and ablate both focal tachycardias and macroreentrant circuits. Recent studies have reported high success rates for catheter ablation of atrial tachycardias.[2,6] Novel mapping systems with automated electrogram analysis should continue to improve the efficiency and accuracy of such procedures.

ANALYSIS OF CHALLENGING INTRACARDIAC
ELECTROGRAMS: CASE II—FOCAL VERSUS
MACROREENTRANT ATRIAL TACHYCARDIA

SECTION II
CASE STUDIES IN SUPRAVENTRICULAR
TACHYCARDIA

105

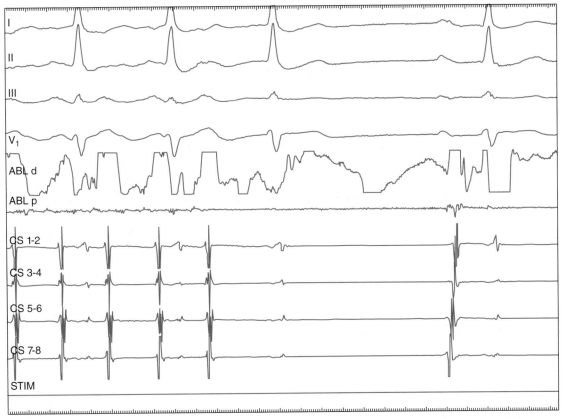

FIGURE 15-6 Termination of the atrial tachycardia to sinus rhythm during ablation at the junction of the left atrial roof and left superior pulmonary vein. ABL = ablation; CS = coronary sinus; d = distal, p = proximal.

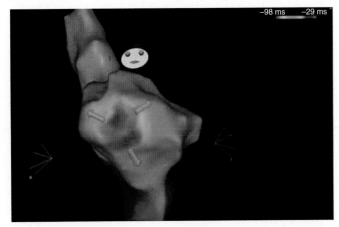

FIGURE 15-7 Electroanatomic mapping during a focal atrial tachycardia reveals centrifugal atrial activation emanating from a single location.

REFERENCES

1. Saoudi N, Cosio F, Waldo A, et al. Classification of atrial flutter and regular atrial tachycardia according to electrophysiologic mechanism and anatomic bases: a statement from a joint expert group from the Working Group of Arrhythmias of the European Society of Cardiology and the North American Society of Pacing and Electrophysiology. *J Cardiovasc Electrophysiol*. 2001;12(7):852-866.

2. Yokokawa M, Latchamsetty R, Ghanbari H, et al. Characteristics of atrial tachycardia due to small vs large reentrant circuits after ablation of persistent atrial fibrillation. *Heart Rhythm*. 2013;10(4):469-476.

3. Goldreyer BN, Gallagher JJ, Damato AN. The electrophysiologic demonstration of atrial ectopic tachycardia in man. *Am Heart J*. 1973;85(2):205-215.

4. Colombowala IK, Massumi A, Rasekh A, et al. Variability in post-pacing intervals predicts global atrial activation pattern during tachycardia. *J Cardiovasc Electrophysiol*. 2008;19(2):142-147.

5. Veenhuyzen GD, Mitchell LB. Distinguishing focal from macroreentrant atrial tachycardias: has this job just become easier? *J Cardiovasc Electrophysiol*. 2008;19(2):148-149.

6. Wasmer K, Mönnig G, Bittner A, et al. Incidence, characteristics, and outcome of left atrial tachycardias after circumferential antral ablation of atrial fibrillation. *Heart Rhythm*. 2012;9(10):1660-1666.

7. Michaud GF, Tada H, Chough S, et al. Differentiation of atypical atrioventricular node re-entrant tachycardia from orthodromic reciprocating tachycardia using a septal accessory pathway by the response to ventricular pacing. *J Am Coll Cardiol*. 2001;38(4):1163-1167.

8. Chen SA, Chiang CE, Yang CJ, et al. Sustained atrial tachycardia in adult patients. Electrophysiological characteristics, pharmacological response, possible mechanisms, and effects of radiofrequency ablation. *Circulation*. 1994;90(3):1262-1278.

SUPRAVENTRICULAR TACHYCARDIA WITH
CONGENITAL HEART DISEASE

SECTION II
CASE STUDIES IN SUPRAVENTRICULAR
TACHYCARDIA

107

16 SUPRAVENTRICULAR TACHYCARDIA WITH CONGENITAL HEART DISEASE

Naomi J. Kertesz, MD

CASE PRESENTATION

The patient is a 38-year-old woman with the diagnosis of transposition of the great arteries. She underwent an atrial switch operation at 2 years of age (Figure 16-1). Her first episode of atrial flutter occurred at 11 years of age. She required multiple medications and ultimately underwent pacemaker implantation due to bradycardia secondary to antiarrhythmic management. She continued to have recurrent flutter requiring multiple cardioversions. She underwent an EP study with attempted ablation at 26 years of age. Multiple circuits were found, and the procedure was unsuccessful. She recently had an episode of atrial flutter while taking sotalol 120 mg BID and metoprolol 12.5 mg daily. She was walking up stairs and noted the onset of flutter (Figure 16-2). She became dizzy and could not make it up the stairs. Her ventricular response was greater than 200 bpm. She underwent cardioversion, and her metoprolol was increased to 25 mg daily. She did not tolerate the increased dose, and she was referred to for repeat attempt at ablation.

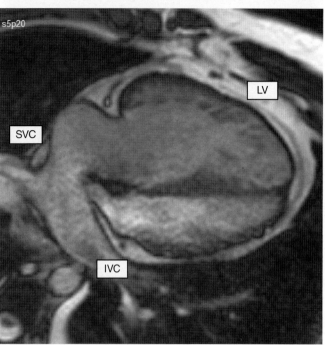

FIGURE 16-1 MRI of transposition of the great arteries following atrial switch operation. Note the baffling of the superior vena cava (SVC) and inferior vena cava (IVC) towards the mitral valve and left ventricle (LV). There is no access to the tricuspid valve from the systemic venous side or the IVC.

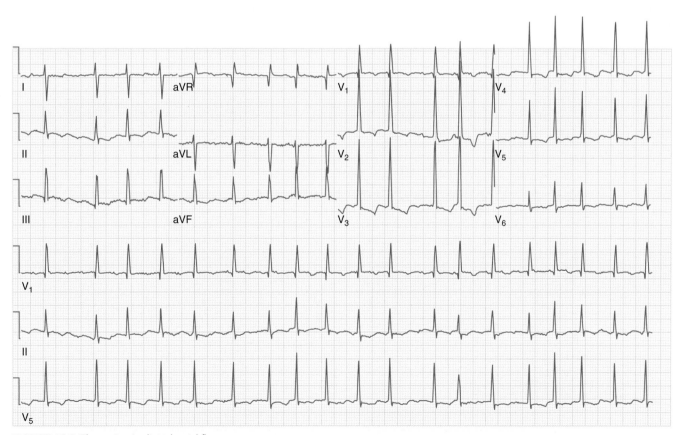

FIGURE 16-2 The patient's clinical atrial flutter.

As is all too common in this population two separate arrhythmias were induced: an atrial tachycardia that had not been seen clinically (Figure 16-3) and atrial flutter (Figures 16-4 and 16-5). Mapping was initially performed on the systemic venous side, and the atrial tachycardia location was identified and ablated. In order to map the atrial flutter, a transbaffle puncture was performed to access the tricuspid valve and the pulmonary venous side (Figure 16-6). Entrainment mapping was used to identify the circuit (see Figure 16-5). The atrial flutter was successfully ablated (Figure 16-7) by placing lesions from the IVC to the baffle on the systemic venous side and then from the baffle to the tricuspid valve on the pulmonary venous side (Figure 16-8). She has had no recurrence of her atrial flutter.

EPIDEMIOLOGY

- Over one million adult congenital heart disease (CHD) patients are living in the United States.[1]
- Forty-five percent have simple defects (atrial septal defect, ventricular septal defect, valve stenosis).
- Forty percent have moderately complex heart disease (tetralogy of Fallot).
- Fifteen percent have severely complex deflects (single ventricle anatomy, Fontan palliation, atrial switch procedure for transposition of the great arteries).
- Any patient who has had an atriotomy incision is at risk for supraventricular arrhythmias.
- Thirty-four percent of older patients with TOF develop symptomatic supraventricular arrhythmias.[2]
- Older style Fontans, that is, atriopulmonary, have up to a 50% incidence of atrial arrhythmias due to atrial dilation and suture lines.[3]

DIAGNOSIS AND MANAGEMENT

Atrioventricular Reentry and Twin AV Nodes

The embryological abnormalities that cause congenital heart defects may also have a direct impact on the conduction system. The AV node and the His bundle may only be displaced, or there may be accessory or duplicated AV connections with the possibility of reentrant arrhythmias.

Atrioventricular Reentry

- Common in some types of congenital heart disease.
- Ebstein anomaly (Figure 16-9) is associated with Wolf-Parkinson-White syndrome in 20% of cases. Nearly half of these patients will have multiple accessory pathways.
- Patients with L-TGA, that is, corrected transposition, also have a high incidence of accessory pathways; many of these patients also have Ebstein anomaly of their left-sided tricuspid valve.
- Given the atrial dilation in these patients the risk of atrial fibrillation with rapid conduction is becoming increasingly problematic in adolescence and adulthood (Figure 16-10).
- Catheter ablation is considered the standard of care for management of accessory pathways.
- It should be recognized that long-term recurrence is higher in patients with Ebstein anomaly. These ablations are complicated by distorted landmarks, difficulty in identifying the true AV groove, and the high incidence of multiple pathways.[4]

Twin AV Nodes

- This is a rarer anomaly typically seen in single ventricles of the heterotaxy variety.

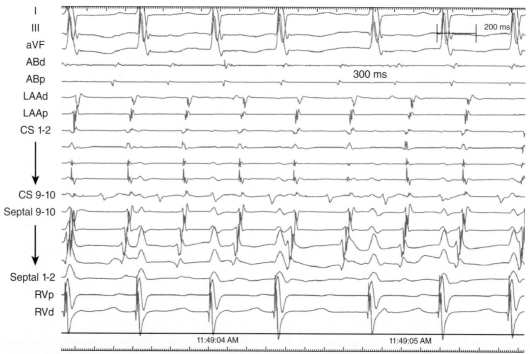

FIGURE 16-3 Atrial tachycardia induced in the EP laboratory.

SUPRAVENTRICULAR TACHYCARDIA WITH
CONGENITAL HEART DISEASE

SECTION II
CASE STUDIES IN SUPRAVENTRICULAR
TACHYCARDIA

109

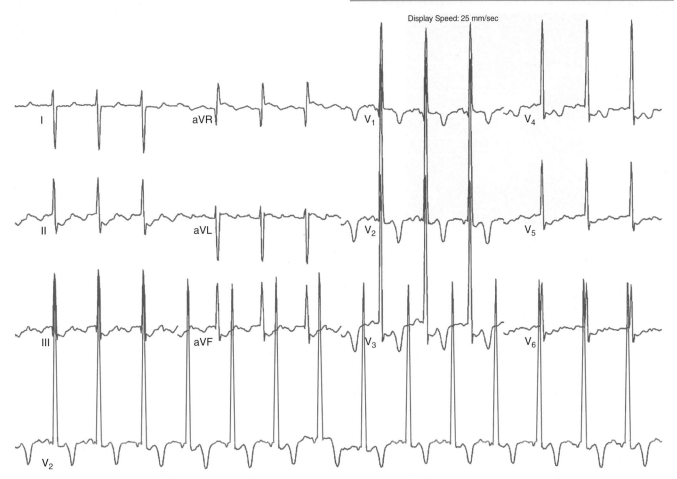

FIGURE 16-4 Atrioventricular block was induced during catheter manipulation, which makes the flutter waves easier to identify.

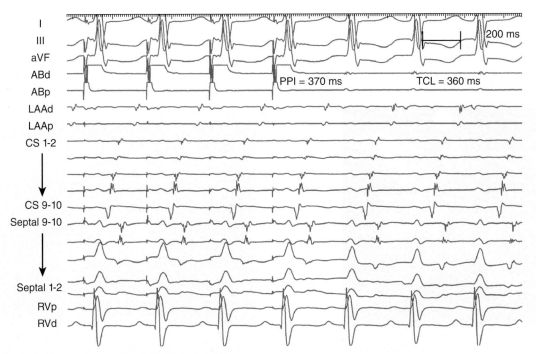

FIGURE 16-5 Entrainment mapping used to define flutter circuit.

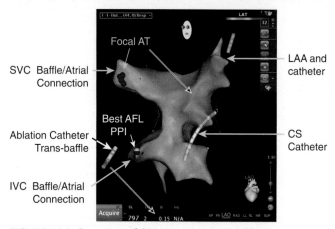

FIGURE 16-6 Carto map of the systemic venous baffle. Note the site of successful atrial tachycardia ablation. The ablation catheter is on the pulmonary venous side of the baffle.

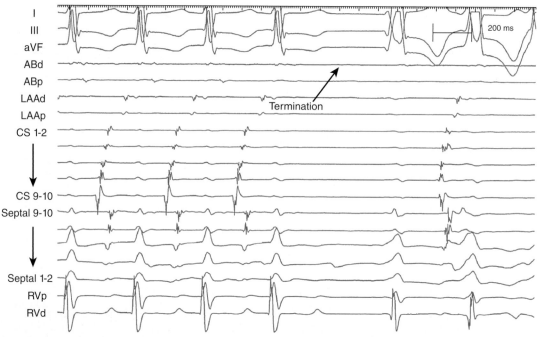

FIGURE 16-7 Atrial flutter terminated with radiofrequency ablation.

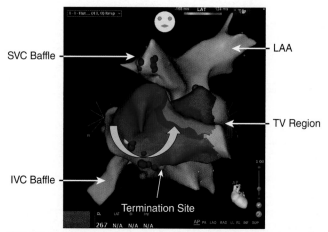

FIGURE 16-8 Both systemic and venous baffles are outlined. In order to completely ablate the flutter isthmus it was necessary to cross the baffle and ablate from the IVC to the tricuspid valve.

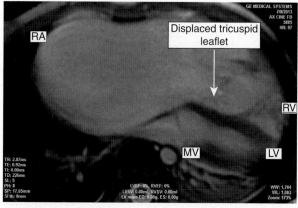

FIGURE 16-9 MRI of Ebstein anomaly of the tricuspid valve. Note the diminutive right ventricle, the displaced tricuspid valve, and the large right atrium.

SUPRAVENTRICULAR TACHYCARDIA WITH
CONGENITAL HEART DISEASE

SECTION II
CASE STUDIES IN SUPRAVENTRICULAR
TACHYCARDIA

111

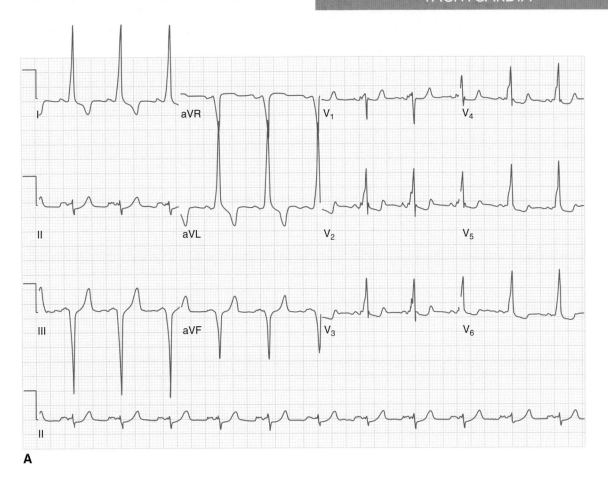

A

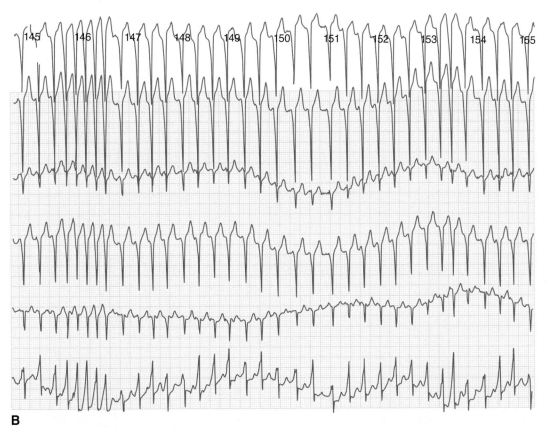

B

FIGURE 16-10 (A) Baseline ECG in an adult with Ebstein anomaly and WPW. (B) Atrial fibrillation in a 20-year-old woman with Ebstein anomaly and WPW.

- There are two AV nodes with 2 discrete His bundles with evidence of a connecting fiber.[5]

- Treatment is focused on ablation of one of the limbs of the duplicate system.

INTRA-ATRIAL REENTRANT TACHYCARDIA (IART)

- Most common mechanism of symptomatic arrhythmia in the adult CHD patient.

- IART or incisional tachycardia are customary labels to distinguish this arrhythmia from typical atrial flutter (Figures 16-11 and 16-12). It is a macroreentrant circuit within atrial muscle caused by atrial dilation, thickening, and scarring.

- Other risk factors for IART include concomitant sinus node dysfunction with tachy-brady syndrome and older age at the time of surgery.[3]

- IART is seen in 30% of patients following an atrial switch operation (Mustard or Senning) (see Figure 16-3); or 50% of patients following a Fontan palliation (Figure 16-13) though IART can occur in any patient who has undergone an atriotomy incision.

- The route of propagation varies depending on the anatomic defect and the surgical repair and is modulated by fibrosis of suture lines or patches.

- It is common to have multiple circuits in one patient. When a tricuspid valve is present the cavotricuspid isthmus is often part of the circuit.

- The IART rate is generally slower than classic flutter with atrial rates of 150 to 250 bpm. The P waves are small and separated by a flat baseline and are masked by the QRS and T waves (Figures 16-14 and 16-15). There may be 1:1 or variable AV conduction.

- One must have high index of suspicion in older CHD patients, as the P waves are so difficult to see. Adenosine may be useful to unmask the arrhythmia (see Figure 16-12).

- IART can lead to hemodynamic instability, including cardiac arrest, or in the subacute setting cause heart failure and thromboembolic phenomena.

Treatment

- IART can be reliably terminated with electrical cardioversion and sometimes with overdrive pacing.

- Many patients with underlying sinus node dysfunction may be significantly bradycardic following cardioversion.

- Consideration should be given to placing cardioversion pads over sternum and back to have the vector of energy travel through the atrium to increase the success rate.

- Patients have a high incidence of thrombus formation and need anticoagulation.

- Long-term therapeutic options include antiarrhythmic drugs, pacemakers, catheter ablation, and surgical intervention.

- Pacemakers are useful for treating tachy-brady syndrome, allowing use of antiarrhythmics in patients with underlying sinus node dysfunction, and antitachycardia pacing. One must be careful with anti-

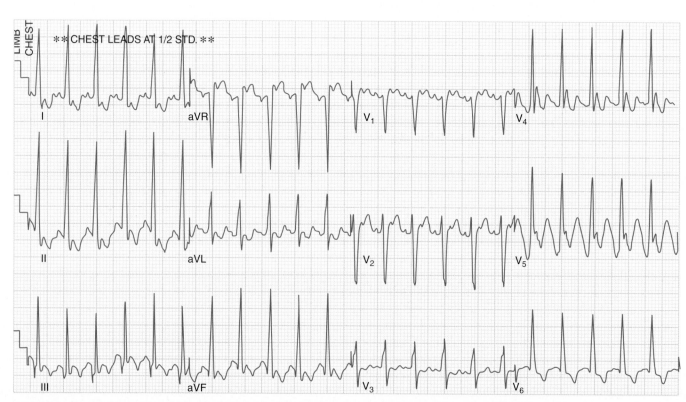

FIGURE 16-11 Atrial flutter in an adult with unrepaired single ventricle.

SUPRAVENTRICULAR TACHYCARDIA WITH
CONGENITAL HEART DISEASE

SECTION II
CASE STUDIES IN SUPRAVENTRICULAR
TACHYCARDIA

113

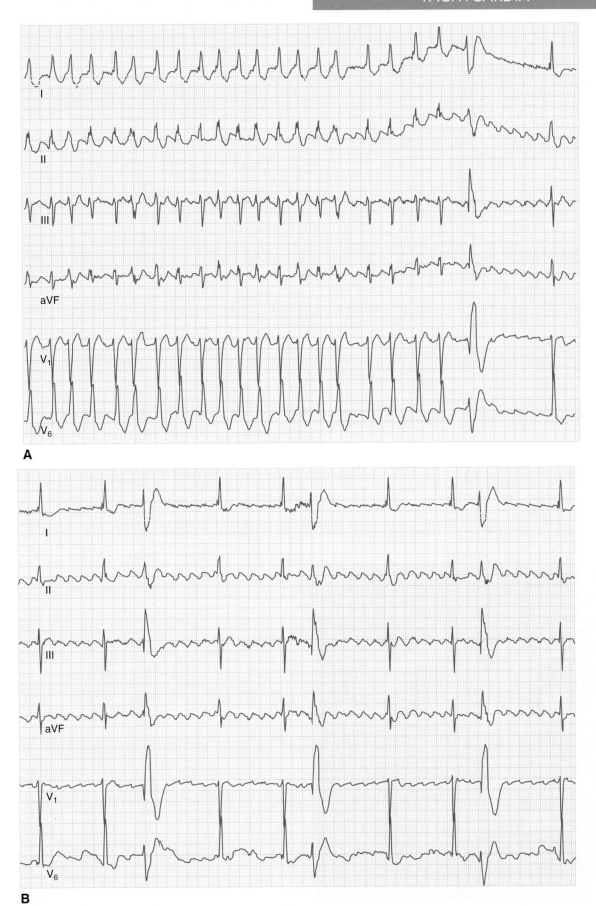

FIGURE 16-12 Nineteen-year-old with Fontan who presented with palpitations. Adenosine administration (A and B) makes classic flutter waves easily seen, which was unexpected given the type of heart disease and baseline ECG (C).

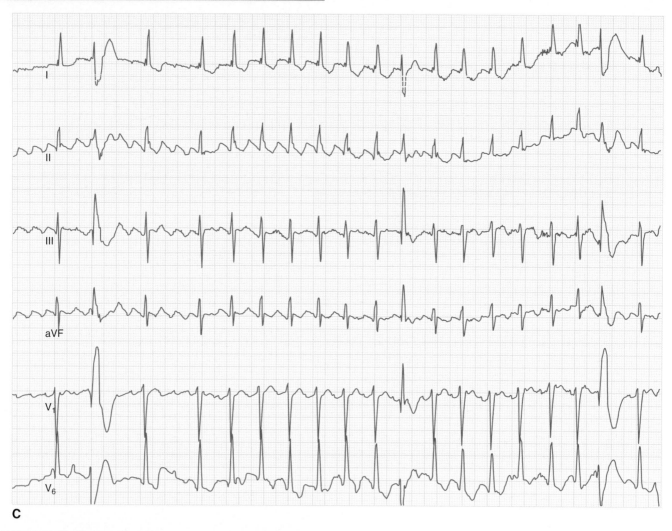

C

FIGURE 16-12 (*Continued*)

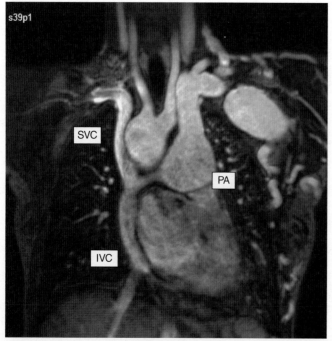

FIGURE 16-13 Lateral tunnel Fontan. Note the SVC and IVC directly connected to the pulmonary arteries (PA).

SUPRAVENTRICULAR TACHYCARDIA WITH
CONGENITAL HEART DISEASE

SECTION II
CASE STUDIES IN SUPRAVENTRICULAR
TACHYCARDIA

115

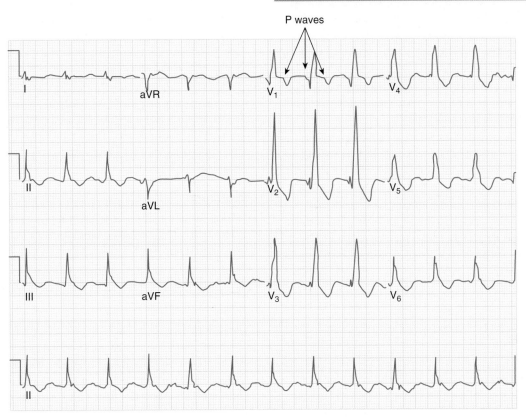

FIGURE 16-14 Thirty-year-old with history of Mustard operation who presented with complaints of tachycardia. She was originally discharged from the ER until ECG reviewed by cardiology. The ECG demonstrates IART with 2:1 AV conduction. Note short PR and P wave buried in T wave.

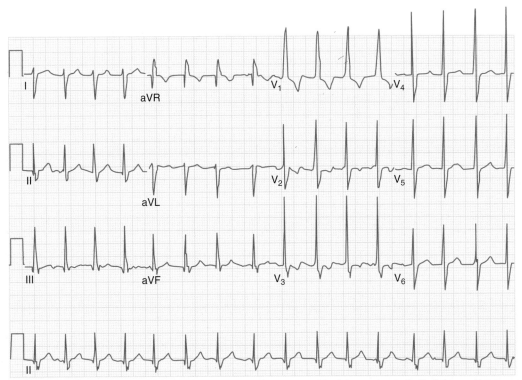

FIGURE 16-15 Twenty-six-year-old status post-Senning operation with AAIR pacemaker due to sinus node dysfunction. He presented to ER with palpitations. Pacemaker interrogation demonstrated that this was IART with 2:1 AV conduction. P waves virtually unable to be seen.

tachycardia pacing as this may cause a shift to a different and faster IART circuit or cause degeneration into atrial fibrillation.

- Catheter ablation using 3-D mapping and irrigated-tip or large-tip catheters has a short term success rate of nearly 90%.[6,7] It is important to remember that in patients with atrial switch procedures the cavotricuspid annulus is in the pulmonary venous atrium and only accessible prograde via transbaffle puncture.

- Recurrence risk is particularly high—nearly 40% in Fontan patients due to the large number of IART circuits and the thickness and size of the atrium. However, ablation still may be useful as it may reduce the frequency of episodes or make drug therapy more effective.[4]

- Surgical ablation is an option and consists of a right atrial maze procedure particularly in the Fontan population. Many times this is combined with a revision of the Fontan connection from an older atriopulmonary anastomosis to a cavopulmonary anastomosis or extracardiac Fontan.

ATRIAL FIBRILLATION

- Atrial fibrillation arises in response to hemodynamic stress in the left atrium (Figure 16-16) and is most commonly associated with aortic stenosis, mitral valve deformities, and unrepaired single ventricles.

- Patients with isolated right-sided heart lesions are at a higher risk of developing atrial arrhythmias than those with isolated left heart lesions. The 30-year risk of developing atrial arrhythmias in an 18-year-old patient with right-sided heart disease (ASD, Ebstein anomaly, Fontan, tricuspid valve abnormality) is 18% in comparison to 11% in one with left-sided disease (VSD, aortic, or mitral valve disease).[8]

- Issues regarding hemodynamic instability, heart failure, and stroke are seen in this population just as in those patients with structurally normal hearts. There is no difference in morbidity or mortality between those with right- or left-sided heart lesions.

Treatment

- Management is similar to atrial fibrillation in adults without CHD and consists of cardioversion, antiarrhythmics for rate control, and anticoagulation.

- Antiarrhythmic therapy is only marginally successful.

- Pacemaker insertion may reduce recurrence in those with sinus node dysfunction.

- Surgical ablation with a right- and left-sided maze is possible.

- Catheter ablation with pulmonary vein isolation has been reported in the presence of congenital heart disease with the most common defect being an ASD. However, pulmonary vein isolation has also been reported in patients, status post-Fontan operation.[9]

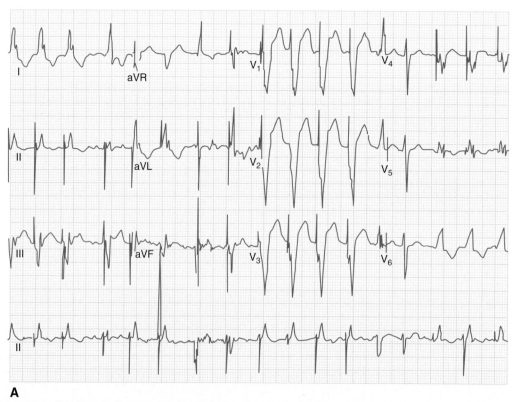

A

FIGURE 16-16 (A and B) Surface ECG and rhythm strip of patient with dual chamber pacemaker and atrial fibrillation. (C) Rhythm strip with atrial wires hooked up to right and left arm; ECG leads therefore displaying on lead I.

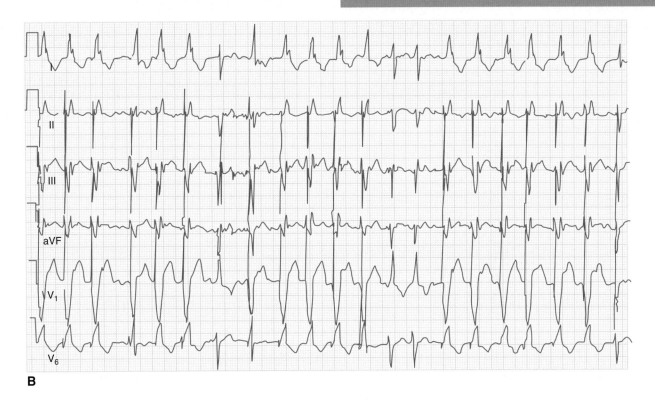

B

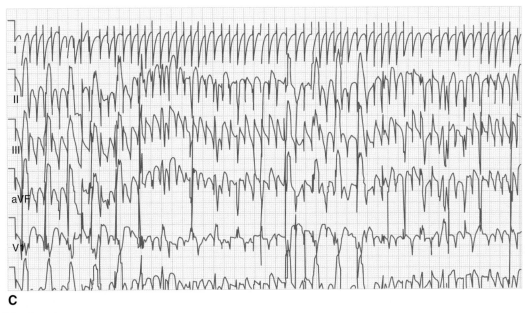

C

FIGURE 16-16 *(Continued)*

REFERENCES

1. Warnes CA, Liberthson R, Danielson GK, et al. Task force 1: the changing profile of congenital heart disease in adult life. *J Am Coll Cardiol.* 2001;37(5):1170-1175.

2. Roos-Hesselink J, Perlroth MG, McGhie J, Spitaels S. Atrial arrhythmias in adults after repair of tetralogy of Fallot. Correlations with clinical, exercise, and echocardiographic findings. *Circulation.* 1995;91(8):2214-2219.

3. Fishberger SB, Wernovsky G, Gentles TL, et al. Factors that influence the development of atrial flutter after the Fontan operation. *J Thorac Cardiovasc Surg.* 1997;113(1):80-86.

4. Lam W, Friedman RA. Electrophysiology issues in adult congenital heart disease. *Methodist Debakey Cardiovasc J.* 2011;7(2): 13-17.

5. Walsh E, Cecchin F. Arrhythmias in adult patients with congenital heart disease. *Circulation.* 2007;115(4):534-545.

6. Triedman JK, Alexander MA, Love BA, et al. Influence of patient factors and ablative technologies on outcomes of radiofrequency ablation of intra-atrial tachycardia in patients with congenital heart disease. *J Am Coll Cardiol*. 2002;39:1827-1835.

7. Jais P, Shah DC, Haissaguerre M, et al. Prospective randomized comparison of irrigated-tip versus conventional-tip catheters for ablation of common flutter. *Circulation*. 2000;101:772-776.

8. Vernier M, Marelli AJ, Pilote L, et al. Atrial arrhythmias in adult patients with right versus left sided congenital heart disease anomalies. *Am J Cardiol*. 2010;106(4):547-551.

9. Philip F, Muhammad KI, Agarwal S, et al. Pulmonary vein isolation for the treatment of drug-refractory atrial fibrillation in adults with congenital heart disease. *Congenit Heart Dis*. 2012;7:392-399.

SECTION III

CASE STUDIES IN VENTRICULAR TACHYCARDIA

17 THE EVALUATION AND MANAGEMENT OF NON-SUSTAINED VENTRICULAR TACHYCARDIA IN PATIENTS AFTER MYOCARDIAL INFARCTION

Yehoshua C. Levine, MD, and Alfred E. Buxton, MD

CASE PRESENTATION

A 57-year-old man with a history of untreated hypertension presented to the emergency department with crushing substernal chest pain and diaphoresis lasting 6 hours. A 12-lead ECG upon arrival showed sinus tachycardia with 3 mm ST-segment elevations in leads V_2-V_5. The patient was emergently transported to the cardiac catheterization laboratory where coronary angiography demonstrated a subtotal occlusion of the proximal left anterior descending coronary artery. Percutaneous coronary intervention was performed, with export thrombectomy and drug-eluting stenting of the culprit vessel and immediate resolution of symptoms. Serum levels of Troponin-T peaked at 3.3 ng/mL. He was admitted to the coronary intensive care unit, where echocardiography the following day showed left ventricular (LV) hypertrophy with moderate hypokinesis of the anteroseptal and anterior walls and an estimated left ventricular ejection fraction (LVEF) of 35% to 40%. He remained asymptomatic and hemodynamically stable and was transferred to the floor later that day, where his cardiac medications were optimally titrated and cardiac rehabilitation planning was begun.

On the fourth hospital day, during the discharge planning process, the patient's telemetry alarmed during a 14-beat run of a wide-complex tachycardia with heart rate approximately 250 bpm (Figure 17-1). He reported no symptoms during the episode. No further episodes of nonsustained ventricular tachycardia (NSVT) were observed for the duration of his hospitalization. The patient and nursing staff are concerned about the telemetry findings and wonder whether his hospital discharge should be delayed so that further evaluation can be performed. What is the significance of these findings on telemetry? Should they influence ongoing clinical management of this patient?

CASE EXPLANATION AND OVERVIEW

This patient has had an episode of NSVT 4 days after an acute anterior myocardial infarction (MI) in the setting of LV dysfunction documented on echocardiogram. Management considerations for this patient include determining the prognostic significance of his NSVT and determining whether further therapy is indicated either while he is still an inpatient or during outpatient follow-up.

Historically, NSVT has been defined in a number of ways based on the duration and rate of the observed arrhythmia.[1] The standard definition is three or more consecutive ventricular premature depolarizations at a rate of at least 100 beats/min, lasting up to a maximum duration of 30 seconds before spontaneous termination.[2] The rate cutoff of 100 beats/min is based on the observation that tachycardias slower than this rate do not generally confer adverse prognostic significance in patients who have a history of MI.[3]

The prevalence and prognostic significance of NSVT in a given patient depends upon the presence and extent of structural heart disease. Up to 3% of asymptomatic patients with no evidence of heart disease have been shown to experience runs of NSVT over the course of 24 hours of monitoring, but the prognostic significance of this finding remains unclear.[4] In contrast, NSVT occurring in patients who have suffered an MI or have a history of idiopathic dilated cardiomyopathy,[5] valvular heart disease such as mitral valve prolapse,[6] longstanding hypertension and left ventricular hypertrophy,[7] and hypertrophic cardiomyopathy[8] is more common and may function as an independent predictor of mortality under certain situations. However, this does not mean that NSVT independently predicts arrhythmic death. NSVT in the post-MI period, such as that which occurred in the Case Presentation, portends a worse overall prognosis, but the incidence of sudden cardiac death (SCD) in patients with NSVT is not increased out of proportion to the increase in total mortality in this patient population.

In the following sections, we will outline the prognostic significance and management considerations of NSVT in patients with a history of MI.

ETIOLOGY AND PATHOPHYSIOLOGY

Unlike sustained tachyarrhythmias, NSVT is usually not associated with symptoms in patients with structural heart disease (because most episodes are brief); rather, it is usually discovered incidentally during electrocardiographic monitoring. Early studies that identified NSVT

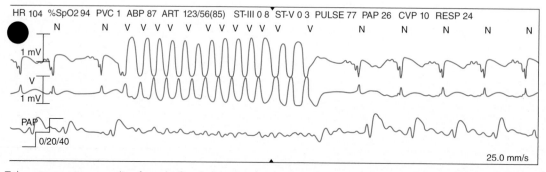

FIGURE 17-1 Telemetry monitor recording from the fourth day after the patient's acute myocardial infarction (MI). Nonsustained ventricular tachycardia (NSVT) is demonstrated on the telemetry strip.

THE EVALUATION AND MANAGEMENT OF NONSUS-
TAINED VENTRICULAR TACHYCARDIA IN PATIENTS
AFTER MYOCARDIAL INFARCTION

SECTION III
CASE STUDIES IN VENTRICULAR
TACHYCARDIA

121

as a risk factor for the development of sudden death in patients with a recent MI were based on the observation that ventricular fibrillation in the acute phase of MI was often preceded by escalating frequency of ventricular ectopy and NSVT. Later studies demonstrated an association between the presence of NSVT discovered in the early postinfarction period and risk of SCD in patients with reduced left ventricular ejection fraction (LVEF).[9] With rare exception, most data suggest that NSVT within the first 48 hours after an MI does not carry prognostic significance.[10] By contrast, NSVT occurring after the first 48 hours after an MI has been linked with an increased risk of both SCD and total mortality in pre-reperfusion era studies,[11] and NSVT was accordingly used as a qualifying characteristic in early implantable cardioverter-defibrillator (ICD) trials in patients with prior MI and LV systolic dysfunction.[12,13] It is important to note, however, that the increased risk of SCD in patients with NSVT is due to the increased risk of total mortality in these patients and not due to any specific predilection to sustained ventricular arrhythmias. Indeed, in a subgroup analysis of the first 1480 patients enrolled in the MUSTT study, Buxton et al found that electrocardiographic characteristics of spontaneous NSVT in patients with coronary artery disease cannot differentiate between patients with and those without sustained VT inducible by programmed stimulation.[14,15] In these patients, NSVT portends a worse overall prognosis, but the risk of SCD is not increased out of proportion to the risk of total mortality. A post-hoc analysis of the relation of LVEF and inducible VT to mode of death in MUSTT-enrolled patients (who all had significant LV dysfunction and spontaneous asymptomatic NSVT) demonstrated a significantly higher risk of mortality in those patients whose LVEF was <30%, regardless of the presence or absence of inducible sustained VT that might predict risk for VT. In these patients, it is the presence and severity of heart failure that serves as a major determinant of total mortality. Furthermore, the percent of total mortality accounted for by arrhythmic events was similar regardless of whether the LVEF was <30% or ≥30% and would likely also be similar whether or not there was a history of documented NSVT.[16]

In the reperfusion era, the presence of NSVT has become a less significant risk stratification tool following an MI, as newer data have not identified an independent association between NSVT and worse prognosis in many situations.[17,18] In the absence of other risk factors such as low LVEF, NSVT predicts neither inducibility of sustained monomorphic VT nor total mortality in patients post-MI. The reason for this is probably multifactorial and has to do with the fact that early reperfusion strategies and the ubiquitous use of β-blocker therapy have reduced both the incidence of NSVT and postinfarction scar burden even in patients who do have NSVT.

MANAGEMENT

The patient described in the Case Presentation has been noted to have asymptomatic NSVT in the setting of an LVEF estimated to be between 35% and 40% after his acute MI. The first question is whether this observation portends worse prognosis. As discussed in the previous section, the more significant issue is his LV dysfunction (reflected both by EF and clinical evidence of heart failure), and he will require optimal medical management and follow-up echocardiography as an outpatient to determine his long-term total mortality. Demonstrating persistent LV dysfunction during follow-up

2 to 3 months after his MI is likely to have greater prognostic utility than observing episodes of NSVT. If LV dysfunction persists in the months-to-years after his MI, his total mortality risk will be higher, but his risk of SCD requires other prognostic variables for accurate risk stratification. Unfortunately, while the LVEF correlates with overall survival, it tells us nothing about how patients die (suddenly versus nonsuddenly).

The next issue is whether the presence of NSVT on routine monitoring should alter medical management for this patient. The historical approach of suppressing NSVT with class I or III antiarrhythmic medications in patients after MI in an effort to reduce the incidence of malignant arrhythmias and SCD has become extinct, as controlled trials showed no evidence that pharmacologic antiarrhythmic therapy reduces overall mortality in this population.[19] Importantly, the CAMIAT trial found that although amiodarone reduced the annual rate of arrhythmic death or resuscitated ventricular tachyarrhythmias in patients who have frequent ventricular premature depolarizations or at least one episode of NSVT between 6 and 45 days post-MI, it did not affect all-cause or cardiac mortality in these patients.[20] β-Blockers are recommended to reduce total mortality in the post-MI period, but do not benefit patients who have NSVT more than patients who do not have NSVT. Therefore, in asymptomatic patients with a history of MI who have NSVT on cardiac monitoring, no medication adjustment is indicated based on the presence of NSVT alone.

The most important practical consideration for this patient is whether to perform an electrophysiology study (EPS) to determine inducibility of sustained monomorphic VT. Indeed, determining the utility of EPS in preparation for possible primary prophylactic ICD implantation is the only way that documenting NSVT might change management. Patients with NSVT in the context of LVEF ≤40% who have inducible sustained monomorphic VT at EPS have a significantly higher risk of SCD and total mortality at 2 years than patients without inducible VT, as demonstrated in the MUSTT trial. Furthermore, noninducible patients in the MUSTT trial had a significantly lower risk of SCD compared with inducible patients at 2 and 5 years (12% versus 18% and 24% versus 32%, respectively).[13,21] There is also evidence that inducibility of ventricular arrhythmias is predictive of subsequent appropriate ICD therapies for VT/VF in patients who undergo ICD implantation.[22] EPS is often performed in borderline-risk patients to determine whether their level of risk justifies ICD implantation, and many of these patients have NSVT. Indeed, a recent National Cardiovascular Data Registry (NCDR) ICD Registry analysis of patients undergoing EPS for improved risk stratification of SCD observed that patients undergoing EPS more often had NYHA class I symptoms and NSVT than patients who did not undergo EPS prior to ICD implantation.[23] If our patient's LVEF remains 35% to 40% at least 3 months after his MI—or if his LVEF becomes 30% to 35% at that point but he has New York Heart Association (NYHA) class I symptoms—NSVT justifies further risk stratification with an EPS to determine whether he is likely to derive improved survival with an ICD.

Whether this patient should be discharged with a wearable cardiac defibrillator (WCD) during this 3-month period is not clearly indicated from an evidence-based perspective. An ongoing randomized clinical trial is evaluating the ability of the WCD to reduce mortality in the first 3 months after MI. It is important to remember that although this period is the single time when patients with MI have highest risk of SCD, many of the SCD occurring during this period appear not to result from arrhythmias. A substudy of the VALIANT trial reviewed autopsy records of patients who suffered SCD early after acute MI and found that at 3 months after the MI, only approximately 30% to 35% of the sudden deaths were considered presumed arrhythmic.[24] These data suggest that a defibrillator, which would terminate ventricular arrhythmias, may not reduce mortality in many patients who experience sudden death early after an acute MI. While current evidence does not demonstrate a reduction in mortality with a WCD, it is nonetheless reasonable to discharge such a patient with this temporary device if the physician is concerned about the patient's risk of arrhythmic SCD.

There are two special situations that should be highlighted:

1. NSVT morphology may be prognostically and diagnostically important. With repeated episodes of NSVT, a 12-lead ECG should be performed to characterize the morphology of VT and to evaluate for an idiopathic VT, most commonly arising from the right ventricular outflow tract (Figure 17-2). In patients with a history of MI whose NSVT morphology suggests right ventricular outflow tract origin, the NSVT is probably not related to the MI and does not carry adverse prognostic significance.

2. Management differs for patients with symptoms (such as palpitations, lightheadedness) that are attributable to NSVT, or patients who develop cardiomyopathy as a direct result of frequent episodes of NSVT. Patients with symptomatic NSVT are more likely to have structurally normal hearts and may not already be treated with β-blockers. By contrast, patients with cardiomyopathy attributable to high NSVT burden will likely already have been started on β-blocker therapy for management of their cardiomyopathy, and the β-blockers may aid in controlling the NSVT burden. Patients in these categories may benefit from antiarrhythmic therapy and/or catheter ablation for symptom relief and/or for optimal treatment of their cardiomyopathy[25] (Figure 17-3). Note that the reason to treat NSVT is for symptom relief, not to reduce mortality risk.

CONCLUSIONS AND RECOMMENDATIONS

The patient presented has had NSVT incidentally noted a few days after his acute MI. As discussed, the more significant prognostic indicator of adverse cardiovascular events is his LV dysfunction, reflected by an LVEF of 35% to 40%. Having had documented NSVT should not affect his post-MI medication regimen and should not result in further monitoring or risk stratification at the current time. However, if he remains a borderline candidate for ICD implantation for primary prevention of SCD in 3 months, that is, if his LVEF remains 35% to 40% or if his LVEF becomes 30% to 35% and he has NYHA class I symptoms—the presence of NSVT would justify further risk stratification with an EPS to determine his candidacy for ICD implantation.

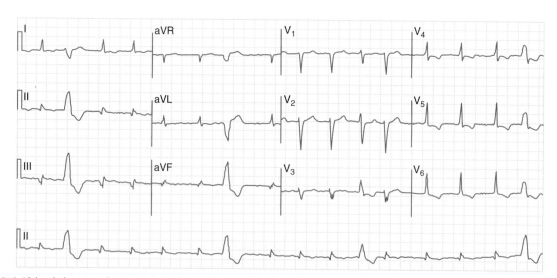

FIGURE 17-2 A 12-lead electrocardiogram tracing from a 60-year-old man with a history of a remote inferior MI who was hospitalized for pneumonia and was incidentally noted to have evidence of ventricular ectopy during his hospitalization. The premature ventricular depolarizations captured on this tracing—and the NSVT documented on cardiac monitoring—arose from the right ventricular outflow tract and had no relation to his prior inferior MI.

THE EVALUATION AND MANAGEMENT OF NONSUS-
TAINED VENTRICULAR TACHYCARDIA IN PATIENTS
AFTER MYOCARDIAL INFARCTION

SECTION III
CASE STUDIES IN VENTRICULAR
TACHYCARDIA

123

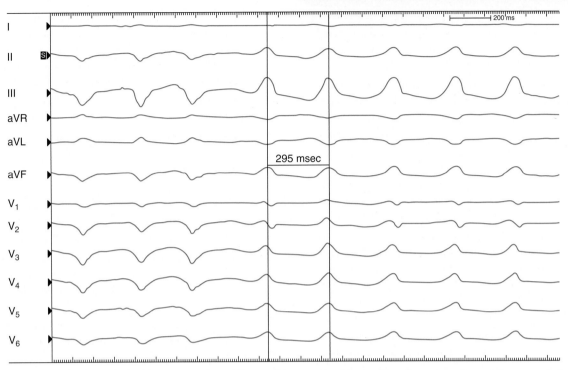

FIGURE 17-3 Induction of NSVT with double extrastimuli in a 76-year-old man with a history of coronary artery disease who presented with NSVT in the setting of presyncope and palpitations and was referred to for ablation.

REFERENCES

1. Buxton AE. Nonsustained ventricular tachycardia: clinical significance and mechanisms. In: Josephson ME, Wellens HJJ, eds. *Tachycardias: Mechanisms and Management*. Mount Kisco, NY: Futura Publishing Co Inc; 1993;353-361.

2. Buxton AE, Calkins H, Callans DJ, et al. ACC/AHA/HRS 2006 key data elements and definitions for electrophysiological studies and procedures: a report of the American College of Cardiology/American Heart Association Task Force on Clinical Data Standards (ACC/AHA/HRS Writing Committee to Develop Data Standards on Electrophysiology). *Circulation*. 2006;114:2534-2570.

3. Anderson KP, DeCamilla J, Moss AJ. Clinical significance of ventricular tachycardia (3 beats or longer) detected during ambulatory monitoring after myocardial infarction. *Circulation*. 1978;57:890.

4. Hinkle LE, Carver ST, Stevens M. The frequency of asymptomatic disturbances of cardiac rhythm and conduction in middle-aged men. *Am J Cardiol*. 1969;24:629-650.

5. Doval HC, Nul DR, Grancelli HO, et al. Nonsustained ventricular tachycardia in severe heart failure. Independent marker of increased mortality due to sudden death. GESICA-GEMA Investigators. *Circulation*. 1996;94:3198-3203.

6. Kligfield P, Hochreiter C, Kramer H, et al. Complex arrhythmias in mitral regurgitation with and without mitral valve prolapse: contrast to arrhythmias in mitral valve prolapse without mitral regurgitation. *Am J Cardiol*. 1985;55:1545.

7. McLenaghan JM, Henderson E, Morris KL, et al. Ventricular arrhythmias in patients with hypertensive left ventricular hypertrophy. *N Engl J Med*. 1987;317:787-792.

8. McKenna WJ, England D, Doi YL, et al. Arrhythmia in hypertrophic cardiomyopathy: influence on prognosis. *Br Heart J*. 1981;46:168.

9. Buxton AE, Marchlinski FE, Waxman HL, et al. Prognostic factors in nonsustained ventricular tachycardia. *Am J Cardiol*. 1984;53:1275-1279.

10. Heidbuchel H, Tack J, Vanneste L, et al. Significance of arrhythmias during the first 24 hours of acute myocardial infarction treated with alteplase and effect of early administration of a beta-blocker or a bradycardic agent on their incidence. *Circulation*. 1994;89:1051-1059.

11. Bigger JT Jr, Fleiss JL, Rolnitzky LM. Prevalence, characteristics and significance of ventricular tachycardia detected by 24-hour continuous electrocardiographic recordings in the late hospital phase of acute myocardial infarction. *Am J Cardiol*. 1986;58(13):1151.

12. Buxton AE, Lee KL, Fisher JD, et al. A randomized study of the prevention of sudden death in patients with coronary artery disease. Multicenter Unsustained Tachycardia Trial Investigators. *N Engl J Med*. 1999;341(25):1882.

13. Moss AJ, Hall WJ, Cannom DS, et al. Improved survival with an implanted defibrillator in patients with coronary disease at high risk for ventricular arrhythmia. Multicenter Automatic Defibrillator Implantation Trial Investigators. *N Engl J Med*. 1996;335(26):1933-1940.

14. Buxton AE, Lee KL, DiCarlo L, et al. Nonsustained ventricular tachycardia in patients with coronary artery disease: relationship to inducible sustained ventricular tachycardia. *Ann Intern Med*. 1996;125:35-39.

15. Buxton AE, Hafley GE, Lehmann MH, et al. Prediction of sustained ventricular tachycardia inducible by programmed stimulation in patients with coronary artery disease: utility of clinical variables. *Circulation*. 1999;99:1843-1850.

16. Buxton AE, Lee KL, Hafley GE, et al. Relation of ejection fraction and inducible ventricular tachycardia to mode of death in patients with coronary artery disease: an analysis of patients enrolled in the Multicenter Unsustained Tachycardia Trial. *Circulation*. 2002;106:2466-2472.

17. Hohnloser SH, Klingenheben T, Zabel M, et al. Prevalence, characteristics and prognostic value during long-term follow-up of nonsustained ventricular tachycardia after myocardial infarction in the thrombolytic era. *J Am Coll Cardiol*. 1999;33(7):1895.

18. Bloch Thomsen PE, Jons C, Raatikainen MJ, et al. Long-term recording of cardiac arrhythmias with an implantable cardiac monitor in patients with reduced ejection fraction after acute myocardial infarction: the Cardiac Arrhythmias and Risk Stratification After Acute Myocardial Infarction (CARISMA) study. *Circulation*. 2010;122:1258-1264.

19. Echt DS, Liebson PR, Mitchell LB, et al. Mortality and morbidity in patients receiving encainide, flecainide, or placebo. The Cardiac Arrhythmia Suppression Trial. *N Engl J Med*. 1991;324(12):781.

20. Cairns JA, Connolly SJ, Roberts R, Gent M. Randomised trial of outcome after myocardial infarction in patients with frequent or repetitive ventricular premature depolarisations: CAMIAT. Canadian Amiodarone Myocardial Infarction Arrhythmia Trial Investigators. *Lancet*. 1997;349(9053):675.

21. Katritsis DG, Zareba W, Camm AJ. Nonsustained ventricular tachycardia. *J Am Coll Cardiol*. 2012;60(20):1993.

22. Daubert JP, Winters SL, Subacius H, et al. Ventricular arrhythmia inducibility predicts subsequent ICD activation in nonischemic cardiomyopathy patients: a DEFINITE substudy. *Pacing Clin Electrophysiol*. 2009;32:755-761.

23. Cheng A, Wang Y, Berger RD, et al. Electrophysiology studies in patients undergoing ICD implantation: findings from the NCDR®. *Pacing Clin Electrophysiol*. 2012;35(8):912-918.

24. Pouleur AC, Barkoudah E, Uno H, et al. Pathogenesis of sudden unexpected death in a clinical trial of patients with myocardial infarction and left ventricular dysfunction, heart failure, or both. *Circulation*. 2010;122:597-602.

25. Chen T, Koene R, Benditt DG, Lu F. Ventricular ectopy in patients with left ventricular dysfunction: should it be treated? *J Card Fail*. 2013;19(1):40-49.

18 PVC AND CARDIOMYOPATHY

Frank Bogun, MD

CASE PRESENTATION 1

A 10-year-old boy was seen for a routine physical examination by his primary care physician (PCP). He was found to have an irregular rhythm. A 12-lead ECG showed a bigeminal rhythm with premature ventricular contractions (PVCs) that displayed a left bundle branch block, inferior axis morphology. A 24-hour Holter monitor demonstrated a PVC burden of 32%. An echocardiogram demonstrated normal left ventricular function and dimensions. The boy and his parents were told not to worry about it and to be checked out again when the boy reached 18 years of age. At the age of 18, the boy, still without any symptoms returned to his PCP and got another ECG, which again showed a bigeminal rhythm (Figure 18-1). Holter monitor now showed a PVC burden of 33%, and the echocardiogram showed an EF of 30% with increased LV dimensions. The patient was started on β-blocker therapy and angiotensin-converting enzyme inhibitors and was referred to a pediatric electrophysiologist, who confirmed that the PVC burden was not suppressed by β-blocker therapy. He thereafter was referred to for an ablation procedure. During the ablation procedure, intracardiac echo was used in combination with an electroanatomic mapping system (Figure 18-2). Activation mapping was performed in the right ventricular outflow tract (RVOT) and identified a site in the posterior RVOT that preceded the onset of the PVC-QRS complex by −27 ms (Figure 18-3A). Pacing at this location reproduced a similar but not identical pace-map compared to the spontaneous PVC (Figure 18-3B). Radiofrequency energy was delivered at this location for a total of 2 minutes, and subsequently the PVC was no longer seen. A repeat echocardiogram 3 months postablation showed an ejection fraction of 40% and reduced LV dimensions. Six months postablation, the left ventricular ejection fraction had normalized to an ejection fraction of 60%, and the LV dimensions improved further. A Holter documented the absence of PVCs.

PVC MECHANISM

Triggered activity via delayed after depolarizations is the most likely mechanism of frequent PVCs, although reentry, especially in patients with structural heart disease and frequent PVCs, has been suggested as a possible mechanism as well.[1] Reentry as a mechanism for PVCs has thus far only been demonstrated in animal models.[2]

PVC CARDIOMYOPATHY: AGGRAVATING FACTORS

Several features in this patient are associated with PVC cardiomyopathy. First, the PVC's burden is >24%. This cut-off value best separated patients with PVC-induced cardiomyopathy from patients without PVC-mediated cardiomyopathy.[3] Of note is that although based on ROC curves this cut-off value could be determined, not

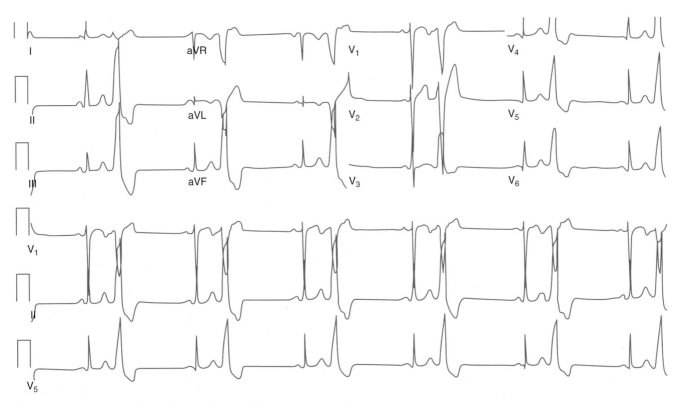

FIGURE 18-1 Shown is a 12-lead ECG with frequent PVCs in a bigeminal rhythm.

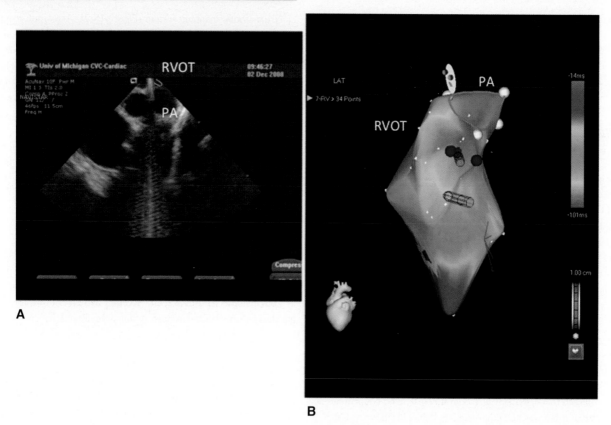

FIGURE 18-2 (A) Illustrates a view of the intracardiac echocardiogram with the ablation catheter located in the right ventricular outflow tract (RVOT; green icon) just below the pulmonary valve. (B) Illustrates an electroanatomic activation map of the RVOT from a left anterior oblique view. Brown tags indicate ablation lesions. The pulmonary annulus is marked (PA).

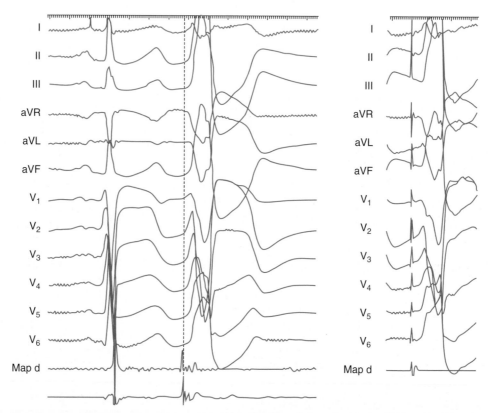

FIGURE 18-3 (A) Shown is the 12-lead ECG tracings and intracardiac recordings from the earliest endocardial site obtained during activation mapping of the PVC in the RVOT. (B) Shown is the 12-lead of the pace-map when pacing is performed from this location.

everyone with a PVC burden >24% had evidence of PVC-induced cardiomyopathy. About 25% of the patients with a higher PVC burden had normal left ventricular function. On the other hand, patients with a lower PVC burden were also at risk for PVC-induced cardiomyopathy, and the lowest PVC burden associated with PVC-induced cardiomyopathy was 10%.

By history, this patient's PVCs were present for at least 10 years. Despite the fact that there is no documentation that the patient's PVC burden was constant, data from Niwano et al suggest that a particular PVC burden often persists over several years.[4] Multivariate analysis has recently demonstrated that a history of palpitations persisting more than 60 months was independently associated with PVC cardiomyopathy.[5] In this study, the duration of palpitations was used as a surrogate for the amount of time a patient was exposed to PVCs.

Finally, this patient was asymptomatic, which appears to be another factor predisposing patients to PVC-induced cardiomyopathy.[5] It is likely that asymptomatic patients seek medical attention later than symptomatic patients, thereby prolonging the exposure time to frequent PVCs.

PVC CARDIOMYOPATHY: NATURAL HISTORY

Not much data is available for the long-term natural history of patients with idiopathic PVCs, that is, in the absence of structural heart disease. In many prior reports where PVCs were associated with adverse outcome, the absence of structural heart disease was not well established.[6] Niwano et al[4] followed 239 patients without structural heart disease (confirmed by echocardiography and MRI) for at least 4 years. During follow-up, a decline in left ventricular function (>6%) was found in 13 patients. Most of these patients had very frequent PVCs that were defined as >20,000/24 hours in this study.

PVC CARDIOMYOPATHY: MECHANISM

The mechanism of PVC-induced cardiomyopathy is not known. Short-term animal research does not support fibrosis as a mechanism. This is supported by clinical studies confirming the absence of scar detected by MRI in patients with PVC-induced cardiomyopathy.[7] A form of tachycardia-mediated cardiomyopathy is also unlikely, since the average heart rate in patients with PVC-induced cardiomyopathy is usually not different from patients with frequent PVCs without cardiomyopathy.[8]

PVC CARDIOMYOPATHY: THERAPY

PVC suppression by either medical therapy or ablation usually results in improvement and normalization of left ventricular function and dimensions.[9,10] In the majority of patients, LV function normalizes within 4 months after an effective ablation, but this case illustrates that the process can take a longer period of time,[11] possibly depending on the length of exposure to frequent PVCs.

PVCs: MAPPING AND ABLATION

Activation mapping is the preferred mapping modality over pace-mapping. This case illustrates that at the earliest endocardial mapping site no perfect match of the pace-map with the spontaneous PVC was demonstrated. In theory, pacing at the site of origin of a ventricular arrhythmia should result in a perfect replication of the targeted ventricular

arrhythmia morphology, provided that the pacing cycle length is equal to the cycle length of the ventricular arrhythmia (for VT) or equal to the coupling interval in the setting of PVCs. Perfect pace-maps, however, are not always present, even when the ventricular arrhythmia can be eliminated within seconds of a radiofrequency energy application. A pace-map score of ≥10/12 leads when comparing the paced QRS morphology to the targeted ventricular arrhythmia QRS-morphology is often used to indicate a "matching pace-map." With intramural foci, there is an early activation at the endocardial breakthrough site; however, the pace-map does not match the targeted morphology of the ventricular arrhythmia, similar to the case illustrated here. The PVC focus was successfully eliminated at the location of the earliest endocardial activation. The earliest site was on the interventricular septum, arguing for an intramural focus. Intramural septal foci can be effectively ablated from one side of the septum, but may require ablation from the other side as well.[12] This was not necessary in this patient.

CASE PRESENTATION 2

A 19-year-old woman presented with syncope and rapid palpitations to the emergency department. She had undergone a failed VT ablation procedure 2 weeks ago and was treated with verapamil. She was transferred to our hospital for further treatment. Prior to the initial ablation, a 24-hour Holter monitor showed frequent PVCs with a PVC burden of 12% and frequent runs of repetitive, nonsustained VT (ns VT; 1100 runs). After the initial ablation procedure, during which an RVOT focus was targeted, her PVC burden was 30%, with only 69 runs of nsVT. The PVCs (Figure 18-4A) had a similar morphology when compared with the VT (Figure 18-4B). The patient was taken to the EP laboratory; with isoproterenol infusion she developed frequent PVCs and easily inducible, sustained, and nonsustained VT. The VT morphology was a right bundle branch block, inferior axis morphology. The mapping procedure was started within the coronary venous system that was mapped with a multipolar catheter documenting the earliest activation time of −25 ms within the distal great cardiac vein (Figure 18-5). Pacing from poles 9/10 produced a similar pace-map (Figure 18-6). Mapping of the aortic cusp using an open irrigated-tip catheter with an electroanatomic mapping system and with intracardiac ultrasound was performed subsequently. A site in the left cusp was identified where a sharp potential preceded the onset of the QRS complex by 35 ms. Radiofrequency energy was delivered. This, however, failed to eliminate the VT. The catheter was moved more cephalad, closer to the left main ostium, and a site with a prematurity of −37 ms was identified (Figure 18-7). Pacing at this site failed to reproduce the same morphology of the targeted VT (see Figure 18-7). The ostium of the left main coronary artery was identified by intracardiac ultrasound and was marked in the 3-D echocardiographic reconstruction of the aortic cusp and the left ventricle (Figure 18-8). The left main coronary artery was canalized with a diagnostic catheter and felt to be about 1 cm away from this site (Figure 18-9). Radiofrequency energy was delivered during VT, while repeated injections into the left main coronary artery were performed in order to ensure continued patency of the vessel (see Figure 18-9). The VT terminated during RF energy delivery and could no longer be induced subsequently. At this point the procedure was terminated. The patient had no recurrence of her VT or PVCs.

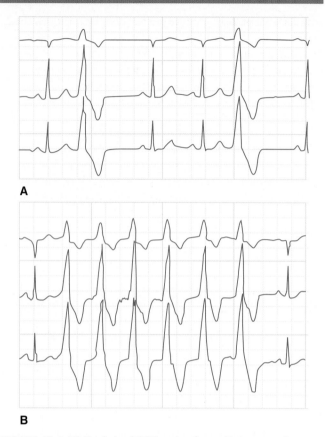

A

B

FIGURE 18-4 (A) Single lead ECG tracing from a Holter recording showing a trigeminal rhythm. (B) Same single lead tracing showing nonsustained VT. The single lead tracing of the PVC is very similar to the nonsustained VT.

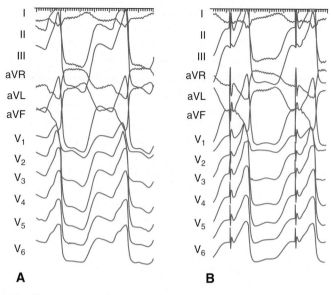

A   **B**

FIGURE 18-6 (A) Twelve-lead ECG morphology of the targeted VT. (B) Pace-map from within the coronary venous system from the earliest site displayed in Figure 18-5.

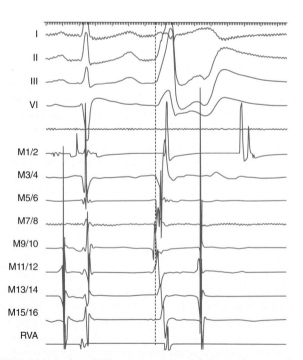

FIGURE 18-5 Surface ECG tracings I, II, III, and V₁ as well as recordings from a multipolar catheter that is deployed within the great cardiac vein. The earliest timing within the coronary venous system was an activation time of −25 ms.

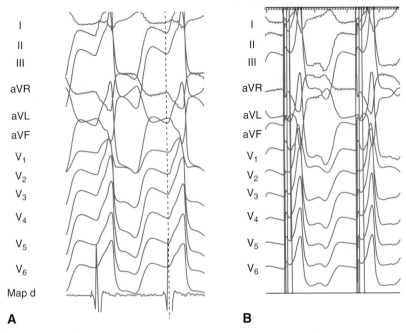

FIGURE 18-7 (A) Twelve-lead ECG of the targeted VT and intracardiac tracings illustrating the earliest activation time recorded from the left aortic cusp. (B) Pacing from this location failed to reproduce the same morphology of the targeted VT. Pacing was performed with a high output (20 mA) in order to achieve capture.

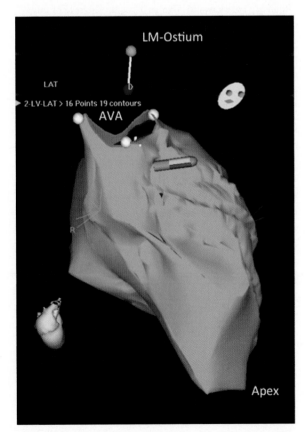

FIGURE 18-8 Three-dimensional reconstruction of the left ventricular cavity by intracardiac echocardiography. The left ventricle is displayed from a right anterior oblique view. The left main ostium is marked (olive tag) as well as the aortic valve annulus (AVA) and the left ventricular apex. The distance of the site where radiofrequency energy was delivered to the left main ostium measured 12.6 mm.

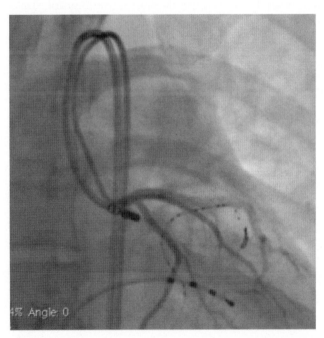

FIGURE 18-9 Shown is a right anterior oblique view of the ablation catheter within the left aortic cusp. A diagnostic coronary catheter is placed in the left main coronary artery while radiofrequency energy is delivered.

PATHOPHYSIOLOGY AND MECHANISM

Triggered activity is the etiology of most outflow tract ventricular tachycardias. Most often, outflow tract tachycardias originate from the right ventricular outflow tract, but can also originate from the aortic cusps, the epicardium, or the pulmonary arteries.

DIAGNOSIS AND MAPPING

The 12-lead ECG is critical in identifying the site of origin of an outflow tract VT. An early transition in lead V_3 and a broad R wave in lead V_1 and V_2 points toward the aortic cusps, the mitral annulus, or the basal left ventricular epicardium. A multipolar catheter within the great coronary vein (see Figures 18-6 and 18-8) demonstrated early activation in the epicardium. However, within the left aortic cusp, a site with even earlier timing was identified. Intracardiac echocardiography helped in identifying critical structures like the left main ostium, and in determining the approximate distance of the left main ostium to the target site within the cusp. The pace-map of the multipolar catheter (electrodes 9/10, the site of the earliest activation within the coronary venous system) that was placed in the great cardiac vein showed a better pace-map compared to the site where the VT was actually ablated, which had a substantially earlier activation time. Unfortunately, pace-mapping in the aortic cusps often requires a high output to capture myocardial tissue, resulting in a mismatch of the pace-map with the targeted ventricular arrhythmia. This was the case in this patient as well.

THERAPY

Delivery of radiofrequency energy was performed after identification of the left main coronary artery and confirmation that the target site was at a safe distance (ie, >7 mm) from the ostium of the left main coronary artery. Simultaneous injection of the left main coronary artery as radiofrequency energy was delivered was performed, since the earliest site of activation appeared closer to the left main coronary artery than expected (see Figure 18-9). A 3.5-mm irrigated-tip catheter was used for this purpose using a power of up to 30 watts.

REFERENCES

1. Bogun F, Crawford T, Chalfoun N, et al. Relationship of frequent postinfarction premature ventricular complexes to the reentry circuit of scar-related ventricular tachycardia. *Heart Rhythm.* 2008;5(3):367-374.

2. El-Sherif N, Scherlag BJ, Lazzara R, Hope RR. Re-entrant ventricular arrhythmias in the late myocardial infarction period. 1. Conduction characteristics in the infarction zone. *Circulation.* 1977;55(5):686-702.

3. Baman TS, Lange DC, Ilg KJ, et al. Relationship between burden of premature ventricular complexes and left ventricular function. *Heart Rhythm.* 2010;7(7):865-869.

4. Niwano S, Wakisaka Y, Niwano H, et al. Prognostic significance of frequent premature ventricular contractions originating from the ventricular outflow tract in patients with normal left ventricular function. *Heart.* 2009;95(15):1230-1237.

5. Yokokawa M, Kim HM, Good E, et al. Relation of symptoms and symptom duration to premature ventricular complex-induced cardiomyopathy. *Heart Rhythm.* 2011;**9**(1):92-5.

6. Lee V, Hemingway H, Harb R, Crake T, Lambiase P. The prognostic significance of premature ventricular complexes in adults without clinically apparent heart disease: a meta-analysis and systematic review. *Heart.* 2012;98(17): 1290-1298.

7. Yokokawa M, Kim HM, Good E, et al. Impact of QRS duration of frequent premature ventricular complexes on the development of cardiomyopathy. *Heart Rhythm.* 2012;**9**(9):1460-4.

8. Olgun H, Yokokawa M, Baman T, et al. The role of interpolation in PVC-induced cardiomyopathy. *Heart Rhythm.* 2011;8(7):1046-1049.

9. Bogun F, Crawford T, Reich S, et al. Radiofrequency ablation of frequent, idiopathic premature ventricular complexes: comparison with a control group without intervention. *Heart Rhythm.* 2007;4(7):863-867.

10. Duffee DF, Shen WK, Smith HC. Suppression of frequent premature ventricular contractions and improvement of left ventricular function in patients with presumed idiopathic dilated cardiomyopathy. *Mayo Clin Proc.* 1998;73(5):430-433.

11. Yokokawa M, Good E, Crawford T, et al. Recovery from left ventricular dysfunction after ablation of frequent premature ventricular complexes. *Heart Rhythm.* 2013;10(2):172-175.

12. Yokokawa M, Good E, Chugh A, et al. Intramural idiopathic ventricular arrhythmias originating in the intraventricular septum: mapping and ablation. *Circ Arrhythm Electrophysiol.* 2012;5(2):258-263.

VENTRICULAR TACHYCARDIA AND CARDIAC
ANATOMY: AORTIC CUSP

SECTION III
CASE STUDIES IN VENTRICULAR
TACHYCARDIA

131

19 VENTRICULAR TACHYCARDIA AND CARDIAC ANATOMY: AORTIC CUSP

Jorge Romero, MD, Luigi Di Biase , MD, PhD, FACC, FHRS, Pasquale Santangeli, MD, Alessandro Paoletti Perini, MD, Francesco Santoro, MD, Rong Bai, MD, J. David Burkhardt, MD, Andrea Natale, MD, FHRS, FESC, FACC

CASE PRESENTATION

A 48-year-old man without any significant past medical history was brought to the emergency department with severe dyspnea and dizziness. He reported similar symptoms for the past 4 months. Electrocardiogram (ECG) revealed monomorphic ventricular tachycardia (VT) at 180 bpm with a left bundle branch block (LBBB) morphology, inferior axis, early transition in lead V_2 and R/S wave amplitud >0.3 and R-wave duration index (R/QRS) > 0.5. Amiodarone was administered with restoration of normal sinus rhythm. Patient underwent electrophysiology study (EPS) with ECG showing only ventricular bigeminy right before the procedure (Figure 19-1A) and sporadic premature ventricular contractions (PVCs) during EPS. Mapping of the right ventricular outflow tract (RVOT) did not reveal

early local activation or similar pace maps. By retrograde approach, the aortic root and coronary cusps were mapped. Earliest depolarization was noted at the commissure between the right and the left aortic cusp (Figure 19-1B), and pace-mapping produced a similar QRS morphology (Figure 19-1C). After aortic angiogram was performed to visualize the coronary arteries, multiple radiofrequency energy applications were given at the commissure with suppression of spontaneous PVCs. Complete suppression was obtained at the end of the procedure. Patient has been asymptomatic for 6 years on no medical therapy without any recurrence of ventricular ectopy by ambulatory event monitoring.

EPIDEMIOLOGY

Ventricular tachycardia (VT) originating from the left ventricular outflow track (LVOT) particularly from the aortic cusp is part of the large family of the so-called "idiopathic ventricular arrhythmias" (IVT), which occur mostly in structurally normal hearts. Aortic cusp VT is rare, given that RVOT VT accounts for almost 80% to 85% of IVTs, whereas it accounts for only 30% of LVOT VTs.[1] It has no gender preference; it might occur at any age and mostly on exertion given its catecholamine-induced nature, but it can also occur at rest. Although, thought to have a benign course, patients with frequent premature ventricular contractions (PVCs) or episodes of VT might develop tachycardia-induced cardiomyopathy and sudden cardiac death. The first case series reporting, patients with VT arising from the aortic sinus of Valsalva was published in 2001. This included 12 patients with LBBB and inferior axis VT with characteristic ECG findings with previously failed ablation, all of whom were successfully ablated from the aortic root.[2]

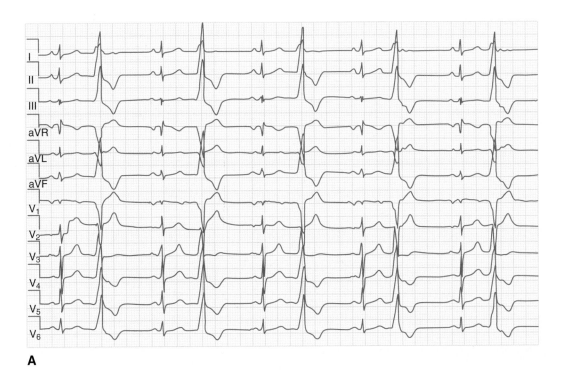

A

FIGURE 19-1A A 12-lead electrocardiogram (25 mm/sec) depicting ventricular bigeminy with an inferior axis and LBBB morphology premature ventricular contractions (PVCs). Notice a QS morphology in lead V_1 with notching on the downward deflection with precordial early transition in lead V_3 that suggests PVCs originating in the commissure between the left and right aortic cusps.

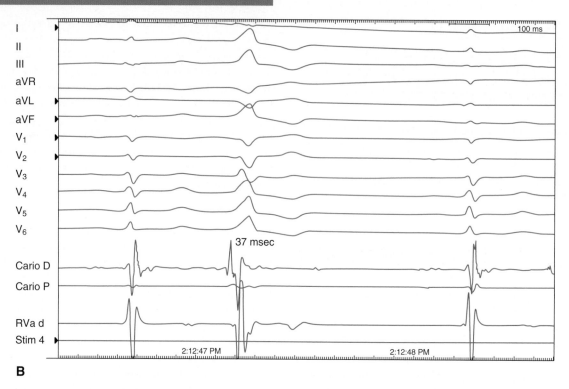

B

FIGURE 19-1B Activation mapping of the same patient using a bipolar catheter. Notice intracardiac electrograms revealing the earliest activation (ie, 37 msec) preceding the QRS complex (PVC) at the commissure between the right and the left aortic cusp.

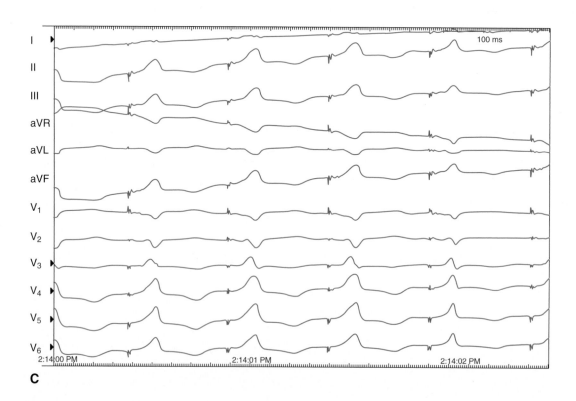

C

FIGURE 19-1C Pace-mapping demonstrating identical PVC morphology at the commissure between the right and the left aortic cusp.

VENTRICULAR TACHYCARDIA AND CARDIAC
ANATOMY: AORTIC CUSP

SECTION III
CASE STUDIES IN VENTRICULAR
TACHYCARDIA

133

ANATOMY OF THE AORTIC ROOT

The aortic valve is the "heart" of the heart. Almost every single structure is directly related to this valve including all four chambers and the rest of the cardiac valves. Its area is approximately 3 to 4 cm^2. Generally, it has three leaflets attached to the aortic annulus but in 1% to 2% of the population the aortic valve might be unicuspid, bicuspid, or quadricuspid. Right above these semilunar (crescent-shape) leaflets are the Valsalva sinuses (VS), which are small dilatation of the ascending aorta. Two of them (ie, left and right) give rise to the left main coronary artery (LMCA) and right coronary artery (RCA) from their superior aspects. They are mainly made up of connective tissue with some muscular bundles from the ventricle. The coronary ostia diameters are 2 to 5 mm for RCA and 4 to 7 mm for LMCA.

The aortic root is an anterior cardiac structure, but it is anatomically posterior and somewhat rightward related to the RVOT. The left aortic sinus is in close contact with left atrium, pulmonary artery, and aorto-mitral continuity. The right sinus is posterior to the RVOT and close proximity to the tricuspid valve, and the noncoronary sinus is anterior to the lower portion of the interatrial septum, which is of critical importance when performing transseptal punctures (Figure 19-2).

ETIOLOGY AND PHYSIOPATHOLOGY

The origin of this type of VT is mostly located at the bottom of any of the sinuses of Valsalva, most commonly from the left followed by the right and rarely from the noncoronary cusps (NCC). Pathology reports have shown that this arrhythmia arises from sleeves of myocardium in the cusps, which are most likely extensions of ventricular muscle into the base of the aortic cusps.[3] The lack of muscular tissue in the NCC renders it without a substrate for arrhythmia formation. Another hypothesis is that in patients with idiopathic dilated cardiomyopathy the basal left ventricular scar may extend into to the aortic sinus of Valsalva, providing the substrate for aortic cusp VT.[4]

Accumulating evidence has suggested that this arrhythmia is related to cAMP-mediated triggered activity with an increase of intracellular calcium, which causes early or delayed after-depolarizations. Consequently, similarly to RVOT VT and other forms of LVOT VT, aortic cusp VT is sensitive to substances (ie, adenosine, acetylcholine, β-blockers) that directly interact with adenylyl cyclase by inhibiting the production of cAMP through G proteins.[5] Likewise, verapamil might also terminate this arrhythmia by direct blocking of calcium receptors and in turn diminishing the available calcium to the sarcoplasmic reticulum.

DIAGNOSIS

Clinical Presentation

• Broad spectrum from monomorphic premature ventricular contractions (PVCs) to repetitive nonsustained VT (NSVT) or paroxysmal sustained monomorphic VT (SMVT).

• Programmed stimulation during EPS can induce and terminate it, especially in patients presenting with SMVT.

Diagnostic Tests

• ECG at rest, signal average electrocardiogram (SAECG), and microvolt T-wave alternans (TWA) are usually unremarkable.

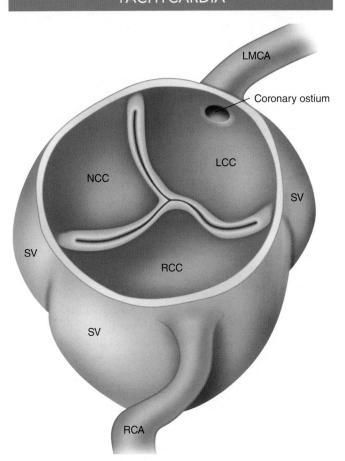

FIGURE 19-2 Aortic root with a transverse section at the level of the sinotubular junction depicting each of the three aortic sinuses of Valsalva (SV), the left coronary cusp (LCC), the right coronary cusp (RCC), and the noncoronary cusp (NCC). The left main coronary artery (LMCA) and the right coronary artery (RCA) are also noted.

- Exercise testing might induce VT in the vast majority of patients who present with SMVT but only a small percentage of patients with NSVT or PVCs.[6]

- Based on its mechanism of action (ie, cAMP-triggered activity), this arrhythmia can be initiated and terminated by programmed stimulation with either atrial or ventricular rapid pacing during EPS, sometimes requiring isoproterenol infusion.

- Entrainment is not feasible due to lack of a reentry loop.

- Adenosine, verapamil, and vasovagal maneuvers usually terminate this arrhythmia.

- For those patients presenting with frequent PVCs, 24-hour Holter monitoring should be considered to assess PVC burden.

Electrocardiography

The 12-lead ECG during episodes of VT is of paramount importance since it might narrow the differential diagnosis and guide the approach of VT ablation. Specific ECG patterns have been recognized in order to localize the exact place where the studied VT is originating. The PVC/VT usually has a LBBB morphology and inferior axis (positive deflection in inferior leads). The main and most helpful criterion to differentiate among the large variety of VT coming from the "ventricular outlet track" is the QRS transition zone in the precordial leads, in which QRS complex becomes positive. The basic approach is as follows:

- The more anterior the VT source is, the later the transition in the precordial leads is going to be (ie, leads V_4-V_5).

- Conversely, the more posterior the structure, the earlier the transition zone will be (ie, V_1-V_2).

- Consequently, RVOT-VT and LVOT-VT usually have transition zones in V_4-V_5 and V_1-V_2, respectively. There are more specific criteria in order to further localize each arrhythmia in each outlet track.

RVOT

- Transition zone V_3 or later + QRS duration <140 msec favors the septum.

- Transition zone V_4 or later + QRS >140 msec favors the free wall.

- To discern from left to right within the RVOT, QS complex amplitude in aVR and aVL is usually analyzed.
  - If aVR > aVL favors a right location.
  - If aVR < aVL favors a left location.

- To discern a superior origin within the RVOT:
  - a high R-wave amplitude in V_1 indicates a superior origin.
  - a low R-wave amplitude in V_1 indicates an inferior location.[7]

Pulmonary Artery

- Transition zone in V_3-V_4

- High amplitude R waves in inferior leads since it is superior to RVOT

- QS in aVL > aVR (leftward of RVOT)

- qR in lead I[8]

Tricuspid Valve

The vast majority of VTs in tricuspid annulus originate in the proximity to His-bundle (para-Hisian or anteroseptal).

- Transition zone V_2-V_3.

- Low amplitude R waves in inferior leads since it is inferior to RVOT.

- a RR' or RsR' pattern in aVL.

- No R wave in V_1.[9]

Aortic Cusp

- Transition zone in V_2-V_3 with rS morphology in V_1-V_2.

- R/S wave amplitude index >0.3 and R-wave duration index (R/QRS) >0.5 examined in V_1-V_2 favors VT originating from sinuses of Valsalva.

- An earlier R/S transition zone (V2) and higher R-wave amplitude and duration for VTs from the left coronary cusp (LCC) when compared to the VTs coming from the right coronary cusp (RCC).[10]
  - In LCC VT, inferior leads have a pointed and tall positive QRS, notched QRS in V_6, and rS pattern in lead I.

- VTs from the commissure between the left and right aortic cusps generally have a qrS pattern in leads V_1-V_3 and/or have a QS morphology in lead V_1 with notching on the downward deflection with precordial transition at lead V_3.[11,12]

Epicardial Sites (Great Cardiac and Anterior Interventricular Veins)

- Early transition zone V_2-V_3 (generally RBBB)

- aVL/aVR wave amplitude index >1.4

- S wave in V_1 >1.2 mV

- A useful ECG parameter to differentiate this origin from aortic cusp VTs is the intrinsicoid deflection (R-wave peak time/QRS) >55% indicating a slowed initial precordial QRS activation.[13]

Aortic Valve–Mitral Valve Continuity (AV-MV)

- Transition zone V_1-V_2 almost simulating a RBBB morphology.

- Broad monophasic R-waves throughout the precordial leads.

- S wave in V_6 particularly if the source is the anterolateral, lateral, or posterior portion of the mitral annulus[14] (Figures 19-3A and 19-3B).

DIFFERENTIAL DIAGNOSIS

As mentioned in the diagnosis section, there are a myriad of distinct VTs that can mimic aortic cusp VT. Besides different types of IVT originating from RVOT, pericardium and mitral, or tricuspid annuli, it is worth mentioning that arrhythmogenic right ventricular dysplasia/cardiomyopathy (ARVD/C) sometimes presents with a similar ECG pattern (ie, LBBB and inferior axis). Nevertheless, the ECG in this inherited cardiomyopathy is often accompanied by T-wave inversion in the right precordial leads and rarely with the pathognomonic epsilon wave. Magnetic resonance with delayed enhancement and endomyocardial biopsy might help in the diagnosis by identification of myocardial fibro-fatty infiltration.

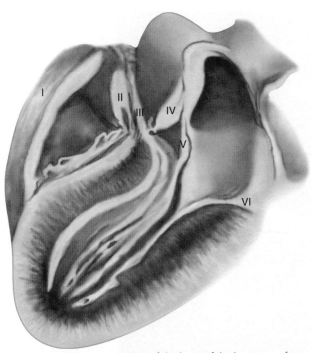

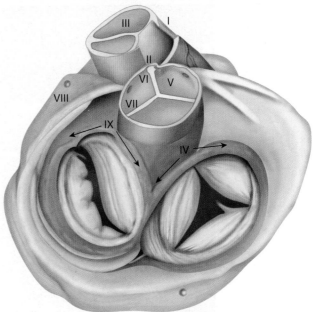

FIGURE 19-3B Short axis view of the heart seen from left to right. (I) Right ventricular outflow track (RVOT) anterior wall; (II) RVOT posterior wall; (III) right coronary cusp (RCC); (IV) left coronary cusp (LCC); (V) Aortic valve-mitral valve continuity (AV-MV) and mitral annulus.

FIGURE 19-3A Long axis view of the base of the heart seen from above. Note the close relationship between the aortic valve and the RVOT, pulmonary, and mitral valves. The roman numerals indicate possible sites of origin of VT and their relationship with the aortic sinus of Valsalva: (I) Right ventricular outflow track (RVOT) anterior wall; (II) RVOT posterior wall; (III) pulmonary valve; (IV) tricuspid valve; (V) right coronary cusp (RCC); (VI) commissure between the left and right aortic cusps; (VII) left coronary cusp (LCC); (VIII) interventricular vein (Epicardial site); (IX) Aortic valve-mitral valve continuity (AV-MV).

MANAGEMENT

Pharmacological Therapy

Acute Management

In the acute setting, aortic cusp VT responds very well to escalating doses of adenosine starting with 6 mg and up to 18 mg every 2 minutes. Verapamil IV and lidocaine drip might also be reasonable options.

Chronic Management

Asymptomatic or mildly symptomatic patients are mostly treated with β-blockers with minimal suppression of ventricular ectopy. Moreover, nondihydropyridine calcium channel blockers (CCB) such as diltiazem and verapamil can be added to refractory cases as an adjuvant therapy. Antiarrhythmic medications (eg, amiodarone, sotalol) have also been implemented in the management of these patients with satisfactory results. However, several permanent side effects of these medications, particularly of amiodarone, outweigh their potential therapeutic benefits.

Invasive Therapy

Catheter ablation (CA) is usually reserved for the management of symptomatic patients with frequent episodes of NSVT/SMVT, for patients with significant PVC burden quantified by ambulatory monitoring, or for patients with history of presyncope or syncope.

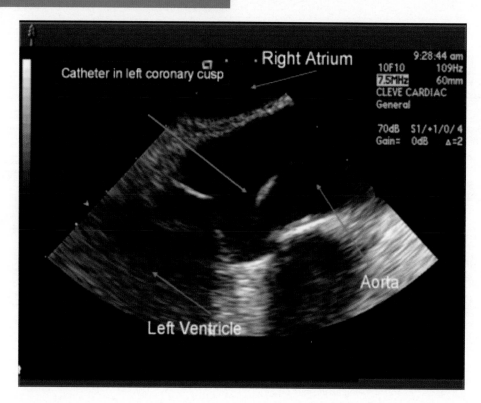

FIGURE 19-4 Ablation of the left coronary cusp guided by intracardiac echocardiography (ICE). Direct and constant visualization of the left main coronary artery (LMCA) significantly reduces the risk of severe complication while performing this procedure.

If quantification of burden of PVCs is greater than 20% to 25% even in asymptomatic patients, CA is strongly recommended in order to prevent or correct LV dysfunction.[15]

CA is highly effective with success rates ranging from 90% to 95%. CA of aortic cusp VT may be challenging due to the complex anatomy. Several structures within the LVOT and RVOT are only separated by millimeters, and completely different approaches might be needed in order to map and ablate any specific type of IVT. Nevertheless, once mapping is performed and the exact localization of the VT source is achieved, CA is relatively simpler than in patients with VT due to structural heart disease since the area to be ablated is significantly smaller and more superficial.

Frequently, induction of the ventricular arrhythmia being studied during EPS may be cumbersome and infusion of isoproterenol alone or in combination with phenylephrine may be necessary. Subsequently, heavy sedation or general anesthesia should be avoided if feasible.

Activation mapping is thought to be the most accurate way to identify the earliest site of activation during spontaneous or induced PVC/VT and subsequently the best modality to obtain high success (see Figure 19-1B). The mapping is completed via a retrograde approach through the femoral arteries, usually after having mapped the RVOT and coronary sinus meticulously.

Although pace-mapping has been widely used, it might yield inadequate sites for ablation because similar VT maps can be obtained with a radius of 10 mm from the VT source (see Figure 19-1C). Yamada et al demonstrated that VT originating from the aortic cusps

often (25%) shows preferential conduction to the RVOT with both closer match of QRS morphology from the RVOT than pacing from within the aortic cusp and significantly longer stimulus-QRS interval from aortic cusp than from RVOT, which renders pace-mapping less reliable.[16] Nevertheless, Azegami et al compared the special resolution and specificity of both pacing and activation mapping using three-dimensional mapping technologies. They reported that the mean area of myocardium activated within the first 10 msec was 3.0 ± 1.6 cm^2, concluding that neither of these two techniques yields perfect targets for ablation since the special resolution of each technique is only modest. Hence, the integration of both of them might be the best approach and it was the approach used for the case presented in this review.

Identification of the right coronary artery (RCA) and left main coronary artery (LMCA) ostia is routinely performed by most electrophysiology laboratories. This might be achieved by different imaging modalities, including aortic root angiography and intracardiac echocardiography (ICE) (Figure 19-4). LMCA or RCA can be cannulated for guidance and protection during CA. The mean distance between the coronary ostia and ablation site is in general 11 millimeters.

CA frequently uses radiofrequency energy, which is maintained for 100 to 120 seconds to reach a temperature of 131°F (55°C), generally low power (15-30 watts) is enough at this area. CA should preferably be performed with simultaneous fluoroscopy to assess catheter position at all times. Cryoablation has been proposed and tested for aortic cusp ablation to prevent potential complication particularly damage of the coronary arteries with less favorable success rates.

VENTRICULAR TACHYCARDIA AND CARDIAC
ANATOMY: AORTIC CUSP

SECTION III
CASE STUDIES IN VENTRICULAR
TACHYCARDIA

137

COMPLICATIONS

Coronary artery thombosis, stenosis, rupture, or dissection may occur in a minority of cases. Likewise, either aortic rupture with cardiac effusion/tamponade or fistulae to left or right atria and aortic dissection have been reported. Aortic insufficiency and aortic leaflet perforation can also occur.

REFERENCES

1. Iwai S, Cantillon DJ, Kim RJ, et al. Right and left ventricular outflow tract tachycardias: evidence for a common electrophysiologic mechanism. *J Cardiovasc Electrophysiol.* 2006;17(10):1052-1058.

2. Kanagaratnam L, Tomassoni G, Schweikert R, et al. Ventricular tachycardias arising from the aortic sinus of valsalva: an underrecognized variant of left outflow tract ventricular tachycardia. *J Am Coll Cardiol.* 2001;37(4):1408-1414.

3. Hasdemir C, Aktas S, Govsa F, et al. Demonstration of ventricular myocardial extensions into the pulmonary artery and aorta beyond the ventriculo-arterial junction. *Pacing Clin Electrophysiol.* 2007;30(4):534-539.

4. Yokokawa M, Good E, Crawford T, et al. Ventricular tachycardia originating from the aortic sinus cusp in patients with idiopathic dilated cardiomyopathy. *Heart Rhythm.* 2011;8(3):357-360.

5. Lerman BB. Response of nonreentrant catecholamine-mediated ventricular tachycardia to endogenous adenosine and acetylcholine. Evidence for myocardial receptor-mediated effects. *Circulation.* 1993;87(2):382-390.

6. Gill JS, Prasad K, Blaszyk K, Ward DE, Camm AJ. Initiating sequences in exercise induced idiopathic ventricular tachycardia of left bundle branch-like morphology. *Pacing Clin Electrophysiol.* 1998;21(10):1873-1880.

7. Kamakura S, Shimizu W, Matsuo K, et al. Localization of optimal ablation site of idiopathic ventricular tachycardia from right and left ventricular outflow tract by body surface ECG. *Circulation.* 1998;98(15):1525-1533.

8. Sekiguchi Y, Aonuma K, Takahashi A, et al. Electrocardiographic and electrophysiologic characteristics of ventricular tachycardia originating within the pulmonary artery. *J Am Coll Cardiol.* 2005;45(6):887-895.

9. Tada H, Tadokoro K, Ito S, et al. Idiopathic ventricular arrhythmias originating from the tricuspid annulus: prevalence, electrocardiographic characteristics, and results of radiofrequency catheter ablation. *Heart Rhythm.* 2007;4(1):7-16.

10. Ouyang F, Fotuhi P, Ho SY, et al. Repetitive monomorphic ventricular tachycardia originating from the aortic sinus cusp: electrocardiographic characterization for guiding catheter ablation. *J Am Coll Cardiol.* 2002;39(3):500-508.

11. Yamada T, Yoshida N, Murakami Y, et al. Electrocardiographic characteristics of ventricular arrhythmias originating from the junction of the left and right coronary sinuses of Valsalva in the aorta: the activation pattern as a rationale for the electrocardiographic characteristics. *Heart Rhythm.* 2008;5(2):184-192.

12. Bala R, Garcia FC, Hutchinson MD, et al. Electrocardiographic and electrophysiologic features of ventricular arrhythmias originating from the right/left coronary cusp commissure. *Heart Rhythm.* 2010;7(3):312-322.

13. Daniels DV, Lu YY, Morton JB, et al. Idiopathic epicardial left ventricular tachycardia originating remote from the sinus of Valsalva: electrophysiological characteristics, catheter ablation, and identification from the 12-lead electrocardiogram. *Circulation.* 2006;113(13):1659-1666.

14. Kumagai K, Fukuda K, Wakayama Y, et al. Electrocardiographic characteristics of the variants of idiopathic left ventricular outflow tract ventricular tachyarrhythmias. *J Cardiovasc Electrophysiol.* 2008;19(5):495-501.

15. Takemoto M, Yoshimura H, Ohba Y, et al. Radiofrequency catheter ablation of premature ventricular complexes from right ventricular outflow tract improves left ventricular dilation and clinical status in patients without structural heart disease. *J Am Coll Cardiol* 2005;45(8):1259-1265.

16. Yamada T, Murakami Y, Yoshida N, et al. Preferential conduction across the ventricular outflow septum in ventricular arrhythmias originating from the aortic sinus cusp. *J Am Coll Cardiol.* 2007;50(9):884-891.

20 MAPPING AND ABLATION OF VENTRICULAR TACHYCARDIA: VOLTAGE MAPPING

Haris M.Haqqani, MBBS (Hons), PhD, and David J. Callans, MD

CASE PRESENTATION

A 33-year-old construction worker with nonischemic dilated cardiomyopathy (DCM) presented with multiple implantable cardioverter-defibrillator (ICD) shocks due to recurrent monomorphic ventricular tachycardia (VT). He had mild global left ventricular (LV) systolic dysfunction with an ejection fraction (EF) of 40% and basal septal intramural delayed gadolinium enhancement (DGE) on magnetic resonance imaging (MRI). He had failed medical therapy with amiodarone and mexiletine and underwent catheter ablation. Three unmappable VT morphologies were induced, including a left bundle branch block (LBBB) morphology, VT of 325 ms cycle length that corresponded to the clinical VT on cycle length, and ICD electrogram analysis (VT 1). Electroanatomic voltage mapping was then performed to define the VT substrate with a 3.5-mm tip open-irrigated catheter using a point-by-point contact mapping technique (Figure 20-1). Endocardial bipolar voltage was normal (>1.5 mV) in both the left and right ventricles (RV) (Figure 20-1A).[1] Epicardial bipolar volt-

age mapping showed normal voltage (>1.0 mV) in all areas except those overlying the coronary arteries in the interventricular and atrioventricular sulci (Figure 20-1B).[2] This corresponds to the expected location of epicardial fat, which exerts an electrogram-attenuating effect on the signal generated by the underlying epimyocardium. No fractionated or isolated late potentials were seen to suggest the presence of epicardial fibrosis.[2] Unipolar electrogram analysis of the RV endocardial map suggested a normal RV free-wall voltage (>5.5 mV) (Figure 20-1C).[3] Unipolar electrogram analysis of the LV did not suggest the presence of any basolateral LV intramural substrate; however, the basal septum exhibited low unipolar signal amplitude (<8.3 mV) from both the LV and RV aspect.[4] This very likely corresponded to the septal area of DGE seen on the MRI (Figure 20-1D, arrows).[4] The putative exit of all three VTs was mapped to the basal septal region using pace-mapping, and extensive substrate ablation here rendered the patient noninducible (Figure 20-2).

CASE EXPLANATION

Catheter ablation of scar-related VT is often beset by the problem of multiple poorly tolerated, unstable VT morphologies that cannot be defined by entrainment mapping. These unmappable VTs need to be targeted in sinus rhythm, and their critical circuit components are invariably located in zones of fibrosis. The various forms of structural heart disease that cause scar-related VT usually display confluent areas of myocardial surface fibrosis. This involves the endocardium in ischemic (postinfarct) cardiomyopathy or the epicardium in arrhythmogenic right ventricular dysplasia. The various forms of nonischemic dilated cardiomyopathy (DCM) are characterized by diffuse interstitial and replacement fibrosis, and

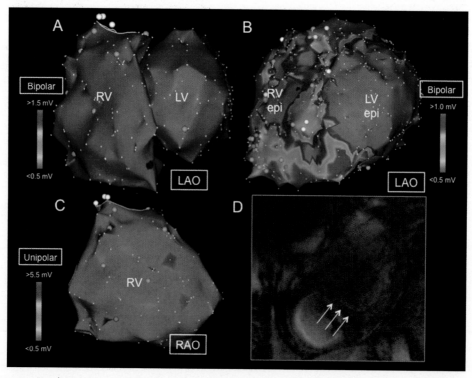

FIGURE 20-1 Electroanatomic voltage maps in a 33-year-old man with nonischemic idiopathic dilated cardiomyopathy.

MAPPING AND ABLATION OF VENTRICULAR
TACHYCARDIA: VOLTAGE MAPPING

SECTION III
CASE STUDIES IN VENTRICULAR
TACHYCARDIA

139

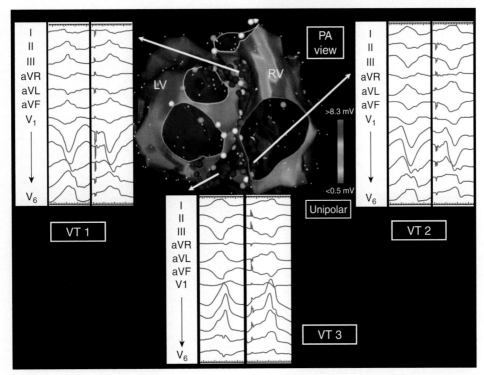

FIGURE 20-2 Posteroanterior projection of unipolar biventricular voltage maps showing periannular septal and infundibular substrate. The three inducible VTs were pace-mapped to this region where radiofrequency ablation rendered them noninducible.

this may result in a basolateral, predominantly epicardial pattern scarring. However, the normal endocardial and epicardial bipolar surface voltage maps in a VT patient with DCM strongly suggested the presence of intramural substrate. Unipolar electrograms have a wider "field-of-view" and may be sensitive to deeper layers of fibrosis within the myocardium. In this case, substrate mapping disclosed the presence of unipolar low voltage on basal septum, suggestive of intramural scarring that corresponded to the DGE-defined fibrosis seen with MRI.

VENTRICULAR ELECTROGRAM RECORDING AND DEFINITIONS

Contact intracardiac electrograms are recorded from the ventricles by placing the distal recording electrodes of a mapping catheter at sequential endocardial or epicardial sites. Typical mapping catheters in current use employ a 3.5-mm distal tip electrode, a 2-mm ring electrode on the shaft, with a 1-mm interelectrode spacing. Unipolar electrograms can be recorded from each of these two electrodes using either Wilson's central terminal or an indifferent electrode in the inferior vena cava. Bipolar electrograms are recorded between the tip and ring electrodes by vector summation of their individual unipolar signals. The signals are digitized and amplified and then subject to high and low pass filtration to remove the effects of low-frequency respiratory noise and high-frequency electrical noise from the final processed electrogram.

Cassidy et al found that normal ventricular bipolar electrograms recorded from healthy myocardial tissue (with a 10-mm bipole, filtered at 30-500 Hz) exhibit characteristic properties (Figure 20-3A). They have sharp, biphasic, or triphasic deflections with peak-to-peak amplitude ≥ 3 mV, duration <70 ms, and/or amplitude:duration ratio >0.045.[5] As they are acquired, normal and abnormal electrograms

can be plotted onto color-coded three-dimensional voltage maps using an electroanatomic mapping system.

All forms of ventricular scarring cause disruption to the normal myocardial syncytial architecture, variably replacing necrotic or apoptotic cardiomyocytes with collagen. In dense sheets of scar, surviving myocyte bundles may be present with abnormally slow and circuitous electrical activation due to the insulating effects of confluent fibrotic zones as well as the loss of normal cell-to-cell coupling. This slow conduction can be also caused by more diffuse interstitial and replacement fibrosis. In either case, electrograms recorded from such regions display reduced peak-to-peak amplitude due to lesser action potential summation from the lower surviving myocyte mass. Additionally, the slow conduction caused by shards of fibrosis results in electrogram prolongation, with multiple deflections commonly seen due to adjacent myocyte bundles being sequentially activated in delayed fashion, rather than rapidly in parallel. These electrogram changes are known as fractionation, and fractioned ventricular electrograms display multiple deflections from baseline, an amplitude ≤ 0.5 mV, a duration ≥ 133 ms, and/or amplitude:duration ratio <0.005 (Figure 20-3B). If delayed conduction occurs into surviving myocyte bundles that are well insulted by surrounding collagen sheets, late components of the local electrogram may be inscribed at a discernible interval (with an isoelectric duration of >20 ms) after the initial electrogram component, which is usually a far-field signal (Figure 20-3C). In very slow conduction regions, these potentials may occur well after the surface QRS complex (Figure 20-3D). These are known variably as late potentials (LP) or isolated late potentials (ILP) and likely represent depolarization of anatomically constrained surviving fiber bundles within dense sheets of scar.[6] Local abnormal ventricular activities (LAVA) is another term used to describe similar electrogram abnormalities within scar.[7]

BIPOLAR ENDOCARDIAL VOLTAGE MAPPING

Electrogram amplitude and morphology analysis and interpretation is greatly facilitated by the use of electroanatomic mapping systems. These systems all localize the tip of the mapping catheter in 3-dimensional space and can use this to create a virtual geometric shell of the ventricle. Electrogram information can be incorporated into this shell using color coding to generate 3-dimensional voltage maps (Figure 20-4).[8] Using an electroanatomic mapping system and detailed point-by-point sinus rhythm mapping in patients without structural heart disease, Marchlinski et al were able to define the normal LV and RV endocardial bipolar voltage limits.[1] They found that the mean bipolar electrogram amplitude in these normal ventricles was 4.8 ± 3.1 mV with 95% of LV recordings displaying a bipolar voltage >1.55 mV. Patients with prior myocardial infarct tend to have a relatively sharp demarcation between the normal ventricle and the area of scar. The border zone of the scar corresponds to the area of bipolar voltage ≤ 1.5 mV, but the majority of most postinfarct scars contain confluent areas of <0.5 mV, the so-called dense-scar region (Figure 20-4).[1,9] Several chronic infarct large animal models have validated bipolar voltage mapping against pathologic analysis and imaging of the infarct scar. Callans et al found that the scar area as imaged using intracardiac echocardiography (ICE) corresponded to the area subtended by bipolar electrogram voltages of ≤ 2.0 mV, with the pathologically defined area correlating best with bipolar signal amplitude of ≤ 1.0 mV. Reddy et al were able to show that the area defined by bipolar electrogram amplitude of ≤ 1.5 mV correlated very well with the pathologically defined infarct ($r = 0.96$, $P = 0.0007$).[10]

EPICARDIAL VOLTAGE MAPPING

The advent of percutaneous epicardial mapping allowed for the successful ablation of VT associated with many nonischemic substrates (eg, Chagasic cardiomyopathy, idiopathic DCM, arrhythmogenic right ventricular dysplasia [ARVD]) in which epicardial VT circuit components are a common finding. While similar substrate mapping criteria could be used on the epicardium as on the endocardium, the presence of epicardial fat can act as a unique confounder by its potential insulating effect, leading to electrogram attenuation. Cano et al analyzed epicardial electrograms in 8 patients without structural heart disease and found a mean bipolar voltage of 3.2 ± 2.5 mV with 95% of all signals having a bipolar amplitude of >0.94 mV when signals over the atrioventricular (AV) grooves and large coronary vessels were excluded.[2] On this basis, they defined a normal epicardial bipolar electrogram voltage to be >1.0 mV (Figure 20-5). More importantly, however, these investigators found that epicardial scar could not be defined on the basis of voltage alone and that electrogram analysis plays a pivotal role. In patients with idiopathic DCM, epicardial scar was strongly suggested by the presence of fractionated or isolated potentials, rather than just low voltage, as such signals were generally not found in the region of the AV grooves or the large coronary vessels (Figure 20-5).[2]

UNIPOLAR VOLTAGE MAPPING

The unipolar ventricular electrogram, recorded between the tip electrode and an indifferent electrode or Wilson's central terminal, potentially has a larger "field of view," and this makes it more susceptible to recording artefacts. Nevertheless, the peak-to-peak amplitude

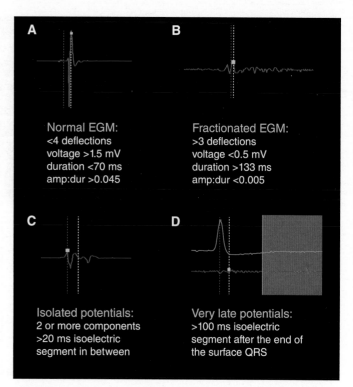

FIGURE 20-3 Characteristics of normal, fractionated, isolated, and very late ventricular electrograms.

MAPPING AND ABLATION OF VENTRICULAR
TACHYCARDIA: VOLTAGE MAPPING

SECTION III
CASE STUDIES IN VENTRICULAR
TACHYCARDIA

141

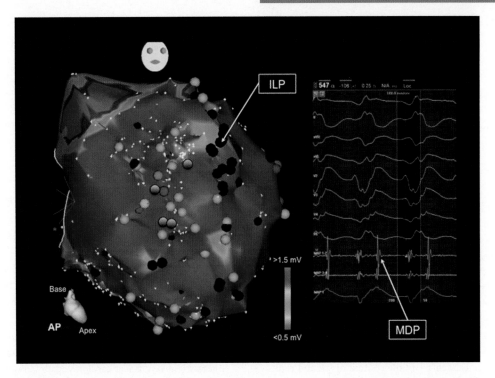

FIGURE 20-4 Endocardial left ventricular substrate map of a 68-year-old man with severe ischemic cardiomyopathy (with three prior infarcts and bypass graft surgery), ejection fraction 20%, who presented in near incessant VT requiring multiple ICD shocks. He has a large area of anteroapicoseptal scar with multiple isolated late potentials (ILP) found throughout. In VT, the labeled ILP corresponded to a mid-diastolic potential (MDP) that was proven to be an entrance site to the common central isthmus. Ablation here terminated the tachycardia early, and further ablation rendered it noninducible.

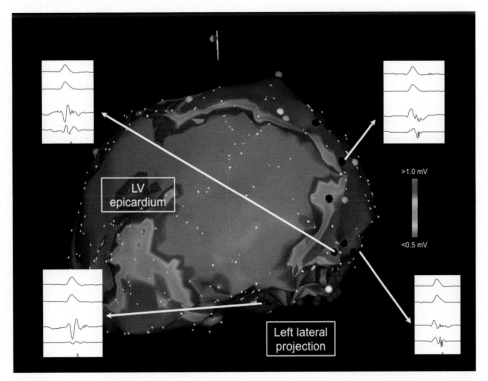

FIGURE 20-5 Epicardial voltage map of a 48-year-old man with dilated cardiomyopathy showing a periannular substrate distribution with isolated and fractionated electrograms recorded within basal low-voltage (bipolar voltage <1.0 mV) areas.

TABLE 20-1 Normal Ventricular Electrogram Voltage Criteria

LV endocardium	>1.5 mV	>8.3 mV
RV endocardial free wall	>1.5 mV	>5.5 mV
RV endocardial septum	>1.5 mV	>8.3 mV
Epicardium	>1.0 mV	

LV = left ventricular; RV = right ventricular.

of the initial unipolar forces may allow the effects of deeper layers of fibrosis to be manifest when the bipolar signal is normal. Hutchinson et al found that the mean unipolar left ventricular electrogram voltage recorded from normal ventricles in patients without structural heart disease was 19.6 ± 6.9 mV and 95% of signals were of amplitude >8.27 mV.[4] In the right ventricle, with its smaller myocardial mass, the same group was able to define that 95% of normal RV signals have a unipolar voltage >5.5 mV.[3]

Having defined the ventricle-specific reference values for unipolar voltage in the absence of scar (Table 20-1), these investigators analyzed patients with scar-related VT in the context of left and right ventricular nonischemic cardiomyopathies. Hutchinson et al found that in the absence of endocardial bipolar abnormalities, regions of low endocardial unipolar voltage predicted the presence of overlying epicardial substrate in all patients, with a 61% area overlap.[4] Polin et al published similar findings in patients with ARVD in whom endocardial RV free-wall unipolar signal attenuation predicted the presence and extent of overlying epicardial scar in patients with minimal abnormalities of endocardial bipolar signals.[3] Hence unipolar endocardial voltage mapping can be used to predict the presence of epicardial substrate, and the potential requirement for obtaining percutaneous pericardial access for VT ablation, in the free walls of both the LV and RV.

Since unipolar signals may be influenced by the presence of fibrosis deep to the endocardial recording surface, they may also, when they are abnormally attenuated in the absence of overlying epicardial scar, predict the presence of intramural substrate. This is of particular relevance in the group of nonischemic DCM patients who have septal fibrosis. Of DCM patients with monomorphic VT undergoing catheter ablation, around 12% have isolated septal substrate without the usual basolateral fibrosis being present.[11] As demonstrated in the case study, these patients sometimes have completely normal endocardial bipolar voltage and a paucity of epicardial substrate, generally only in the preaortic LV summit region. MRI characteristically displays an intramural layer of DGE deep in the ventricular septum. Bipolar biventricular voltage mapping of the septum is not surprisingly normal in such situations due to the normal RV and LV septal endomyocardium overlying the intramural fibrosis. Unipolar mapping should be performed with a normal voltage cut-off of >8.27 mV for both the RV as well as the LV septum due to its greater muscle mass than the RV free wall. Once an area of septal fibrosis is identified, mapping efforts, particularly pace-mapping, can be directed to this region, but ablation of VT associated with septal substrate remains challenging with currently available techniques and energy sources.[11]

SUMMARY

Substrate-based strategies are frequently required for successful ablation of scar-related VT as the majority of patients have unmappable VT morphologies. Voltage mapping underpins these strategies as it is the first and often most crucial step in defining the regions where VT circuit components reside. Depending on the particular form of structural heart disease present, both endocardial and epicardial mapping may be required, and both bipolar and unipolar voltage analysis may be pivotal.

REFERENCES

1. Marchlinski FE, Callans DJ, Gottlieb CD, Zado E. Linear ablation lesions for control of unmappable ventricular tachycardia in patients with ischemic and nonischemic cardiomyopathy. *Circulation.* 2000;101(11):1288-1296.

2. Cano O, Hutchinson MD, Lin D, et al. Electroanatomic substrate and ablation outcome for suspected epicardial ventricular tachycardia in left ventricular nonischemic cardiomyopathy. *J Am Coll Cardiol.* 2009;54(9):799-808.

3. Polin GM, Haqqani HM, Tzou W, et al. Endocardial unipolar voltage mapping to identify epicardial substrate in arrhythmogenic right ventricular cardiomyopathy/dysplasia. *Heart Rhythm.* 2011;8(1):76-83.

4. Hutchinson MD, Gerstenfeld EP, Desjardins B, et al. Endocardial unipolar voltage mapping to detect epicardial ventricular tachycardia substrate in patients with nonischemic left ventricular cardiomyopathy. *Circ Arrhythm Electrophysiol.* 2011;4(1):49-55.

5. Cassidy DM, Vassallo JA, Marchlinski FE, Buxton AE, Untereker WJ, Josephson ME. Endocardial mapping in humans in sinus rhythm with normal left ventricles: activation patterns and characteristics of electrograms. *Circulation.* 1984;70(1):37-42.

6. Bogun F, Good E, Reich S, et al. Isolated potentials during sinus rhythm and pace-mapping within scars as guides for ablation of post-infarction ventricular tachycardia. *J Am Coll Cardiol.* 2006;47(10):2013-2019.

7. Jais P, Maury P, Khairy P, et al. Elimination of local abnormal ventricular activities: a new end point for substrate modification in patients with scar-related ventricular tachycardia. *Circulation.* 2012;125(18):2184-2196.

8. Gepstein L, Hayam G, Ben-Haim SA. A novel method for nonfluoroscopic catheter-based electroanatomical mapping of the heart. In vitro and in vivo accuracy results. *Circulation.* 1997;95(6):1611-1622.

9. Haqqani HM, Marchlinski FE. Electrophysiologic substrate underlying postinfarction ventricular tachycardia: characterization and role in catheter ablation. *Heart Rhythm.* 2009;6(8):S70-76.

10. Reddy VY, Wrobleski D, Houghtaling C, Josephson ME, Ruskin JN. Combined epicardial and endocardial electroanatomic mapping in a porcine model of healed myocardial infarction. *Circulation.* 2003(25);107:3236-3242.

11. Haqqani HM, Tschabrunn CM, Tzou WS, et al. Isolated septal substrate for ventricular tachycardia in nonischemic dilated cardiomyopathy: incidence, characterization, and implications. *Heart Rhythm.* 2011;8(8):1169-1176.

21 MAPPING AND ABLATION OF VENTRICULAR TACHYCARDIA:LOCAL ABNORMAL VENTRICULAR ACTIVITY

Benajmin Berte, MD, F Sacher, MD, Pierre Jaïs, MD

BACKGROUND OF VT ABLATION

Catheter ablation of ventricular tachycardia (VT) is effective and particularly useful in patients with frequent defibrillator interventions.[3,4] Various substrate modification techniques have been described for unmappable or hemodynamically intolerable VT. Noninducibility is the most frequently used end point but is associated with significant limitations, so the optimal end point remains unclear. Elimination of late potentials and/or local abnormal ventricular activities (LAVAs) during sinus rhythm or ventricular pacing recently showed to be a useful and effective end point for substrate-based VT ablation.[1,2,3,5]

DEFINITION OF LAVA

LAVA is the abbreviation for local abnormal ventricular activity. These potentials are due to surviving bundles in fibrotic scar, poorly coupled to the healthy myocardium. We prefer to use this term to include the abnormal signals critical to VT that are occurring during the QRS because abnormal activity is not always late: it can occur anytime during the far-field QRS complex. It is a collective term for all abnormal ventricular signals; all late potentials (LPs) are LAVAs but not all LAVAs are LPs. LAVA lateness is measured from the onset of QRS to the end of the LAVA signal.

TABLE 21-1 Characteristics of LAVA

Characteristics	LAVA Signal	Healthy Myocardium
Amplitude (peak-to-peak) (mV)	>90% of LAVA <1.5 mV bipolar. Amplitude epicardial often > endocardial LAVA (median 0.37 mV versus 0.11 mV).[1]	>1.5 mV bipolar (caveat epicardial fat mapping of >2.8 mm thickness).
Slope (dV/dT)	Higher dV/dT (cfr PV potential) than far-field signal.	Lower dV/dT than local LAVA. High dV/dT if rising from normal conduction system (His, RBB, LBB, healthy Purkinje).
Lateness according to QRS onset (till end of signal) (ms)	>99% of LAVAs occur between QRS onset and 200 ms after QRS. Early at septal sites (43% after QRS complex) and late at lateral (81% after QRS complex) and epicardial sites (epi versus endo: 91% versus 66% after QRS complex (Figure 21-1). Very late (>200 ms) within dense scar (76%).	Inside the QRS.
Number of peaks (n)/fragmentation	Double potentials/split signal. More fragmented deeply inside dense scar.	One signal without fragmentation.
Duration (ms)	Single sharp potential of short duration can be abnormal. >95 ms is pathologic and sign of slow conduction.	<95 ms.
Consistency	Consecutive beats with same activation (excluding PVC and fusion beats).	Consecutive beats with same activation.
Electrical coupling	Poorly coupled (delay in sinus rhythm, different responses to pacing, cfr lower).	Normal coupling.

Important: Early LAVA needs to be distinguished from normal signals coming from the conduction system (His, RBB, LBB, normal Purkinje). RV pacing is required to uncouple LAVA from far-field signal.

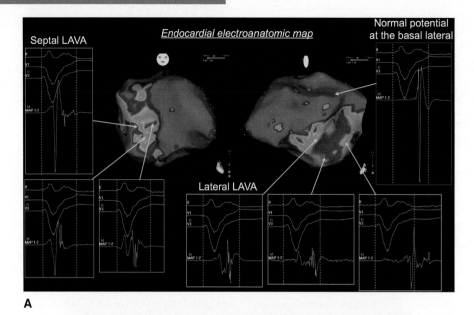

A

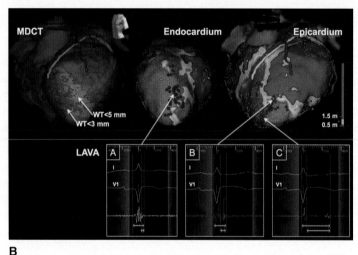

B

FIGURE 21-1 (A) Late LAVA lateral and early LAVA septal. (B) Earlier LAVA endocardial and later LAVA epicardial. This also illustrates the longest delays in the dense scar. Reproduced with permission from Komatsu Y, Daly M, Sacher F, et al. Electrophysiologic characterization of local abnormal ventricular activities in postinfarction ventricular tachycardia with respect to their anatomic location. Heart rhythm : the official journal of the Heart Rhythm Society 2013:Nov;10(11):1630-1637.

PREPROCEDURAL IMAGING AND LAVA CHARACTERISTICS

Preprocedural imaging can help identify a scar region through delayed gadolinium enhancement on magnetic resonance imaging (DE-MRI), or wall thinning using multidetector CT (MDCT), indicating the need for epicardial access and preventing potential complications by accurate localization of the coronaries and the phrenic nerve. Scar identified as DE-MRI and wall thinning on MDCT scan are well correlated with the low voltage area on the EAM system and the appearance of LAVA[6]. DE-MRI is ideal to depict the scar versus healthy myocardium, except in the presence of ICD, which precludes good quality images. This is why MDCT can be used as a surrogate, especially when wall thinning is present at the scar area. Different image possibilities are shown in Table 21-2. LAVA probability differs by disease entity. In ischemic cardiomyopathy (ICM) we observed LAVA predominantly endocardially, with epicardial involvement depending on the degree of transmurality. Ninety percent of LAVA

is seen in zones with wall thinning of <5 mm with very late LAVA occurring almost exclusively in a <3 mm wall thinning area.[7] No LAVAs are seen >20 mm outside the scar border zone, and most LAVAs appear in the border zone.[6,7] Nonischemic cardiomyopathy (NICM) is a more heterogeneous entity. Dilated cardiomyopathy (DCM) shows most LAVA perivalvular. Postmyocarditis patients typically present with only epicardial LAVA and complete normal endocardial mapping.[7] Arrhythmogenic right ventricular cardiomyopathy (ARVC) shows most LAVA at the epicardial site with some endocardial LAVA because of wall thinning.

TECHNIQUES TO UNMASK LAVA

The signal recorded with a mapping catheter is always a combination of far-field and near-field potentials. Figure 21-2 shows the difference between far-field and near-field signals. In order to unmask local abnormal activity, several different pacing techniques can be used, as explained in Table 21-3.

MAPPING AND ABLATION OF VENTRICULAR
TACHYCARDIA:LOCAL ABNORMAL
VENTRICULAR ACTIVITY

SECTION III
CASE STUDIES IN VENTRICULAR
TACHYCARDIA

145

TABLE 21-2 Preprocedural Imaging

Imaging Tool	Scar Characteristics	Other	Typical Disease
DE-MRI	Scar visualisation (nl, gray zone, and scar) reveals focal fibrosis % of transmurality, subendo, or subepicardial scar. Contrast uptake in pappilary muscle. Apical aneurysm, LVEF, wall motion.	Real anatomy with endo and epi-cardial segmentation. Scar map for EAM.	Ischemic CM. Dilated CM. Postmyocarditis.
MDCT	Wall thinning (nl, <5 mm and >3 mm). Calcification. Fibro-fatty replacement. Coronary lesions.	Real anatomy with endo and epi-cardial segmentation. Phrenic nerve. Papillary muscle. Coronary arteries/aortic root/CS. Wall thinning map for EAM.	Ischemic CM. ARVC.
Body surface mapping	Zones of slow conduction in SR. Periprocedural mapping of VT circuit/PVC.		All types, also idiopathic.

The MDCT wall thinning area tends to be smaller than the low voltage area on EAM, and the MRI scar area tends to be larger.

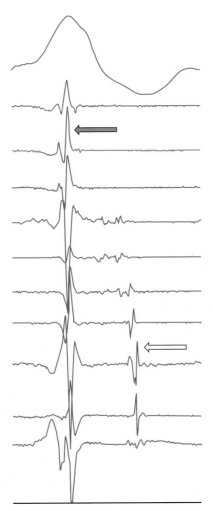

FIGURE 21-2 Differentiation between far-field and near-field signals: ECG shows ventricular QRS signal. Multipolar catheter recording shows far-field and near-field signals. Far-field signals are synchronous, of higher amplitude, have lower dV/dT (black arrow). In contrast, near-field signals are delayed as they are generated by local, poorly coupled surviving bundles (white arrow). They have sharper dV/dT and lower amplitude.

MAPPING OF LAVA DURING SR OR VT

In sinus rhythm, most centers perform automatic substrate mapping with an electroanatomic mapping (EAM) system. Different cut-offs for normal and abnormal myocardium are used in unipolar or bipolar mode. Epicardial fat can make epicardial substrate mapping more difficult; it can mimic low voltage areas but will not show fragmentation or delayed activation. Therefore, some centers include special EGM characteristics together with low voltage as criteria for defining scar regions such as wide, split, late, and fragmented signals to the low voltage area.[8] True intramural or septal scar can be difficult to identify and preprocedural imaging, pacing maneuvers (delayed transmural conduction time [>40 ms] and fractionated, late, split, and wide [>95 ms] potentials on the left-sided septum during RV pacing), and/or unipolar voltage map (<8.3 mV unipolar septal mapping from inside the LV) can be helpful.[8-14] It is our practice to create a high density endocardial (and epicardial) substrate-based voltage map with special annotation of all LAVA points and sites with good pace-maps. We perform automatic mapping in most ICM patients, but in NICM, we tend to manually adapt the substrate map toward the near-field (LAVA) signal in order to create better scar delineation, especially during epicardial mapping, as automatic bipolar and unipolar mapping can be normal in those cases. Some operators change the color scale of the substrate map to visualize (critical or bystander) channels.[15]

During VT, activation mapping and entrainment mapping is performed. In certain cases, LAVA can be recorded during the whole VT cycle length to define the entire VT circuit and isthmus (Figure 21-3). Ideal ablation sites are within the critical isthmus with demonstration of mid-diastolic LAVA, concealed entrainment with PPI-TCL<30 ms, Stim-QRS interval >40 to 70 ms, and cessation of VT during ablation. But ablation would be continued after VT termination to reach the end point of LAVA elimination.

ABLATION OF LAVA

Over the years, different VT ablation strategies have been investigated: circular lesions around the whole scar, lines to connect islands of surviving tissue in order to block channels, critical isthmus ablation,

TABLE 21-3 Techniques to Unmask LAVA Activity

Pacing Site/Maneuver	Far-Field Signal versus Near-Field (LAVA) Signal
RV apex pacing	No change (no LAVA?).
	Unmasked LAVA with delay of local signal.
	Changed or reversed activation (QRS-LAVA towards LAVA-QRS).
	Variable degree of conduction block (2:1 or more or disappearance).
	Particularly useful to unmask early septal LAVA and differentiate from healthy conduction system.
Extrastimulus pacing	Increased local delay or block.
Local pacing (or ectopics)	Same possibilities as above.
Fixed amplitude or decreasing output	Loss of far-field capture can result in changes in Stim-QRS delay and QRS morphology of the paced beats.
	Within dense scar, local capture can unmask previously hidden LAVA activity.
Pacing at endo/epifacing sites	Different activation sequences.
	Change in conduction delays.
Spontaneous PVC	Reversed activation or local delay.

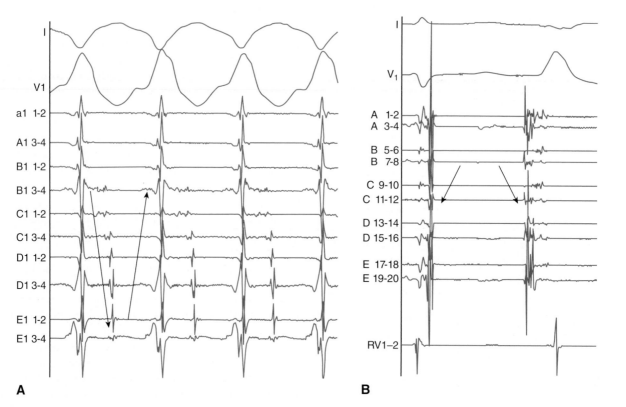

A

B

FIGURE 21-3 (A) Multipolar mapping of LAVA covering almost whole cycle length during VT. (B) Reversed activation sequence between sinus beat and ectopic beat. (C) 2:1 block of a LAVA signal.

MAPPING AND ABLATION OF VENTRICULAR
TACHYCARDIA:LOCAL ABNORMAL
VENTRICULAR ACTIVITY

SECTION III
CASE STUDIES IN VENTRICULAR
TACHYCARDIA

147

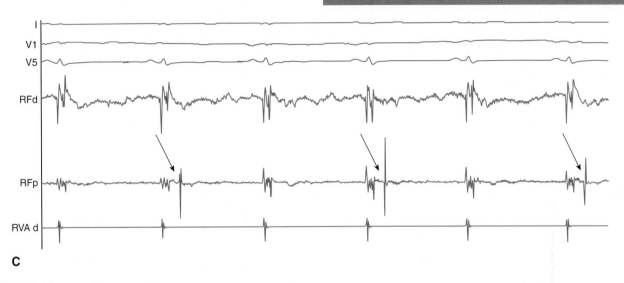

FIGURE 21-3 (Continued)

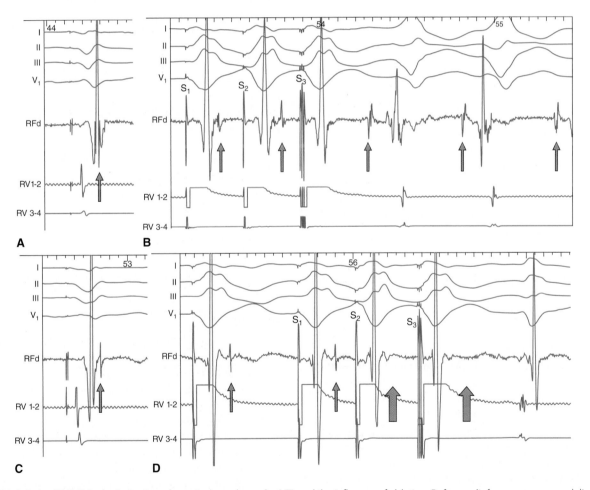

FIGURE 21-4 Role of LAVA in the induction of ventricular tachycardia (VT) and the influence of ablation. Before radiofrequency energy delivery (RF): (A) At first sight, the local ventricular electrogram during baseline-paced rhythm looks simple. However, in the terminal portion of this simple-looking signal, a very high-frequency component (LAVA) can be identified. (B) Programmed electric stimulation from the right ventricle (RV) unmasks the LAVA potential by increasing the delay from the far-field signal. The delay observed during RV pacing suggests poor coupling of the muscle bundle generating the LAVA signal. The delay is maximal with S_3, which is associated not only with a change in the polarity of LAVA but also with the induction of VT. Post-RF energy delivery: (C). After delivery of RF energy, there is a remarkable delay (see A) between the far-field ventricular signal and LAVAs during baseline-paced rhythm. (D) Repeat programmed electric stimulation from the RV results in the absence of LAVA signals after the far-field ventricular potential during S_2 and S_3 (open arrows). The absence of LAVAs is associated with an inability to induce the VT. Although ablation has rendered VT noninducible, further RF energy application is indicated to completely eliminate the LAVAs. Reproduced with permission from Jais P, Maury P, Khairy P, et al. Elimination of local abnormal ventricular activities: a new end point for substrate modification in patients with scar-related ventricular tachycardia. Circulation 2012;May 8;125(18):2184-2196.

TABLE 21-4 Different Voltage Criteria for Substrate-Based Mapping

	Marchlinski et al	Cano et al	Zeppenfeld et al
Normal endocardium	>1.5 mV bipolar >8.27 mV unipolar LV >5.5 mV unipolar RV	>1.5 mV bipolar	>1.5 mV bipolar
Normal epicardium	>1 mV bipolar	>1 mV bipolar + split, late, or wide potentials (>80 ms duration)	>1.81 mV bipolar >7.95 mV unipolar if fat ≥2.8mm: + split, late, or wide potentials
Border zone	<0.5 mV-1.5 mV bipolar	<0.5 mV-1.5 mV bipolar	<0.5 mV-1.5 mV bipolar
Dense scar	<0.5 mV bipolar	<0.5 mV bipolar	<0.5 mV bipolar

and recently, scar homogenization and LAVA ablation.[16-18] These techniques can be complementary.

STANDARDIZED APPROACH FOR VT ABLATIONS

Preparation

First, the usual interrogation and examination of the patient is performed. Imaging is performed to exclude intraventricular thrombus, delineate the scar, and provide further anatomical information. In absence of ICD, MRI is systematically performed, if possible associated with MDCT imaging. In others, MDCT imaging only is performed. The ICD logs are examined and the ICD deactivated. Twelve-lead ECG of the clinical VT is evaluated to acquire information about the exit site, cycle length, and possible multiple morphologies. Preprocedural imaging helps to plan the access needed (endocardial only, combined endocardial, and epicardial or epicardial only) and is imported in the EAM system for image integration purposes (location of scar, phrenic nerve, coronary arteries, papillary muscles). Hemodynamic stability and the need for circulatory support is assessed. Contraindications for pericardial access is evaluated (low platelet count <50.000, uninterrupted NOAC use, prior cardiac surgery, prasugrel/clopidogrel use).

Endo and/or Epicardial Access

If epicardial access is planned, an RV apex catheter (check threshold for RV pacing) is positioned before performing a subxyphoidal anterior percutaneous puncture with a tuohy needle, fluoroscopy in left lateral projection and using minimal doses of contrast (Figure 21-6).[1] A long guidewire is inserted, and after careful checking of correct pericardial position (inserting about 40 cm confirms that the guidewire is not in a cardiac chamber), a steerable sheath (epicardial Agilis or short curved Agilis) is inserted in the pericardial space. Heparin is commenced after the pericardial puncture. Endocardial access is obtained with transseptal or retrograde aortic access, depending on cases.

Substrate Mapping

An endocardial and/or epicardial anatomical and substrate map is made with a bipolar cut-off of <0.5 mV (scar), 0.5-1.5 mV (border zone), and above >1.5 mV (normal) used as automatic standard settings for endo- and epicardial mapping. In NICM with

subepicardial scar only, manual adjustment of the voltage map toward the near-field LAVA signal is performed. All LAVA signals are annotated on the EAM system, and maneuvers to unmask LAVA are performed. Multipolar mapping (Pentaray catheter) allows quick and high-density mapping (off-label use epicardially) of possible LAVA.

VT Induction

After the completion of the substrate map in sinus rhythm, an attempt to induce VT is performed. Figure 21-7 shows an induced monomorphic VT. Depending on the hemodynamic stability, activation mapping and entrainment mapping is performed (cf LAVA ablation). LAVA sites in sinus rhythm may match with mid-diastolic activity during VT. Figure 21-8 shows an activation map in sinus rhythm and during VT. Figure 21-9 shows LAVA in almost the entire VT cycle length on the mapping catheter. The mid-diastolic LAVA signal is ablated. and VT terminates at that site. Ablation is continued in SR to eliminate all LAVA.

Ablation During VT

LAVA sites are ablated during VT. Figure 21-9 shows LAVA in almost the whole VT cycle length on the mapping catheter. The mid-diastolic LAVA signal is ablated, and VT terminates at that site.

Ablation in SR

After ablation during VT, if VT cannot be induced or if only rapid hemodynamically unstable VT is induced (with need for DC shock), substrate ablation is performed during sinus rhythm.

All LAVAs are targeted aiming at elimination or isolation. LAVAs are first ablated at the border zone—where they are shortly coupled—before considering ablation deeper inside the scar. This strategy may result in the elimination of the late LAVA inside the dense scar with less ablation than a systematic RF delivery at the entire scar surface would require.[19] Ideal ablation sites show local LAVA, have a good or perfect pace-map compared to the VT morphology (>10/12), and demonstrate local capture with long Stim-QRS time >40 to 70 ms (sign of slow conduction). The procedural end point is complete elimination of all LAVA.

Checking the Ablation End Point

After all possible LAVA elimination, a new substrate map is made, and multipolar mapping is repeated to check for persisting LAVA signals. Further ablation is performed if needed. Inducibility is checked at the end of the procedure.

MAPPING AND ABLATION OF VENTRICULAR
TACHYCARDIA:LOCAL ABNORMAL
VENTRICULAR ACTIVITY

SECTION III
CASE STUDIES IN VENTRICULAR
TACHYCARDIA

149

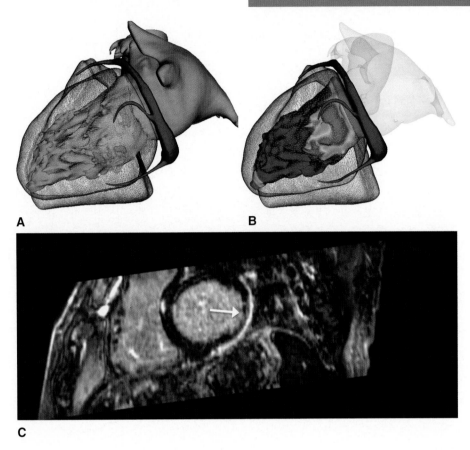

FIGURE 21-5 Patient with a known history of an earlier acute coronary syndrome and LAD lesion in whom an endocardial-only approach was planned. DE-MRI a day before the procedure showed subepicardial basal scar only. A new patent interrogation was performed and suggestive for a postmyocarditis scar. A combined endo- and epicardial approach was then decided, and only epicardial LAVA was found and ablated. (A) MDCT wall-thinning imaging. (B) Color-coded 3-D wall thickness map. (C) DE-MRI short axis view shows subepicardial scar only (white arrow).

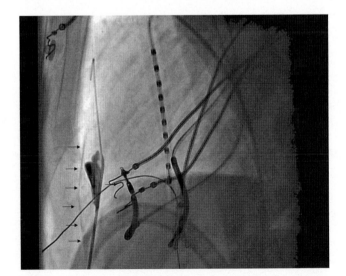

FIGURE 21-6 Lateral fluoroscopic projection showing the subxiphoid pericardial puncture with a Tuohy needle. The course of the needle in the substernal space is almost tangential to the posterior border of the sternum. It penetrates the parietal layer of the pericardium anteriorly as visualized from the contrast staining the anterior pericardium. Intra-pericardial entry is confirmed with contrast trickling into the pericardial space (arrows). The guidewire is then inserted. Reproduced with permission from Jais P, Maury P, Khairy P, et al. Elimination of local abnormal ventricular activities: a new end point for substrate modification in patients with scar-related ventricular tachycardia. Circulation 2012;125:2184-96.

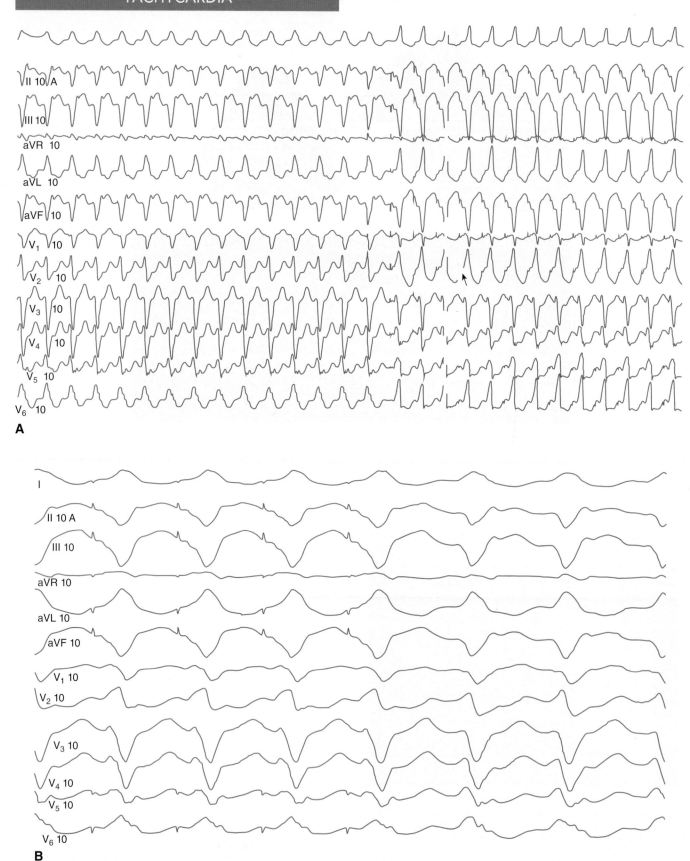

FIGURE 21-7 Patient with a previous inferior myocardial infarction and scar-related VT. (A) Clinical VT and entrainment/pace-mapping shows manifest fusion with short Stim-QRS <40 ms. (B) Almost perfect pace-map 11/12 with clinical VT, Stim-QRS >40 ms. (C) Ablation during stable clinical VT with prolongation and restoration of sinus rhythm during ablation.

MAPPING AND ABLATION OF VENTRICULAR
TACHYCARDIA:LOCAL ABNORMAL
VENTRICULAR ACTIVITY

SECTION III
CASE STUDIES IN VENTRICULAR
TACHYCARDIA

151

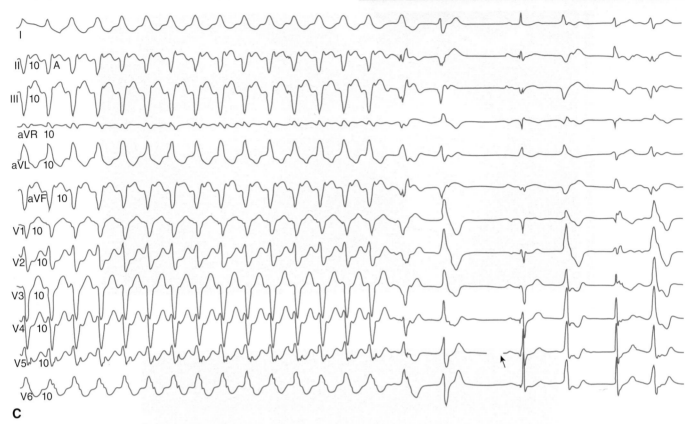

C

FIGURE 21-7 (Continued)

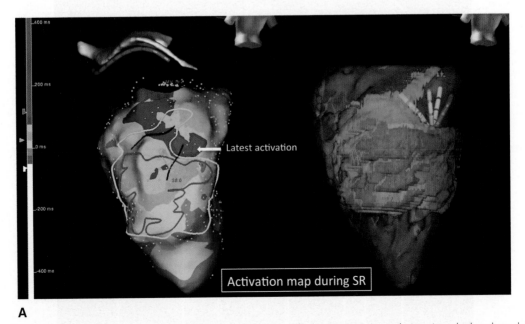

A

FIGURE 21-8 Patient with a previous inferior myocardial infarction. (A) On the left, the activation map during sinus rhythm shows latest activation inside the isthmus toward the exit site (purple zone), deep inside the scar in the laterobasal region. The figure on the right shows a three-dimensional MDCT wall thinning area of <2 mm in red and <4 mm in yellow. (B) On the left, the activation map during clinical VT shows short, funnel-shaped isthmus with "figure-of-eight" activation. Ablation is performed at mid isthmus. On the right, a three-dimensional MDCT segmentation model is shown. The red area shows wall thinning of <2 mm. On the left in both A and B, encircling of the wall thinning areas <2 mm (in red) and <4 mm (in yellow <4 mm) are shown. Wall thinning underestimates the scar area.

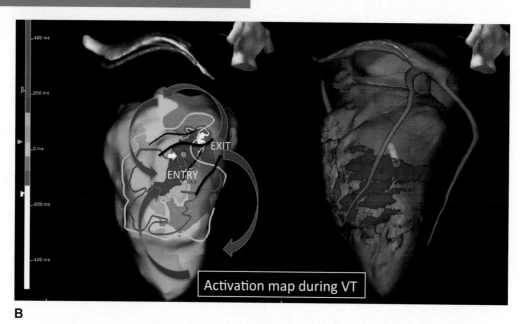

FIGURE 21-8 (*Continued*)

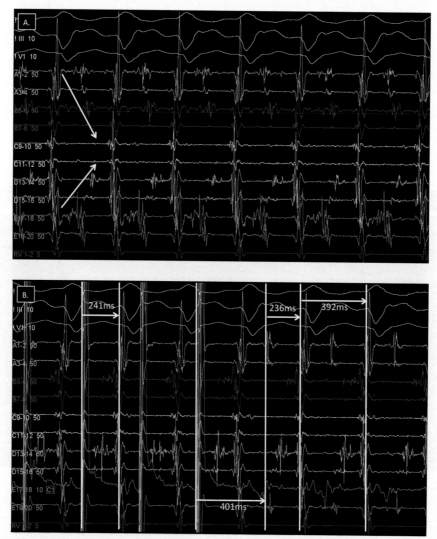

FIGURE 21-9 Same patient with previous myocardial infarction. (A) Multipolar mapping during clinical VT shows LAVA during almost whole cycle length (entry-isthmus-exit: arrows). (B) Entrainment with long Stim-QRS 241 ms, concealed fusion, Stim–QRS = EGM–QRS and PPI–TCL = 401–392 = 9 ms: entry site inside isthmus. (C) Ablation midway isthmus still shows mid-diastolic potentials (white arrow) and stops VT with prolongation (not PVC) in 2 sec.

MAPPING AND ABLATION OF VENTRICULAR
TACHYCARDIA:LOCAL ABNORMAL
VENTRICULAR ACTIVITY

SECTION III
CASE STUDIES IN VENTRICULAR
TACHYCARDIA

153

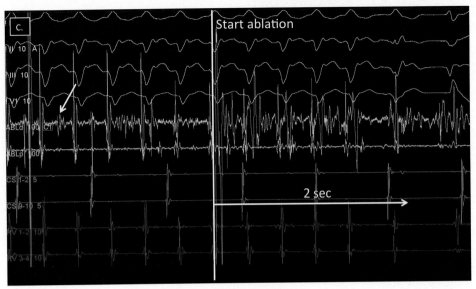

FIGURE 21-9 (*Continued*)

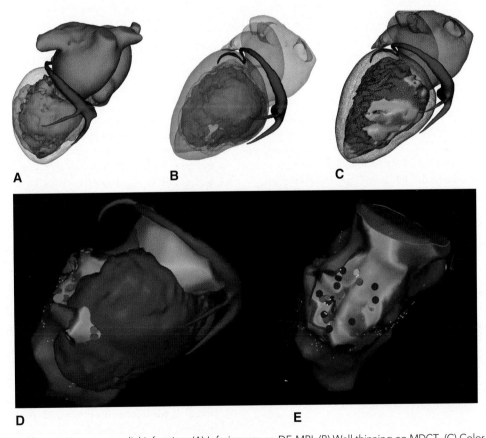

FIGURE 21-10 Patient with a previous myocardial infarction. (A) Inferior scar on DE-MRI. (B) Wall thinning on MDCT. (C) Color-coded wall thickness map. All are integrated in the EAM system using the MUSIC platform. (D) Image integration into the EAM system with merge of MDCT/MRI model with DE scar visualization and an endocardial bipolar voltage map. (E) Good correlation between scar on MRI and low voltage on EAM. LAVA points are tagged in purple and ablation points in red. Mid-diastolic LAVAs are tagged in green.

Postprocedural Management

In case of uncomplicated pericardial puncture, the pericardial sheath is withdrawn at the end. Some authors give intrapericardial corticoids systematically, and others leave a pericardial pigtail for 24 hours.[20,21]

END POINT OF LAVA ABLATION

The only clear end point for LAVA ablation is complete LAVA elimination. In our experience, all LAVAs are eliminated in 60% to 70% of the patients.[1] Endo and epi LAVA elimination requires epicardial

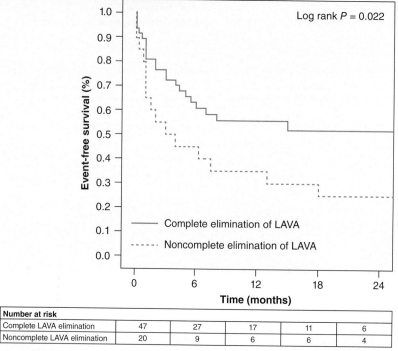

FIGURE 21-11 Kaplan-Meier curves depict freedom from recurrent ventricular tachycardia or death in patients with and without complete elimination of local abnormal ventricular activities (LAVAs). Jaïs et al, with permission.[1]

ablation in 58% of ICM patients and 82% of NICM patients (paper submitted). Incomplete LAVA elimination is accepted if the patient is hemodynamically unstable. A high risk of complications is expected because of LAVA sites <5 mm from a coronary artery or the phrenic nerve or because LAVA cannot be eliminated with high power, particularly in the case of intraseptal or intramural scar. These complications can often been prevented; preprocedural image integration of CS, coronary arteries, phrenic nerve and periprocedural systematic coronary angiogram, and phrenic pace-mapping if epicardial ablation is used are very helpful.

PROGNOSIS OF LAVA ABLATION

Emerging data demonstrate that complete LAVA elimination has a significantly better prognosis and mortality benefit compared to incomplete elimination, irrespective of VT inducibility (Figure 21-11).

CONCLUSION

LAVA ablation with the aim for complete LAVA elimination is feasible and associated with a better clinical outcome. It has the advantage offering a clear end point with the ability to work in sinus rhythm.

REFERENCES

1. Jais P, Maury P, Khairy P, et al. Elimination of local abnormal ventricular activities: a new end point for substrate modification in patients with scar-related ventricular tachycardia. *Circulation.* 2012;125(18):2184-2196.

2. Komatsu Y, Daly M, Sacher F, et al. Electrophysiologic characterization of local abnormal ventricular activities in postinfarction ventricular tachycardia with respect to their anatomic location. *Heart Rhythm.* 2013;10(11):1630-7.

3. Aliot EM, Stevenson WG, Almendral-Garrote JM, et al. EHRA/HRS Expert Consensus on Catheter Ablation of Ventricular Arrhythmias: developed in a partnership with the European Heart Rhythm Association (EHRA), a Registered Branch of the European Society of Cardiology (ESC), and the Heart Rhythm Society (HRS); in collaboration with the American College of Cardiology (ACC) and the American Heart Association (AHA). *Heart Rhythm.* 2009;6:886-933.

4. Zipes DP, Camm AJ, Borggrefe M, et al. ACC/AHA/ESC 2006 guidelines for management of patients with ventricular arrhythmias and the prevention of sudden cardiac death—executive summary: a report of the American College of Cardiology/American Heart Association Task Force and the European Society of Cardiology Committee for Practice Guidelines (Writing Committee to Develop Guidelines for Management of Patients with Ventricular Arrhythmias and the Prevention of Sudden Cardiac Death). Developed in collaboration with the European Heart Rhythm Association and the Heart Rhythm Society. *Eur Heart J.* 2006;27:2099-2140.

5. Arenal A, Glez-Torrecilla E, Ortiz M, et al. Ablation of electrograms with an isolated, delayed component as treatment of unmappable monomorphic ventricular tachycardias in patients with structural heart disease. *J Am Coll Cardiol.* 2003;41:81-92.

6. Cochet H, Komatsu Y, Sacher F, et al. Integration of merged delayed-enhanced magnetic resonance imaging and multidetector computed tomography for the guidance of ventricular tachycardia ablation: a pilot study. *J Cardiovasc Electrophysiol.* 2013;24:419-426.

7. Komatsu Y, Cochet H, Jadidi A, et al. Regional myocardial wall thinning at multidetector computed tomography correlates to

MAPPING AND ABLATION OF VENTRICULAR
TACHYCARDIA:LOCAL ABNORMAL
VENTRICULAR ACTIVITY

SECTION III
CASE STUDIES IN VENTRICULAR
TACHYCARDIA

155

arrhythmogenic substrate in postinfarction ventricular tachycardia: assessment of structural and electrical substrate. *Circ Arrhyth Electrophysiol.* 2013;6:342-350.

8. Cano O, Hutchinson M, Lin D, et al. Electroanatomic substrate and ablation outcome for suspected epicardial ventricular tachycardia in left ventricular nonischemic cardiomyopathy. *J Am Coll Cardiol.* 2009;54:799-808.

9. Haqqani HM, Tschabrunn CM, Tzou WS, et al. Isolated septal substrate for ventricular tachycardia in nonischemic dilated cardiomyopathy: incidence, characterization, and implications. *Heart Rhythm.* 2011;8:1169-1176.

10. Garcia FC, Bazan V, Zado ES, Ren JF, Marchlinski FE. Epicardial substrate and outcome with epicardial ablation of ventricular tachycardia in arrhythmogenic right ventricular cardiomyopathy/dysplasia. *Circulation.* 2009;120:366-375.

11. Hutchinson MD, Gerstenfeld EP, Desjardins B, et al. Endocardial unipolar voltage mapping to detect epicardial ventricular tachycardia substrate in patients with nonischemic left ventricular cardiomyopathy. *Circ Arrhythm Electrophysiol.* 2011;4:49-55.

12. Liuba I, Marchlinski FE. The substrate and ablation of ventricular tachycardia in patients with nonischemic cardiomyopathy. *Circ J.* 2013;77:1957-1966.

13. Polin GM, Haqqani H, Tzou W, et al. Endocardial unipolar voltage mapping to identify epicardial substrate in arrhythmogenic right ventricular cardiomyopathy/dysplasia. *Heart Rhythm.* 2011;8:76-83.

14. Wijnmaalen AP, van der Geest RJ, van Huls van Taxis CF, et al. Head-to-head comparison of contrast-enhanced magnetic resonance imaging and electroanatomical voltage mapping to assess post-infarct scar characteristics in patients with ventricular tachycardias:

real-time image integration and reversed registration. *Eur Heart J.* 2011;32:104-114.

15. Perez-David E, Arenal A, Rubio-Guivernau JL, et al. Noninvasive identification of ventricular tachycardia-related conducting channels using contrast-enhanced magnetic resonance imaging in patients with chronic myocardial infarction: comparison of signal intensity scar mapping and endocardial voltage mapping. *J Am Coll Cardiol.* 2011;57:184-194.

16. Marchlinski FE, Callans DJ, Gottlieb CD, Zado E. Linear ablation lesions for control of unmappable ventricular tachycardia in patients with ischemic and nonischemic cardiomyopathy. *Circulation.* 2000;101:1288-1296.

17. Reddy VY, Neuzil P, Taborsky M, Ruskin JN. Short-term results of substrate mapping and radiofrequency ablation of ischemic ventricular tachycardia using a saline-irrigated catheter. *J Am Coll Cardiol.* 2003;41:2228-2236.

18. Carbucicchio C, Ahmad Raja N, Di Biase L, et al. High-density substrate-guided ventricular tachycardia ablation: Role of activation mapping in an attempt to improve procedural effectiveness. *Heart Rhythm.* 2013.

19. Tung R, Mathuria NS, Nagel R, et al. Impact of local ablation on interconnected channels within ventricular scar: mechanistic implications for substrate modification. *Circ Arrhythm Electrophysiol.* 2013;6:1131-1138.

20. Sacher F, Roberts-Thomson K, Maury P, et al. Epicardial ventricular tachycardia ablation a multicenter safety study. *J Am Coll Cardiol.* 2010;55:2366-2372.

21. Sarkozy A, Tokuda M, Tedrow UB, et al. Epicardial ablation of ventricular tachycardia in ischemic heart disease. *Circ Arrhythm Electrophysiol.* 2013.

22 ABLATION OF VENTRICULAR TACHYCARDIA WITH NONISCHEMIC CARDIOMYOPATHY

Haris M.Haqqani, MBBS (Hons), PhD, and
David J.Callans, MD

CASE PRESENTATION

A 35-year-old previously well man with no family history of cardiac disease presented with dyspnea, cough, recurrent palpitations, and syncope due to sustained monomorphic ventricular tachycardia (VT).

He was in sinus rhythm with right bundle branch block (RBBB) and had moderate segmental left ventricular (LV) systolic dysfunction with an ejection fraction (EF) of 35%. Coronary angiography showed normal coronary arteries, and three monomorphic VTs were induced at EP study. Standard medical therapy was commenced and uptitrated for nonischemic cardiomyopathy (NICM), and a single chamber implantable cardioverter-defibrillator (ICD) was placed.

The patient was referred to after sustaining multiple shocks due to monomorphic VT despite treatment with amiodarone. He had unchanged LV systolic dysfunction and global right ventricular (RV) hypokinesis. Bilateral perihilar and mediastinal adenopathy was seen on thoracic CT, and cardiac PET scan showed uptake here as well as in the ventricles in a distribution consistent with sarcoidosis. Gluococortiocoids were commenced, and the patient underwent catheter ablation for ongoing episodes of VT.

Endocardial substrate mapping showed preserved LV voltage but a confluent area of anterior and septal RV scarring with widespread isolated and fractionated potentials (Figure 22-1A to C).

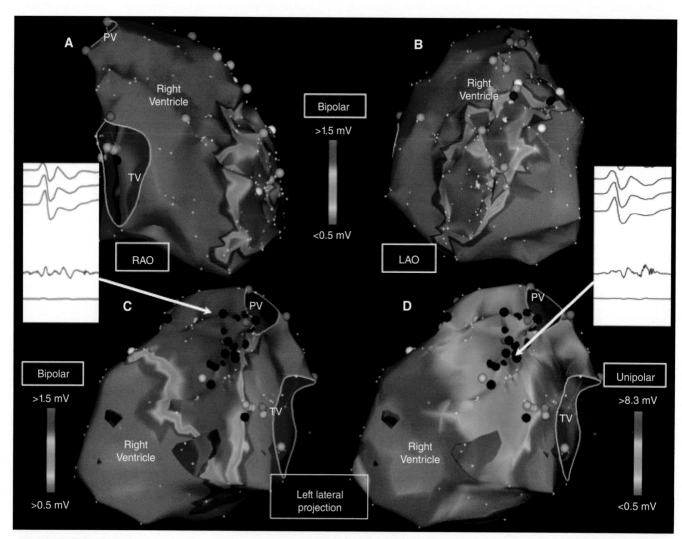

FIGURE 22-1 Bipolar right ventricular endocardial voltage maps from the patient in the case example are displayed in the right anterior oblique (RAO), left anterior oblique (LAO), and left lateral projections (A to C). A large confluent area of low bipolar voltage containing widespread isolated late potentials (black dots) is seen consistent with scarring. This is present in the anterior right ventricle and extends to the basal and mid septum. The unipolar right ventricular endocardial voltage map is displayed (D) and is adjusted for left ventricular septal wall thickness, rather than right ventricular free wall, with normal peak to peak amplitude defined as >8.3 mV. This suggests a much larger area of basal septal involvement.

ABLATION OF VENTRICULAR TACHYCARDIA
WITH NONISCHEMIC CARDIOMYOPATHY

SECTION III
CASE STUDIES IN VENTRICULAR
TACHYCARDIA

157

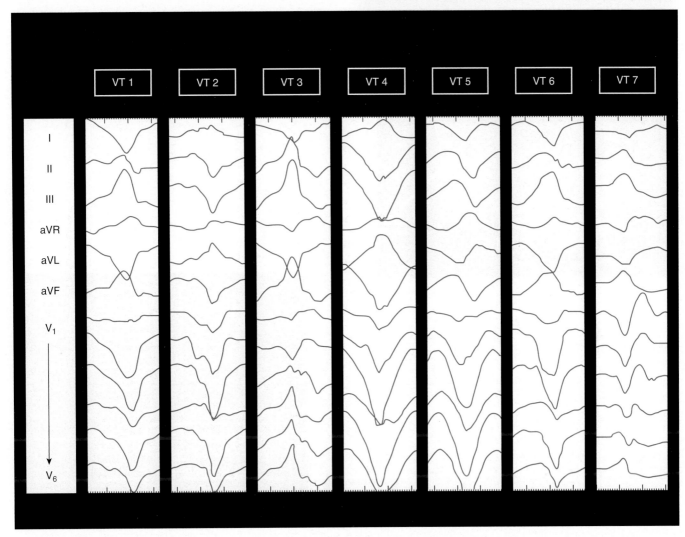

FIGURE 22-2 The seven ventricular tachycardia (VT) morphologies induced in this patient are displayed. VT 3 and VT 7 have left bundle branch block morphology. Only VT 2 was mappable.

Unipolar voltage analysis suggested a significantly larger area of intramural septal substrate (Figure 22-1D). Seven distinct VTs were inducible with programmed stimulation, only two of which were of RBBB configuration (Figure 22-2). Due to frequently changing morphologies as well as hemodynamic intolerance, only one of the VTs was mappable: VT 2, which had a cycle length of 431 ms. Entrainment mapping showed this VT to be a large macroreentrant circuit with an exit site on the infundibular septum of the RV and an entrance site on the inferoseptal RV (Figure 22-3). Central isthmus circuit components were seen on the septal RV in confluent area of endocardial scarring containing widespread isolated and fractionated potentials. Ablation here terminated VT, but other VTs were still inducible. Extensive substrate ablation was then performed from both sides of the interventricular septum, targeting these potentials and sites of good pace-maps with long stimulus to QRS delay. Following this, VT 3 was still inducible with a right bundle right inferior axis morphology and precordial transition pattern break in V_2, strongly suggestive of a preaorticepicardial exit. Percutaneous pericardial

access was obtained, and epicardial substrate mapping showed preserved voltages over the LV and RV free walls with the expected low-voltage area over the interventricular groove due to pericoronary fat. However, at the anteroseptal LV and at the LV summit, on either side of the left anterior descending artery, a cluster of isolated and fractioned potentials were seen, and pace-maps here, while not perfect, recreated the precordial and limb lead vectors of VT 3 (Figure 22-4). Extensive ablation here (after coronary angiography defined the LAD to be >5 mm from lesion sites) and in the preaortic region of the LV endocardium rendered this VT noninducible. Rapid VT, similar to VT 5, was still inducible with triple extra stimuli at the end of the procedure.

After this procedure, no ICD shocks occurred over short-term follow-up.

CASE EXPLANATION

This patient with NICM due to cardiac sarcoidosis highlights some of the considerable challenges in dealing with VT in this context.

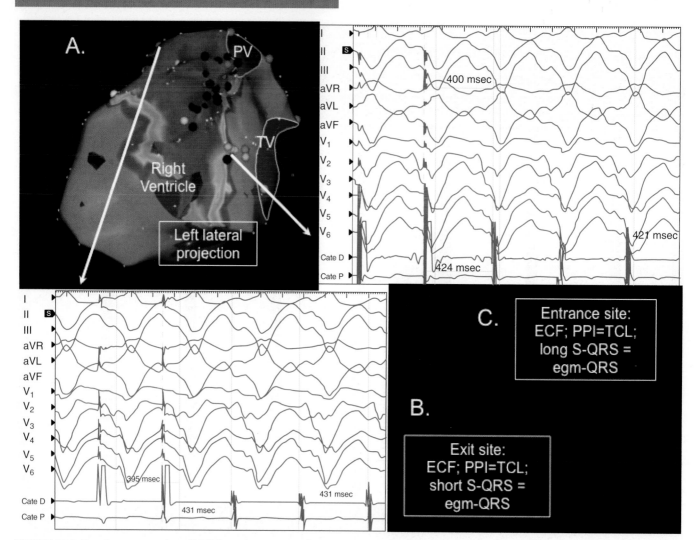

FIGURE 22-3 Entrainment mapping of VT 2 from the patient in the case example, proving this VT to be due to a large loop reentrant circuit located in septal substrate. (A) This figure displays the endocardial right ventricular bipolar voltage map showing confluent septal scarring. (B) Exit site response is demonstrated, showing entrainment with concealed fusion (ECF), postpacing interval (PPI) equaling the tachycardia cycle length (TCL), and short stimulus to QRS (S-QRS) interval equaling the electrogram to QRS (egm-QRS). (C) Entrance site response is shown with concealed entrainment, PPI=TCL, and long S-QRS equaling the egm-QRS.

The initial consideration of establishing a secondary cause for the NICM is well demonstrated as some etiologies other than idiopathic dilated cardiomyopathy (DCM) may have specific management or prognostic considerations. In the case of cardiac sarcoidosis, immunosuppression may be considered although even with treatment, prognosis is guarded with a considerable proportion of patients progressing to death or cardiac transplantation. Establishment of the diagnosis may require, in addition to a detailed clinical assessment, evaluation with biomarkers, serology, cardiac magnetic resonance imaging (MRI), PET scanning, and endomyocardial biopsy.

As seen in this patient, multiple VT morphologies are the rule in the setting of cardiac sarcoidosis, and indeed with any NICM, with the majority generally being unmappable by entrainment. Given the usually widespread, disparate regions of patchy, often subepicardial inflammation and fibrosis, both LBBB and RBBB VT configurations are seen. This patient displayed a less common pattern of confluent septal scarring, primarily manifest from the RV side of the septum

with a patchier continuation to the epicardial aspect of the septum in the preaortic LV summit region. Such confluent scarring forms the electrophysiologic milieu necessary for the establishment of large-loop reentrant VT circuits, such as those that were proved by entrainment mapping in this patient. After ablating mappable tachycardias, extensive substrate ablation is necessary to target the usually widespread regions of endocardial, epicardial, and intramural scarring seen in these patients. Even after successful VT ablation, the prognosis for transplant-free survival is guarded in cardiac sarcoidosis and is worse than in other etiologies of NICM due to progressive heart failure and recurrent VT.[1,2]

EPIDEMIOLOGY AND CLINICAL SIGNIFICANCE

Although sustained monomorphic VT is an uncommon presentation in NICM, sudden death due to presumed ventricular arrhythmias is well described. The risk of this rises with worsening LV systolic function as the burden of ventricular fibrosis increases and the capacity

ABLATION OF VENTRICULAR TACHYCARDIA
WITH NONISCHEMIC CARDIOMYOPATHY

SECTION III
CASE STUDIES IN VENTRICULAR
TACHYCARDIA

159

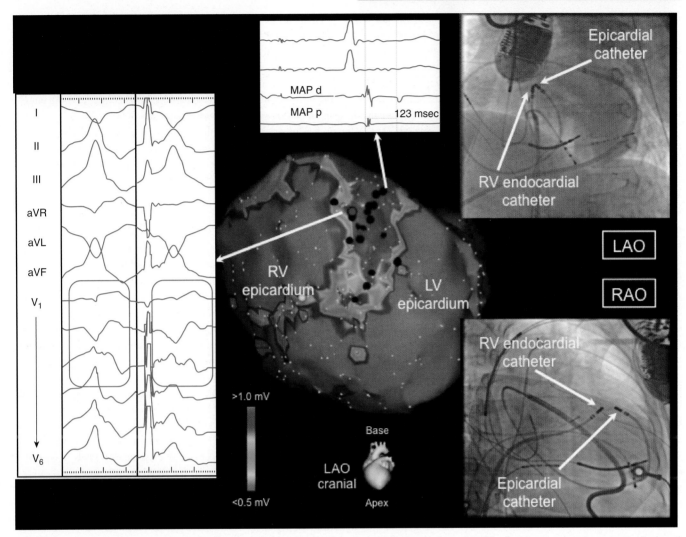

FIGURE 22-4 The epicardial voltage map from the patient in the case example is displayed. A small patch of midanteroseptal scarring is displayed with networks of isolated late potentials (one is highlighted) in addition to low bipolar voltage (<0.5 mV), distinguishing it from epicardial pericoronary fat. VT 3 was pacemapped to this region as shown. The fluoroscopic proximity of the endocardial and epicardial catheters mapping VT 3 is shown. Only epicardial pacemapping was able to recreate the V1-V3 precordial transition pattern break as shown.

to hemodynamically tolerate VT declines. The search for better risk stratifying tools remains the focus of much current investigation as this will lead to better targeted ICD therapy. Monitoring studies in patients suffering sudden death have demonstrated that monomorphic VT is the antecedent arrhythmia in many of these cases.[3] Although sudden death can be effectively prevented with ICDs, such devices are not a cure for VT, and multiple shocks can confer considerable morbidity on patients and possibly even increase mortality.[4-6] Antiarrhythmic drug therapy has not proven to be an effective management option to eliminate shocks and comes with a significant risk of adverse events, particularly with the use of amiodarone.[7]

ETIOLOGY AND PATHOPHYSIOLOGY OF VT IN NICM

In the context of NICM and in direct comparison to the postinfarct situation, catheter ablation of scar-related VT can be a difficult procedure with poorer outcomes in general.[2] Compared to other contexts, VT in NICM is more likely to be focal and to involve the His-Purkinje system.[8] These latter VTs include typical and atypical forms of

bundle-branch reentry and are very important to recognize as they are readily amenable to catheter ablation.[9] Myocardial reentrant VT is seen when the interstitial and replacement fibrosis typically present in the early stages of NICM has progressed to the point of forming more confluent regions of scarring that allow for the fixed and functional barriers of VT circuits to be formed. Unlike a mature infarct scar, which extends inward from the endocardium, the scarring in NICM may lie deep to the myocardium surface, where it can be effectively shielded from currently available mapping and ablation technologies.

ENDOCARDIAL ELECTROPHYSIOLOGIC SUBSTRATE

Although patients with NICM often have diffuse interstitial and replacement fibrosis as well as variable degrees of myocyte hypertrophy and myofibril disarray,[10] those presenting with monomorphic VT generally have confluent areas of scar which form the substrate for reentrant and triggered arrhythmias.[8] Remarkably, in a theme echoed across the various etiologies of nonischemic left and right ventricular cardiomyopathies, the fibrosis is generally centered around the basal, periannular regions.[11,12] However, it is important to highlight the marked heterogeneity observed, with some patients having no detectable endocardial abnormality at all. The precise characteristics of this electrophysiologic substrate can be defined with the use of electroanatomic mapping as demonstrated in the previous case example. Normal bipolar voltage parameters are extrapolated from mapping completed in ischemic cardiomyopathy, and normal voltage is measured as peak-to-peak signal amplitude of >1.5 mV, although pathologic correlation studies have not been performed in NICM. On the resulting electroanatomic substrate map, fractionated and isolated late potentials (ILPs) are tagged, and areas of slow conduction and putative VT exits are located by pace-mapping. In LV NICM, the basolateral periannular regions are much more commonly involved than the basal septal areas.[11] The pathologic process may progress apically as the disease evolves, thus generating apical VT morphologies, and this may predict a worse prognosis as the total scar burden rises.[13]

EPICARDIAL ELECTROPHYSIOLOGIC SUBSTRATE

Although there is considerable heterogeneity, many patients with NICM-related VT have a greater burden of scarring on the epicardium than on the endocardium.[14] This characteristically mirrors the regional pattern seen on the endocardium with a predilection for the basolateral areas overlying the endocardial scarring, as well as the preaortic region of the LV summit. The presence of epicardial fat, particularly near the coronary arteries in the atrioventricular and interventricular sulci, confounds the assessment of epicardial fibrosis due to the attenuating effect it has on signal amplitude. Consequently, a bipolar voltage cutoff for epicardial substrate of <1.0 mV has been shown to be a better discriminator, in addition to requiring the low voltage area to contain fractionated and isolated late potentials (which are not caused by fat but are reflective of slow conduction within scar).[14] The summated effects of the endocardial and epicardial substrate in the basolateral LV can be seen on the surface ECG in the R:S ratios of V_1 and V_6.[15]

ELECTROCARDIOGRAPHIC CLUES TO EPICARDIAL VT EXIT

The predilection for the electrophysiologic substrate in NICM to involve the epicardium means that a considerable proportion of the VTs seen in these patients will have epicardial origins. In the case of VT due to intramyocardial reentry, this means that some or all of the circuit components may be epicardial.[16] If the exit of the reentrant wavefront from the constrained diastolic isthmus is located on the epicardium, several characteristic surface ECG features may be seen during VT. Broadly, these can be divided into two categories: (1) interval criteria and (2) morphology criteria. The former are QRS onset criteria and include a pseudo-delta wave duration of ≥34 ms, a V_2 intrinsicoid deflection of ≥85 ms, and a shortest RS complex duration of ≥121 ms.[17] These are based on the assumption that epicardial VT exits are relatively late in engaging the His-Purkinje system compared to endocardial exit sites. The second group, the morphology criteria, is based on the fact that the ventricular myocardium is thick enough for its transmural depolarization to register on the surface ECG. In sinus rhythm, this can be seen as small Q waves in V_6 reflective of left-to-right transmural septal activation. The presence of QS waves in focus leads during VT (lead I for basal, and the inferior leads for inferior sites of origin) suggest an epicardial site of

VT circuit exit. With epicardial VT exits on the basolateral LV, the inferior leads do not register a small initial Q wave because all activation is directed toward them, with no initial endocardial-to-epicardial basolateral LV vector as is seen with an endocardial exit (Figure 22-5). Similar morphology criteria can be applied to other exit regions.[18] Valles et al described an algorithm combining both interval and morphology criteria with an accuracy of 90%.[19]

It is important to stress that all the ECG criteria predicting epicardial VT origins are only able to give information about VT exit sites. The absence of such criteria does not exclude the possible presence of other critical VT circuit components on the epicardium (or intramurally), even with endocardial exit sites.

SEPTAL AND INTRAMURAL SUBSTRATE

While some degree of septal scarring is probably present in the majority of NICM patients with VT, a small but important minority of patients display only isolated septal substrate with sparing of the basolateral LV (Figure 22-6).[20] These patients may have low bipolar voltage with abnormal electrograms on either the LV or RV aspects of the interventricular septum (or both), as well as on the epicardial surfaces at the top and bottom of the septum, namely the preaortic region on the LV summit or at the crux. Rarely, there may be no bipolar voltage abnormality on any cardiac surface in patients with intramurally confined substrate, but low unipolar voltage may suggest its presence deep to the endocardial surface.[21] Patches of intramural septal delayed gadolinium enhancement are a well-described finding on cardiac MRI in NICM, and the electrophysiologic substrate described in this subgroup of NICM VT patients is likely to correspond to the same pathology as visualized on MRI.[22]

PROCEDURAL MANAGEMENT

The most common indication for catheter ablation of VT in the setting of NICM remains recurrent appropriate ICD therapies despite medical therapy, often including high-dose amiodarone. There is some data to suggest that earlier ablation may be associated with better outcomes and lower VT recurrences.[23] The risks of both endocardial and epicardial ablation are discussed with the patient, including death, stroke, myocardial infarction, groin complications, tamponade, valvular damage, atrioventricular block with septal ablation, abdominal or pericardial bleeding with pericardial access, and phrenic nerve or coronary artery injury with epicardial ablation.[24] Adequate procedural preparation is essential including an analysis of all surface ECGs and ICD electrograms from clinical VTs. Intracardiac thrombus is excluded with echocardiography prior to the procedure. Patients can be studied under general anaesthesia or conscious sedation, but the latter has the distinct advantage of allowing more induced VTs to be mapped as hemodynamic tolerance is improved. Additional depth of sedation or conversion to general anesthetic may be required for percutaneous pericardial access. Depending on the degree of LV systolic dysfunction and dilatation, consideration should be given to mechanical hemodynamic support with an intraaortic balloon pump or, less frequently, with a percutaneous left ventricular assist device. Also, intracardiac echocardiography may be useful to define anatomy (valvular, papillary muscle, etc.), image ventricular scarring,[25] monitor for catheter contact and lesion formation, exclude complications such as tamponade, and potentially assist with pericardial access.

ABLATION OF VENTRICULAR TACHYCARDIA
WITH NONISCHEMIC CARDIOMYOPATHY

SECTION III
CASE STUDIES IN VENTRICULAR
TACHYCARDIA

161

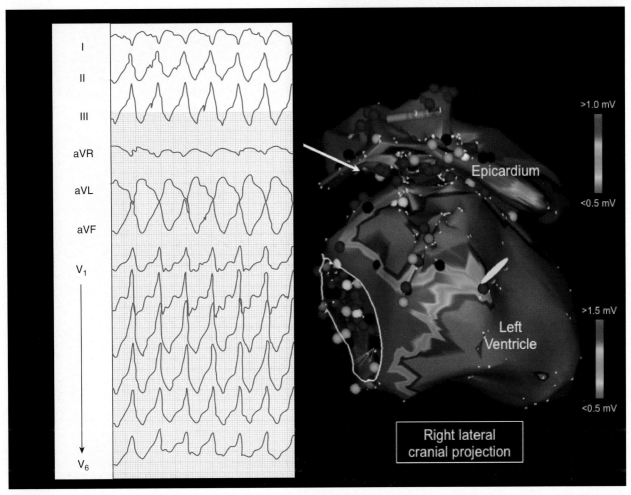

FIGURE 22-5 A 68-year-old man with idiopathic NICM who had undergone three prior endocardial and epicardial VT ablations and one surgical VT ablation presented with the clinical VT shown. Both interval and morphology criteria strongly suggest an epicardial exit from the basolateral left ventricle with long intrinsicoid deflections, pseudo-delta waves, and RS complexes in the precordium, as well as the absence of inferior Q waves and the absence of R waves in lead I and aVL. Extensive adhesions from prior sternotomy and VT ablation were encountered, limiting epicardial mapping, but the clinical VT was pace-mapped to the region shown and successfully ablated there.

After vascular access is obtained, systemic anticoagulation is achieved with heparin and endocardial substrate mapping commences, often of both LV and RV. Any sustained VTs induced during this process are mapped by entrainment if hemodynamically and morphologically stable, or else they are terminated by overdrive pacing or DC cardioversion. During the substrate mapping process, endocardial low voltage zones are defined, both bipolar and unipolar, and isolated and fractioned potentials are tagged. Pacing at these sites during sinus rhythm is used to define potential slow zones, anatomically constrained conducting channels, and regions of good pace-maps. Programmed ventricular stimulation is then performed, and induced VTs are compared for cycle length and morphology (both on surface ECG and ICD electrograms) to clinical tracings. Bundle branch and interfascicular reentry VT mechanisms are excluded upfront by His bundle electrogram and Purkinje potential analysis, as well as RV apical entrainment. Mappable VTs have their circuit components (entrance, central isthmus, exit) defined by entrainment and ablated at critical sites. Unmappable VTs have their putative critical machinery defined in sinus rhythm by analysis of the voltage map and by pace-mapping. Extensive endocardial substrate ablation is then performed. In some

cases, VT circuit components may be best ablated from the left aortic sinus of Valsalva.[26] Programmed stimulation is then repeated, and ongoing inducibility of sustained monomorphic VT (particularly clinical morphologies) is an indication to proceed to epicardial mapping.

Systemic anticoagulation must first be fully reversed with protamine, and a normalized activated clotting time must be documented. Percutaneous pericardial access is obtained in the manner first described by Sosa et al,[27] and after an intracardiac wire position has been excluded by fluoroscopy in the left anterior oblique projection, a deflectable sheath is introduced into the pericardial space and aspirated to assess for pericardial bleeding. Epicardial substrate mapping is then performed, and VT induction, mapping, and ablation are repeated as on the endocardium. Phrenic nerve capture with high output pacing must be assessed prior to ablation at sites on the LV free wall. Likewise, coronary artery imaging is necessary to ensure lesions are delivered a safe distance from major epicardial coronary vessels.

If minimal epicardial substrate is found or if no VT circuit components can be mapped to the epicardium, a detailed assessment for the presence of intramural scarring is important, particularly on

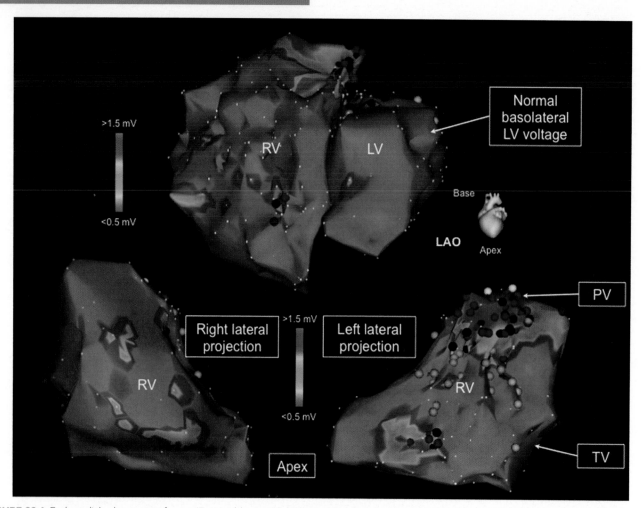

FIGURE 22-6 Endocardial voltage maps from a 47-year-old man with NICM and isolated septal scarring who presented with VT storm and 52 appropriate ICD shocks. Left ventricular endocardial voltage was essentially preserved, but septal infundibular RV scarring was seen. Epicardial substrate map (not shown) was normal. Pre-ICD MRI had suggested septal delayed enhancement with LV free wall sparing. His clinical and four other induced VT morphologies were all mapped to the septum and successfully ablated. He was noninducible at the end of the case and has had no further VT over a 15-month follow-up period.

the septum.[20] In these cases, conventional irrigated radiofrequency ablation may be ineffective in creating lesions of sufficient depth to abolish conduction through deep intramural VT isthmuses. Bipolar radiofrequency energy delivery or intracoronary ethanol ablation may both be considered in such instances.

Despite significant limitations, the currently accepted end point for the ablation procedure remains VT noninducibility.

OUTCOMES

Compared to the postinfarct context where the substrate is subendocardial in the majority of cases, scar-related VT ablation in NICM is a more difficult undertaking. Monomorphic VT is rarer in this context, thus large series and randomized trials of ablation strategies do not exist. The largest published experiences suggest that the majority of patients can achieve a reasonable VT-free survival and reduction in recurrent ICD shocks, but the outcomes depend significantly on the cause of NICM with sarcoidosis patients faring the worst.[2] If catheter ablation fails, open surgical cryoablation may offer an additional alternative in select cases.[28] Additionally, a substantial number of NICM patients may succumb to progressive congestive cardiac failure, even after successful VT ablation.

REFERENCES

1. Koplan BA, Soejima K, Baughman K, Epstein LM, Stevenson WG. Refractory ventricular tachycardia secondary to cardiac sarcoid: electrophysiologic characteristics, mapping, and ablation. *Heart Rhythm.* 2006;3(8):924-929.

2. Tokuda M, Tedrow UB, Kojodjojo P, et al. Catheter ablation of ventricular tachycardia in nonischemic heart disease. *Circ Arrhythm Electrophysiol.* 2012;5(5):992-1000.

3. Bayes de Luna A, Coumel P, Leclercq JF. Ambulatory sudden cardiac death: mechanisms of production of fatal arrhythmia on the basis of data from 157 cases. *Am Heart J.* 1989;117(1):151-159.

4. Bardy GH, Lee KL, Mark DB, et al. Amiodarone or an implantable cardioverter-defibrillator for congestive heart failure. *N Engl J Med.* 2005;352(3):225-237.

5. Bradfield JS, Buch E, Shivkumar K. Interventions to decrease the morbidity and mortality associated with implantable cardioverter-defibrillator shocks. *Curr Opin Crit Care.* 2012(5);18:432-437.

6. Sweeney MO. The contradiction of appropriate shocks in primary prevention ICDs: increasing and decreasing the risk of death. *Circulation.* 2010(25);122:2638-2641.

ABLATION OF VENTRICULAR TACHYCARDIA
WITH NONISCHEMIC CARDIOMYOPATHY

SECTION III
CASE STUDIES IN VENTRICULAR
TACHYCARDIA

163

7. Connolly SJ, Dorian P, Roberts RS, et al. Comparison of beta-blockers, amiodarone plus beta-blockers, or sotalol for prevention of shocks from implantable cardioverter defibrillators: the OPTIC Study: a randomized trial. *JAMA*. 2006;295(2):165-171.

8. Soejima K, Stevenson WG, Sapp JL, Selwyn AP, Couper G, Epstein LM. Endocardial and epicardial radiofrequency ablation of ventricular tachycardia associated with dilated cardiomyopathy: the importance of low-voltage scars. *J Am Coll Cardiol*. 2004;43(10):1834-1842.

9. Lopera G, Stevenson WG, Soejima K, et al. Identification and ablation of three types of ventricular tachycardia involving the His-Purkinje system in patients with heart disease. *J Cardiovasc Electrophysiol*. 2004;15(1):52-58.

10. Roberts WC, Siegel RJ, McManus BM. Idiopathic dilated cardiomyopathy: analysis of 152 necropsy patients. *Am J Cardiol*. 1987;60(16):1340-1355.

11. Hsia HH, Callans DJ, Marchlinski FE. Characterization of endocardial electrophysiological substrate in patients with nonischemic cardiomyopathy and monomorphic ventricular tachycardia. *Circulation*. 2003;108(6):704-710.

12. Marchlinski FE, Zado E, Dixit S, et al. Electroanatomic substrate and outcome of catheter ablative therapy for ventricular tachycardia in setting of right ventricular cardiomyopathy. *Circulation*. 2004;110(16):2293-2298.

13. Frankel DS, Tschabrunn CM, Cooper JM, et al. Apical ventricular tachycardia morphology in left ventricular nonischemic cardiomyopathy predicts poor transplant-free survival. *Heart Rhythm*. 2013;10(5):621-626.

14. Cano O, Hutchinson MD, Lin D, et al. Electroanatomic substrate and ablation outcome for suspected epicardial ventricular tachycardia in left ventricular nonischemic cardiomyopathy. *J Am Coll Cardiol*. 2009;54(9):799-808.

15. Tzou WS, Zado ES, Lin D, et al. Sinus rhythm ECG criteria associated with basal-lateral ventricular tachycardia substrate in patients with nonischemic cardiomyopathy. *J Cardiovasc Electrophysiol*. 2011;22(12):1351-1358.

16. Swarup V, Morton JB, Arruda M, Wilber DJ. Ablation of epicardial macroreentrant ventricular tachycardia associated with idiopathic nonischemic dilated cardiomyopathy by a percutaneous transthoracic approach. *J Cardiovasc Electrophysiol*. 2002;13(11):1164-1168.

17. Berruezo A, Mont L, Nava S, Chueca E, Bartholomay E, Brugada J. Electrocardiographic recognition of the epicardial origin of ventricular tachycardias. *Circulation*. 2004;109(15):1842-1847.

18. Bazan V, Gerstenfeld EP, Garcia FC, et al. Site-specific twelve-lead ECG features to identify an epicardial origin for left ventricular tachycardia in the absence of myocardial infarction. *Heart Rhythm*. 2007;4(11):1403-1410.

19. Valles E, Bazan V, Marchlinski FE. ECG criteria to identify epicardial ventricular tachycardia in nonischemic cardiomyopathy. *Circ Arrhythm Electrophysiol*. 2010;3(1):63-71.

20. Haqqani HM, Tschabrunn CM, Tzou WS, et al. Isolated septal substrate for ventricular tachycardia in nonischemic dilated cardiomyopathy: incidence, characterization, and implications. *Heart Rhythm*. 2011;8(8):1169-1176.

21. Hutchinson MD, Gerstenfeld EP, Desjardins B, et al. Endocardial unipolar voltage mapping to detect epicardial ventricular tachycardia substrate in patients with nonischemic left ventricular cardiomyopathy. *Circ Arrhythm Electrophysiol*. 2011;4(1):49-55.

22. McCrohon JA, Moon JC, Prasad SK, et al. Differentiation of heart failure related to dilated cardiomyopathy and coronary artery disease using gadolinium-enhanced cardiovascular magnetic resonance. *Circulation*. 2003;108(1):54-59.

23. Frankel DS, Mountantonakis SE, Robinson MR, Zado ES, Callans DJ, Marchlinski FE. Ventricular tachycardia ablation remains treatment of last resort in structural heart disease: argument for earlier intervention. *J Cardiovasc Electrophysiol*. 2011;22(10):1123-1128.

24. Sacher F, Roberts-Thomson K, Maury P, et al. Epicardial ventricular tachycardia ablation a multicenter safety study. *J Am Coll Cardiol*. 2010;55(21):2366-2372.

25. Bala R, Ren JF, Hutchinson MD, et al. Assessing epicardial substrate using intracardiac echocardiography during VT ablation. *Circ Arrhythm Electrophysiol*. 2011;4(5):667-673.

26. Yokokawa M, Good E, Crawford T, et al. Ventricular tachycardia originating from the aortic sinus cusp in patients with idiopathic dilated cardiomyopathy. *Heart Rhythm*. 2011;8(3):357-360.

27. Sosa E, Scanavacca M, d'Avila A, Pilleggi F. A new technique to perform epicardial mapping in the electrophysiology laboratory. *J Cardiovasc Electrophysiol*. 1996;7(6):531-536.

28. Anter E, Hutchinson MD, Deo R, et al. Surgical ablation of refractory ventricular tachycardia in patients with nonischemic cardiomyopathy. *Circ Arrhythm Electrophysiol*. 2011;4(4):494-500.

23 ABLATION OF VENTRICULAR TACHYCARDIA IN PATIENTS WITH LEFT VENTRICULAR ASSIST DEVICES

Troy Rhodes, MD, PhD, FHRS, CCDS

CASE PRESENTATION

A 63-year-old man with ischemic cardiomyopathy (Class IV, Stage D, LVEF 10%) was admitted with decompensated heart failure requiring vasopressor and mechanical (IABP) support. He underwent implantation of a HeartMate II left ventricular assist device (LVAD) as a bridge to transplantation. His postoperative course was uneventful except for paroxysmal atrial fibrillation (AF) for which he was started on amiodarone. Prior to discharge, he underwent implantation of a primary prevention implantable cardioverter-defibrillator (ICD). He presented several weeks later with multiple ICD shocks for sustained monomorphic ventricular tachycardia (SMVT) at 170 bpm that did not terminate with antitachycardia pacing (ATP). He was referred to for VT ablation with the assistance of anesthesia. He was accompanied to the EP lab by a LVAD-support nurse.

Right femoral venous and arterial accesses were obtained for vascular access and hemodynamic monitoring. Quadripolar catheters were placed in the right atrium and right ventricular apex, and a deflectable catheter was placed at the His bundle. Despite burst and programmed ventricular stimulation at baseline and with isoproterenol, his clinical VT was not inducible, and he underwent a substrate-based ablation.

Given severe aortic atheroma, a transseptal approach to the left ventricle was taken (Figure 23-1). He received a heparin bolus and infusion titrated to maintain an activated clotting time (ACT) between 300 and 350 seconds. Electroanatomic mapping was performed with a CARTO navigation system (Johnson & Johnson, New Brunswick, NJ; Biosense-Webster, Diamond Bar, CA) and radiofrequency (RF) ablation was performed with an irrigated, deflectable mapping-ablation catheter. Intracardiac ultrasound catheter was used for transseptal access, to identify catheter-tissue interface and anatomical landmarks such as the LVAD inflow cannula, and to monitor for pericardial effusion.

Electroanatomical mapping showed endocardial scar (<0.5 mV) involving the mid to apical anteroseptum and the posterolateral walls with border zone surrounding the LVAD cannula. The endocardial scar seen was out of proportion to his cardiomyopathy. Linear ablation lines were extended from the LVAD cannula through both scar zones; the posterolateral line was extended to the mitral valve annulus while the anteroseptal line was limited to sites below the His-Purkinje system (Figure 23-2).

Postablation, he had recurrent VT, and mexiletin was added to amiodarone. He initially did well on this regimen, but several months

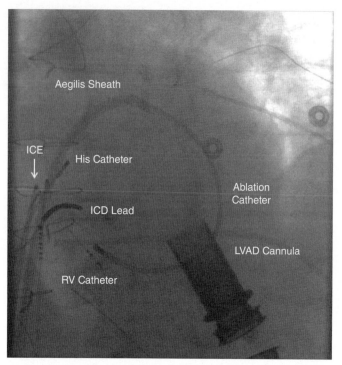

FIGURE 23-1 Left anterior oblique (LAO 35°) image during transseptal VT ablation.

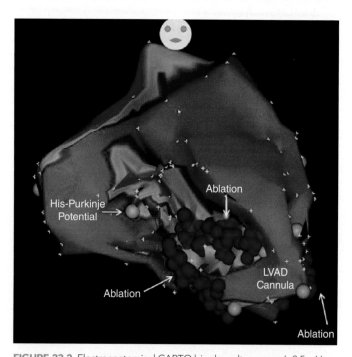

FIGURE 23-2 Electroanatomical CARTO bipolar voltage map (<0.5 mV and 1.5 mV color range). Orange dot shows most inferior His-Purkinje potential. Yellow dots depict apical LVAD cannula. Linear ablation lines extending from anteroseptal LVAD cannula to mid septum. The apical aspect of the posterior lateral ablation line is also seen.

ABLATION OF VENTRICULAR TACHYCARDIA IN
PATIENTS WITH LEFT VENTRICULAR ASSIST DEVICES

SECTION III
CASE STUDIES IN VENTRICULAR
TACHYCARDIA

165

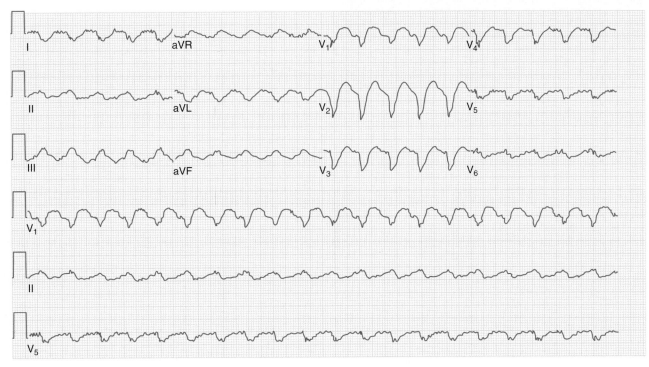

FIGURE 23-3 Surface ECG showing left bundle inferior axis morphology VT 122 bpm. The artifact seen throughout the ECG is noise from the LVAD.

later he had recurrent slow VT 120 bpm below his detection limit (Figure 23-3) and was referred to the EP lab for repeat VT ablation. With programmed ventricular stimulation, his clinical VT (left bundle inferior axis CL 520 ms) was induced and hemodynamically tolerated. Activation and entrainment mapping was performed throughout the LV via a transseptal approach without sites of early activation being detected. Mapping of the right ventricle showed earliest activation with concealed entrainment (Figure 23-4) at 12 o'clock on the tricuspid annulus. During ablation, there was prolongation of the CL with termination of VT. Postablation, VT was no longer inducible.

VENTRICULAR TACHYCARDIA DURING VAD SUPPORT

As seen with this patient, over one-third of patients will have ventricular tachyarrhythmia events (VTEs) within 30 days following LVAD implantation.[1,2] While concomitant ICD implantation has increased survival in VAD supported patients, there is a 25% incidence of appropriate ICD therapies.[3] The highest rates of VTEs are seen within the first 2 weeks following VAD support,[1,4-7] and recurrent VTEs are common with an average of 5 events per patient during VAD support.[8] Unfortunately, a lack of VTEs early following VAD support does not preclude late VTEs. While VTEs may be hemodynamically tolerated in the setting of VAD support,[9,10] they are associated with increased hospitalization rates, need for antiarrhythmic drug therapy, and increased mortality.[1,9,11-13]

Several factors predict the likelihood of VTEs during VAD support. The most consistent risk factor for VTEs is a history of VTEs prior to VAD support which doubles the risk of VTEs during VAD support.[13] Early studies showed patients with ischemic heart disease had a greater risk for VTEs during VAD support,[1,5]

while a more recent study in patients with continuous support found that those with nonischemic heart disease had a 2.3-fold greater risk of VTEs.[8]

MECHANISMS OF VT

Inflow cannula effects, pathologic fibrosis of the failing heart, and electrical remodeling within the VAD-supported heart are mechanisms for ventricular arrhythmias in VAD patients. With continuous-flow VADs, increased VAD speed, increased pulmonary venous return,[14] and transient changes in venous return[15] can cause negative pressure at the inflow cannula drawing the interventricular septum or left ventricular free wall toward the cannula causing arrhythmias due to mechanical stimulation (suction events). Antecedent myocardial fibrosis and localized myocardial injury and fibrosis at the cannula insertion site are proarrhythmic in VAD patients.

There are also molecular and cellular electrophysiologic adaptations that occur in the setting of VAD support. Changes in both QRS and QT interval are seen in the acute and chronic phase of VAD support and affect arrhythmic risk.[13] In VAD patients who experienced VTEs, decreased expression of connexin-43 can lead to decreased electrical conduction velocity and increased risk of ventricular arrhythmias.[16,17] But no study has shown a correlation between QRS duration and VTEs.[13] One study showed an early increase in QTc following initiation of VAD support correlated with the higher rate of VTEs early in VAD support.[4] Altered myocyte calcium handling with upregulation of the sodium-calcium exchanger (NCX) can lead to delayed afterpotentials and VTEs in VAD patients.[13] A recent study showed higher NCX gene expression in VAD patients with VTEs than those without VTEs.[2]

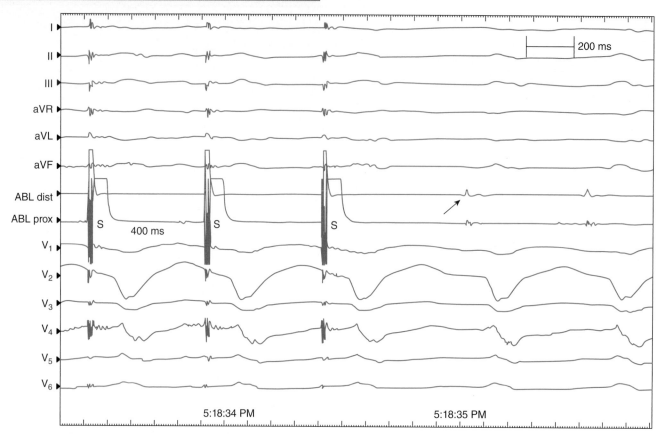

FIGURE 23-4 Concealed fusion during ventricular pacing during VT. The 12-lead ECG and intracardiac recordings from the proximal and distal electrodes of the ablation catheter are shown. Ventricular pacing stimuli (S) are delivered from the distal electrode of the ablation catheter at a cycle length of 400 ms showing concealed fusion. Ablation at this site (arrow) leads to slowing and then termination of the VT.

VT ABLATION

Typically, VT ablation reflects a second-line approach following failure of antiarrhythmic and heart failure therapies. The American College of Cardiology/American Heart Association/European Society of Cardiology guidelines recommend catheter ablation be considered for patients with drug refractory ventricular arrhythmias and recurrent ICD therapies.[18] VT ablation has been shown to be safe and effective in VAD patients.[19-23] Ventricular tachyarrhythmias are generally hemodynamically tolerated in VAD-supported patients,[9,10] making VT ablation via activation and entrainment mapping more feasible. A large series of VT ablation in VAD patients showed scar-related VT in 75% of cases, 14% arising from the apical inflow, 2.7% due to focal or micro reentry, and 1.4% due to bundle branch reentry.[22]

There are several technical issues that require special consideration during VT ablation in VAD patients. Vascular access can be challenging due to the lack of pulsatile arterial flow and concurrent anticoagulation which may increase the risk of vascular-related complications (hematoma, pseudoaneurysm, retroperitoneal bleed). The use of ultrasound-guided vascular access may reduce this risk.[22,23]

Preprocedural evaluation of the aorta and aortic valve by transesophageal echocardiography (TEE) and/or intracardiac echocardiography (ICE) should be performed. If the aortic valve is immobile, thrombosed, oversewn, or greater-than-moderate aortic atheroma is present, then a transseptal approach to the LV should be taken; in other cases, a retrograde aortic approach is utilized. Transiently decreasing the LVAD flow to allow normal aortic valve opening may facilitate crossing the aortic valve. Inadvertent catheterization of the outflow cannula in the ascending aorta and the apical inflow cannula should be avoided.[23]

In some cases, LV unloading by the LVAD may lead to smaller LV volumes making catheter manipulation more challenging.[23]

Unfortunately, VAD patients may also have hemodynamically intolerant VTs likely due to RV dysfunction, leading to decreased LV preload and reduced cardiac output[22,23] and requiring a substrate approach for ablation.

REFERENCES

1. Ziv O, Dizon J, Thosani A, Naka Y, Magnano AR, Garan H. Effects of left ventricular assist device therapy on ventricular arrhythmias. *J Am Coll Cardiol.* 2005;45(9):1428-1434.

2. Refaat M, Chemaly E, Lebeche D, Gwathmey JK, Hajjar RJ. Ventricular arrhythmias after left ventricular assist device implantation. *Pacing Clin Electrophysiol.* 2008;31(10):1246-1252.

3. Cantillon DJ, Tarakji KG, Kumbhani DJ, Smedira NG, Starling RC, Wilkoff BL. Improved survival among ventricular assist device recipients with a concomitant implantable cardioverter-defibrillator. *Heart Rhythm.* 2010;7(4):466-471.

4. Harding JD, Piacentino V 3rd, Rothman S, Chambers S, Jessup M, Margulies KB. Prolonged repolarization after ventricular assist

device support is associated with arrhythmias in humans with congestive heart failure. *J Card Fail.* 2005;11(3):227-232.

5. Bedi M, Kormos R, Winowich S, McNamara DM, Mathier MA, Murali S. Ventricular arrhythmias during left ventricular assist device support. *Am J Cardiol.* 2007;99(8):1151-1153.

6. Raasch H, Jensen BC, Chang PP, et al. Epidemiology, management, and outcomes of sustained ventricular arrhythmias after continuous-flow left ventricular assist device implantation. *Am Heart J.* 2012;164(3):373-378.

7. Kuhne M, Sakumura M, Reich SS, et al. Simultaneous use of implantable cardioverter-defibrillators and left ventricular assist devices in patients with severe heart failure. *Am J Cardiol.* 2010;105(3):378-382.

8. Oswald H, Schultz-Wildelau C, Gardiwal A, et al. Implantable defibrillator therapy for ventricular tachyarrhythmia in left ventricular assist device patients. *Eur J Heart Fail.* 2010;12(6):593-599.

9. Oz MC, Rose EA, Slater J, Kuiper JJ, Catanese KA, Levin HR. Malignant ventricular arrhythmias are well tolerated in patients receiving long-term left ventricular assist devices. *J Am Coll Cardiol.* 1994;24(7):1688-1691.

10. Busch MC, Haap M, Kristen A, Haas CS. Asymptomatic sustained ventricular fibrillation in a patient with left ventricular assist device. *Ann Emerg Med.* 2011;57(1):25-28.

11. Ambardekar AV, Allen LA, Lindenfeld J, et al. Implantable cardioverter-defibrillator shocks in patients with a left ventricular assist device. *J Heart Lung Transplant.* 2010;29(7):771-776.

12. Brenyo A, Rao M, Koneru S, et al. Risk of mortality for ventricular arrhythmia in ambulatory LVAD patients. *J Cardiovasc Electrophysiol.* 2012;23(5):515-520.

13. Pedrotty DM, Rame JE, Margulies KB. Management of ventricular arrhythmias in patients with ventricular assist devices. *Curr Opin Cardiol.* 2013;28(3):360-368.

14. Reesink K, Dekker A, Van der Nagel T, et al. Suction due to left ventricular assist: implications for device control and management. *Artif Organs.* 2007;31(7):542-549.

15. Vollkron M, Voitl P, Ta J, Wieselthaler G, Schima H. Suction events during left ventricular support and ventricular arrhythmias. *J Heart Lung Transplant.* 2007;26(8):819-825.

16. Saez JC, Nairn AC, Czernik AJ, Fishman GI, Spray DC, Hertzberg EL. Phosphorylation of connexin43 and the regulation of neonatal rat cardiac myocyte gap junctions. *J Mol Cell Cardiol.* 1997;29(8):2131-2145.

17. Gutstein DE, Morley GE, Fishman GI. Conditional gene targeting of connexin43: Exploring the consequences of gap junction remodeling in the heart. *Cell Commun Adhes.* 2001;8(4-6):345-348.

18. European Heart Rhythm Association, Heart Rhythm Society, Zipes DP, et al. ACC/AHA/ESC 2006 guidelines for management of patients with ventricular arrhythmias and the prevention of sudden cardiac death: a report of the American College of Cardiology/American Heart Association task force and the European Society of Cardiology committee for practice guidelines (writing committee to develop guidelines for management of patients with ventricular arrhythmias and the prevention of sudden cardiac death). *J Am Coll Cardiol.* 2006;48(5):e247-346.

19. Dandamudi G, Ghumman WS, Das MK, Miller JM. Endocardial catheter ablation of ventricular tachycardia in patients with ventricular assist devices. *Heart Rhythm.* 2007;4(9):1165-1169.

20. Osaki S, Alberte C, Murray MA, et al. Successful radiofrequency ablation therapy for intractable ventricular tachycardia with a ventricular assist device. *J Heart Lung Transplant.* 2008;27(3):353-356.

21. Herweg B, Ilercil A, Sheffield CD, Caldeira CC, Rinde-Hoffman D, Barold SS. Ablation of left ventricular tachycardia via transeptal approach and crossing of a mechanical mitral valve prosthesis. *Pacing Clin Electrophysiol.* 2010;33(7):900-903.

22. Cantillon DJ, Bianco C, Wazni OM, et al. Electrophysiologic characteristics and catheter ablation of ventricular tachyarrhythmias among patients with heart failure on ventricular assist device support. *Heart Rhythm.* 2012;9(6):859-864.

23. Herweg B, Ilercil A, Kristof-Kuteyeva O, et al. Clinical observations and outcome of ventricular tachycardia ablation in patients with left ventricular assist devices. *Pacing Clin Electrophysiol.* 2012;35(11):1377-1383.

24 REMOTE MAGNETIC NAVIGATION ABLATION OF IDIOPATHIC EPICARDIAL PREMATURE VENTRICULAR COMPLEXES

Mahmoud Houmsse, MD

CASE PRESENTATION

A 42-year-old man has severe symptoms of palpitations, fatigue, and dyspnea on exertion attributable to frequent premature ventricular contractions (PVCs) and was referred to for ablation of the PVCs after failing medical therapy with a β-blocker and a calcium channel blocker. Surface echocardiography found no structural heart disease and normal left ventricular ejection fraction (LVEF). A 24-hour Holter monitor showed 31% unifocal PVCs, with a morphology of right bundle, inferior axis, with presence of Q waves in lead aVL and I (Figure 24-1), suggestive of an epicardial origin. The hemodynamic impact of the PVCs is reflected by the absent cardiac output with each PVC, thus the effective heart rate is 35 bpm (Figure 24-2). The maximal deflection index (MDI), calculated by dividing the maximum deflection of the PVC complex in precordial leads by the PVC duration,[1] is prolonged (>0.55) (Figure 24-3). Pseudo-delta waves in precordial leads are another feature of an epicardial origin of the PVC[2-4] (Figure 24-3). At electrophysiologic testing, there was no inducible supraventricular or ventricular tachycardia. Mapping of the PVC began in the left ventricle and then aortic cusp, but there was no early presystolic electrocardiogram (EGM) or optimal pace-mapping in any of these regions. It was then attempted to map the coronary sinus (CS); however, multiple manual catheter manipulations to cannulate the CS were unsuccessful. Therefore, it was decided to utilize remote magnetic navigation to access the CS ostium (Figure 24-4). This process was achieved by positioning the remote navigation mapping catheter at the infero-medial aspect of tricuspid annulus, and then a posterolateral vector navigated the catheter into the CS os with successful access, which was confirmed by the typical EGM of the CS. Further superior then anterior vector via the magnets allowed navigation of the mapping catheter to be smoothly advanced into the CS system. Electroanatomic mapping in the distal CS disclosed the earliest presystolic EGM of 31 milliseconds (ms) (Figure 24-5) and 12/12-pace map match (Figure 24-6). In the CS, the catheter impedance was quite high (170-180 Ω) consistent with the catheter wedged within the CS. The impedance was too elevated to use a conventional ablation catheter, so an irrigated catheter was used, and power was limited to a maximum of 20 watts. There was the expected drop in impedance during delivery of the RF current, and the PVC source was eliminated (Figure 24-7). During follow up, the patient had significant improvement in his symptoms, and the PVC burden on the postablation 24-hour Holter monitor was only 1.3%.

EPIDEMIOLOGY OF EPICARDIAL IDIOPATHIC PVCs

Diagnosis of idiopathic PVCs or ventricular tachycardia (VT) is feasible only after excluding structural heart disease. In the United States, 10% of VTs are idiopathic.[5] The majority of patients with idiopathic PVCs will undergo electrophysiologic testing and attempt at radiofrequency ablation because of either symptomatic high burden PVCs with normal heart function,[6] or ineffective antiarrhythmic therapy or tachycardia-induced cardiomyopathy,[7] which has been reported to reverse by elimination of a high burden of PVCs.[8]

ELECTROCARDIOGRAPHIC CRITERIA OF IDIOPATHIC EPICARDIAL PVCs

Numerous studies have described the electrocardiographic features, pharmacologic intervention, and electrophysiologic mapping and

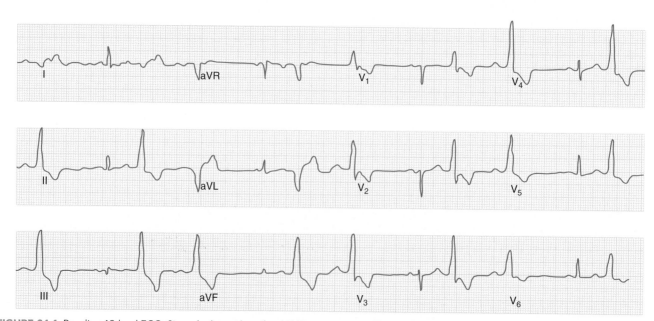

FIGURE 24-1 Baseline 12-lead ECG. Sinus rhythm with unifocal PVCs in a pattern of bigeminy.

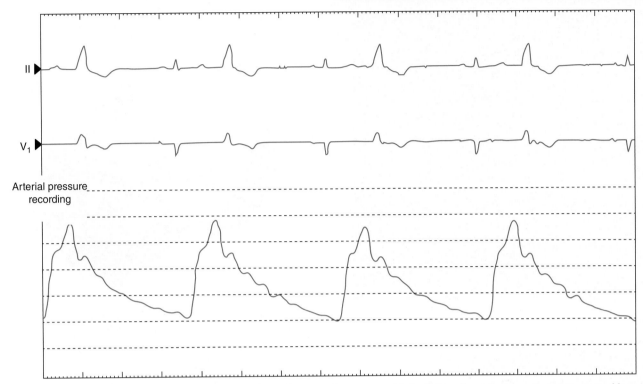

FIGURE 24-2 Arterial pressure recording during bigeminy. The absent cardiac output with the PVCs reflects the hemodynamic impact of frequent PVCs and that the effective heart rate is only about 35 bpm.

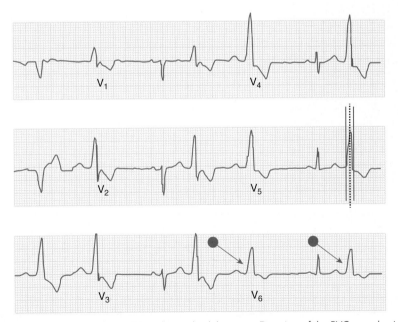

FIGURE 24-3 Assessment of maximal deflection index (MDI) and pseudo-delta wave. Duration of the PVC complex in V_5 = 134 ms (red line to red line); duration of maximum deflection, V_5 = 76 ms (first red line to dashed blue line), thus the maximum deflection index = 76/134 = .57. The pseudo-delta wave is denoted by red arrows in V_6. The upstroke of the PVC is slowed, *as if* the activation is due to conduction over an accessory pathway, yet this ECG pattern is due to slow conduction when the ectopic beat originates from the epicardium and conducts toward the endocardium with late involvement of the His-Purkinje system.

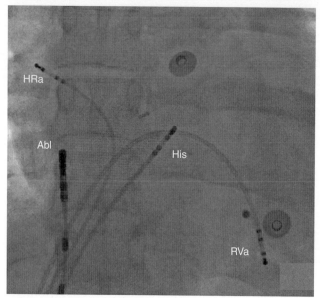

A

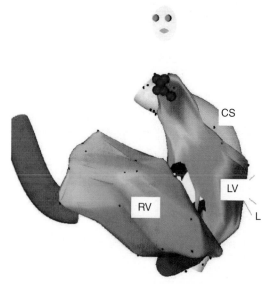

FIGURE 24-5 Pace-map of the PVC when pacing from the ablation catheter at the distal coronary sinus. Twelve-lead ECG: pace-mapping and spontaneous PVC from distal coronary sinus, 12/12 pace-map match.

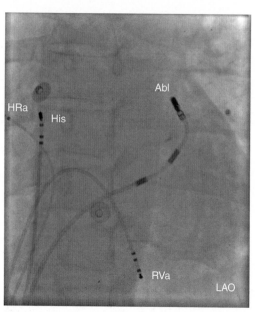

B

FIGURE 24-4 Fluoroscopic image of catheters during ablation procedure. HRa = quadripolar catheter in the high rate atrium catheter; Abl = magnetic-guided irrigated-tip ablation catheter; His = quadripolar catheter in the His position; RVa = quadripolar catheter in the right ventricular apex. (A) Anterior-posterior fluoroscopic image of the magnetic-guided irrigated-tip ablation catheter (Abl) in the right atrium. (B) Left anterior oblique (LAO) fluoroscopic image of the irrigated-tip ablation catheter (Abl), advanced using remote magnetic navigation, into the distal coronary sinus.

REMOTE MAGNETIC |NAVIGATION ABLATION OF
IDIOPATHIC EPICARDIAL PREMATURE VENTRICULAR
COMPLEXES

SECTION III
CASE STUDIES IN VENTRICULAR
TACHYCARDIA

171

Paced QRS versus Native PVC

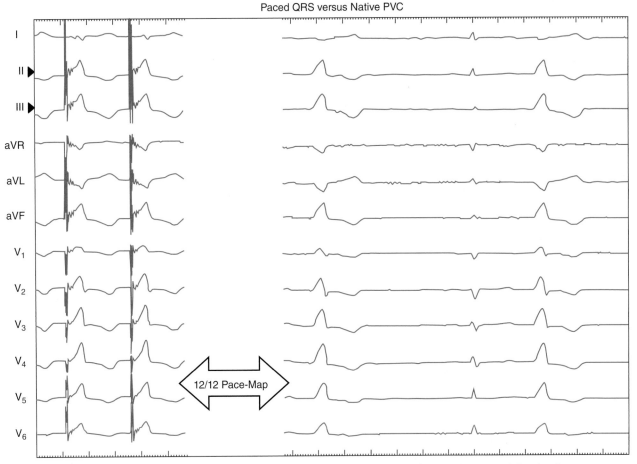

FIGURE 24-6 LAO image of electroanatomic map of PVC, including right ventricle (RV), left ventricle (LV), and the distal coronary sinus (CS). Successful ablation site of PVC denoted by red dots.

ablation of epicardial PVC/VT.[5,9-12] Electrocardiographic criteria of epicardial left ventricular origin include:

- Prolonged maximum deflection index (MDI) (Figure 24-3)—more than 0.55 is an important predictor of epicardial LVT arising from perivascular origin.[1]
- Pseudo-delta wave pattern noted with the PVC morphology (Figure 24-3)[2]—related to slower activation that originates from the epicardium toward the endocardium and late involvement of the His-Purkinje conduction system.[3,4]

The common approach to mapping a presumed left ventricular tachycardia is to first complete endocardial mapping and then to map the aortic cusp and coronary sinus of Valsalva, followed by the CS.[13,14] If these sites have poor mapping criteria, then mapping of the epicardium is completed via percutaneous epicardial access.[12]

REMOTE MAGNETIC NAVIGATION ABLATION OF EPICARDIAL PVCs

Mapping and ablation of epicardial PVC/VT arising from perivascular origin via CS system has been successfully completed even in patients with history of cardiac surgery.[15] Open-irrigated tip radiofrequency catheter ablation is utilized because of high impedance within the CS and has been demonstrated, as in our case, to be successful and safe, including unusual sites like the anterior interventricular coronary vein.[16,17]

CS venous system access is an important step to be performed when mapping idiopathic PVC, especially if ECG criteria are suggestive for epicardial origin. However, access of the CS system can be difficult with manual manipulation. Lack of access to the CS can then result in extra, unnecessary steps, including mapping of the left ventricular endocardium and aortic cusp via femoral artery puncture, with the associated risk of arterial access and catheter manipulation in the left heart. Also, the operator may then decide to cannulate the epicardial space via percutaneous pericardial puncture. Therefore, the additional effort to cannulate and map the CS, including use of a remote navigation system, is quite important. Also, remote magnetic navigation system offers other advantages over manual manipulation including catheter stability, meticulous detailed mapping, and reduced fluoroscopy.[18,19]

Delivery of RF current within the CS system requires careful attention to power and impedance. Because of high impedance within the CS, the power is quite limited when using conventional nonirrigated RF catheters. Therefore, the ablation catheter to use within the CS is an irrigated-tip, which will cool the tip-myocardium interface, allowing delivery of RF current without further increase in impedance. The suggested settings are to start at low energy (15 watts) and high flow rates of 20 to 30 cc/minute, and to titrate up the power with close monitoring of impedance changes, reduction in EGM amplitude, and elimination of the PVC source. If RF ablation with an

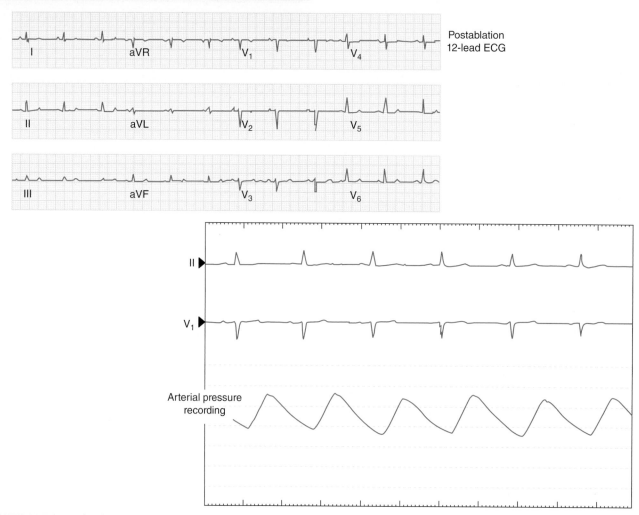

Postablation
12-lead ECG

II

V₁

Arterial pressure
recording

FIGURE 24-7 Immediately postablation, the 12-lead ECG shows sinus rhythm without PVCs (top) and the immediate hemodynamic improvement noted by the change in the arterial pressure line (bottom).

irrigated-tip catheter is not successful or limited, then an alternative is cryoablation.[20,21]

CONCLUSION

Idiopathic left ventricular outflow tract PVC that is most likely arising from a perivascular origin is best mapped first endocardially, then via the CS venous system. When manual manipulation fails, remote magnetic navigation facilitates an access of the CS as well as stability of the RF ablation catheter. Because of the unique CS anatomy and ablation within a venous structure, an irrigated-tip ablation catheter should be utilized using low energy and high irrigation flow rate, with increase in energy until achieving the desired result.

REFERENCES

1. Daniels DV, Lu YY, Morton JB, et al. Idiopathic epicardial left ventricular tachycardia originating remote from the sinus of Valsalva: electrophysiological characteristics, catheter ablation, and identification from the 12-lead electrocardiogram. *Circulation.* 2006;113(13):1659-1666.

2. Rodriguez LM, Smeets JL, Timmermans C, Wellens HC. Predictors for successful ablation of right- and left-sided idiopathic ventricular tachycardia. *Am J Cardiol.* 1997;79:309-314.

3. Burgess MJ, Lux RL, Ershler PR, Menlove R. Determination of transmural location of onset of activation from cardiac surface electrograms. *Circulation.* 1990;82:1335-1342.

4. Josephson ME, Miller JM. Endocardial and epicardial recordings: correlation of twelve-lead electrocardiograms at the site of origin of ventricular tachycardia. *Ann N Y Acad Sci.* 1990;601:128-147.

5. Lerman BB, Stein KM, Markowitz SM, Mechanisms of idiopathic left ventricular tachycardia. *J Cardiovasc Electrophysiol.* 1997;5:571-583.

6. Dixit S. Idiopathic premature ventricular complexes causing tachycardia-induced cardiomyopathy: benign arrhythmia with sinister implications. *Heart Rhythm.* 2007;7:868-869.

7. Chugh SS, Shen WK, Luria DM, Smith HC. First evidence of premature ventricular complex-induced cardiomyopathy: a potentially reversible cause of heart failure. *J Cardiovasc Electrophysiol.* 2000;ii:328-329.

REMOTE MAGNETIC |NAVIGATION ABLATION OF
IDIOPATHIC EPICARDIAL PREMATURE VENTRICULAR
COMPLEXES

SECTION III
CASE STUDIES IN VENTRICULAR
TACHYCARDIA

173

8. Bogun F, Crawford T, Reich S, et al. Radiofrequency ablation of frequent, idiopathic premature ventricular complexes: comparison with a control group without intervention. *Heart Rhythm.* 2007;7:863-867.

9. Callans DJ, Menz V, Schwartzman D, Gottlieb CD, Marchlinski FE. Repetitive monomorphic tachycardia from the left ventricular outflow tract: electrocardiographic patterns consistent with a left ventricular site of origin. *J Am Coll Cardiol.* 1997;29:1023-1027.

10. Yeh SJ, Wen MS, Wang CC, Lin FC, Wu D. Adenosine-sensitive ventricular tachycardia from the anterobasal left ventricle. *J Am Coll Cardiol.* 1997;30:1339-1345.

11. Ouyang F, Cappato R, Ernst S, et al. Electroanatomic substrate of idiopathic left ventricular tachycardia: unidirectional block and macro-reentry within the Purkinje network. *Circulation.* 2002;105:462-469.

12. Nogami A. Idiopathic left ventricular tachycardia: assessment and treatment. *Cardiac Electrophysiol Rev.* 2002;6:448-462.

13. Tada H, Naito S, Ito S, et al. Significance of two potentials for predicting successful catheter ablation from the left sinus of valsalva for left ventricular epicardial tachycardia. *Pacing Clin Electrophysiol.* 2004;8:1053-1059.

14. Tada H. Idiopathic epicardial ventricular arrhythmias: diagnosis and ablation technique from the aortic sinus of valsalva. *Indian Pacing Electrophysiol J.* 2005;5:96-105.

15. Najjar Jl, Bortone A, Boveda S, Albenque JP. Radiofrequency ablation of an epicardial ventricular tachycardia through the great cardiac vein in a patient with mitro-aortic mechanical prostheses. *Europace.* 2007;9:1069-1072.

16. Mantica M, De Luca L, Fagundes R, Tondo C. Transcatheter ablation through the cardiac veins in a patient with a biventricular device and left ventricular epicardial arrhythmias. *Europace.* 2006;8:980-983.

17. Hirasawa Y, Miyauchi Y, Kiiwasaki Y, Kobayashi Y. Successful radiofrequency catheter ablation of epicardial left ventricular outflow tract tachycardia from the anterior interventricular coronary vein. *J Cardiovasc Electrophysiol.* 2005;16:1378-1380.

18. Schmidt B, Chun KRJ, Tilz RR, Koektuerk B, Ouyang F, Kuck KH. Remote navigation systems in electrophysiology. *Europace.* 2008;10:iii57-iii61.

19. Saliba W, Reddy VY, Wazni O, et al. Atrial fibrillation ablation using a robotic catheter remote control system: initial human experience and long-term follow-up results. *J Am Coll Cardiol.* 2008;51;2407-2411.

20. Houmsse M, Daoud EG. Techniques to ablate premature ventricular ectopy arising from the coronary sinus system. *Pacing Clin Electrophysiol.* 2010;34:e74-e77.

21. Di Biase L, Saliba W, Natale A. Successful ablation of epicardial arrhythmias with cryoenergy after failed attempts with radiofrequency energy. *Heart Rhythm.* 2009;6,109-112.

25 BUNDLE BRANCH REENTRANT VENTRICULAR TACHYCARDIA

Emile G. Daoud, MD

CASE PRESENTATION

A 68-year-old woman is admitted for an evaluation of sudden syncope resulting in a head laceration. She has a 4-year history of a nonischemic cardiomyopathy with stable NYHA class II symptoms and left ventricular ejection fraction of 40%, treated with lisinopril and Toprol XL. Laboratory studies were unremarkable, and surface echocardiography demonstrates no change in the ejection fraction. The 12-lead ECG shows sinus bradycardia with a left bundle branch block (LBBB) pattern (Figure 25-1).

EXPERT OPINION

This is a worrisome history. Sudden syncope associated with an injury, especially in the setting of structural heart disease, implies an abrupt drop in blood pressure with subsequent cerebral hypoperfusion and loss of consciousness. The evaluation should be based on the assumption that the mechanism is a malignant dysrhythmia.

- *Differential*: Ventricular tachycardia (VT); findings from the ECG suggests sinus node disease, infra-Hisian conduction block.

- Neurological etiologies and vasodepressor mechanisms of syncope are unlikely in the absence of prior neurologic disease or symptoms of vagal discharge.

- *Evaluation*: Electrophysiology study (EPS) to evaluate for a mechanism of syncope. Since the accuracy of electrophysiology testing in the setting of a nonischemic cardiomyopathy is low, if the EPS does not reveal the etiology of syncope, there should be a consideration for empiric implantation of a defibrillator (ICD).

PATHOPHYSIOLOGY AND MANAGEMENT

At EPS, VT was reproducibly induced with programmed stimulation of the ventricle. The tracing (Figure 25-2) shows surface leads V_1 and aVF and intracardiac tracings from the His catheter and the radiofrequency ablation (RFA) catheter, positioned at the right bundle. The mechanism of the tachycardia is bundle branch reentrant ventricular tachycardia (BBR-VT). The hallmark features are:

- VA dissociation. The single atrial beat is marked with an A on the His mid electrode.

- QRS morphology during the VT is identical to the QRS morphology of the patient's native LBBB during sinus rhythm.

- There is significant infra-Hisian conduction delay during the VT with an H-V interval of 124 ms.

- The activation sequence is from His bundle→right bundle→right ventricular myocardium. The right bundle potential is highlighted with an arrow.

- Changes in the H-H interval precede changes in the V-V interval (compare the H-H interval measurements on His ds to V-V intervals on the RFA recording).

The mechanism of BBR-VT is significant conduction disease within the His-Purkinje system establishing the substrate for reentry. The most common form of BBR-VT utilizes antegrade conduction over the right bundle (Figure 25-3). The tachycardia is often initiated by retrograde block in the right bundle, slow concealed retrograde conduction over the left bundle-His (curved dashed line), allowing adequate time for recovery and then antegrade conduction over the right bundle. Activation of the myocardium (the asterisk *) is with a QRS morphology identical to a left bundle branch block pattern. The VT was successfully eliminated by ablation of the right bundle. Postablation, infranodal conduction was unreliable, and a biventricular pacing ICD was subsequently implanted.

Features of Bundle Branch Reentrant VT

- BBR-VT is an unusual reentrant VT utilizing both bundles and is due to conduction disease within the His-Purkinje system; it is

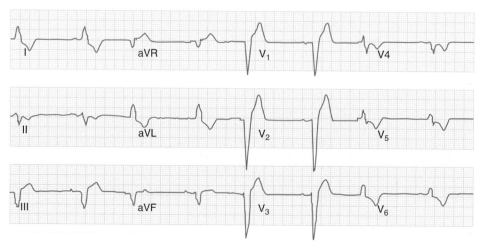

FIGURE 25.1 Sinus bradycardia with a left bundle branch block pattern.

BUNDLE BRANCH REENTRANT VENTRICULAR
TACHYCARDIA

SECTION III
CASE STUDIES IN VENTRICULAR
TACHYCARDIA

175

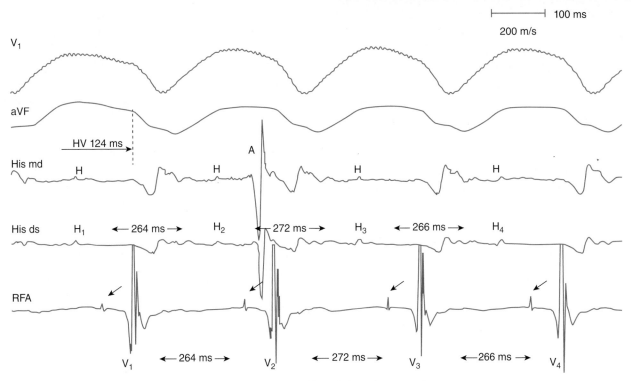

FIGURE 25.2 Surface and intracardiac tracing during induced sustained bundle branch reentry VT.

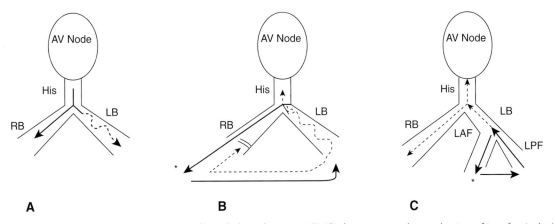

A   **B**   **C**

FIGURE 25.3 (A) and (B) demonstrate the mechanism of bundle branch reentry VT; (C) demonstrates the mechanism of interfascicular VT.

more commonly induced in patients with nonischemic CM (up to 40%) than ischemic CM (4%-6%).

- Also reported in patients with prior aortic/mitral valve surgery due to proximity of surgery to conduction system, myotonic dystrophy, and with a Class I sodium channel-blocking antiarrhythmic medication. Each of these can result in slow conduction in the His-Purkinje system.

- Patients often present with syncope, near-syncope, or sudden cardiac death.

- The morphology of the VT is usually a LBBB pattern with an identical morphology as the patient's native QRS conduction during sinus rhythm; it can also be a right bundle branch block VT.

- Findings at EPS often include: (1) prolongation of the HV interval; (2) tachycardia induction is dependent upon critical prolongation of

the V-H interval; (3) during VT, the HV interval is usually longer than baseline conduction, but can be unchanged or slightly shorter; (4) during VT, a stable His potential is recorded prior to each QRS and changes in the H-H interval precede changes in the V-V interval (Figure 25-2).

- Tachycardia can be eliminated by ablation of one of the bundles—most often and easily the right bundle. Successful ablation, however, may result in complete or high-grade AV block.

- Another form of His-Purkinje VT is interfascicular VT. This reentrant circuit is contained within the left anterior and left posterior fascicles. Thus, the VT morphology often has a right bundle/left anterior or posterior fascicular block pattern (Figure 25-3).

REFERENCES

1. Akhtar M, Gilbert C, Wolf F, et al. Reentry within the His-Purkinje system. Elucidation of reentrant circuit using right bundle branch and His bundle recordings. *Circulation.* 1978;58(2):295-304.

2. Cohen TJ, Chien WW, Lurie KG, et al. Radiofrequency catheter ablation for treatment of bundle branch reentrant ventricular tachycardia: results and long-term follow-up. *J Am Coll Cardiol.* 1991;18:1767-1773.

3. Merino JL, Peinado R, Fernandez-Lozano I, et al. Bundle-branch reentry and the postpacing interval after entrainment by right ventricular apex stimulation: a new approach to elucidate the mechanism of wide-QRS-complex tachycardia with atrioventricular dissociation. *Circulation.* 2001;103:1102-1108.

4. Crijns HJ, Smeets JL, Rodriguez LM, et al. Cure of interfascicular reentrant ventricular tachycardia by ablation of the anterior fascicle of the left bundle branch. *J Cardiovasc Electrophysiol.* 1995;6:486-492.

5. Mazur A, Kusniec J, Strasberg B. Bundle branch reentrant ventricular tachycardia. *Indian Pacing Electrophysiol J.* 2005;5:86-95.

VENTRICULAR TACHYCARDIA
IN CONGENITAL HEART DISEASE

SECTION III
CASE STUDIES IN VENTRICULAR
TACHYCARDIA

177

26 VENTRICULAR TACHYCARDIA IN CONGENITAL HEART DISEASE

Naomi J. Kertesz, MD

CASE PRESENTATION

The patient is a 26-year-old man with past medical history of tetralogy of Fallot, status post complete repair at 9 months of age with a large transannular RV outflow patch in addition to ASD and VSD closure. The repair included a ventriculotomy. This is the only surgical intervention BW has undergone.

BW has had palpitations for the past 5 years. He also describes 4 syncopal episodes over the past 7 years. All episodes were associated with painful stimuli. He was given an event monitor that demonstrated SVT at 150 bpm (Figure 26-1). As part of his normal follow-up he underwent an MRI and was found to have right ventricular ejection fraction of 36% and a right ventricular end diastolic volume of 161 mL/m^2 (Figure 26-2). As part of a prepulmonary valve replacement protocol, he underwent a hemodynamic catheterization (Figure 26-3) and programmed ventricular stimulation (Figure 26-4). There was reproducibly inducible monomorphic VT with double and triple extra stimuli at baseline from the RV apex that was able to be pace-terminated (Figures 26-5 and 26-6). The VT circuit was mapped using 3-D mapping, and an array catheter and was found to be a macroreentrant circuit around the right ventricular free wall which corresponded to his prior right ventriculotomy site (Figure 26-7). He underwent a slow pathway modification for his atrioventricular node reentry. He went to the operating room the following day and underwent surgical pulmonary valve replacement and cryoablation to isolate the area of the right ventricular outflow tract. He underwent a repeat electrophysiology study 8 months later and had no inducible arrhythmias with or without isoproterenol.

EPIDEMIOLOGY

- Congenital heart disease (CHD) is the most common form of birth defect with an incidence of 8 significant defects per 1000 live births.[1] Due to advances in both diagnosis and treatment the majority of children live to adulthood. Over one million adult congenital heart disease patients are living in the United States.[2] There are now a greater number of adults than children with congenital heart disease living in the United States.[3]

- Forty-five percent of these adults have simple defects (atrial septal defect, ventricular septal defect, valve stenosis).

- Forty percent have moderately complex heart disease (tetralogy of Fallot).

- Ventricular arrhythmias are rare among CHD patients during the first or second decade of life.

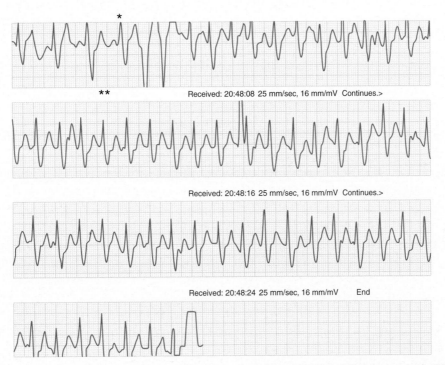

*

** Received: 20:48:08 25 mm/sec, 16 mm/mV Continues.>

Received: 20:48:16 25 mm/sec, 16 mm/mV Continues.>

Received: 20:48:24 25 mm/sec, 16 mm/mV End

FIGURE 26-1 Transtelephonic monitor (TTM) tracing demonstrating SVT. At first glance, the TTM demonstrates a wide QRS tachycardia. On further inspection, the QRS in sinus rhythm (*) is the same as the QRS in tachycardia (**). Patients with congenital heart disease commonly have a bundle branch block at baseline due to VSD repair. Therefore, it is important to determine not only the QRS duration but to determine whether the morphology is the same or different as that which is seen in sinus rhythm.

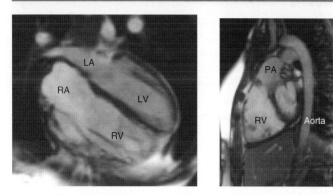

FIGURE 26-2 MRI of patient with TOF. This patient has a dilated RV and PA due to severe pulmonary regurgitation following TOF repair. Many patients require pulmonary valve replacement during late adolescence or early adulthood.

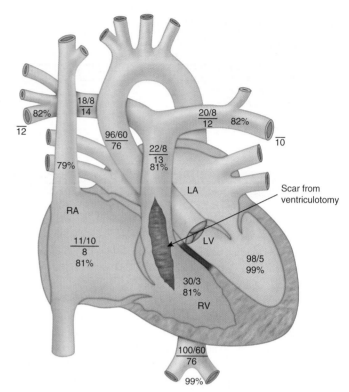

FIGURE 26-3 Cardiac catheterization diagram. The ventriculotomy incision was used to enlarge the RVOT, pulmonary valve, and MPA.

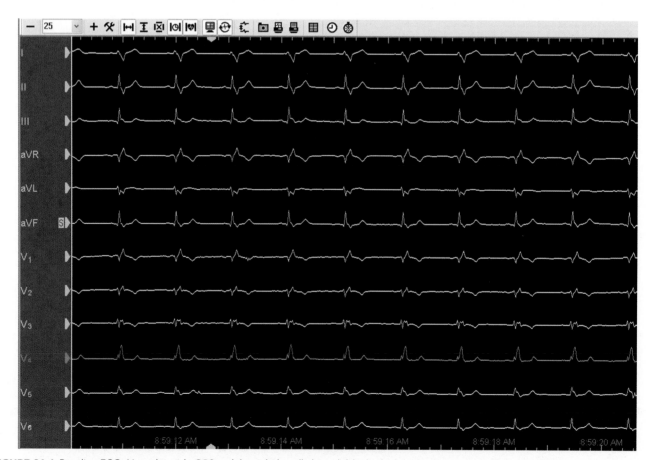

FIGURE 26-4 Baseline ECG. Note the wide QRS and the right bundle branch block which is classic in patients following TOF repair.

VENTRICULAR TACHYCARDIA
IN CONGENITAL HEART DISEASE

SECTION III
CASE STUDIES IN VENTRICULAR
TACHYCARDIA

179

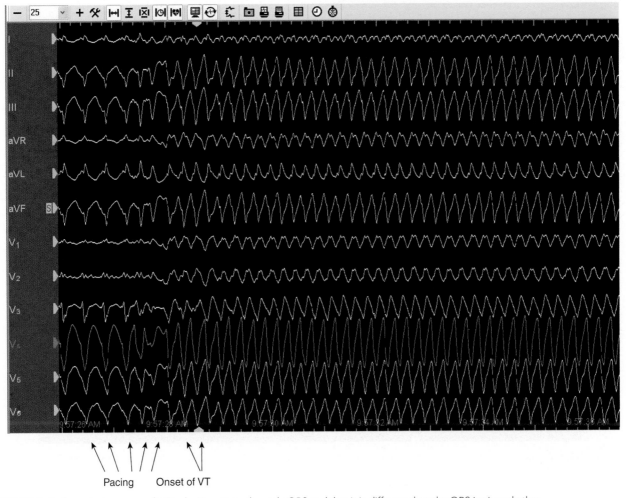

Pacing   Onset of VT

FIGURE 26-5 Surface electrograms of VT induction. Note the wide QRS and that it is different than the QRS in sinus rhythm.

- Patients at highest risk for developing ventricular tachycardia are those who have undergone a ventriculotomy or patching of certain ventricular septal defects.

- Historically sudden cardiac death (SCD) in patients with CHD has been observed most often among patients with TOF and transposition of the great arteries (TGA) who are status post a Mustard or Senning operation[4] (Figure 26-8).

- However, due to advances in surgical technique and timing of repair, a substantial shift in the epidemiology of mortality in CHD patients has occurred over the past 25 years. A comparison of mortality due to CHD between 1987 and 1988 and between 2004 and 2005 showed that the overall mortality rate had decreased by 31%.[5] There has been a 40% reduction in annualized death rates for TOF and a 71% reduction for TGA between 1979 and 2005 in the United States.[6] In patients with noncyanotic defects such as ventricular septal defects and coarctation of the aorta, arrhythmias were the leading cause of death before 1990, but after 1990 myocardial infarction was the leading cause of overall mortality. In those with cyanotic defects, ie, TOF and TGA, arrhythmias remain the leading cause of late death.

- Sustained VT appears to be the single biggest contributor to the 2% per decade incidence of sudden death in TOF.[2]

ETIOLOGY AND PATHOPHYSIOLOGY

- There are two main causes of ventricular arrhythmias in congenital heart disease. One is the result of the surgical scars from the repair, and the other is due to long-standing abnormal hemodynamics resulting from volume or pressure overload. Understanding the causes of the arrhythmia is only half the battle. One should understand that the surgical repairs have changed over time and the age at which these repairs are performed has also changed. This has contributed to the changing incidence of sudden cardiac death.

- The mechanism for VT resulting from scar is reminiscent of the intra-arterial reentry atrial tachycardia (scar atrial flutter). It is due to a macroreentrant circuit involving narrow conduction corridors defined by the regions of surgical scar and natural conduction barriers such as the rim of a ventricular septal defect and the edge of a valve annulus. Tetralogy of Fallot is a classic example of congenital heart disease that results in this type of VT. The prevalence of VT after TOF repair has been estimated to be between 3% and 14%.[2]

- Ventricular arrhythmias can also develop due to long standing hemodynamic overload, which causes advanced ventricular dysfunction or hypertrophy. Examples of CHD lesions that can eventually lead to this myopathic variety of VT include aortic valve

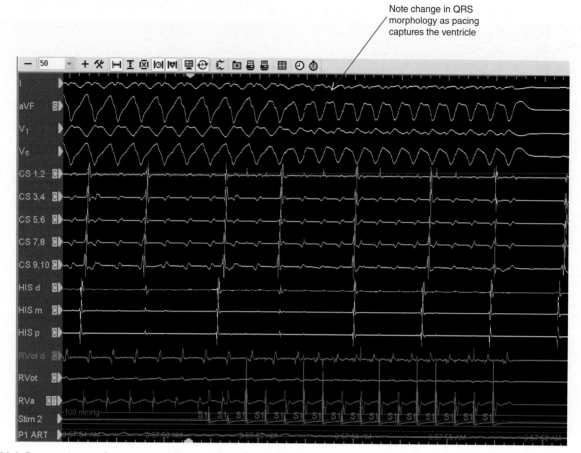

FIGURE 26-6 Burst pacing used to terminate VT. Note onset of pacing as seen as S_1 on the Stim channel. Note the change in QRS morphology as pacing captures the ventricle.

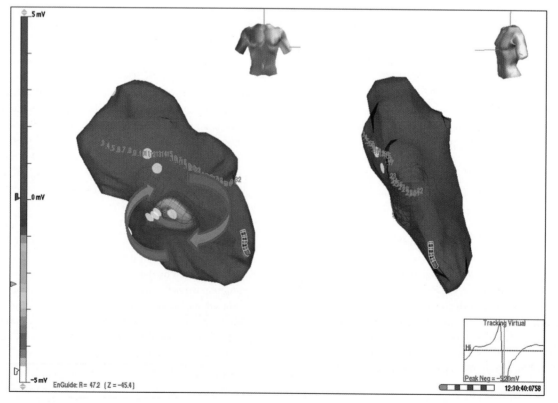

FIGURE 26-7 AP and lateral projections of right ventricle. In the image on the left, the white dots represent area of scar from ventriculotomy incision, and the blue arrows represent the circuit of the VT traveling between two areas of scar.

VENTRICULAR TACHYCARDIA
IN CONGENITAL HEART DISEASE

SECTION III
CASE STUDIES IN VENTRICULAR
TACHYCARDIA

181

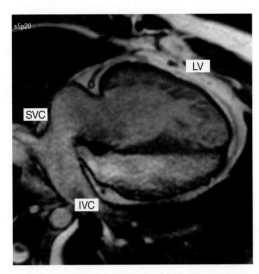

FIGURE 26-8 Transposition status post atrial baffle repair (Mustard or Senning repair). Note that the SVC and IVC blood is directed to the mitral valve and left ventricle, which is connected to the pulmonary artery. The pulmonary veins, not shown, are directed to the right ventricle, which is connected to the aorta.

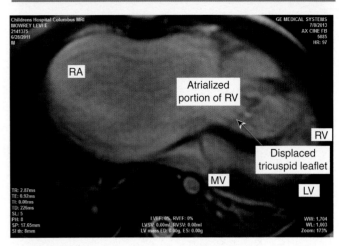

FIGURE 26-9 MRI of Ebstein anomaly. Note large amount of atrialized right ventricle due to displaced tricuspid leaflets. The functional RV is now significantly smaller due to a large part becoming atrialized (above the TV).

disease; LTGA or DTGA following atrial repair when the right ventricle is the systemic ventricle; severe Ebstein anomaly (Figure 26-9); single ventricle physiology (Figure 26-10); and Eisenmengers syndrome.[2]

DIAGNOSIS AND MANAGEMENT

- While sustained VT can lead to sudden cardiac death or syncope, some patients present with palpitations. As many of them have an underlying bundle branch block, it is important to realize that the presence of a wide QRS tachycardia does not mean it is ventricular in etiology. Alternatively, if a patient does not faint, it does not mean that it is SVT. Distinguishing VT from SVT can be challenging in young adults in whom a baseline ECG is not available. Due to the relatively healthy AV node, it is not uncommon for there to be one-to-one ventriculoatrial (VA) conduction retrograde in VT (Figure 26-11). Adenosine and/or the use of a transesophageal lead can be very helpful to produce transient VA dissociation to prove that the AV node is not part of the arrhythmia circuit (Figures 26-12 and 26-13).

- While patients may present with sustained ventricular arrhythmias, it is far more common for individuals to present with nonsustained VT.

- The value of programmed ventricular stimulation (VSTIM) in patients with CHD was demonstrated by Alexander et al in 1999.[7] VSTIM identified a subgroup with significantly increased mortality and sudden arrhythmic events. A negative VSTIM was a favorable prognostic sign; however, the frequency of false-negative studies was high.

- The value of VSTIM was then evaluated in patients following TOF.[8] Inducible monomorphic VT and polymorphic VT predicted future clinical VT and SCD. In a multivariate analysis, inducible sustained VT was an independent risk factor for subsequent events (Figure 26-14).

- As many patients with TOF have significant pulmonary regurgitation, it was thought that if the underlying hemodynamic abnormalities were corrected the patients would no longer be at risk of SCD. Harrild demonstrated that the incidence of VT or sudden death was

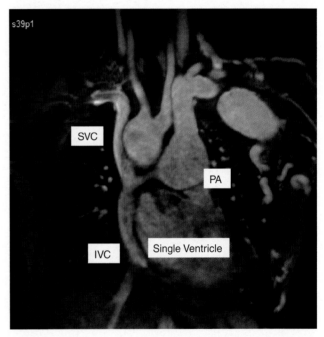

FIGURE 26-10 Single ventricle patient status post-Fontan procedure. Note SVC and IVC with direct connection to pulmonary artery with no intervening ventricle. Note the large dilated single ventricle.

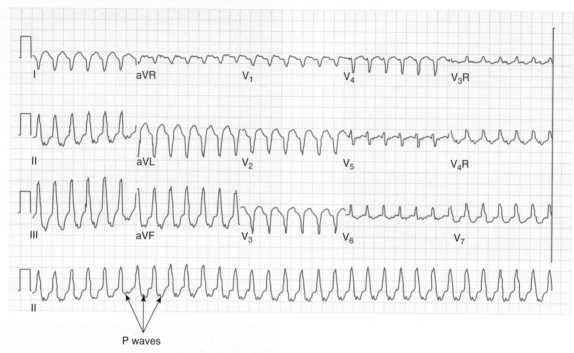

FIGURE 26-11 Wide QRS tachycardia in an 18-year-old with 1:1 VA conduction. This could be either SVT or VT. It is unlikely to be SVT in a patient with TOF because the tachycardia has a LBBB morphology rather than a RBBB.

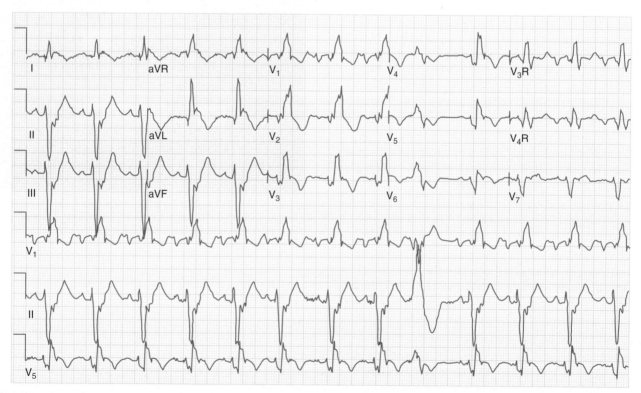

FIGURE 26-12 Baseline ECG in a 44-year-old with TOF. Note RBBB morphology of QRS.

VENTRICULAR TACHYCARDIA
IN CONGENITAL HEART DISEASE

SECTION III
CASE STUDIES IN VENTRICULAR
TACHYCARDIA

183

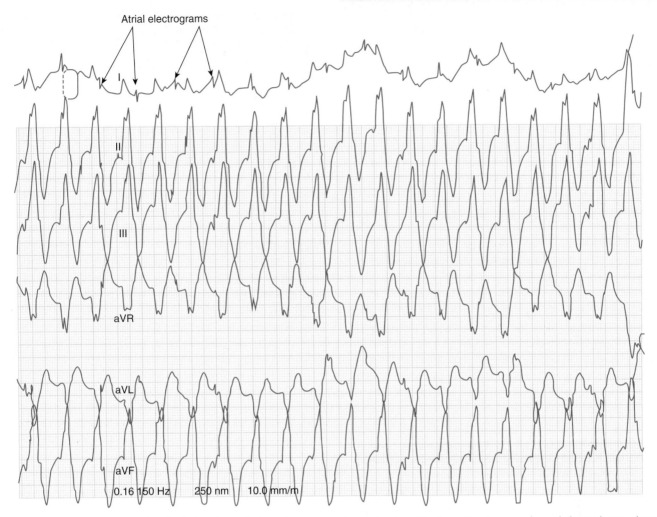

FIGURE 26-13 Same patient with wide QRS tachycardia. In order to prove the mechanism of tachycardia a transesophageal electrode was placed that demonstrated VA dissociation.

not reduced by pulmonary valve replacement and improvement of hemodynamics.[9]

- Attention was then focused on the determining the indications for primary prevention of sudden cardiac death. The largest study to identify independent predictors of sudden death included 793 patients with repaired TOF from six centers. Four independent predictors were identified: older age at repair, QRS interval of 180 msec or longer, transannular patch, and annual increase QRS interval.[10]

- In Khairy's study evaluating VSTIM in TOF, the independent risk factors for inducible VT were age 18 or older at the time of testing, palpitations, prior palliative surgery, modified Lown classification of premature ventricular beats of two or higher, and a CT ratio of 0.6 or higher on CXR.[8] Inducible sustained VT had a sensitivity of 77% and specificity of 79.5% in predicting sudden cardiac death or clinical ventricular tachycardia.

- Given the low rate of sudden cardiac death in TOF of 0.15%, the decision of whether to implant an ICD can be difficult. In a study

evaluating the role of ICDs in patients with TOF, the only two independent predictors of appropriate shocks were nonsustained VT and a left ventricular end-diastolic pressure higher than 12 mm Hg. A risk score was developed on the basis of regression coefficients of the variables retained in the final multivariate model (Table 26-1). Patients were into low (0-2), intermediate (3-5), and high risk (6-12) groups based on their risk of sudden death as shown in Fig 15.[11]

- The risk of ICD implantation, however, is not zero. When evaluating patients with both ICD and CHD, inappropriate shocks were observed in 30% of patients predominantly because of atrial tachyarrhythmias. Related complications were seen in 29% of patients with ICD implantation.[12] In patients with TOF and ICDs, inappropriate shocks were observed in 5.8% of patients per year. Complications other than inappropriate shocks occurred in 30% and were predominantly late-lead related.[11]

- Risk stratification for sudden death in TOF remains imperfect and incomplete. Figure 26-15 summarizes a generalized algorithmic

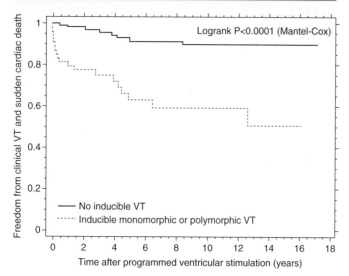

FIGURE 26-14 Value of programmed ventricular stimulation in tetralogy of Fallot. Kaplan-Meier event-free survival curves are plotted and compared according to whether patients did or did not have inducible sustained VT on electrophysiology testing. Those patients with inducible VT had significantly higher risk of either clinical VT or sudden cardiac death. (Reproduced with permission from Kairy P, Landzberg MJ, Gatzoulis MA, et al. Value of programmed ventricular stimulation after tetralogy of Fallot repair. *Circulation.* 2004;109:1994-2000. Figure 2B:1998.)

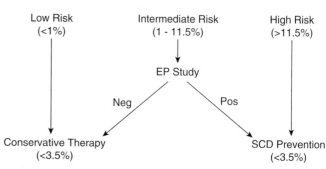

Risk Score	Risk Category	Sudden Death Risk
0 - 2	Low	<1%
3 - 5	Intermediate	1 - 11.5%
6 - 12	High	>11.5%

FIGURE 26-15 Risk stratification approach by Khairy et al[13] in tetralogy of Fallot. Risk score is calculated based on variables in Table 26-1. Based on the risk category, the decision can be made whether an EP study with ventricular extrastimulus protocol would increase the risk of sudden cardic death to justify ICD implantation.

TABLE 26-1 Risk Score for Appropriate Implantable Cardioverter-Defibrillator Shocks in Primary Prevention

Variable	Points Attributed
Prior palliative shunt	2
Inducible sustained VT	2
QRS duration ≥180 ms	1
Ventriculotomy incision	2
Nonsustained VT	2
LVEDP ≥12	3
Total Points	12

Abbreviations: LVEDP, left ventricular end diastolic pressure; VT = ventricular tachycardia.

approach by Khairy et al[13] that is based on a quantitative assessment of the current state of knowledge.

• While there is a great body of literature demonstrating the risk factors associated with sudden death in TOF, this is not true about DTGA status post atrial switch procedure. Currently, the only documented risk factors for sudden death in this population are symptoms of arrhythmia or heart failure or documented atrial flutter or fibrillation. This data makes the decision to place ICDs for primary prevention difficult.

VENTRICULAR TACHYCARDIA
IN CONGENITAL HEART DISEASE

SECTION III
CASE STUDIES IN VENTRICULAR
TACHYCARDIA

185

REFERENCES

1. Hoffman JL, Kaplan Silberthson RR. Prevalence of congenital heart disease. *Am Heart J.* 2004;147(3):425-439.

2. Walsh E, Cecchin F. Arrhythmias in adult patients with congenital heart disease. *Circulation.* 2007;115(4):534-545.

3. Perloff JK, Warnes CA. Challenges posed by adults with repaired congenital heart disease. *Circulation.* 2001;103(21):2637-2643.

4. Silka M, Bar-Cohen. A contemporary assessment of the risk for sudden cardiac death in patients with congenital heart disease. *Pediatr Cardiol.* 2012;33(3):452-460.

5. Khairy P, Ionescu-Ittu R, Mackie AS, Abrahmaowicz M, Pilote L, Marelli AJ. Changing mortality in congenital hear disease. *J Am Coll Cardiol.* 2010;56(14):1149-1157.

6. Pillutla P, Shetty KD, Foster E. Mortality associated with adult congenital heart disease: trends in the U.S. population from 1979 to 2005. *Am Heart J.* 2009;158(5):874-879.

7. Alexander ME, Walsh EP, Saul JP, Epstein MR, Triedman JK. Value of programmed ventricular stimulation in patients with congenital heart disease. *J Cardiovasc Electrophysiol.* 1999;10(8):1033-1044.

8. Kairy P, Landzberg MJ, Gatzoulis MA, et al. Value of programmed ventricular stimulation after tetralogy of Fallot repair. *Circulation.* 2004;109(16):1994-2000.

9. Harrild DM, Berul CI, Cecchin F, et al. Pulmonary valve replacement in tetralogy of Fallot: impact on survival and ventricular tachycardia. *Circulation.* 2009(3);119:445-451.

10. Gatzoulis MA, Balaji, Webber SA, et al. Risk factors for arrhythmia and sudden cardiac death late after repair tetralogy of Fallot: a multicenter study. *Lancet.* 2000;256(9234):975-981.

11. Khairy P, Harris L, Landzberg MJ, et al. Implantable cardioverter–defibrillators in tetralogy of Fallot. *Circulation.* 2008;117(3):363-370.

12. Koyak Z, de Groot JR, Van Gelder IC, et al. Implantable cardioverter defibrillator therapy in adults with congenital heart disease: who is at risk of shocks? *Circ Arrhythm Electrophysiol.* 2012;5(1):101-110.

13. Khairy P, Dore A, Poirier N, et al. Risk stratification in surgically repaired tetralogy of Fallot. *Expert Rev Cardiovasc Ther.* 2009;7(7):755-762.

SECTION IV

PREVENTION OF THROMBOEMBOLISM RELATED TO ATRIAL FIBRILLATION

27 PREVENTION OF THROMBOEMBOLISM IN ATRIAL FIBRILLATION: COUMADIN

Zhenguo Liu, MD, PhD

CASE PRESENTATION

A 67-year-old woman with medical history of hypertension and type 2 diabetes was evaluated at the emergency department for sudden onset of right facial dropping and slurred speech. No other complaints. Her blood pressure was 146/82 mm Hg with heat rate 78 bpm and irregular. Her 12-lead ECG upon arrival in the emergency room showed atrial fibrillation with ventricular rate of 74. A head CT scan and carotid ultrasound examination were unremarkable. Her symptoms were resolved 12 hours later. A transesophageal echocardiogram revealed a dilated left atrium, moderate mitral regurgitation, and mild global left ventricular hypokinesis with an estimated ejection fraction of 45%. No apparent thrombus was identified in her left atrial appendage. No right to left shunt was present. A subsequent coronary angiogram demonstrated non–flow-limiting lesions. Attempts were made to convert her to normal sinus rhythm without success. She was sent home with a β-blocker, ACE inhibitor, baby ASA, and Coumadin (warfarin). The patient has been doing well since then.

COMMENTS AND DISCUSSION

Atrial fibrillation (AF) is the most common cardiac arrhythmia with a growing prevalence due to an aging population. One of the major issues for AF is stroke and systemic embolism in patients at high risk that are associated with significant morbidity and mortality as well as medical cost. Existing data demonstrate that oral anticoagulation is highly cost-effective for the prevention of stroke and systemic embolism in high-risk patients, but not for those with a low risk of stroke. Coumadin or warfarin is one of the commonly used oral anticoagulation agents for the prevention and treatment of thromboembolism in patients with AF or atrial flutter.[1,2]

MECHANISM OF ACTION, PHARMACODYNAMICS, AND PHARMACOKINETICS FOR COUMADIN

- Coumadin or warfarin acts by inhibiting the synthesis of vitamin K-dependent clotting factors, including factors II, VII, IX, and X, and the anticoagulant proteins C and S.

- Anticoagulation effect generally occurs within 24 hours after oral administration. Its peak anticoagulant effect may be delayed for 72 to 96 hours. The duration of action of a single dosing is 2 to 5 days. The effective half-life ranges from 20 to 60 hours with a mean of about 40 hours.

- Coumadin is essentially absorbed completely after oral administration, with its peak concentration usually within 4 hours of administration. Approximately 99% of the drug is bound to plasma proteins with a small distribution volume.

- The elimination of coumadin is almost entirely by hepatic cytochrome P-450 enzymes that may vary based on patient's age and ethnic background. Asian patients may require lower initiation and maintenance doses.

INDICATIONS FOR COUMADIN THERAPY IN AF PATIENTS

- Due to significant risk for stroke and systemic embolism, anticoagulation therapy is recommended for high-risk AF patients. Patient characteristics and risk factors have been used for stroke risk stratification, known as **CHADS$_2$** (1 point for each of the following: **C**ongestive heart failure, **H**ypertension, **A**ge $\geq$75 years, **D**iabetes, and 2 points for previous **S**troke or transient ischemic attack) and recently **CHA$_2$DS$_2$-VASc** (1 point for **C**ongestive heart failure, **H**ypertension, 2 points for **A**ge $\geq$75 years, 1 point for **D**iabetes, 2 points for previous **S**troke, transient ischemic attack, or thromboembolism, 1 point for **V**ascular disease, **A**ge 65 to 75 years, and female **S**ex category) as shown in Table 27-1. The ACC/AHA/HRS/ESC recommends that AF patients with a CHADS$_2$ score of $\geq$1 should be treated with oral anticoagulation (such as Coumadin with international normalized ratio [INR] 2-3) if no contraindications exist.[1-5]

- Oral anticoagulation therapy (such as Coumadin with INR 2-3) is recommended for AF patients before and after cardioversion for at least 4 weeks regardless of their CHADS$_2$ score.

- Systemic anticoagulation such as Coumadin with INR 2-3 is recommended for all patients for at least 2 months following an AF ablation procedure. Continuation of systemic anticoagulation more than 2 months following ablation should be based on the patient's risk factors, including assessment with CHADS$_2$ or CHA$_2$DS$_2$VASc score, and other risk factors for stroke and *not* on the amount of AF or type (paroxysmal, persistent or long-standing persistent AF) of AF.

MANAGEMENT OF PATIENTS WITH HIGH INR

If a patient's INR is high ($\geq$4.0) or Coumadin therapy needs to be reversed clinically, an algorithm could be followed as suggested by Garcia and Crowther[6] and as shown in Figure 27-1.

TABLE 27-1 Factors for Establishing the Risk of Stroke in AF Patients

Risk Factor	CHADS$_2$ Score	CHA$_2$DS$_2$-VASc Score
Congestive heart failure	1	1
Hypertension	1	1
Age $\geq$75	1	2
Type 2 diabetes	1	1
Stroke/TIA/thromboembolism	2	2
Vascular disease	N/A	1
Age 65 to 74	N/A	1
Female Sex	N/A	1
Maximum score	6	9

PREVENTION OF THROMBOEMBOLISM IN ATRIAL
FIBRILLATION: COUMADIN

SECTION IV
PREVENTION OF THROMBOEMBOLISM
RELATED TO ATRIAL FIBRILLATION

189

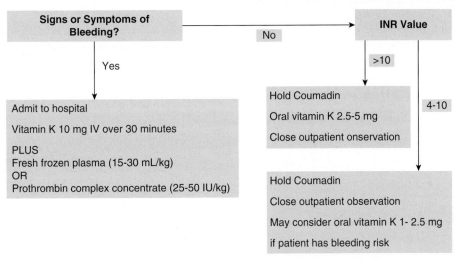

FIGURE 27-1 Suggested algorithm for the management of patients with international normalized ratio (INR) over 4. Abbreviation: IV, intravenously. (Modified with permission from Garcia DA, Crowther MA. Reversal of warfarin: case-based practice recommendations. Circulation. 2012;Jun 12;125(23):2944-2947).

ALTERNATIVES TO ANTICOAGULATION WITH COUMADIN

- Dabigatran (Pradaxa) and rivaroxaban (Xarelto) are new anticoagulants approved for the prevention of thromboembolic events in AF patients. There is no need for laboratory monitoring for INR or dietary restrictions. However, these agents carry the bleeding risks similar to that of Coumadin and are without a reliable reversal agent.[7]

- Combined therapy with clopidogrel (Plavix) and aspirin may occasionally be considered if the patient is not a suitable candidate for Coumadin or dabigatran or rivaroxaban. But this dual antiplatelet therapy is less effective for the prevention of thromboembolic events.

CONCOMITANT TREATMENT WITH COUMADIN AND ANTIPLATELET AGENTS

- Triple therapy with Coumadin and aspirin plus clopidogrel has increased risk for bleeding with no significant benefit on reducing thromboembolic risk in AF patients.[8,9]

- Double therapy with Coumadin and one antiplatelet agent (aspirin or clopidogrel) increases the risk for early bleeding (within 90 days after initiation).

REFERENCES

1. Calkins H, Kuck KH, Cappato R, et al. 2012 HRS/EHRA/ECAS expert consensus statement on catheter and surgical ablation of atrial fibrillation: recommendations for patient selection, procedural techniques, patient management and follow-up, definitions, endpoints, and research trial design: a report of the Heart Rhythm Society (HRS) Task Force on Catheter and Surgical Ablation of Atrial Fibrillation. Developed in partnership with the European Heart Rhythm Association (EHRA), a registered branch of the European Society of Cardiology (ESC) and the European Cardiac Arrhythmia Society (ECAS); and in collaboration with the American College of Cardiology (ACC), American Heart Association (AHA), the Asia Pacific Heart Rhythm Society (APHRS), and the Society of Thoracic Surgeons (STS). Endorsed by the governing bodies of the American College of Cardiology Foundation, the American Heart Association, the European Cardiac Arrhythmia Society, the European Heart Rhythm Association, the Society of Thoracic Surgeons, the Asia Pacific Heart Rhythm Society, and the Heart Rhythm Society. *Heart Rhythm*. 2012;9(4):632-696.e21.

2. Fuster V, Rydén LE, Cannom DS, et al. 2011 ACCF/AHA/HRS focused updates incorporated into the ACC/AHA/ESC 2006 Guidelines for the management of patients with atrial fibrillation: a report of the American College of Cardiology Foundation/American Heart Association Task Force on Practice Guidelines developed in partnership with the European Society of Cardiology and in collaboration with the European Heart Rhythm Association and the Heart Rhythm Society. *J Am Coll Cardiol*. 2011;57(11):e101-198.

3. Lip GY, Nieuwlaat R, Pisters R, et al. Refining clinical risk stratification for predicting stroke and thromboembolism in atrial fibrillation using a novel risk factor-based approach: the Euro heart survey on atrial fibrillation. *Chest*. 2010;137(2):263-272.

4. Olesen JB, Torp-Pedersen C, Hansen ML, Lip GY. The value of the CHA2DS2-VASc score for refining stroke risk stratification in patients with atrial fibrillation with a CHADS2 score 0-1: a nationwide cohort study. *Thromb Haemost*. 2012;107(6):1172-1179.

5. Taillandier S, Olesen JB, Clémenty N, et al. Prognosis in patients with atrial fibrillation and CHA2DS2-VASc Score = 0 in a community-based cohort study. *J Cardiovasc Electrophysiol*. 2012;23(7):708-713.

6. Garcia DA, Crowther MA. Reversal of warfarin: case-based practice recommendations. *Circulation*. 2012;125(23):2944-2947.

7. Brem E, Koyfman A, Foran M. Review of recently approved alternatives to anticoagulation with warfarin for emergency clinicians. *J Emerg Med*. 2013;45(1):143-149.

8. Dans AL, Connolly SJ, Wallentin L, et al. Concomitant use of antiplatelet therapy with dabigatran or warfarin in the Randomized Evaluation of Long-Term Anticoagulation Therapy (RE-LY) trial. *Circulation.* 2013;127(5):634-640.

9. Lamberts M, Olesen JB, Ruwald MH, et al. Bleeding after initiation of multiple antithrombotic drugs, including triple therapy, in atrial fibrillation patients following myocardial infarction and coronary intervention: a nationwide cohort study. *Circulation.* 2012;126(10):1185-1193.

PREVENTION OF THROMBOEMBOLISM
IN ATRIAL FIBRILLATION: FACTOR XA AND
THROMBIN INHIBITORS

SECTION IV
PREVENTION OF THROMBOEMBOLISM
RELATED TO ATRIAL FIBRILLATION

191

28 PREVENTION OF THROMBOEMBOLISM IN ATRIAL FIBRILLATION: FACTOR XA AND THROMBIN INHIBITORS

J. Michael Boyd, PharmD, BCPS

CASE PRESENTATION

A 67-year-old woman presents to the clinic for evaluation of her atrial fibrillation (AF). Her medical history is significant for hypertension and diabetes mellitus. Atrial fibrillation was diagnosed 2 years ago and has been managed with sotalol and warfarin to this point. Her $CHADS_2$ score is 2, and thus her estimated annual stroke risk is 4%. Recent laboratory studies are notable only for an international normalized ratio (INR) of 1.7. An electrocardiogram demonstrates sinus rhythm with a QT interval of 460 ms. The patient notes that there has been considerable variation in her INR values and that she is concerned about her stroke risk, as well as risk for bleeding. She inquires regarding alternative anticoagulants.

EPIDEMIOLOGY

The prevalence of AF in the United States is estimated to be between 2.7 and 6.1 million in 2010.[1,2] Patients with AF are nearly 5 times as likely to suffer an ischemic stroke as those without AF.[3] In patients

with AF deemed to have considerable risk for thromboembolism, treatment has traditionally meant a vitamin K antagonist, such as warfarin. Though proven to be highly effective in the prevention of thromboembolic events, warfarin has many undesirable properties. These drawbacks include:

- Required monitoring of the INR to maintain a narrow therapeutic goal
- Multiple drug and dietary interactions
- Delayed onset and dissipation of effect due to mechanism of action
- Unpredictable dosing in part related to genetic polymorphisms

The worldwide approval of novel oral anticoagulants has provided alternatives to warfarin that may prove attractive for many patients with AF.

FACTOR Xa AND THROMBIN INHIBITORS

Rivaroxaban (Xarelto) and apixaban (Eliquis) are the first factor Xa inhibitors approved for the prevention of stroke and thromboembolism in patients with nonvalvular AF. Several other agents (edoxaban, darexaban, betrixaban, otamixaban) are in various stages of development.[4] Whereas warfarin inhibits thrombus formation through inhibition of clotting factor synthesis, factor Xa inhibitors exert their activity through direct inhibition of activated clotting factor X in the common pathway of the clotting cascade (Figure 28-1). Differences in mechanism of action, pharmacokinetic properties (Table 28-1), and drug interactions (Table 28-2) give factor Xa inhibitors several advantages compared to warfarin (Table 28-3).

Dabigatran (Pradaxa) is the first direct thrombin inhibitor available for thromboembolic prevention in nonvalvular AF. Dabigatran directly blocks free and clot-bound thrombin (Factor II) in the final step of the clotting

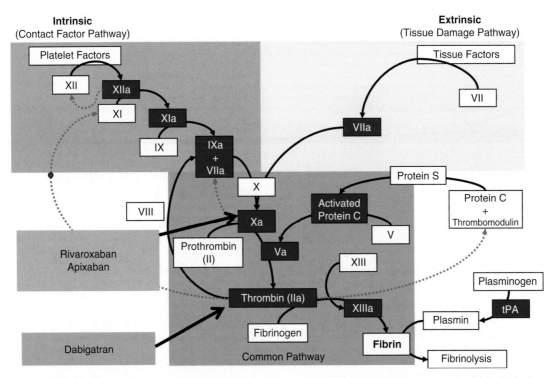

FIGURE 28-1 Clotting cascade depicting site of action of factor Xa and thrombin inhibitors. (Used with permission of Erik Abel, PharmD, BCPS.)

TABLE 28-1 Pharmacokinetic Properties of Novel Anticoagulants

	Dabigatran	Rivaroxaban	Apixaban
Bioavailability	3%-7%	60%-80%	50%
t_{max}	1 h	2-4 h	3-4 h
$t_{1/2}$	12-17 h	5-9 h	12 h
Protein-binding	35%	92%-95%	87%
Metabolism	Minimal, P-gp substrate	CYP 3A4, P-gp substrate	CYP 3A4, P-gp substrate
Clearance	80% renal	66% renal, 28% biliary	27% renal

Abbreviations: CYP = cytochrome P-450; P-gp = P-glycoprotein.

TABLE 28-2 Serious Drug Interactions of Novel Anticoagulants

Dabigatran	Rivaroxaban	Apixaban
Ketoconazole	Ketoconazole	Ketoconazole
Itraconazole	Itraconazole	Itraconazole
Dronedarone	Lopinavir/ritonavir	Lopinavir/ritonavir
Rifampin	Ritonavir	Ritonavir
Antiplatelet agents	Indinavir/ritonavir	Indinavir/ritonavir
Anticoagulants	Conivaptan	Antiplatelet
Nonsteroidal anti-inflammatory drugs (NSAIDs)	Carbamazepine	agents
	Phenytoin	Phenytoin
	Rifampin	Carbamazapine
	St. John's wort	Rifampin
	Dronedarone	St. John's wort
	Antiplatelet agents	Anticoagulants
	Anticoagulants	NSAIDs
	NSAIDs	

TABLE 28-3 Advantages and Disadvantages of Anticoagulants for Prevention of Thromboembolism in Patients with Atrial Fibrillation

	Vitamin K Antagonists	Factor Xa and Thrombin Inhibitors
Advantages	• Inexpensive • Clinician familiarity • Reversible	• Fixed dosing • No need for therapeutic monitoring • Rapid, predictable effect • Quick resumption of clotting function after discontinuation • Few drug interactions • No diet interactions • Increased efficacy[*] • Equal or less bleeding[*]
Disadvantages	• Variable dosing • INR monitoring required • Delayed onset/offset of effect • Many drug interactions • Many diet interactions	• Expensive • No reliable antidote established • Avoidance/adjustment needed in renal failure • No reliable way to monitor effects

[*]Agent and/or dose-dependent, compared to warfarin.

PREVENTION OF THROMBOEMBOLISM
IN ATRIAL FIBRILLATION: FACTOR XA AND
THROMBIN INHIBITORS

SECTION IV
PREVENTION OF THROMBOEMBOLISM
RELATED TO ATRIAL FIBRILLATION

193

cascade (See Figure 28-1). Similar to factor Xa inhibitors, mechanistic and pharmacokinetic properties of dabigatran offer many advantages compared to warfarin (see Tables 28-1 to 28-3).

Similar to warfarin, the primary adverse effect of factor Xa and thrombin inhibitors is increased risk of bleeding. Though clinical trials suggest similar or lower rates of bleeding compared to warfarin, management of severe bleeding presents more challenges with the new agents. Poor sensitivity of clinically available laboratory tests (PT, INR, aPTT) and lack of a specific antidote for the new agents make assessment and reversal of the anticoagulant effect difficult in the setting of acute hemorrhage.

CLINICAL TRIALS

In patients with AF, each of the new anticoagulants has been compared to warfarin for stroke and systemic embolism prevention in large, randomized, noninferiority trials. Dabigatran was assessed by the RE-LY trial, rivaroxaban in the ROCKET-AF trial, and apixaban in the ARISTOTLE study.[5-7] Notable similarities of these trials include:

- Large sample sizes
- Common end points—combination of stroke and systemic embolism (efficacy) and similarly defined major bleeding (safety)
- Exclusion of patients with severe renal insufficiency, significant valvular heart disease, or prosthetic heart valves
- Duration of follow-up of about 2 years

Significant differences in the design of these trials include:

- Patients randomized to warfarin were unblinded to treatment in RE-LY but were blinded in ROCKET-AF and ARISTOTLE.
- Adjustments for renal insufficiency were made in ROCKET-AF and ARISTOTLE, but not in RE-LY.
- Higher stroke-risk patients (CHADS$_2$ ≥2) were enrolled in the ROCKET-AF trial.

In RE-LY, patients were randomized to one of 2 doses of dabigatran (110 mg or 150 mg twice daily) or open-label warfarin with an INR goal of 2 to 3. Time in therapeutic INR range for the warfarin group was roughly 65%. Approximately two-thirds of the patients were considered high risk for stroke (CHADS$_2$ ≥2). For the preven-

tion of stroke and systemic embolism, the results of RE-LY demonstrate noninferiority for both doses of dabigatran compared to warfarin as well as superiority for the 150 mg dose (Table 28-4). Compared with warfarin, major bleeding was reduced with the 110 mg dose and similar with the 150 mg dose (Table 28-5). Of note, both doses of dabigatran showed reduced rates of life-threatening bleeding and intracranial hemorrhage versus warfarin while the 150 mg dose was associated with an increased rate of gastrointestinal (GI) bleeding.

The ROCKET-AF study compared rivaroxaban 20 mg daily (15 mg daily for CrCl 30 to 49 mL/min) with blinded adjusted-dose warfarin (goal INR 2 to 3). Warfarin patients had INR values within the therapeutic range 55% of the time. Patients at low or intermediate risk of stroke (CHADS$_2$ 0 to 1) were excluded from ROCKET-AF. The primary outcome of this study by the intention-to-treat analysis revealed that rivaroxaban was noninferior to warfarin for the prevention of stroke and systemic embolism in this patient population (see Table 28-4). Importantly, a reduction in events in the rivaroxaban group during treatment was offset by a significant increase in events in the rivaroxaban group after discontinuation of study drug. This suggests that patients may be at risk for stroke when discontinuing rivaroxaban in the absence of adequate alternative anticoagulation. Additionally, similar rates of major bleeding were reported for both groups while less intracranial hemorrhage and more GI bleeding was noted with rivaroxaban (see Table 28-5).

Apixaban at a dose of 5 mg twice daily was compared to blinded dose-adjusted warfarin (goal INR 2 to 3) in ARISTOTLE. A reduced apixaban dose of 2.5 mg twice daily was used for patients with 2 or more of the following: age of at least 80 years, weight of 60 kilograms or less, or serum creatinine of 1.5 mg per deciliter or more. Two-thirds of patients had a CHADS$_2$ score of at least 2, and the mean time in therapeutic range for warfarin patients was 62.2%. The results of ARISTOTLE reveal superiority of apixaban compared to warfarin for the combined end point of stroke and systemic embolism (see Table 28-4). Additionally, for the predefined secondary end point of death from any cause, apixaban became the first new agent to show reduced mortality compared to warfarin (3.52% versus 3.94% per year; hazard ratio, 0.89; 95% CI, 0.80 to 0.998; P = 0.047). For safety end points, apixaban reduced all types of bleeding with

TABLE 28-4 Intention-to-Treat Efficacy Results of the Major Clinical Trials of New Oral Anticoagulants Compared to Warfarin for the Combined Primary Endpoint of Stroke or Systemic Embolism[5,6,7]

| Study | Event Rate per 100 Patient Years | | Hazard Ratio (95% CI) | P-value | |
	Study Drug	Warfarin		Noninferiority	Superiority
RE-LY- (dabigatran 110 mg)	1.53	1.69	0.91 (0.74-1.11)	<0.001	0.34
RE-LY- (dabigatran 150 mg)	1.11	1.69	0.66 (0.53-0.82)	<0.001	<0.001
ROCKET-AF (rivaroxaban)	2.1	2.4	0.88 (0.75-1.03)	<0.001	0.12
ARISTOTLE (apixaban)	1.27	1.60	0.79 (0.66-0.95)	<0.001	0.01

TABLE 28-5 Bleeding Endpoint Results of the Major Clinical Trials of New Oral Anticoagulants Compared to Warfarin[5,6,7]

Study	Event Rate per End Points 100 Patient Years		Harard Ratio (95% CI)	P-value
	Study Drug	Warfarin		
RE-LY (dabigatran 110 mg)				
Major bleeding	2.71	3.36	0.80 (0.69-0.93)	0.003
Intracranial	0.23	0.74	0.31 (0.2-0.47)	<0.001
Gastrointestinal	1.12	1.02	1.10 (0.86-1.41)	0.43
RE-LY (dabigatran 150 mg)				
Major bleeding	3.11	3.36	0.93 (0.81-1.07)	0.31
Intracranial	0.3	0.74	0.40 (0.27-0.60)	<0.001
Gastrointestinal	1.51	1.02	1.50 (1.19-1.89)	<0.001
ROCKET-AF (rivaroxaban)				
Major bleeding	3.6	3.4	1.04 (0.90-1.20)	0.58
Intracranial	0.5	0.7	0.67 (0.47-0.93)	0.02
Gastrointestinal	2.0	1.2	NR	<0.001
ARISTOTLE (apixaban)				
Major bleeding	2.13	3.09	0.69 (0.60-0.80)	<0.001
Intracranial	0.33	0.8	0.42 (0.3-0.58)	<0.001
Gastrointestinal	0.76	0.86	0.89 (0.7-1.15)	0.37

Major bleeding: clinically overt bleeding with accompanying decrease in hemoglobin of ≥2 g/dL or transfusion of ≥2 units of blood, occurring at a critical site, or resulting in death.

the exception of GI bleeding for which it showed similar rates (see Table 28-5).

SPECIFIC CLINICAL ISSUES

Holding novel anticoagulants for invasive procedures requires consideration of multiple factors including:

- Thromboembolic risk of the patient in the absence of anticoagulation—may be assessed using the CHADS$_2$ or CHA$_2$DS$_2$-VASc risk assessment tools (Table 28-6). For either tool, a score of 0 is considered low risk, 1 is intermediate, and 2 or higher is high risk for thromboembolism.

- Bleeding risk of the procedure/surgery—generally any procedure that could result in bleeding in a non-compressible organ (intracranial, intraspinal, intraocular, retroperitoneal, intrathoracic, or pericardial) should be deemed high risk.[10]

- Pharmacokinetic properties of the specific agent—most importantly elimination half-life ($t_{1/2}$) and patient characteristics which may affect $t_{1/2}$ such as renal function (see Table 28-1).

General recommendations for holding the new oral anticoagulants are presented in Table 28-7. Because there are no available specific reversal agents, it is advisable to consider holding doses for longer periods for procedures with high bleeding risk. Considering the rapid onset of the new agents, anticoagulant therapy should be resumed after hemostasis and when bleeding risk has declined, generally 24 to 48 hours after the procedure/surgery. No bridge therapy with parenteral anticoagulants should be administered.

- Management of bleeding
  ○ Minor bleeding may be managed by holding the anticoagulant.
  ○ Major or life-threatening bleeding requires the initiation of general resuscitative measures including:
    ■ Stopping the anticoagulant, giving activated charcoal if last dose is recent (<1-2 hours).
    ■ Manage hemodynamic compromise—administer fluid, blood, and vasopressors as needed to maintain tissue perfusion.
    ■ Apply topical thrombin as appropriate.
    ■ Correct deficiencies in essential components of clot formation (ie, fibrinogen, platelets).

PREVENTION OF THROMBOEMBOLISM
IN ATRIAL FIBRILLATION: FACTOR XA AND
THROMBIN INHIBITORS

SECTION IV
PREVENTION OF THROMBOEMBOLISM
RELATED TO ATRIAL FIBRILLATION

195

TABLE 28-6 CHADS$_2$ and CHA$_2$DS$_2$-VASc Stroke Risk Assessment Tools for Patients with Atrial Fibrillation[8,9]

	Condition	Points	Score	Annual Risk (95% CI)
CHADS$_2$				
C	Congestive heart failure	1	0	1.9 (1.2-3.0)
H	Hypertension (BP >140/90 or on antihypertensive drug)	1	1	2.8 (2.0-3.8)
A	Age ≥75 y	1	2	4.0 (3.1-5.1)
D	Diabetes mellitus	1	3	5.9 (4.6-7.3)
S$_2$	Prior stroke or TIA	2	4	8.5 (6.3-11.1)
			5	12.5 (8.2-17.5)
			6	18.2 (10.5-27.5)
CHA$_2$DS$_2$-VASc				
C	Congestive heart failure	1	0	0
H	Hypertension (BP >140/90 or on antihypertensive drug)	1	1	0.7
A$_2$	Age ≥75 y	2	2	1.9
D	Diabetes mellitus	1	3	4.7
S$_2$	Prior stroke or TIA	2	4	2.3
V	Vascular disease (PAD, MI, aortic plaque)	1	5	3.9
A	Age 65-74 y	1	6	4.5
Sc	Sex category (female)	1	7	10.1
			8	14.2
			9	100

Abbreviations: BP = blood pressure, MI = myocardial infarction, PAD = peripheral artery disease, TIA = transient ischemic attack. Annual risk is defined for patients with atrial fibrillation who are not taking anticoagulants. Risk is modified for aspirin use.

- For dabigatran only, consider hemodialysis—low protein binding allows for removal via dialysis.
- Consider the administration of prothrombin complex concentrates (PCCs). Information on the use of PCCs for the reversal of the effects of factor Xa and thrombin inhibitors is limited with variable results.[11,12] The clotting factor content of the numerous PCC products varies considerably. Generally, for treatment of major bleeding due to factor Xa inhibitors nonactivated 4-factor PCCs (factors II, VII, IX, X) are preferred over nonactivated 3-factor PCCs (which have very small amounts of factor VII). The use of anti-inhibitor coagulant complex, which is similar to 4-factor PCC with the exception that factor VII is in the activated form, may be useful for the treatment of bleeding associated with dabigatran. Of note, the most safe and effective dose of PCC for the reversal of factor Xa and thrombin inhibitors remains to be determined, and caution should be used in the administration of PCC due to the risk of thrombosis.

PATIENT EDUCATION

- Patients with AF treated with anticoagulants should be counseled to recognize the signs and symptoms of stroke. Facial droop, aphasia, slurred speech, and unilateral arm weakness are all signs of focal neurological deficit caused by a stroke. Patients should be encouraged to seek immediate medical attention at the earliest sign of stroke.

- As the most common adverse effect of thrombin and Xa inhibitors is bleeding, patients must be aware of the signs and symptoms of bleeding. Overt hemorrhage, including hematochezia, hematemesis, retinal hemorrhage, intractable epistaxis, and trauma-induced hemorrhage, requires emergency medical attention. Gastrointestinal adverse effects (dyspepsia, gastritis) may occur with dabigatran likely due to tartaric acid being present in the capsules.

- Patients must be strongly encouraged to avoid abrupt discontinuation of any of the novel anticoagulants. Short half-lives leading to relatively quick dissipation of effect may increase the risk of

TABLE 28-7 Manufacturer-Suggested Factor Xa and Thrombin Inhibitor

Dabigatran	Hold Time	Rivaroxaban	Hold Time	Apixaban	Hold Time
CrCl ≥50 mL/min	1-2 d	Consider holding for longer period for moderate/high bleeding risk procedures	≥24 h	Low bleeding risk procedure	≥24 h
CrCl <50 mL/min	3-5 d			Moderate/high bleeding risk procedure	≥48 h

Abbreviation: CrCl = creatinine clearance.

thromboembolism in the absence of bridging therapy when any of the new agents are discontinued. This is particularly true of rivaroxaban given its short half-life. Post-hoc analysis of the ROCKET-AF trial demonstrated that patients randomized to rivaroxaban had an inordinately high incidence of stroke when they stopped taking the medication in the absence of bridging anticoagulant therapy.[13]

• Proper storage of dabigatran is critical, and patients should be advised of such. Dabigatran is highly susceptible to hydrolysis and should be stored in its original packaging to minimize moisture exposure. Improper storage, such as in patient pill organizers, could lead to excessive degradation and potential ineffectiveness of dabigatran.

• Due to saturable absorption with rivaroxaban, patients should be told to take doses ≥ 15mg with a large meal (usually dinner). Food slows absorption of rivaroxaban allowing for more complete absorption and better bioavailability.

REFERENCES

1. Go AS, Hylek EM, Phillips KA, et al. Prevalence of diagnosed atrial fibrillation in adults: national implications for rhythm management and stroke prevention: the AnTicoagulation and Risk Factors in Atrial Fibrillation (ATRIA) study. *JAMA.* 2001;285(18):2370-2375.

2. Miyasaka Y, Barnes ME, Gersh BJ, et al. Secular trends in incidence of atrial fibrillation in Olmstead County, Minnesota, 1980 to 2000, and implications on the projections for future prevalence [published correction appears in *Circulation.* 2006;114:e498]. *Circulation.* 2006;114(2):119-125.

3. Wolf PA, Abbott RD, Kannel WB. Atrial fibrillation as an independent risk factor for stroke: The Framingham Study. *Stroke.* 1991;22:983-988.

4. De Caterina R, Husted S, Wallentin L, et al. New oral anticoagulants in atrial fibrillation and acute coronary syndromes: ESC Working Group on Thrombosis—Task Force on Anticoagulants

in Heart Disease position paper. *J Am Coll Cardiol.* 2012;59: 1413-1425.

5. Connolly SJ, Ezekowitz MD, Yusuf S, et al. Dabigatran versus warfarin in patients with atrial fibrillation. *N Engl J Med.* 2009;361:1139-1151.

6. Patel MR, Mahaffey KW, Garg J. et al. Rivaroxaban versus warfarin in nonvalvular atrial fibrillation. *N Engl J Med.* 2011;365:883-891.

7. Granger CB, Alexander JH, McMurray JJV, et al. Apixaban versus warfarin in patients with atrial fibrillation. *N Engl J Med.* 2011;365:981-992.

8. Gage BF, Waterman AD, Shannon W, et al. Validation of clinical classification schemes for predicting stroke: results from the National Registry of Atrial Fibrillation. *JAMA.* 2001;285:2864-2870.

9. Lip GY, Nieuwlaat R, Pisters R, Lane DA, Crijns HJ. Refining clinical risk stratification for predicting stroke and thromboembolism in atrial fibrillation using a novel risk factor-based approach: The Euro Heart Survey on Atrial Fibrillation. *Chest.* 2010;137:263-272.

10. Baron TH, Kamath PS, McBane RD. Management of antithrombotic therapy in patients undergoing invasive procedures. *N Engl J Med.* 2013;368:2113-2124.

11. Kaatz S, Kouides PA, Garcia DA, et al. Guidance on the emergent reversal of oral thrombin and factor Xa inhibitors. *Am J Hematol.* 2012;87: Suppl 1: S141-S145. [Erratum, *Am J Hematol.* 2012;87:748.]

12. Dzik WS. Reversal of drug-induced anticoagulation: old solutions and new problems. *Transfusion.* 2012;52:Suppl 1:45S-55S.

13. Patel MR, Hellkamp AS, Lokhnygina Y, et al. Outcomes of discontinuing rivaroxaban compared with warfarin in patients with nonvalvular atrial fibrillation: analysis from the ROCKET AF trial (Rivaroxaban Once-Daily, Oral, Direct Factor Xa Inhibition Compared With Vitamin K Antagonism for Prevention of Stroke and Embolism Trial in Atrial Fibrillation). *J Am Coll Cardiol.* 2013;61:651-658.

SECTION V

ANTIARRHYTHMIC MEDICAL THERAPY FOR ATRIAL FIBRILLATION

29 CLASS I ANTIARRHYTHMIC MEDICATIONS

M. Rizwan Sardar, MD, Wajeeha Saeed, MD, Kar-Lai Wong, MD, FACC

CASE PRESENTATION

The patient is a 52-year-old white man who presented with recurrent atrial fibrillation (AF). He first suffered AF 5 years ago. The episode lasted for 4 hours and spontaneously terminated shortly after presentation to the emergency department. He had been maintained on β-blockers. In the past 5 years he had 3 episodes of AF; all of them converted spontaneously within 1 to 3 hours. The frequency of AF has increased, and this was the third episode that he had suffered in the past 6 months. The duration of AF also lasted longer, and one episode required cardioversion. During AF, the patient complained of palpitations and fatigue but no lightheadedness or chest pain.

The patient is otherwise healthy and without other medical problems, specifically denying hypertension, diabetes, or peripheral vascular disease. He exercises by running three miles daily. He is not taking any medication besides a β-blocker. His previous workup, including echocardiogram, stress test, and thyroid function test, was normal. He was placed on flecainide 100 mg bid. On flecainide, he remained free of AF for 3 years.

CLASSIFICATION

- Under the modified Singh-Vaughan Williams classification, sodium channel blocking drugs are class I drugs that further subdivide into three classes (See Table 29-1).

Class IA Agents

Qunidine

- Quinidine has a direct suppressant effect on the sinus node, AV node, and His-Purkinje system. In the innervated human heart, quinidine also has indirect vagolytic and sympathomimetic effects on sinus node and AV node function.
- Most of quinidine is metabolized in the liver with 20% of the parent drug and metabolites being excreted via kidney. Elimination is reduced in patients with congestive heart failure, renal disease, or liver disease.

- The blood pressure may decrease from the α-blocking property, but it does not have any significant negative inotropic action.
- Quinidine is effective in the treatment of supraventricular tachycardias (SVT) including AF, but its utility is limited secondary to an increase in mortality from proarrhythmia most commonly due to torsades de pointes.
- It is also effective in suppressing ventricular premature complexes (VPCs) and ventricular tachycardia (VT) by decreasing cardiac conduction velocity and increasing repolarization duration.
- Gastrointestinal side effects such as diarrhea are common. Central nervous system symptoms such as hearing loss and cinchonism have been reported; thrombocytopenia and immune-mediated reactions may also occur.
- Polymorphic VT is observed in up to 1.5% of patients from torsades de pointes (TdP). Incidence of TdP is not always dose-related and can occur anytime during the treatment course.

Procainamide

- Procainamide has variable effects on sinus node and AV node function. It often increases the HV conduction time and prolongs the QT interval.
- The liver metabolizes 30% to 50% of procainamide into a cardioactive metabolite (N-acetylprocainamide [NAPA]), which is cleared by the kidney. Patients with renal dysfunction have a markedly prolonged half-life of NAPA. Both procainamide and NAPA levels should be monitored to evaluate plasma concentration of the drug.
- Oral procainamide does not significantly affect the blood pressure. Rapid IV injection may result in hypotension, decrease in pulmonary vascular resistance, and decline in cardiac output. Procainamide has a strong negative inotropic effect.
- Procainamide is effective in treatment of AF. It also suppresses antegrade and retrograde conduction over accessory bypass tracts by prolonging the bypass tract refractory period, making it an effective treatment for WPW or bypass tract-related SVT.
- Procainamide increases the effective ventricular refractory and can effectively suppress VPCs, slow down the rate of VT, and terminate VT.
- GI and CNS side effects are common. Pancytopenia and agranulocytosis can be life-threatening. Systemic lupus erythematosus syndrome is observed in 15% to 20% of patients taking procainamide for more than a year, especially in slow acetylators.

Disopyramide

- Disopyramide has a variable effect on sinus node function because of its strong anticholinergic effect in addition to its sodium channel blocking property.

TABLE 29-1 Harrison Modification of Class I Agents

	Action Potential	Refractory Period	Repolarization	Agents
IA	↑	↑	↑	Procainamide; quinidine; disopyramide
IB	↓	↓	↓	Lidocaine; mexiletine
IC	—	↑	—	Flecainide; propafenone

Adapted with permission from Harrison DC: Antiarrhythmic drug classification: New science and practical applications. Am J Cardiol 1985; Jul 1;56(1):185-187.

- The liver eliminates 15% of disopyramide in the first pass. It is then cleared by renal excretion.

- Disopyramide has a substantial negative inotropic effect and decreases cardiac output significantly. It should be avoided in patients with ventricular dysfunction.

- Disopyramide is effective in preventing AF. Due to its vagolytic properties it is especially effective in young patients with vagally mediated AF.

- It has been shown that disopyramide is effective in suppressing VPCs and sustained VT. Its use in treatment of ventricular tachyarrhythmia is limited because of its strong negative inotropic effect.

- Anticholinergic side effects such as dry mouth, urinary retention, and dry eyes are common. TdP has been reported from QT prolongation, but the incidence is less compared to quinidine or procainamide. Avoid the drug in patients with glaucoma, benign prostatic hypertrophy, and congestive heart failure (CHF).

Class IB Agents

Lidocaine

- Lidocaine has minimal effect on the sinus node, AV node, or His-Purkinje system function. It does not affect the ventricular refractory period.

- Lidocaine undergoes rapid extensive first pass elimination by liver and then is bound to adipose tissue. It can only be used in intravenous form, and the dosage should be adjusted in patients with hepatic dysfunction or congestive heart failure.

- Hepatic enzyme inducers like phenytoin, rifampin, and barbiturates lower the levels.

- At therapeutic levels, lidocaine causes minimal hemodynamic effect and is generally well tolerated even in patients with ventricular dysfunction or CHF.

- Lidocaine increases the ventricular fibrillation threshold and thus is effective in treatment of ventricular fibrillation in the setting of ischemia. It has minimal effect in on either the atrial or ventricular refractory period, and its use in treatment of atrial tachyarrhythmias and monomorphic VT is limited.

- Prophylactic use of Lidocaine for post-MI VPCs is no longer supported.

- CNS side effects such as tremor, confusion, and seizures can occur, especially in elderly patients. It does not prolong the QT interval, and it is not common to see ventricular proarrhythmic side effects. Lidocaine levels should be checked if used more than 24 hours.

Mexiletine

- Similar to lidocaine, mexiletine has no significant effects on the sinus node, AV node function, or atrial and ventricular refractory periods.

- Mexiletine is well absorbed in the GI tract without significant first pass elimination. It has a large volume distribution. The liver metabolizes 90% of mexiletine.

- Mexiletine has minimal hemodynamic effects and is usually well tolerated in patients with ventricular dysfunction.

- Mexiletine is effective in the treatment of VT but has limited utility for treating atrial tachyarrhythmias.

- GI and CNS side effects, similar to lidocaine, are common with mexiletine. When compared to other antiarrhythmic drugs, the risk of ventricular proarrhythmic side effects is low.

Class IC Agents

Flecainide

- Flecainide slows conduction in all cardiac tissues, and thus the PR and QRS are often both lengthened. There is minimal QT prolongation.

- Seventy-five percent of the drug is eliminated hepatically with 25% eliminated unchanged by kidneys.

- Flecainide is very effective in suppressing VPCs and nonsustained ventricular tachycardia. Its utility in treatment of ventricular tachyarrhythmias is limited because of an increase in mortality when it is used in patients with cardiomyopathy.[2]

- In patients with a structurally normal heart, flecainide is effective in preventing paroxysmal AF. When 300 mg of oral flecainide is given within 2 hours of onset of atrial fibrillation, 92% of atrial fibrillation is terminated within 3 hours. This makes flecainide an acceptable antiarrhythmic drug to be used as a pill in a pocket treatment for patients with sporadic rare occurrences of atrial fibrillation.[3]

- Flecainide has a significant negative inotropic effect and may exacerbate congestive heart failure in patients with underlying ventricular dysfunction. It should be avoided in patients with cardiomyopathy because of increasing cardiac mortality in this subgroup of patients.

- Flecainide may convert AF into atrial flutter with a fast ventricular response, and therefore the concomitant use of an AV nodal blocking agent is generally recommended.

- CNS side effects such as headache and tremor are the most common noncardiac side effects, but are usually not severe.

Propafenone

- Propafenone, like flecainide, increases both PR and QRS intervals. It has both β-blocker and calcium channel blocker properties and thus should be used cautiously in patients with underlying sick sinus syndrome, conduction disease, or asthma.

- Propafenone is rapidly metabolized in the liver by the P-450 system into two active metabolites, 5-hydroxypropafenone and N-depropylpropafenone. The active metabolites are eliminated by renal clearance. The dosage of the drug needs to be reduced in patients with severe hepatic and renal insufficiency.

- Propafenone is very effective in suppressing VPCs and nonsustained ventricular tachycardia. Although it was not studied in the CAST trial, given its similarity to flecainide, propafenone should not be used in patients with a structurally abnormal heart.

- Propafenone is effective in maintaining sinus rhythm in patients with paroxysmal atrial fibrillation when compared to placebo. It decreases both antegrade and retrograde conduction via accessory bypass tracts and can be considered for treatment of bypass-related supraventricular tachycardia.

- Propafenone causes mild CNS side effects such as nausea, vomiting, and metallic taste.

Tables 29-2 to 29-5 discuss the pharmacokinetics, interactions, and various effects of class I drugs.

TABLE 29-2 Typical Effects on ECG and Intracardiac Intervals

	AA	PR	QRS	QT	AH	HV
Procainamide	↔	↑	↑	↑	↑	↑
Quinidine	↔↓	0	↑	↑↑	↓	↑
Disopyramide	↔	↔	↔	↔↓	↔	↔↑
Lidocaine	↔	↔	↔	↓	↔	↔
Mexiletine	↔	↔	↔	↓	↔	↔
Flecainide	↔	↑	↑	↔↑	↑	↑↑
Propafenone	↔↑	↑	↑	↔↑	↑	↑↑

TABLE 29-3 Pharmacokinetics of Class I Antiarrhythmic Drugs

Drug	Major Route of Elimination	Half-Life (Hours)	Active Metabolite
Quinidine	Hepatic (50-90) Renal (10-30)	7-18	3-Hydroxy quinidine
Procainamide	Hepatic (40-70) Renal (30-60)	3-5	N-acetyl procainamide
Disopyramide	Hepatic (10-35) Renal (35-80)	7-9	Mono-N-dealkyl disopyramide
Lidocaine	Hepatic (90) Renal (minimal)	2-4	None
Mexiletine	Hepatic (90) Renal (10)	8-12	None
Flecainide	Hepatic (70) Renal (25)	11	Meta-O-dealkylated flecainide
Propafenone	Hepatic (>90) Renal (minimal)	2-32*	5-Hydroxy propafenon

*Inherited variability in metabolism.

TABLE 29-4 Interaction with Common Cardiovascular Drugs

Drug	Digoxin	Verapamil/ Diltiazem
Quinidine	↑ Digoxin level	—
Procainamide	—	—
Disopyramide	—	+ Negative ionotropic effect
Lidocaine	—	—
Mexiletine	—	—
Flecainide	↑ Digoxin level	+ Negative ionotropic effect
Propafenone	↑ Digoxin level	+ Negative ionotropic effect

+ Additive effect.

TABLE 29-5 Effect of Class I Antiarrhythmic Drugs on Thresholds

Drug	Pacing Thresholds	Defibrillation Thresholds
Lidocaine	↔	↑
Quinidine	↑	↑
Procainamide	↑	↔↑
Flecainide	↑	↑
Propafenone	↔	↔
Mexiletine	↔	↔/↑
Disopyramide	↔	↔

REFERENCES

1. Harrison DC. Antiarrhythmic drug classification: new science and practical applications. *Am J Cardiol.* 1985;56(1):185-187.

2. Echt DS, Liebson PR, Mitchell LB, et al. Mortality and morbidity in patients receiving encainide, flecainide, or placebo— The Cardiac Arrhythmia Suppression Trial. *N Engl J Med.* 1991;324:781-788.

3. Alboni P, Botto GL, Baldi N, et al. Outpatient treatment of recent-onset atrial fibrillation with the "pill-in-the-pocket" approach. *N Engl J Med.* 2004;351:2384-2391.

30 CLASS III ANTIARRHYTHMIC DRUGS

Roi Altit, MD, Agnieszka Mochon, MD, Steven Rothman, MD

CASE PRESENTATION

An 82-year-old man was admitted to the hospital for treatment of recurrent atrial arrhythmias. He had a past medical history of a nonischemic cardiomyopathy and was status postplacement of a biventricular implantable cardioverter-defibrillator (BiV-ICD). His most recent ejection fraction was 45% (20% prior to BiV-ICD implantation). He had complained of malaise, dyspnea on exertion, and lightheadedness for the past couple of weeks, and his ECG on admission showed recurrence of atrial flutter with 2:1 AV conduction (Figure 30-1). The patient was started on dofetilide, and after his second dose he converted spontaneously to an atrial paced rhythm with biventricular pacing. An ECG at that time showed a significantly longer corrected QT interval (Figure 30-2). Soon afterward, the patient developed recurrent episodes of polymorphic ventricular tachycardia resulting in multiple ICD shocks (Figure 30-3). He received intravenous magnesium to suppress his ventricular arrhythmias, and the dofetilide

was discontinued. He was eventually placed on amiodarone and was discharged from the hospital in sinus rhythm.

BACKGROUND

Class III Antiarrhythmic Agents

Vaughan-Williams class III drugs are membrane active antiarrhythmic agents that affect the potassium channels located on the surface of myocytes during the plateau and repolarization phases of the action potential (Figure 30-4). The duration of these phases are a direct result of the balance between the inward calcium currents and the outward potassium currents. Blocking of the potassium currents during repolarization causes a prolongation in the action potential duration with a resultant increase in the QT interval on the surface ECG. The most commonly used agents in this class are amiodarone, dronedarone, sotalol, dofetilide, and ibutilide. In addition to their predominant potassium channel effect, some of these drugs exhibit effects on other channels and/or receptors (Table 30-1). A comparison of their pharmacokinetic profiles is shown in Table 30-2.

Class III Antiarrhythmic Drugs—General Indications and Usage

- All class III agents can be used for conversion and/or maintenance of sinus rhythm in patients with atrial fibrillation and atrial flutter.

- Amiodarone and sotalol also have indications in the treatment and prevention of ventricular arrhythmias.

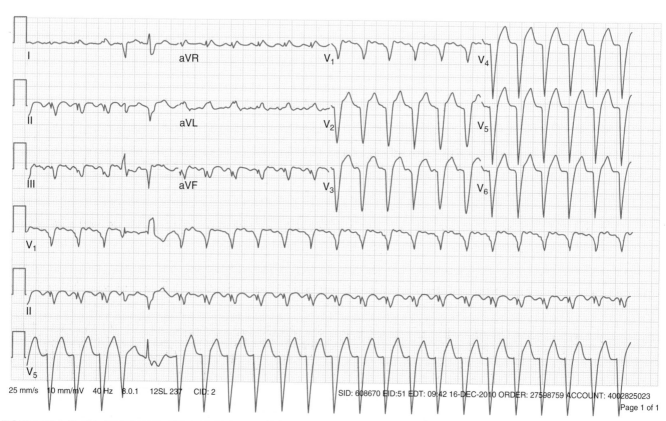

FIGURE 30-1 Twelve-lead electrocardiogram showing atrial flutter with 2:1 conduction. The corrected QT interval is 490 msec in the presence of a complete left bundle branch block.

CLASS III
ANTIARRHYTHMIC DRUGS

SECTION V
ANTIARRHYTHMIC MEDICAL THERAPY
FOR ATRIAL FIBRILLATION

203

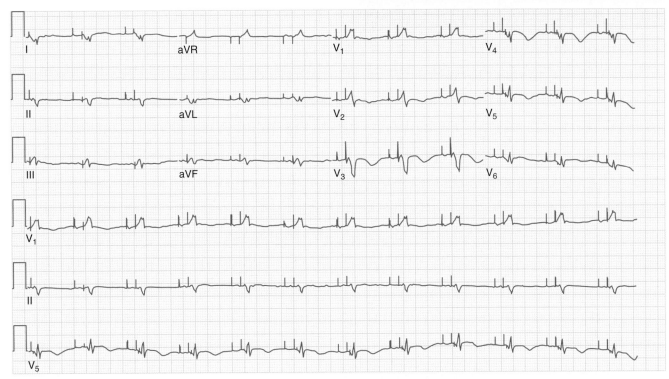

FIGURE 30-2 Twelve-lead electrocardiogram obtained after two doses of dofetilide and spontaneous restoration of an AV sequentially paced rhythm. The corrected QT interval is 650 msec in the presence of biventricular pacing.

- Drugs with predominantly class III effects (dofetilide, sotalol, ibutilide) may decrease defibrillation thresholds and can be used to facilitate direct-current cardioversions.

Proarrhythmic Effects of Class III Antiarrhythmic Agents

- The major side effect of this class of drugs is the risk of torsades de pointes (TdP), a type of polymorphic ventricular tachycardia associated with prolongation of the QT interval.

- Class III agents with predominant potassium channel blocking activity (sotalol, ibutilide, dofetilide) are more likely to cause TdP than those agents with multiple channel blocking activity (amiodarone, dronedarone).

- Patient factors that increase the risk of TdP include hypokalemia, hypomagnesemia, bradycardia, severe left ventricular dysfunction, impaired drug metabolism, and/or elimination and coadministration with other QT prolonging medications.

- Sotalol, dofetilide, and ibutilide demonstrate reverse-use dependence, resulting in a more potent potassium channel blocking effect at slower heart rates. This results in a longer QT interval with bradycardia and a higher risk of TdP.[1]

SPECIFIC AGENTS

Dofetilide

Dofetilide is a highly specific blocker of the rapid component of the delayed rectifier potassium current (Ikr), causing prolongation of the atrial and ventricular effective refractory periods. The drug is cleared predominantly through renal excretion and is contraindicated in patients with a creatinine clearance (CrCl) less than 20 mL/min. There are several drugs that significantly increase the plasma level of dofetilide and are contraindicated in its use. These include verapamil and trimethoprim, which increase the peak plasma concentrations of dofetilide, cimetidine, which inhibits renal tubular secretion of dofetilide, and ketoconazole, which is a significant inhibitor of the cytochrome p450 CYP3A4 isoenzyme, used in the hepatic metabolism of dofetilide. Hydrochlorothiazide is also contraindicated with the use of dofetilide due to both an increase in dofetilide's serum plasma concentration and a reduction in serum potassium, the combination of which can result in a marked increase in the QT interval.

Indications

Dofetilide is currently indicated for the treatment of atrial fibrillation. In the SAFIRE-D trial,[2] up to 29% of patients with persistent atrial fibrillation converted to sinus rhythm, most within the first 36 hours, and up to 58% of patients were able to maintain sinus rhythm for 1 year. In another study assessing the acute efficacy of dofetilide, Cotiga et al reported cardioversion rates ranging from 20% to 85% depending on the CrCl-based dosage.[3] The risk of proarrhythmia, including TdP, in this same trial was 1.2%.

Current guidelines recommend dofetilide as a second line agent in patients with atrial fibrillation and no structural heart disease.[4] In patients with depressed left ventricular function and congestive heart failure, however, dofetilide is a first-line agent as it has been shown

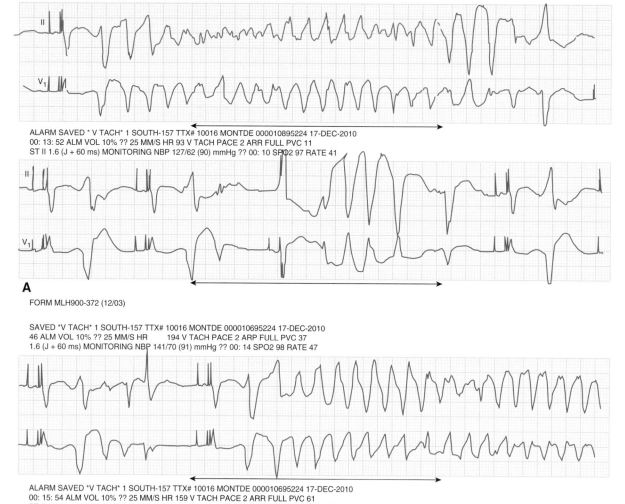

ALARM SAVED *VFIB/VTAC* 1 SOUTH-157 TTX# 10016 MONTDE 000010695224 17-DEC-2010
00: 14: 02 ALM VOL 10% ?? 25 MM/S HR 0 VFIB/VTAC PACE 2 ARR FULL PVC 24
ST II 1.3 (J + 60 ms) MONITORING NBP 127/62 (90) mmHg ?? 00: 10 SPO2 97 RATE 40

ALARM SAVED * V TACH* 1 SOUTH-157 TTX# 10016 MONTDE 000010895224 17-DEC-2010
00: 13: 52 ALM VOL 10% ?? 25 MM/S HR 93 V TACH PACE 2 ARR FULL PVC 11
ST II 1.6 (J + 60 ms) MONITORING NBP 127/62 (90) mmHg ?? 00: 10 SPO2 97 RATE 41

A

FORM MLH900-372 (12/03)

SAVED *V TACH* 1 SOUTH-157 TTX# 10016 MONTDE 000010695224 17-DEC-2010
46 ALM VOL 10% ?? 25 MM/S HR   194 V TACH PACE 2 ARP FULL PVC 37
1.6 (J + 60 ms) MONITORING NBP 141/70 (91) mmHg ?? 00: 14 SPO2 98 RATE 47

ALARM SAVED *V TACH* 1 SOUTH-157 TTX# 10016 MONTDE 000010695224 17-DEC-2010
00: 15: 54 ALM VOL 10% ?? 25 MM/S HR 159 V TACH PACE 2 ARR FULL PVC 61
ST II 1.6 (J + 60 ms) MONITORING NBP 141/70 (91) mmHg ?? 00: 14 SPO2 99 RATE 49

B

FIGURE 30-3 Telemetry strips showing polymorphic ventricular tachycardia in association with marked QT prolongation (torsade de pointes). Top strips (A) show nonsustained episodes of TdP and the bottom strip (B) shows an episode of TdP degenerating into ventricular fibrillation, terminated by an ICD discharge.

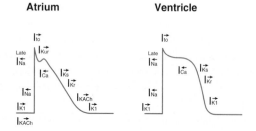

FIGURE 30-4 Atrial and ventricular action potentials are shown along with their major ionic currents. Arrows denote direction of current (left = inward current; right = outward current). Class III antiarrhythmic agents block the potassium ion currents I(K).

CLASS III
ANTIARRHYTHMIC DRUGS

SECTION V
ANTIARRHYTHMIC MEDICAL THERAPY
FOR ATRIAL FIBRILLATION

205

TABLE 30-1 Class III Antiarrhythmic Channel/Receptor Effects

	Channels								Receptors			
	Na (Fast)	Na (Med)	Na (Slow)	Ca	Kr	Ks	Kur	I_f	α	β	M2	A1
Amiodarone	x			x	x	x	x		x	X		
Sotalol										X		
Dronedarone	x			x	x	x	x		x	X		
Dofetilide					x							
Ibutilide			x		x							

TABLE 30-2 Comparison of the Pharmacokinetics of Class III Antiarrhythmic Drugs

	Amiodarone	Dronedarone	Sotalol	Dofetilide	Ibutilide
Form	IV and PO	PO	PO	PO	IV
Bioavailability	35%-65% (PO)	70%-90%	90%-100%	90%	
Time to peak plasma conc. (PO Only)	3-7 h after oral dose	3-4 h	2.5-4 h	2-3 h	
Half-life	56 d	13-19 h	12 h	7-13 h	2-12 h
Metabolism	Hepatic	Hepatic	No liver metabolism	Hepatic (only 20%)	Hepatic
Major route of elimination	Liver	Liver	Kidneys	Kidneys	Kidneys

to have a neutral effect on mortality in this patient population.[5,6] Like other predominant potassium channel blockers, however, the use of dofetilide should be avoided in patients with significant hypertrophic cardiomyopathy due to an increased risk of proarrhythmia. While dofetilide is not indicated for use in patients with ventricular arrhythmias, there have been studies demonstrating a decreased incidence of ventricular tachycardia in patients with previously implanted cardioverter defibrillators.[7]

Dosing

- Dosing algorithm for dofetilide is shown in Table 30-3.
- Dofetilide should be discontinued if any QTc interval after the second or subsequent doses exceed 500 msec (550 msec in the presence of a bundle branch block).
- Requires in-hospital initiation.
- Correction of serum potassium and magnesium levels prior to drug initiation.
- Restricted to providers who have completed specialized training.

Side Effects

- No significant hemodynamic effects.
- Major cardiovascular adverse events are related to QT prolongation and risk of TdP (about 1%-3%).
- Risk factors for TdP include high dose, female gender, baseline QT >450 msec, and history of sustained VT.

- Excessive QTc increase during loading calls for immediate discontinuation of the drug.
- Avoid in combination with other QT prolonging agents (antifungals, macrolide antibiotics, and protease inhibitors).

Sotalol

Sotalol is a water-soluble, racemic mixture of L- and D-isomers. While both isomers have class III antiarrhythmic properties, the L-isomer also has mild β-blocker properties. Sotalol prolongs atrial and ventricular repolarization by blocking the rapid component of the Ikr current. ECG changes associated with the use of sotalol result from its β-blocking properties (slowing of the sinus rate and PR prolongation), as well as its class III potassium blocking activity (QT prolongation) in a dose-dependent fashion.

Indications

Sotalol is predominantly used for the treatment of atrial fibrillation and is considered a first-line antiarrhythmic agent in patients without structural heart disease or those with coronary artery disease and normal left ventricular function.[4] It should be avoided in patients with severe left ventricular hypertrophy and also in those with left ventricular dysfunction. While not particularly effective in pharmacologic cardioversion, it is useful in the prevention of recurrent atrial fibrillation, especially at doses of 120 mg or 160 mg BID.[8] Sotalol has also been shown to decrease the recurrence of ventricular arrhythmias in patients with inducible VT and also to decrease the

TABLE 30-3 Initial Dosing Schedule for Dofetilide

Creatinine Clearance	Initial Dose (mcg)	QTc >15% or QTc >500 msec (550 msec in Bundle Branch Block)
>60 mL/min	500 BID	250 BID
40-60 mL/min	250 BID	125 BID
20-39 mL/min	125 BID	125 qD
<20 mL/min	—	—

incidence of ICD shock therapy in patients with a previously implanted cardioverter-defibrillator.[9]

Dosing

- Initiation should occur in the hospital with ECG monitoring and close monitoring of renal function.
- Initial dose 80 to 160 mg/d with therapeutic effect usually at the dose of 160 to 320 mg/d.
- Patients with refractory ventricular arrhythmias may require doses of up to 480 to 640 mg/d (only if benefit outweighs potential proarrhythmic drug effects).
- Dosing intervals should be adjusted depending on CrCl, with 2 times a day dosing for CrCl >60 mL/min and once a day dosing for CrCl 40 to 60 mL/min.
- Two to three days should be allowed between dose adjustments.
- Discontinuation of this medication occurs over a 1 to 2 week taper.
- Avoid the concomitant use of other QT prolonging agents.

Side effects

- Torsades de pointes has been observed in up to 2.3% of patients being treated for the prevention of atrial fibrillation with sotalol.
- Symptoms mostly related to the β-blocker effect: fatigue, dyspnea, bradycardia, and heart failure.

Contraindications

- CrCl <40 mL/min (dose should be adjusted for renal function).
- QTc >500 ms.
- Significant LVH (>1.4 cm).
- Decompensated heart failure.
- Sick sinus syndrome and advanced AV block.
- Severe asthma.

Ibutilide

Ibutilide is a class III agent with potassium channel blocking activity of the rapid Ikr current and also delays the inactivation of the slow inward sodium current. It is metabolized in the liver and has a half-life of approximately 6 hours. There are no significant drug–drug interactions when administered with calcium channel blockers, β-blockers, or digoxin. Proarrhythmic effects include sustained and nonsustained polymorphic VT in up to 4% to 5% of patients.

Indications

Ibutilide is indicated for the pharmacologic cardioversion of atrial fibrillation and atrial flutter. It is effective in terminating atrial fibrillation in approximately 50% of patients and atrial flutter in 65% to 76% of patients.[10] It has been used to facilitate cardioversion in patients already on a sodium channel blocker, such as procainamide, flecainide, or propafenone, and also those on amiodarone. Ibutilide decreases the defibrillation threshold and can be used to enhance the effectiveness of electrical cardioversion in patients with atrial fibrillation.[11]

Dosing

- Dosing algorithm shown in Table 30-4.
- Administer with continuous ECG monitoring due to proarrhythmic effects.
- No dose adjustment in patients with hepatic or renal dysfunction, but drug clearance may be prolonged in patients with hepatic dysfunction.
- Arrhythmia termination occurs within 1 hour of infusion.
- ECG monitoring for 4 hours after drug administration or until QTc returns to baseline is required. Patients with hepatic dysfunction or nonsustained ventricular tachycardia during drug administration should be monitored longer.

Side effects

- ECG effects include QT prolongation and mild slowing of the heart rate.
- May cause transient hypotension and bradycardia.
- Like other class III agents it can trigger TdP.
- Risk of ventricular tachycardia is approximately 4%.

Contraindications

- Avoid in patients with high risk of ventricular arrhythmias (baseline QTc >440 ms, hypokalemia, hypomagnesemia, sinus node dysfunction, low ejection fraction).
- Should not be coadministered with other QT-prolonging medications.

Amiodarone

While classified as a class III antiarrhythmic agent, amiodarone has properties than span across all of the Von Williams classifications.[12] In addition to blocking multiple potassium channels, including IKr, IKs,

TABLE 30-4 Dosing of Ibutilide

Weight	Dose
≥60 kg	1 mg IV over 10 min, can repeat 10 min after the end of initial infusion if arrhythmia has not terminated.
<60 kg	0.01 mg/kg IV over 10 min, can repeat 10 min after the end of initial infusion if arrhythmia has not terminated.

CLASS III
ANTIARRHYTHMIC DRUGS

SECTION V
ANTIARRHYTHMIC MEDICAL THERAPY
FOR ATRIAL FIBRILLATION

207

Ito, IK1, IKACh, and IKNa, amiodarone also has significant sodium channel, calcium channel, and β-receptor blocking activity. As a result, the electrocardiogram may show a slowing of the heart rate, increase in the PR interval, and widening of the QRS and QT prolongation. Amiodarone is primarily metabolized in the liver, and due to its significant lipophilic nature, accumulation in fatty tissue, and large volume of distribution, it has a long and variable half-life of typically 35 to 40 days, though it can be as long as 100 days.

Although amiodarone is a class III antiarrhythmic and can cause significant QT prolongation, it has a relatively low risk of TdP.[13] The exact mechanism for the low risk of TdP is not definitively known, but several theories have been postulated:

- Some evidence suggests that TdP is initiated and/or propagated by calcium-dependant early afterdepolarizations. Amiodarone's ability to block the slow inward calcium current via the L-calcium channels, leads to lower influx calcium availability and therefore a decreased risk of TdP.

- Another theory involves the differential prolongation of the repolarization period between Purkinje fibers and ventricular myocardium amongst different class III agents. Nearly all class III agents other than amiodarone prolong the repolarization of Purkinje fibers, where early afterdepolarizations resulting in TdP appear to be generated, more so than ventricular myocardium. The reverse is true of amiodarone.

- Finally, amiodarone may selectively block the action of triiodothyronine at the myocardial nuclear receptor. This leads to increased homogeneity of repolarization in contiguous myocardial cells and to a significant reduction in QT dispersion on the surface electrocardiogram as opposed to a drug like quinidine, which increases QT dispersion.

Indications

Amiodarone has been used extensively in the treatment of both ventricular and supraventricular arrhythmias, including atrial fibrillation and atrial flutter. Its favorable hemodynamic profile and low risk of proarrhythmia make it the drug of choice in patients with severe cardiomyopathy, heart failure, and recurrent cardiac arrhythmias. Prior to the use of ICDs, amiodarone was shown to decrease sudden cardiac death by up to 30% in high-risk patients.[14] Amiodarone and also been shown to be useful in preventing ICD therapy/shocks in patients with cardiac arrhythmias and prior ICD implantation. It may, however, increase the defibrillation threshold in these patients and can also result in significant slowly of the VT rate.

In patients with atrial fibrillation, it is the most commonly used and most effective antiarrhythmic agent, with over 60% of patients maintaining sinus rhythm in one year.[15] Similar to dofetilide, amiodarone has not been shown to cause an increased mortality in a high-risk patient population with severe LV dysfunction and heart failure.[16] Unfortunately, the drug does have significant long-term side effects and should be limited in its use for patients with non–life-threatening arrhythmias. Therefore, current guidelines recommend the use of amiodarone to maintain sinus rhythm in patients with coronary artery disease who are not candidates for dofetilide or sotalol; patients with heart failure who are not candidates for dofetilide; patients with severe concentric left ventricular hypertrophy; and in patients refractory to other antiarrhythmic drugs as an alternative to ablation.[4] Preventive loading with amiodarone can be considered in high-risk patients (previous AF, valvular surgery) who are undergoing cardiac surgery. Amiodarone is contraindicated in patients with severe lung or liver disease, advanced sinus node dysfunction, and AV conduction disease greater than first-degree AV block.

Dosing

- Amiodarone typically requires a significant loading dose secondary to its large volume of distribution.

- For ventricular arrhythmias, a total loading dose of 8 to 10 grams is usually required while smaller loading doses are used for atrial arrhythmias.

- An algorithm for the initiation of amiodarone (po and IV) is shown in Table 30-5 for both supraventricular and ventricular indications.

Side effects

- Amiodarone can have significant effects on multiple organ systems, many of which are listed in Table 30-6.

- Bradycardia can occur due to both sinus node suppression and AV conduction effects.

- Hypotension may occur during IV administration.

Drug–Drug Interactions

- Increased concentration and effect of warfarin and digoxin.

- Increased risk of bradycardia and AV block with concomitant AV nodal blocking agents.

- Potential proarrhythmic effect in combination with other drugs that prolong the QT interval.

- Increased risk of liver function abnormalities and myopathy with simvastatin and atorvastatin.

TABLE 30-5 Amiodarone Dosing

	Atrial Fibrillation	Ventricular Arrhythmia	Pulseless VT or VF
IV	150 mg bolus, followed by infusion of 1 mg/min × 6 h, then 0.5 mg/min	150 mg bolus, followed by infusion of 1 mg/min × 6 h, then 0.5 mg/min	300 mg, can repeat 150 mg
PO	800 mg daily in 2 doses for 2 wks, followed by 20-400 mg/d and after 3-6 mo: 100-300 mg/d	800-1600 mg daily in 2 doses for 1-3 weeks, followed by 600-800 mg/d in 2 doses for 1 mo, then 400 mg daily	

TABLE 30-6 Side Effects of Amiodarone

Pulmonary	• Diffuse opacities on chest CT • Decrease in DLCO • Follow-up: Chest x-ray at baseline and yearly, PFTs at baseline and when symptoms, CT chest if symptoms
Gastrointestinal tract	• Abnormal liver function panel • Hepatitis and cirrhosis • Follow up: liver function test at baseline and every 6 mo
Thyroid	• Hypo- and hyperthyroidism • Follow up: thyroid function tests at baseline and every 6 mo
Skin	• Discoloration • Photosensitivity
Central nervous system	• Ataxia • Tremor • Peripheral neuropathy
Ocular	• Optic neuropathy • Iris discoloration • Follow-up: ophthalmologic exam at baseline and when symptoms
Cardiovascular	• Bradycardia and AV block • Proarrhythmia • Follow up: ECG at baseline and when clinically indicated
Genitourinary	• Epididymitis • Erectile dysfunction

Dronedarone

Dronedarone is a noniodinated derivative of amiodarone with an added methane sulfonyl group, resulting in a shorter half-life and lower tissue accumulation due to decreased lipophilicity. Similar to amiodarone, dronedarone blocks several multiple potassium currents, the inward sodium currents, L-type calcium currents, and β-adrenergic receptors. The electrocardiographic effects caused by dronedarone are similar to those of amiodarone and include a decrease in the heart rate, an increase in the PR interval, QRS duration, and QT interval.

Indications

Dronedarone is clinically indicated for the maintenance of sinus rhythm in a patient with recurrent paroxysmal or persistent AF and is effective in prolonging the time to recurrence of atrial fibrillation.[17] The ATHENA trial also demonstrated dronedarone to be effective in decreasing cardiovascular hospitalizations in patients with atrial arrhythmias.[18] It is not as effective in maintaining sinus rhythm; however, when compared to amiodarone dronedarone has a low risk of TdP, but unlike amiodarone, the use of dronedarone should be limited to patients without a history of congestive heart failure or significant left ventricular dysfunction, as an increased mortality has been noted in this high-risk population.[19] Although effective in slowing the ventricular response rate during atrial fibrillation, dronedarone should not be used as a rate control agent in patients with permanent atrial fibrillation.[20]

Dosing

• Dronedarone is available in only one dosage form of 400 mg every 12 hours.

• Absorption is increased 2- to 3-fold when taken with food and should therefore be taken with meals.

Side Effects

• Causes dose-dependant QT prolongation, but TdP not reported.

• Much less extra cardiac toxicities than amiodarone.

• GI side effects including abdominal pain, nausea, and diarrhea.

• Transient increase in serum creatinine without reduction in renal function.

Contraindications

• Congestive heart failure

• Permanent atrial fibrillation

• Severe liver impairment

• Bradycardia (HR <50 bpm)

• Sick sinus syndrome

• First degree AV block with PR interval >280 ms or higher AV block

• Prolonged QT (QTc >500 msec) or coadministration with QT prolonging agents (antifungals, macrolide antibiotics, and protease inhibitors)

Drug–Drug Interactions

- Use with verapamil, diltiazem, digoxin, warfarin, and/or statin medications requires caution and dose adjustment due to risk of QT prolongation.

SUMMARY

The Vaughan-Williams class III antiarrhythmic agents provide an important option in the treatment of atrial and ventricular arrhythmias. Those drugs with predominant class III effects, however, are at a higher risk of causing proarrhythmia (TdP) and should be initiated in a monitored setting. While amiodarone and dronedarone appear to have a significantly lower risk of TdP, their use is limited by either noncardiac side effects (amiodarone) or an increased mortality in patients with structural heart disease and heart failure (dronedarone). With careful patient selection and appropriate follow-up, however, all of the class III antiarrhythmics can be used successfully in the treatment of cardiac arrhythmias.

REFERENCES

1. Hondeghem LM, Snyders DJ. Class III antiarrhythmic agents have a lot of potential but a long way to go. Reduced effectiveness and dangers of reverse use dependence. *Circulation.* 1990;81(2):686-690.

2. Singh S, Zoble RG, Yellen L, et al. Efficacy and safety of oral dofetilide in converting to and maintaining sinus rhythm in patients with chronic atrial fibrillation or atrial flutter: the symptomatic atrial fibrillation investigative research on dofetilide (SAFIRE-D) study. *Circulation.* 2000;102(19):2385-2390.

3. Cotiga D, Arshad A, Aziz E, Joshi S, Koneru JN, Steinberg JS. Acute conversion of persistent atrial fibrillation during dofetilide initiation. *Pacing Clin Electrophysiol.* 2007;30(12):1527-1530.

4. Fuster V, Rydén LE, Cannom DS, et al. 2011 ACCF/AHA/HRS focused updates ncorporated into the ACC/AHA/ESC 2006 guidelines for the management of patients with atrial fibrillation: a report of the American College of Cardiology Foundation/American Heart Association Task Force on practice guidelines. *Circulation.* 2011;123(10):e269-e367.

5. Torp-Pedersen C, Moller M, Bloch Thomsen PE, et al.. Dofetilide in patients with congestive heart failure and left ventricular dysfunction. Danish Investigations of Arrhythmia and Mortality on Dofetilide Study Group. *N Eng J Med.* 1999;341(12):857-865.

6. Kober L, Bloch Thomsen PE, Moller M, et al; Danish Investigators of Arrhythmia and Mortality on Dofetilide (Diamond) Study Group. Effect of dofetilide in patients with recent myocardial infarction and left-ventricular dysfunction: a randomised trial. *Lancet.* 2000;356:2052-2058.

7. Boriana G, Lubinski A, Capucci A, et al; Ventricular Arrhythmias Dofetide Investigators. A multicentre, double-blind randomized crossover comparative study on the efficacy and safety of dofetilide vs sotalol in patients with inducible sustained ventricular tachycardia and ischaemic heart disease. *Eur Heart J.* 2001:22(23):2180-2191.

8. Benditt DG, Williams JH, Jin J, et al. Maintenance of sinus rhythm with oral d,l-sotalol therapy in patients with symptomatic atrial fibrillation and/or atrial flutter. d,l-Sotalol Atrial Fibrillation/Flutter Study Group. *Am J Cardiol.* 1999;84(3):270-277.

9. Pacifico A, Hohnloser SH, Williams JH, et al. Prevention of implantable-defibrillator shocks by treatment with sotalol. d,l-Sotalol Implantable Cardioverter-Defibrillator Study Group. *N Eng J Med.* 1999;340(24):1855-1862.

10. Volgman AS, Carberry PA, Stambler B, et al. Conversion efficacy and safety of intravenous ibutilide compared with intravenous procainamide in patients with atrial flutter or fibrillation. *J Am Coll Cardiol.* 1998;31(6):1414-1419.

11. Oral H, Souza JJ, Michaud GF, et al. Facilitating transthoracic cardioversion of atrial fibrillation with ibutilide pretreatment. *N Eng J Med.* 1999;340(24):1849-1854.

12. Goldschlager N, Epstein AE, Naccarelli GV, et al. A practical guide for clinicians who treat patients with amiodarone: 2007. *Heart Rhythm.* 2007;4(9):1250-1259.

13. Amiodarone Trials Meta-Analysis Investigators. Effect of prophylactic amiodarone on mortality after acute myocardial infarction and in congestive heart failure: meta-analysis of individual data from 6500 patients in randomised trials. *Lancet.* 1997;350:1417-1424.

14. Sim I, McDonald KM, Lavori PW, Norbutas CM, Hlatky MA. Quantitative overview of randomized trials of amiodarone to prevent sudden cardiac death. *Circulation.* 1997;96(9):2823-2829.

15. AFFIRM First Antiarrhythmic Drug Substudy Investigators. Maintenance of sinus rhythm in patients with atrial fibrillation: an AFFIRM substudy of the first antiarrhythmic drug. *J Am Coll Cardiol.* 2003;42(1):20-29.

16. Singh SN, Fletcher RD, Fisher SG, et al. Amiodarone in patients with congestive heart failure and asymptomatic ventricular arrhythmia. Survival Trial of Antiarrhythmic Therapy in Congestive Heart Failure. *N Eng J Med.* 1995;333(2):77-82.

17. Singh BN, Connolly SJ, Crijns HJ, et al; EURIDIS and ADONIS Investigators. Dronedarone for maintenance of sinus rhythm in atrial fibrillation or flutter. *N Eng J Med.* 2007;357(10):987-999.

18. Hohnloser SH, Crijns HJ, van Eickels M, et al; ATHENA Investigators. Effect of dronedarone on cardiovascular events in atrial fibrillation. *N Eng J Med.* 2009;360(7):668-678.

19. Kober L, Torp-Pedersen C, McMurray JJ, et al; Dronedarone Study Group. Increased mortality after dronedarone therapy for severe heart failure. *N Eng J Med.* 2008;358(25):2678-2687.

20. Connolly SJ, Camm AJ, Halpern JL, et al. Dronedarone in high-risk permanent atrial fibrillation. *N Eng J Med.* 2011;365(24):2268-2276.

31 DRONEDARONE USE FOR THE TREATMENT OF ATRIAL FIBRILLATION

Gerald Naccarelli, MD, and Talal Moukabary, MD

CASE PRESENTATION

A 59-year-old man with history of coronary artery disease and prior myocardial infarction was referred to for the treatment of paroxysmal atrial fibrillation. He reported recurrent episodes of palpitations during the past 6 months. The episodes last from a few minutes to a few hours. However, he has no chest pain, dyspnea, or syncope. One event was captured on a 12-lead ECG as shown (Figure 31-1), and

he was cardioverted to sinus rhythm with an external shock. Other than his atrial fibrillation he is doing well. He follows a heart-healthy diet and is able to exercise daily with no difficulty. He is anticoagulated with warfarin for stroke prevention. His recent echocardiogram shows normal left ventricular systolic function. Dronedarone therapy was initiated. During a follow-up visit, the patient reported having no more episodes of palpitations. He had diarrhea in the form of loose stools for 1 week after the initiation of dronedarone; however, it resolved spontaneously. His follow-up ECG is shown in Figure 31-2.

INTRODUCTION

Although amiodarone has an unparalleled efficacy in the maintenance of sinus rhythm in patients with atrial fibrillation, its side effect profile is prohibitive. Dronedarone was developed as a noniodinated analog of amiodarone, with the goal of being an antiarrhythmic agent for rhythm control in patients with atrial fibrillation (Table 31-1). It was hypothesized that dronedarone will have fewer thyroid

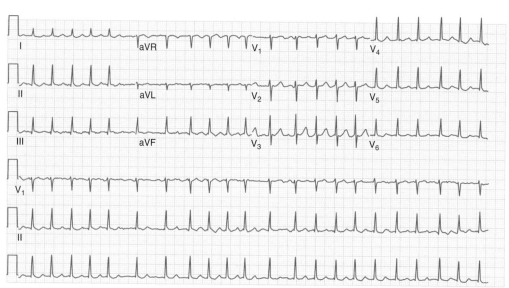

FIGURE 31-1 The 12-lead ECG showing atrial fibrillation.

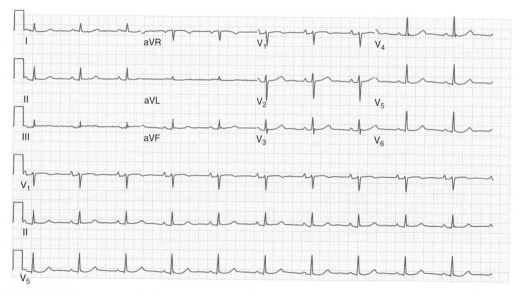

FIGURE 31-2 The 12-lead ECG showing sinus rhythm with slightly prolonged QT interval.

DRONEDARONE USE FOR
THE TREATMENT OF ATRIAL FIBRILLATION

SECTION V
ANTIARRHYTHMIC MEDICAL THERAPY
FOR ATRIAL FIBRILLATION

211

TABLE 31-1 Similarities and Differences between Amiodarone and Dronedarone

	Amiodarone	Dronedarone
Iodine moiety	Yes	No
Elimination half-life	53 d	14-30 h
Lipophilic properties	Strong	Moderate
Tissue accumulation	Yes	No
Blocks IKr; IKs; B1; ICa; Ito; INa	Yes	Yes
Dosing	Daily after loading	Twice daily with meals
Food effect	Yes	Yes
CYP4503A4 metabolism	Yes	Yes
Increases creatinine	Yes	Yes
Increase QT but low TDP	Yes	Yes
Efficacy in suppressing AF	65%	50%
Rate control in AF	Yes	Yes
Efficacy in suppressing ventricular tachyarrhythmias	Yes	Probably
Decreases CV hospitalization	No	Yes
Warfarin interaction	Yes	No
Dabigatran interaction	Yes	Yes
Digoxin interaction	Yes	Yes
Simvastatin interaction	Yes	Yes
Pulmonary/thyroid toxicity	Yes	No
Hepatic toxicity	Yes	Yes
Safety concerns in CHF	SCD-HeFT (NYHA III)	ANDROMEDA

Reproduced with permission from Naccarelli GV, Wolbrette DL, Levin V, et al.: Safety and efficacy of dronedarone in the treatment of atrial fibrillation/flutter. Clin Med Insights Cardiol 2011; 5:103–119.
Modified from Naccarelli et al.[21]
Abbreviations: AF, atrial fibrillation; CHF, congestive heart failure; CV, cardiovascular; TDP, torsades de pointes.

and pulmonary effects than amiodarone due to the elimination of the iodine moiety. Clinical trials showed that dronedarone is more effective than placebo without an increase in the rates of pulmonary toxic effects and of thyroid and liver dysfunction.[1]

MECHANISM OF ACTION AND PHARMACOKINETICS

Similar to amiodarone, dronedarone is a class III antiarrhythmic agent. It blocks multiple repolarizing currents (the delayed rectifier current, the ultra-rapid delayed rectifier current, the inward rectifier current, and the transient outward current) in addition it blocks depolarizing sodium and L-type calcium currents and has an antiadrenergic effect.[2]

Dronedarone is 70% to 94% absorbed after oral administration, but due to significant first pass metabolism its absolute bioavailability is only 15%. Peak plasma concentrations are achieved within 3 to 6 hours. Plasma dronedarone level increases two- and threefold when it is taken with food. Steady-state plasma concentrations are reached within 4 to 8 days following the initiation of dronedarone 400 mg twice daily.[3]

The terminal half-life of dronedarone is 13 to 19 hours, and it is cleared mainly nonrenally. It is highly bound to plasma proteins and does not accumulate significantly in the tissues.[3]

Dronedarone does not affect the glomerular filtration rate, but it significantly decreases renal *creatinine* clearance by about 18%. This is likely due to inhibition of the cationic transport system in a way similar to cimetidine. This effect resolves once the drug is discontinued.[4]

METABOLISM AND INTERACTIONS

Dronedarone is primarily metabolized by the CYP3A4 system in the liver. Accordingly, its clearance may decrease in patients with hepatic impairment, and so it is contraindicated in patients with severe hepatic impairment. There is no requirement for dose adjustment in patients with renal insufficiency.[3]

Dronedarone is a metabolized by CYP3A4 in the liver. Dronedarone is also a moderate inhibitor of CYP3A4. Coadministration of dronedarone and CYP3A4 inhibitors may cause bradycardia and atrioventricular conduction block. Lower doses of dronedarone are recommended when it is coadministered with diltiazem or verapamil (moderate CYP3A4 inhibitors)(Table 31-2).

Dronedarone causes a modest increase in bioavailability of metoprolol in CYP2D6 extensive metabolizers due to CYP2D6 inhibition.[5]

Coadministration of dronedarone with QT prolonging drugs, such as class I and III antiarrhythmic medications, some macrolide antibiotics, some phenothiazines, and tricyclic antidepressants, carries a risk of inducing torsades de pointes-type ventricular tachycardia.[6]

When given with digoxin, dronedarone has the potential for increasing digoxin level by P-glycoprotein-mediated interaction in the kidney.[3,7]

Dronedarone increases serum warfarin exposure, but it does not cause clinically significant prolongation of INR values.[8,9] Similarly it increases dabigatran,[10] rivaroxaban, and apixaban levels. Caution should be used in using dronedarone and dabigatran together, particularly in patients with decreased renal function.[6]

Dronedarone increases simvastatin, rosuvastatin, and atorvastatin exposure, which increases the potential for statin-induced myopathy.[3]

Grapefruit juice is a moderate inhibitor of CYP3A and results in an increase in dronedarone exposure.[3]

TABLE 31-2 Cardiovascular Drug Interactions with Dronedarone

Drug	Mechanism	Effect	Dose Adjustment
Digoxin	P-g P substrate	2.5-fold increase digoxin level	Halve the digoxin dose.
Verapamil, diltiazem	CYP3A inhibitors	1.4- to 1.7-fold increase in dronedarone level	Lower dose of calcium channel blocker.
β-Blockers	CYP2D6 substrate	1.6-fold increase in metoprolol level	Lower β-blocker dose.
Simvastatin	CYP3A substrate	Up to four fold increase in simvastin level	Maximum simvastatin dose 10-40 mg.
Dabigatran	P-g P substrate	1.1-1.9 increase in dabigatran level	Consider lower dose of dabigatran.

Reproduced with permission from Naccarelli GV, Wolbrette DL, Levin V, et al.: Safety and efficacy of dronedarone in the treatment of atrial fibrillation/flutter. Clin Med Insights Cardiol 2011; 5:103–119.
Modified from Naccarelli et al.[21]
Abbreviations: CYP, cytochrome; P-g P, P-glycoprotein.

CLINICAL USE

Dronedarone is primarily used for the maintenance of sinus rhythm in patients with paroxysmal atrial fibrillation without heart failure (Tables 31-3 and 31-4). This is regardless of the presence of coronary artery disease. Dronedarone should not be used as a rate control agent in patients with permanent atrial fibrillation.

Patients treated with dronedarone have significantly longer times to first recurrence of AF and significantly greater chances of remaining in sinus rhythm at 6 and 12 months compared with placebo (ADONIS, EURIDIS, and DAFNE trials).[1,11]

Although dronedarone is more effective than placebo, it is less effective compared to amiodarone (DIONYSOS trial).[12]

The 2011 ACC/AHA/HRS Focused Update on the Management of Patients with Atrial Fibrillation and the 2010 ESC Guidelines for the Management of Atrial Fibrillation list dronedarone among the first line antiarrhythmic agents for maintaining sinus rhythm in patients with recurrent paroxysmal or persistent AF who have no (or minimal) heart disease, hypertensive heart disease without substantial left ventricular hypertrophy, or coronary artery disease, but without heart failure.[13,14] The American guidelines and an updated European statement agree that dronedarone should not be used in patients with heart failure or left ventricular systolic dysfunction.[15]

Dronedarone is rarely able to chemically cardiovert AF or atrial flutter to sinus rhythm (<10%).[11] However, given that there is a potential for cardioversion during drug initiation, it is recommended that patients have therapeutic anticoagulation for at least 3 weeks or a transesophageal echocardiogram for assessment of left atrial thrombus prior to the initiation of dronedarone for patients who are in atrial fibrillation. This scenario is most commonly seen when loading patients with dronedarone in preparation for an electrical cardioversion.

Dronedarone slows the resting ventricular heart rate in patients who develop recurrent AF.[1,7,16] However, dronedarone should NOT be prescribed exclusively as a rate control medication in permanent AF, given that the PALLAS trial demonstrated an increase in cardiovascular mortality when dronedarone was used solely as a rate-controlling agent.[17]

When changing between dronedarone and other antiarrhythmic drugs that have the potential for QT prolongation and torsades des pointes, at least five half-lives should be allowed with the exception of amiodarone. When changing from amiodarone to dronedarone, there are a few approaches. Dronedarone can be started immediately after discontinuation of amiodarone (ADONIS and EURIDIS trials[1]), can be started 1 month after discontinuation of amiodarone (ATHENA[16]), or 2 months after discontinuation of amiodarone (ERATO[5]).

In general, dronedarone can be started promptly after amiodarone discontinuation, except in cases of clinically significant bradycardia or QT prolongation.

Dronedarone was shown to reduce the rates of hospitalization and cardiovascular mortality (post-hoc analysis of EURIDIS and ADONIS[1] and ATHENA[18]). However, it significantly increases the risk of cardiovascular events (cardiovascular death, myocardial infarction, stroke and systemic embolism) and possibly even stroke and hospitalization for heart failure when used for rate control in patients with permanent atrial fibrillation especially those who are older or have heart failure (ANDROMEDA, PALLAS[17,19]).

SIDE EFFECTS AND MONITORING

The most common side effects are relatively benign (crampy abdominal pain, diarrhea, nausea, vomiting). Dronedarone may result in

TABLE 31-3 Appropriate and Inappropriate Clinical Use of Dronedarone

Appropriate	Inappropriate
Paroxysmal or recurrent persistent AF for rhythm control	Permanent AF for rate control
AF with CAD	CHF or LV systolic dysfunction
AF with HTN	Substantial LVH

Abbreviations: AF, atrial fibrillation; CAD, coronary artery disease; CHF, congestive heart failure; HTN, hypertension; LV, left ventricle; LVH, left ventricular hypertrophy.

DRONEDARONE USE FOR
THE TREATMENT OF ATRIAL FIBRILLATION

SECTION V
ANTIARRHYTHMIC MEDICAL THERAPY
FOR ATRIAL FIBRILLATION

213

TABLE 31-4 Clinical Trials Investigating Efficacy of Dronedarone

Trial	Number of Patients and Follow-Up	Inclusion Criteria	Main Exclusion Criteria	Results	Conclusion
DAFNE Placebo versus dronedarone 40, 600, 800 mg BID	270 pts 6 mo f/u	Persistent AF (<12 m) average AF duration only 122 d	AFI, NYHA class III or IV, EF <35%	**First AF recurrence:** 800 mg daily-60 d versus placebo-5.3 d 1200,1600 mg/d-no difference from placebo	Lack of dose effect, modest efficacy in preventing first recurrence in persistent AF, with 400 mg bid/meals
EURIDIS/ADONIS Placebo versus dronedarone 400 mg BID	612 pts in EURIDIS 625 pts in ADONIS 12 mo f/u	Paroxysmal/persistent AF	NYHA class III or IV, PR >0.27 vs, Heart rate <50 bpm; Creatinine >1.6 mg/dL	**First AF recurrence:** D. 116 d P. 53 d **At 12 mo recurrence:** D. 64.1% P. 75.2% P. <0.001	Modest efficacy in preventing AF recurrence in patients with minimal SHD. Good safety over 12 mo f/u.
ERATO Placebo versus dronedarone for rate control	174 pts 6 mo f/u	Permanent AF with resting HR > 80 bpm	NYHA class III or IV	Treatment effect on mean VR on day 14 -11.7 bpm At maximal exercise −24.5 bpm	Rate control properties in addition to digoxin, β-blockers, and Ca-blockers
DIONYSOS Dronedarone versus amiodarone	504 pts 6 mo f/u	Persistent AF	NYHA class III or IV, QTc >500 ms, paroxymal AF/ AFl, high degree AV block, thyroid disorder	AF recurrence or premature drug discontinuation for intolerance or lack of efficacy: D. 75.1% A. 58.8% **AF recurrence at 12 mo:** D. 63.5% A. 42%	Dronedarone significantly less effective than amiodarone but fewer side effects and better tolerated.
ATHENA Dronedarone versus placebo	4648 pts F/U: mean of 21 mo	Elderly patients with paroxysmal or persistent AF/AFl plus risk factors	Permanent AF; Decompensated heart failure	24% RR in cardiovascular hospitalizations (p <0.0001)	Dronedarone reduced hospitalizations in moderate risk, elderly patients with paroxysmal or persistent AF/AFl
PALLAS Dronedarone versus placebo in permanent AF	3236 out of planned 10,800 pts F/U: median 3.6 mo	Permanent AF	Paroxysmal or persistent AF	2.29-fold increase (CI: 1.34-3.94; p = 0.002) in the primary composite CV end point (stroke, MI, systemic embolism, or CV death)	Doubling of CV events with dronedarone in permanent AF

Reproduced with permission from Naccarelli GV, Wolbrette DL, Levin V, et al.: Safety and efficacy of dronedarone in the treatment of atrial fibrillation/flutter. Clin Med Insights Cardiol 2011; 5:103–119.
Modified from Naccarelli et al.[21]
Abbreviations: AF/AFl, atrial fibrillation/flutter; bpm, beats per minute; CV, cardiovascular; D, dronedarone; f/u, follow-up; MI, myocardial infarction; P, placebo; pts, patients.

other side effects including generalized weakness, and dermatologic manifestations such as eczema, pruritus, skin inflammation, rash, and skin photosensitivity.

Although rare, there are potentially life-threatening side effects. In general, dronedarone should not be prescribed in patients with previous lung or liver toxicity due to amiodarone.

Some authors recommend hepatic function testing should be performed at the time of dronedarone initiation and repeated at 3 and 6 months and a electrocardiogram annually and at the time of any clinical change.[6,18,20] Hepatocellular injury, including acute liver failure requiring transplant, has been reported with the use of dronedarone. Since the reported cases have occurred within 6 months of drug initiation, it is reasonable to check hepatic function at baseline and within the first 6 months of treatment. Intermittent long-term surveillance testing may also be reasonable.[6]

Pulmonary toxicity has been reported with dronedarone.[15] Routine lung surveillance is reasonable, but there are formal recommendations as to when and how.

Rare cases of torsades de pointes were reported, and dronedarone should be discontinued in this instance.[18,20] On the other hand, dronedarone causes bradycardia and QT prolongation, neither of which usually requires drug discontinuation.

CONCLUSION

Dronedarone-induced proarrhythmia is rare, and the drug can be safely initiated as an outpatient. Although less efficacious than amiodarone in the prevention of recurrent AF, dronedarone appears to be a safer and better tolerated drug in patients with preserved left ventricular function. The guidelines suggest that dronedarone should be used prior to amiodarone and in patients with or without coronary artery disease, as long as left ventricular function is preserved.

REFERENCES

1. Singh BN, Connolly SJ, Crijns HJGM, et al. Dronedarone for maintenance of sinus rhythm in atrial fibrillation or flutter. *N Engl J Med.* 2007;357(10):987-999.

2. Varró A, Takács J, Németh M, et al. Electrophysiological effects of dronedarone (SR 33589), a noniodinated amiodarone derivative in the canine heart: comparison with amiodarone. *Br J Pharmacol.* 2001;133:625-634.

3. Hoy SM, Keam SJ: Dronedarone. *Drugs.* 2009;69:1647-1663.

4. Tschuppert Y, Buclin T, Rothuizen LE, et al.: Effect of dronedarone on renal function in healthy subjects. *Br J Clin Pharmacol.* 2007;64:785-791.

5. Damy T, Pousset F, Caplain H, Hulot J-S, Lechat P: Pharmacokinetic and pharmacodynamic interactions between metoprolol and dronedarone in extensive and poor CYP2D6 metabolizers healthy subjects. *Fundam Clin Pharmacol.* 2004;18:113-123.

6. Multaq prescribing information (Internet). Accessed September 20, 2014. http://products.sanofi.us/multaq/multaq.pdf

7. Davy JM, Herold M, Hoglund C, et al. Dronedarone for the control of ventricular rate in permanent atrial fibrillation: the Efficacy and safety of dRonedArone for the cOntrol of ventricular rate during atrial fibrillation (ERATO) study. *Am Heart J.* 2008;156:527.e1-9.

8. Shirolkar SC, Fiuzat M, Becker RC: Dronedarone and vitamin K antagonists: a review of drug-drug interactions. *Am Heart J.* 2010;160:577-582.

9. Patel C, Yan GX, Kowey PR: Dronedarone. *Circulation.* 2009;120:636-644.

10. Connolly SJ, Ezekowitz MD, Yusuf S, Reilly PA, Wallentin L. Newly identified events in the RE-LY trial. *N Engl J Med.* 2010;363:1875-1876.

11. Touboul P, Brugada J, Capucci A, Crijns HJGM, Edvardsson N, Hohnloser SH. Dronedarone for prevention of atrial fibrillation: a dose-ranging study. *Eur Heart J.* 2003;24:1481-1487.

12. Le Heuzey JY, De Ferrari GM, Radzik D, Santini M, Zhu J, Davy JM. A short-term, randomized, double-blind, parallel-group study to evaluate the efficacy and safety of dronedarone versus amiodarone in patients with persistent atrial fibrillation: the DIONYSOS study. *J Cardiovasc Electrophysiol.* 2010;21:597-605.

13. Wann LS, Curtis AB, January CT, et al. 2011 ACCF/AHA/HRS focused update on the management of patients with atrial fibrillation (Updating the 2006 Guideline): a report of the American College of Cardiology Foundation/American Heart Association Task Force on Practice Guidelines. *Heart Rhythm.* 2011;8:157-176.

14. Camm AJ, Kirchhof P, Lip GYH, et al. Guidelines for the management of atrial fibrillation: the Task Force for the Management of Atrial Fibrillation of the European Society of Cardiology (ESC). *Eur Heart J.* 2010;31:2369-2429.

15. European Medicines Agency. European Medicines Agency recommends restricting use of Multaq. http://www.ema.europa.eu/ema/index.jsp?curl=pages/news_and_events/news/2011/09/news_detail_001344.jsp&murl=menus/news_and_events/news_and_events.jsp&mid=WC0b01ac058004d5c1. Accessed September 20, 2014.

16. Page RL, Connolly SJ, Crijns HJGM, et al. Rhythm- and rate-controlling effects of dronedarone in patients with atrial fibrillation (from the ATHENA trial). *Am J Cardiol.* 2011;107:1019-1022.

17. Connolly SJ, Camm AJ, Halperin JL, et al. Dronedarone in high-risk permanent atrial fibrillation. *N Engl J Med.* 2011;365:2268-2276.

18. Hohnloser SH, Crijns HJGM, Van Eickels M, et al. Effect of dronedarone on cardiovascular events in atrial fibrillation. *N Engl J Med.* 2009;360:668-678.

19. Kober L, Torp-Pedersen C, McMurray JJV, et al. Increased mortality after dronedarone therapy for severe heart failure. *N Engl J Med.* 2008;358:2678-2687.

20. Kao DP, Hiatt WR, Krantz MJ: Proarrhythmic potential of dronedarone: emerging evidence from spontaneous adverse event reporting. *Pharmacotherapy.* 2012;32(8):767-71.

21. Naccarelli GV, Wolbrette DL, Levin V, et al. Safety and efficacy of dronedarone in the treatment of atrial fibrillation/flutter. *Clin Med Insights Cardiol.* 2011;5:103-119.

32 AMIODARONE

Sunita J. Ferns, MD, MRCPCH, and Gerald V.
Naccarelli, MD, FHRS

CASE PRESENTATION

A 65-year-old patient with diabetes, chronic kidney disease, hypertension, and known ischemic cardiomyopathy status postcoronary artery bypass grafting with an ejection fraction of 35% and no known arrhythmia history had a single chamber implantable cardioverter-defibrillator (ICD) placed for primary prevention. He presented 6 months later with two shocks within 48 hours. Interrogation of his ICD revealed a supraventricular tachycardia with rapid ventricular conduction. The best choice in the management of the above patient would be:

1. Upgrade to a dual chamber device.

2. Initiate treatment with a class IC antiarrhythmic medication.

3. Initiate treatment with tikosyn.

4. Initiate treatment with amiodarone.

5. Turn off ventricular tachytherapies as this is an atrial tachycardia.

COMMENT

Thirty to seventy percent of ICD patients require antiarrhythmic drug therapy for suppression of recurrent ventricular tachycardia (VT) or suppression of prophylaxis against atrial fibrillation (AF) with rapid ventricular rates. The majority of patients with ICDs have structural heart disease and left ventricular dysfunction that would preclude use of IC agents. In this patient with renal dysfunction, amiodarone would be the drug of choice.

HISTORY

Amiodarone was developed in Belgium in 1961 as a treatment for angina.[1] Its antiarrhythmic properties were later confirmed by Mauricio Rosenbaum.[2] Amiodarone has been widely used worldwide since the 1970s and in 1985 received FDA approval for the treatment of life-threatening ventricular tachyarrhythmias.[3]

MECHANISM OF ACTION

Amiodarone has a broad spectrum of antiarrhythmic actions across all four drug classes with effects on Na, K, and Ca channels via perturbation of the lipid environment in the membrane bilayer.[4-8] Additionally, it also has α- and β-blocking properties.[9,10] Like other class III antiarrhythmic medications, amiodarone prolongs the cardiac action potential via inhibition of IK_r with resultant lengthening of the repolarization phase (phase 3) of the action potential.[5,11] By prolongation of the action potential, it increases the wavelength of the wavefront within the reentrant circuit and thereby reduces the excitable gap. If the excitable gap is reduced sufficiently, the leading edge of activation encounters refractory tissue from the tail of the previous wave and cannot propagate further.[12] A delay in repolarization manifests as an increase in the QT interval, which may be proarrhythmic.[13,14] Due to its strong sodium channel blocking effects across all conduction tissue, it can also depress myocardial and His-Purkinje conduction.[13,15] With acute administration, Na and Ca blocking effects predominate with AV node slowing, and with chronic administration, effects on the K channel predominate with predictable lengthening of refractory periods and repolarization.[5,16,17]

PHARMACOLOGY/METABOLISM

Chemically, amiodarone is a highly lipid soluble iodinated benzofuran derivative similar to thyroxine.[18,19] The bioavailability ranges from 22% to 86% with about 50% absorbed from the gut. It has a large volume of distribution due to accumulation to varying degrees in different tissues, especially in fat, and may take many weeks to reach a steady state or be eliminated from the system. The half-life ranges from 30 to 110 days.[3,20] With oral administration, peak plasma levels are reached in 6 to 8 hours, and with higher doses peak effects may be evident in 48 hours. In most cases with lower loading doses, however, effects may be seen only in 2 to 6 weeks. After discontinuation, plasma levels may be seen for 2 to 3 months but may continue to be detected up to 9 months later.[21] Studies have shown that drug effects depend on tissue stores and not on plasma levels, and therefore plasma levels are not used to guide therapy. Because of its slow accumulation, a loading dose is usually prescribed with the aim of using the lowest possible maintenance dose to minimize toxicity. Amiodarone undergoes extensive hepatic metabolism to DEA (desethyl-amiodarone), an active metabolite very similar to amiodarone. It interacts with warfarin and other hepatically metabolized drugs due to interference with CYP2C9 hepatic metabolic pathway.[22] As the kidney is not involved in its metabolism, there are no dose adjustments required in renal failure or dialysis.

INDICATIONS

Ventricular Arrhythmias

Oral Therapy

Due to its minimal arrhythmogenic and negative inotropic effects and its efficacy at preventing sustained VT/VF or death, amiodarone remains the drug of choice in patients with sustained ventricular tachyarrhythmias associated with structural heart disease, especially those with LV dysfunction ventricular dysfunction, who are not candidates for an implantable cardioverter-defibrillator (ICD).[23-25] Its efficacy at 2 years in prevention of sustained VT/VF or death is approximately 60%, and in fact the efficacy of amiodarone is similar to ICD therapy in patients with left ventricular ejection fractions greater than 35%.[26-28] However, in patients with NYHA III in the Sudden Cardiac Death in Heart Failure Trial (SCD-HeFT) trial, amiodarone adversely affected survival.[29] Therefore, it is reserved for patients with nonsustained VT that is symptomatic, refractory to β-blocker therapy, and concerning enough to warrant treatment.[25]

Intravenous Therapy

The intravenous (IV) form is used for prophylaxis and treatment of recurrent VF and hemodynamically unstable VT in patients unresponsive to other antiarrhythmic therapy. The current ACLS guidelines suggest its use in persistent VF or pulseless VT when standard resuscitative measures fail.[30,31]

Atrial Arrhythmias

Oral Therapy

Despite not being FDA approved for atrial fibrillation (AF), amiodarone is frequently used for the management of AF as it has a greater than 60% efficacy rates for maintaining sinus rhythm.[32] The current American College of Cardiology (ACC) guidelines suggest its use for AF in patients postmyocardial infarction or with congestive heart failure, LV dysfunction, or hypertrophy who are not candidates for sotalol or dofetilide; patients who are antiarrhythmic drug-refractory; or symptomatic patients as a medical alternative to catheter ablation.[33] It is not routinely recommended for preoperative prophylaxis.[25]

Intravenous Therapy

The IV form is used to treat various supraventricular arrhythmias especially in the acute and postoperative setting.[34] It can also be used as a rate controlling agent in acute onset AF, and though ineffective in AF conversion in the acute setting, it can help maintain sinus rhythm 1 to 2 days after cardioversion.[25,35]

DOSING

Loading may be initiated on an outpatient basis depending on the situation; however, for high loading doses hospital admission with monitoring of rhythm and the QT interval is advisable.

Oral

A loading dose of up to 1600 mg a day may be started with reduction in maintenance dose to as low as 100 mg a day.[36]

Intravenous

IV boluses may be up to 150 mg followed by a continuous infusion of 1 to 2 mg/min. An IV infusion is administered through a central line as it can cause local phlebitis.[12]

Adverse Effects

Adverse effects that are dose-related are usually seen in the initial phases of therapy and may decrease with down titration of the dose. Close monitoring of these patients is necessary to assess efficacy, adjust dose, and evaluate for toxic effects. Due to the long half-life of the drug, initial visits should be every 3 to 6 months. The diagnosis and management of adverse effects are summarized in Table 32-1.

Cardiac

Cardiac adverse effects are related to amiodarone's effects on the action potential and include bradyarrhythmias, worsening of conduction defects, and ventricular arrhythmias.[37,38] In patients with an ICD, ventricular tachycardias may occur at a lower rate than the detection rate, and arrhythmias may go unrecognized. The defibrillation threshold may be increased, and ICD treatments may be ineffective. Hypotension may be a side effect especially with the IV form and is thought to be related to its α-blocking properties.

Extracardiac

Amiodarone has significant extracardiac effects on multiple organ systems. Because of its high iodine content and close structural association to thyroxine and effects on thyroid metabolism, hypothyroidism may be seen in up to a third of patients.[39] Thyroid screening is indicated at baseline and 6 months after starting therapy as it usually takes a few months for hormonal levels to equilibrate.[25] Hypothyroidism is diagnosed with a high TSH level that reverses after discontinuation of the drug. If hypothyroidism persists, possibly due to intrinsic defects in thyroid synthesis, thyroid supplements are required. Hyperthyroidism is a much less frequent problem but may occur any time during therapy. The typical clinical symptoms of hyperthyroidism may be masked due to the β-blocking effect of the drug. Treatment with antithyroid agents may be needed in addition to discontinuation of the drug.[40]

Pulmonary toxicity can occur in up to 5% to 20% of patients on chronic doses and can manifest as pulmonary fibrosis, chronic interstitial pneumonitis, organizing pneumonia, bronchiolitis obliterans, or ARDS.[41-44] Toxicity involving the lung is usually related to the cumulative dose but may occur any time during the course of therapy, and data supports involvement at both low and higher dose ranges.[45] The usual presentation is an initial cough, followed by progressive dyspnea. A high index of suspicion is required as these may be confused with heart failure symptoms. Pulmonary function tests show restrictive lung disease and a decreased diffusion capacity. Though this is a sensitive test, the specificity is limited and therefore not suggested as a routine monitoring tool.[25] Management includes discontinuing the drug and initiation of steroids. Gastrointestinal symptoms are usually dose-related, though long-term effects on the liver may be seen with chronic accumulation. An increase in transaminase levels may be seen in 10% to 20% of patients, though hepatitis is relatively rare. Corneal microdeposits may be seen in 50% to 100% of patients with prolonged therapy. Although these do not affect vision, the deposits can cause cysts and abscesses, but usually reverse with drug discontinuation. Another reversible side effect, with long term use, is blue gray discoloration of the skin seen in up to 10% of patients.[46] Skin photosensitivity with exposure to sunlight may be seen as an acute or chronic effect. Other side effects include gastrointestinal upset and neurological problems such as headache, proximal muscle weakness, peripheral neuropathy, and ataxia.[24] Due to these numerous side effects, under two-thirds of patients remain on therapy 5 years after treatment.[47]

DRUG INTERACTIONS

Amiodarone has multiple drug interactions especially with drugs that are metabolized in the liver or highly protein bound.[48] The interactions are summarized in Table 32-2.

PREGNANCY AND PEDIATRIC PATIENTS

Amiodarone can cross the placental barrier due to its high lipid solubility and can affect the developing fetus. It should therefore be avoided in pregnancy.[49,50] Despite not being adequately studied in children, the IV form is frequently used in atrial and ventricular tachyarrhythmias after congenital heart surgery. Due to its side effects, it is less commonly used for long-term maintenance therapy.

SUMMARY

In summary, amiodarone is the most effective antiarrhythmic agent for the treatment of AF and ventricular tachycardias. Amiodarone has a

TABLE 32-1 Diagnosis and Management of Adverse Effects

Organ System	Monitoring Test	Frequency of Monitoring	Diagnosis	Treatment
Cardiac	ECG	Baseline; yearly	• History: fatigue, dizziness, syncope, palpitations • ECG • Holter	May need to discontinue drug Permanent pacing
Thyroid	Thyroid function tests	Baseline; 6 monthly	• History: weight changes, changes in activity level, palpitations • TFTs	Hypo: Thyroxine Hyper: Propylthiouracil Methimazole
Pulmonary	Chest radiograph Lung function tests	Baseline; yearly Baseline; depending on clinical suspicion and radiograph abnormalities	• History: new cough, dyspnea • Chest radiograph • Lung function tests	Discontinue drug Corticosteroids in severe cases
Opthalmologic	Opthalmic examination	Baseline if visual impairment	• Opthalmic examination to look for corneal deposits • Optic neuropathy	Discontinue/decrease drug Consult ophthalmology
Skin	As clinically indicated	Clinical visits	• Blue discoloration • Photosensitivity	Reassurance, avoidance of prolonged exposure Decrease dose
Gastrointestinal	Liver function tests	Baseline; 6 monthly	• History: nausea, vomiting, constipation • Liver enzymes >2 times normal	Discontinue drugs Exclude other causes
Neurologic	As clinically indicated	Clinical visits	• History: parasthesias, muscle pain, gait disturbances	Dose adjustment

TABLE 32-2 Drug Interactions with Amiodarone

Drug	Interaction	Intervention
Warfarin	Increased levels and vice versa	Decrease dose of both drugs.
Digoxin	Increases levels and effect	Decrease dose of both drugs.
Quinidine procainamide, disopyramide, propafenone	Increases level and both prolong QTc, precipitate torsades de pointes	Decrease/discontinue drug.
Other QT prolonging drugs	Prolong QTc	Monitor QT, avoid concomitant use with other drugs that prolong QT.
Calcium channel blockers and β-blockers	Severe depression of sinus and AV node function	Monitor, may need to decrease dose of either drug.
Flecainide, phenytoin, dofetilide, theophylline	Increases levels	Decrease dose.
Rifampin	Decreases levels	Increase dose.
Statins	Worsening liver function abnormalities, myalgias	Decrease statin dose.
Potassium losing diuretics	QT prolongation and precipitation of torsades de pointes	Monitoring electrolytes and potassium supplementation.

low propensity for proarrhythmia and can be initiated as an outpatient drug and safely used in most patients with structural heart disease. Due to its potential to cause serious end-organ toxicity, amiodarone should be reserved to treat patients who have not been successfully treated with other antiarrhythmic agents. Close monitoring is essential as side effects can manifest at any time during the course of therapy.

REFERENCES

1. Deltour G, Binon F, Tondeur R, et al. Studies in the benzofuran series. VI. Coronary-dilating activity of alkylated and aminoalkylated derivatives of 3-benzoylbenzofuran. *Arch Int Pharmacodyn Ther.* 1962;139:247-254.

2. Rosenbaum MB, Chiale PA, Halpern MS, et al. Clinical efficacy of amiodarone as an antiarrhythmic agent. *Am J Cardiol.* 1976;38(7):934-944.

3. Mason JW. Drug therapy: amiodarone. *N Engl J Med.* 1987;316(8):455-466..

4. Singh BN, Vaughan Williams EM. The effect of amiodarone, a new anti-anginal drug, on cardiac muscle. *Br J Pharmacol.* 1970;39(4):657-667.

5. Kodama I, Kamiya K, Toyama J. Cellular electropharmacology of amiodarone. *Cardiovasc Res.* 1997;35(1):13-29.

6. Mason JW, Hondeghem LM, Katzung B. Amiodarone blocks inactivated cardiac sodium channels. *Pflugers Arch.* 1983;396(1):79-81.

7. Honjo H, Kodama I, Kamiya K, Toyama J. Block of cardiac sodium channels by amiodarone studied by using Vmax of action potential in single ventricular myocytes. *Br J Pharmacol.* 1991;102(3):651-656.

8. Nishimura M, Follmer CH, Singer DH. Amiodarone blocks calcium current in single guinea pig ventricular myocytes. *J Pharmacol Exp Ther.* 1989;251(2):650-659.

9. Disatnik MH, Shainberg A. Regulation of beta-adrenoceptors by thyroid hormone and amiodarone in rat myocardial cells in culture. *Biochem Pharmacol.* 1991;41(6-7):1039-1044.

10. Chatelain P, Meysmans L, Mattéazzi JR, Beaufort P, Clinet M. Interaction of the antiarrhythmic agents SR 33589 and amiodarone with the beta-adrenoceptor and adenylatecyclase in rat heart. *Br J Pharmacol.* 1995;116(3):1949-1956.

11. Kamiya K, Nishiyama A, Yasui K, et al. Short- and long-term effects of amiodarone on the two components of cardiac delayed rectifier K+ current. *Circulation.* 2001;103(9):1317-1324.

12. Zipes DP. Class III antiarrhythmic drugs: amiodarone, ibutilide, and sotalol. In: Zipes DP, ed. *Cardiac Electrophysiology: From Cell to Bedside: Expert Consult*, 4th ed. Philadelphia, PA: Saunders Elsevier; c2004:932-937.

13. Finerman WB Jr, Hamer A, Peter T, Weiss D, Mandel WJ. Electrophysiologic effects of chronic amiodarone therapy in patients with ventricular arrhythmias. *Am Heart J.* 1982;104(5 Pt 1):987-996.

14. Nademanee K, Singh BN, Hendrickson J, et al. Amiodarone in refractory life-threatening ventricular arrhythmias. *Ann Intern Med.* 1983;98(5 Pt 1):577-584.

15. Hamer AWF, Mandel WJ, Zaher CA, Karagueuzini HS, Peter T. The electrophysiologic basis for the use of amiodarone for treatment of cardiac arrhythmias. *Pacing Clin Electrophysiol.* 1983;6(4):784-794.

16. Singh BN, Venkatesh N, Nademanee K, Josephson MA, Kannan R. The historical development, cellular electrophysiology and pharmacology of amiodarone. *Prog Cardiovasc Dis.* 1989;31(4):249-280.

17. Singh BN, Sarma JSM, Zhanag ZH, Takanaka C. Controlling cardiac arrhythmias by lengthening repolarization: rationale from experimental findings and clinical considerations. *Ann NY Acad Sci.* 1992;644:187-209.

18. Harjai KJ, Licata AA. Effects of amiodarone on thyroid function. *Ann Intern Med.* 1997;126(1):68-73.

19. Guo W, Kamiya K, Toyama J. Evidences of antagonism between amiodarone and triiodothyronine on the K+ channel activities of cultured rat cardiomyocytes. *J Mol Cell Cardiol.* 1997;29(2):617-627.

20. Gillis AM, Kates RE. Clinical pharmacokinetics of the newer antiarrhythmic agents. *Clin Pharmacokinet.* 1984;9(5):375-403.

21. Singh BN. Antiarrhythmic actions of amiodarone: a profile of a paradoxical agent. *Am J Cardiol.* 1997;78(4A):41-53.

22. Ohyama K, Nakajima M, Suzuki M, Shimada N, Yamazaki H, Yokoi T. Inhibitory effects of amiodarone and its N-deethylated metabolite on human cytochrome P450 activities: prediction of in vivo drug interactions. *Br J Clin Pharmacol.* 2000;49(3):244-253.

23. Vorperian VR, Havighurst TC, Miller S, January CT. Adverse effects of low dose amiodarone: a meta-analysis. *J Am Coll Cardiol.* 1997;30(3):791-798.

24. Amiodarone Trials Meta-Analysis Investigators. Effect of prophylactic amiodarone on mortality after acute myocardial infarction and in congestive heart failure: meta-analysis of individual data from 6500 patients in randomised trials. *Lancet.* 1997;350(9089):1417-1424.

25. Goldschlager N, Epstein AE, Naccarelli GV, et al. Practice Guidelines Sub-committee, North American Society of Pacing and Electrophysiology (HRS). A practical guide for clinicians who treat patients with amiodarone: 2007. *Heart Rhythm.* 2007;4(9):1250-1259.

26. Heger JJ, Prystowsky EN, Jackman WM, et al. Amiodarone: clinical efficacy and electrophysiology during long-term therapy for recurrent ventricular tachycardia. *N Engl J Med.* 1981;305(10):539-545.

27. The CASCADE Investigators. Randomized antiarrhythmic drug therapy in survivors of cardiac arrest (the CASCADE study). *Am J Cardiol.* 1993;72(3):280-287.

28. Sim I, McDonald KM, Lavori PW, Norbutas CM, Hlatky MA. Quantitative overview of randomized trials of amiodarone to prevent sudden cardiac death. *Circulation.* 1997;96(9):2823-2829.

29. Bardy GH, Lee KL, Mark DB, et al. Sudden Cardiac Death in Heart Failure Trial (SCD-HeFT) Investigators. Amiodarone or an implantable-cardioverter-defibrillator for congestive heart failure. *N Engl J Med.* 2005;352(3):225-237.

30. Kowey PR, Levine JH, Herre JM, et al. Randomized, double-blind comparison of intravenous amiodarone and bretylium

in the treatment of patients with recurrent, hemodynamically destabilizing ventricular tachycardia or fibrillation. The Intravenous Amiodarone Multicenter Investigators Group. *Circulation*. 1995;92(11):3255-3263.

31. Scheinman MM, Levin JH, Cannom DS, et al. Dose-ranging study of intravenous amiodarone in patients with life-threatening ventricular tachyarrhythmias. The Intravenous Amiodarone Multicenter Investigators Group. *Circulation*. 1995;92(11):3264-3272.

32. Roy D, Talajic M, Dorian P, et al. Canadian Trial of Atrial Fibrillation Investigators. Amiodarone to prevent recurrence of atrial fibrillation. *N Engl J Med*. 2000;342(13):913-920.

33. Fuster V, Ryden LE, Cannom DC, et al. ACC/AHA/ESC guidelines for the management of patients with atrial fibrillation: a report of the American College of Cardiology/American Heart Association Task Force on Practice Guidelines and the European Society of Cardiology Committee for Practice Guidelines. *J Am Coll Cardiol*. 2006;48(4):854-906.

34. Trappe HJ, Brandis B, Weismueller P. Arrhythmias in the intensive care patient. *Curr Opin Crit Care*. 2003;9(5):345-355.

35. Clemo HF, Wood MA, Gilligan DM, Ellenbogen KA. Intravenous amiodarone for acute heart rate control in the critically ill patient with atrial tachyarrhythmias. *Am J Cardiol*. 1998;81(5):594-598.

36. Mahmarian JJ, Smart FW, Moyé LE, et al. Exploring the minimal dose of amiodarone with antiarrhythmic and hemodynamic activity. *Am J Cardiol*. 1994;74(7):681-686.

37. Rankin AC, Pringle SD, Cobbe SM, et al. Amiodarone and torsades de pointes. *Am Heart J*. 1990;120(6 Pt 1):1482.

38. Rankin AC, Pringle SD, Cobbe SM. Acute treatment of torsades de pointes with amiodarone proarrhythmic and antiarrhythmic association of QT prolongation. *Am Heart J*. 1990;119(1):185-186.

39. Harjai KJ, Licata AA. Effects of amiodarone on thyroid function. *Ann Intern Med*. 1997;126 (1):63-73.

40. Martino E, Bartalena L, Bogazzi F, Braverman LE. The effects of amiodarone on the thyroid. *Endocr Rev*. 2001;22(2):240-254.

41. Morady F, Sauve MJ, Malone P, et al. Long-term efficacy and toxicity of high-dose amiodarone therapy for ventricular tachycardia or ventricular fibrillation. *Am J Cardiol*. 1983;52(8):975-979.

42. Singh SN, Fisher SG, Deedwania PC, Rohatgi P, Singh BN, Fletcher RD: for the Congestive Heart Failure-Survival Trial of Antiarrhythmic Therapy (CHFSTAT) Investigators. Pulmonary effect of amiodarone in patients with heart failure. *J Am Coll Cardiol*. 1997;30(2):514-517.

43. Van Mieghem W, Coolen L, Malysse I, Lacquet LM, Deneffe GJ, Demedis MG. Amiodarone and the development of ARDS after lung surgery: *Chest*. 1994;105(6):1642-1645.

44. Kennedy JI, Myers JL, Plumb VJ, Fulder JD. Amiodarone pulmonary toxicity. Clinical, radiologic, and pathologic correlations. *Arch Intern Med*. 1987;147(1):50-55.

45. Kharabsheh S, Abendroth CS, Kozak M. Fatal pulmonary toxicity occurring within two weeks of initiation of amiodarone. *Am J Cardiol*. 2002;89(7):896-898.

46. High WA, Weiss SD. Pigmentation related to amiodarone. *N Engl Med*. 2001;354(20):1464.

47. Herre JM, Sauve MJ, Malone P, et al. Long-term results of amiodarone therapy in patients with recurrent sustained ventricular tachycardia or ventricular fibrillation. *J Am Coll Cardiol*. 1989;13(2):442-9.

48. Almog S, Shafran N, Halkin H, et al. Mechanism of warfarin potentiation by amiodarone: dose and concentration dependent inhibition of warfarin elimination. *Eur J Clin Pharmacol*. 1985;28(3):257-261.

49. Page RL: Treatment of arrhythmias during pregnancy. *Am Heart J*. 1995;130(4):871-876.

50. Widerhorn J, Bhandari AK, Bughi S, Rahimtoola SH, Elkayam U. Fetal and neonatal adverse effects profile of amiodarone treatment during pregnancy. *Am Heart J*. 1991;122(4 Pt 1):1162-1166.

33 LONG-TERM MONITORING OF ANTIARRHYTHMIC DRUG THERAPY

Melissa J., Snider PharmD, BCPS, CLS

CASE PRESENTATION

The patient is a 66-year-old woman with a history of paroxysmal atrial fibrillation and hypertension who presents to clinic for routine antiarrhythmic medication monitoring due to being on long-term therapy with dronedarone. She feels well and is adherent to her medications which include dronedarone, metoprolol, hydrochlorothiazide, and warfarin. Last echocardiogram 4 months ago confirmed ejection fraction of 55% to 60%. A 12-lead ECG is performed and reveals atrial fibrillation, duration unknown. Lab work history confirms therapeutic INRs over the past 4 weeks and normal electrolytes and renal function. The recommendation is made for this patient to undergo direct current cardioversion today. Procedure is successful, and the patient is back in normal sinus rhythm. She is to continue on current medications and continue to be closely monitored.

CASE EXPLANATION

Long-term use of any antiarrhythmic medication warrants outpatient monitoring to some degree. The structure and content of this monitoring can vary, but having a protocol or checklist in place is crucial. In the case of BB, it was especially important in this asymptomatic patient who is on dronedarone to be monitored. This is due to this drug's black box warning regarding the risk of morbidity and mortality in patients with decompensated heart failure or persistent atrial fibrillation, and specific recommendations to cardiovert or discontinue drug if the arrhythmia (atrial fibrillation) recurs. This is one example of many critical interventions that occur through routine monitoring of chronic antiarrhythmic medication therapy.

EPIDEMIOLOGY/ETIOLOGY

- Chronic antiarrhythmic medication for rhythm control is used in nearly one-third of patients with atrial fibrillation in the United States.[1]

- Rhythm control strategy is more likely to be utilized in younger patients with fewer medical comorbidities, and is also more common in patients having undergone cardioversion or electrophysiology intervention.[2]

- Risks or toxicities of antiarrhythmic medications need to be weighed against benefits.
  - Risk may include torsades de pointes, development of heart failure, unwanted effects on heart rate, and organ damage or dysfunction.
  - Benefits may include the potential for improved quality of life and improved long-term outcomes.

PATHOPHYSIOLOGY

With use of chronic antiarrhythmic medications, consider the following:

- Unique patient characteristics (presence of myocardial ischemia, heart failure, LVH, congenital long QT, etc).

- Drug interactions, known or theoretical.

- Electrolytes, specifically potassium and magnesium.

- Renal function.

- Adverse reactions including toxicities or intolerances.

- Risk of proarrhythmias (prolonged QT, TdP, bradycardia, heart block, wide complex tachycardia, etc).

MANAGEMENT/FOLLOW-UP AND LONG-TERM COMPLICATIONS

Clinical Considerations for Management

- Each class of drugs should be monitored according to the prescribing information.

- Patient encounter for monitoring should always include:
  - Patient report of arrhythmia symptoms
  - Medication adherence screening
  - Drug interaction assessment and education
  - Adverse drug reaction screening
  - Completion of objective testing
  - Consideration of strategy for rate control and stroke prophylaxis as indicated
  - Verbal and written patient education

- Defining protocols to guide monitoring allows for improved compliance with adhering to requirements.
  - Example protocols attached (Tables 33-1 and 33-2).
  - Availability of objective testing on site is ideal as it offers comprehensive monitoring and increases patient adherence (eg, ECG, device clinic, monitor placement, laboratory services).

- Flowsheet documentation of results is beneficial for detecting trends in monitoring, including labs, pulmonary function tests, ECG parameters, etc.

- QT prolongation
  - Antiarrhythmic medications, especially class III, carry some risk of QT prolongation at varying degrees.
  - Consider all factors that can increase the QT interval (Table 33-3).
  - QTdrugs.org is an excellent reference for QT-prolonging medications.[7]

Operational Considerations for Management

- Consider the design and structure of how antiarrhythmic medication monitoring will be done.

- Pharmacist monitoring of outpatient antiarrhythmic medication therapy has been shown to improve patient adherence to recommended testing protocols and to help identify adverse events and clinically significant drug interactions.[8]

- Pharmacist monitoring of antiarrhythmic drug therapy in an outpatient clinic provided cost benefits to the patients, cost savings to the institution, and efficiency for the electrophysiology program.[8]
  - Allows electrophysiologists more time in other activities.

LONG TERM MONITORING OF ANTIARRHYTHMIC
DRUG THERAPY

SECTION V
ANTIARRHYTHMIC MEDICAL THERAPY
FOR ATRIAL FIBRILLATION

221

TABLE 33-1 Example Clinical Protocols for Monitoring Long-Term Antiarrhythmic Therapy[3,4,5]

Drug	Monitoring Parameter	Frequency	Management
Amiodarone			
	12-lead ECG	Every 6 mo	Consider dose decrease or discontinuation for second-degree or higher AV block or QT/QTc >600 ms.
	CXR and PFT (specifically DLCO)	Baseline, then every 12 mo as needed, if symptoms develop	If pulmonary fibrosis seen, discontinue amiodarone. If DLCO% reduced by >10%, consider referral to pulmonary.
	TSH and fT4	Baseline, then every 6 mo	If hypothyroid, consider thyroid hormone supplementation. If hyperthyroid, consider amiodarone discontinuation or consideration of antithyroid drug.
	ALT, AST, alkaline phosphatase	Baseline, then every 6 mo	If elevation seen in hepatic transaminases >3xULN, consider amiodarone discontinuation or dose reduction.
	Interview or physical examination	Baseline, then every 6 mo	For neurologic adverse effects (ataxia, tremors, peripheral neuropathy) or for GI adverse effects (nausea or vomiting), consider dose reduction or discontinuation if severe. If photosensitivity or skin discoloration (blue/purple/grey) is occurring, educate patient to prevent with UVa/UVb sunscreen or protective clothing while in sunlight.
	Ophthalmologic examination	Baseline, then every 6 mo	If optic neuritis seen, discontinue amiodarone immediately (corneal deposits do not require intervention).
	Drug interaction screening	Every visit	Common clinical interactions: statins (Simvastatin contraindicated for >20 mg/d dose), digoxin, warfarin. Many other interactions with: CYP450 3A4 inhibitors (ie, protease inhibitors), CYP450 3A4 inducers (ie, rifampin), CYP450 3A4 substrates.
	Heart rate	Every visit	Consider intervention or closer monitoring at heart rate <45 bpm.
	Black box warning		Intended for use only in patients with the indicated life-threatening arrhythmias because its use is accompanied by substantial toxicity.
Dronedarone			
	12-lead ECG	Every 3 mo	Consider dose decrease or discontinuation for second-degree or higher AV block, QT/QTc >500 ms, or PR >280 ms. If atrial fibrillation or atrial flutter is seen, cardioversion should be performed, or dronedarone should be discontinued.
	CXR and PFTs (specifically DLCO)	Baseline, then every 12 mo as needed, if symptoms develop	If pulmonary fibrosis seen, discontinue dronedarone. If DLCO% reduced by >10%, consider referral to pulmonary.
	TSH and fT4	Baseline, then every 6 mo	If hypothyroid seen, consider thyroid hormone supplementation. If hyperthyroid seen, consider dronedarone discontinuation or consideration of antithyroid drug.

TABLE 33-1 Example Clinical Protocols for Monitoring Long-Term Antiarrhythmic Therapy[3,4,5]

Drug	Monitoring Parameter	Frequency	Management
	ALT, AST, alkaline phosphatase	Baseline, then at months 1, 2, 3, 4, 5, 6, 9, and 12, then every 6 mo	If elevation seen in hepatic transaminases >3xULN, consider dronedarone discontinuation or dose reduction.
	Interview or physical examination	Baseline, then every 3 mo	For s/s heart failure consider discontinuation and evaluation. For GI adverse effects (nausea or diarrhea), consider dose reduction or discontinuation if severe.
	Drug interaction screening	Every visit	Statins (avoid simvastatin >10 mg/d), digoxin, grapefruit juice, P-gp inhibitors (ie, dabigatran), β-blockers, calcium channel blockers, CYP450 3A4 inducers, warfarin.
	Heart rate	Every visit	Consider intervention or closer monitoring at heart rate <45 bpm.
	Renal function	Baseline, at 1 mo, then every 6 mo	For SCr >25% increase from baseline and consider discontinuation or referral to nephrology.
	Echocardiogram	At physician discretion	Screening for new onset heart failure.
	Black box warning		Increased risk of death, stroke, and heart failure in patients with decompensated heart failure or permanent atrial fibrillation.
Sotalol			
	12-lead ECG	Every 6 mo	Consider dose decrease or discontinuation for QT/QTc >500 ms.
	Renal function	Every 6 mo	Dose adjust for CrCl per prescribing information (dosing differs for atrial and ventricular arrhythmias).
	Electrolytes	Baseline, then every 6 mo	Consider potassium supplementation for potassium level <4.0 mmol/L. Consider magnesium supplementation for magnesium level <2.0 mg/dL and potassium level <4.0 mmol/L. Consider magnesium supplementation if level <1.5 mg/dL regardless of potassium level.
	Heart rate	Every visit	Consider intervention or closer monitoring at heart rate <50 bpm.
	Interview or physical examination	Baseline, then every 6 mo	For signs or symptoms of heart failure consider discontinuation. For bronchospasm or fatigue, consider dose reduction or discontinuation.
	Drug interaction screening	Every visit	QTc-prolonging drugs, diltiazem, verapamil, β-blockers, citalopram.
	Black box warning		To minimize the risk of induced arrhythmia, patients initiated or reinitiated on sotalol should be placed for a minimum of three days (on their maintenance dose) in a facility that can provide cardiac resuscitation and continuous electrocardiographic monitoring. CrCl should be calculated prior to dosing.
Dofetilide			
	12-lead ECG	Every 3 mo	Consider dose decrease or discontinuation for QT/QTc >500 ms.
	Renal function	Every 3 mo	Dose adjust according to CrCl and QTc per prescribing information.

LONG TERM MONITORING OF ANTIARRHYTHMIC
DRUG THERAPY

SECTION V
ANTIARRHYTHMIC MEDICAL THERAPY
FOR ATRIAL FIBRILLATION

223

TABLE 33-1 Example Clinical Protocols for Monitoring Long-Term Antiarrhythmic Therapy[3,4,5] (*Continued*)

Drug	Monitoring Parameter	Frequency	Management
	Electrolytes	Baseline, then every 3 mo	Consider potassium supplementation for potassium level <4.0 mmol/L. Consider magnesium supplementation for magnesium level <2.0 mg/dL and potassium level <4.0 mmol/L. Consider magnesium supplementation if level <1.5 mg/dL regardless of potassium level.
	Heart rate	Every visit	Consider intervention or closer monitoring at heart rate <50 bpm.
	Drug interaction screening	Every visit	QTc-prolonging drugs, cimetidine, verapamil, ketoconazole, trimethoprim, itraconazole, ketoconazole, prochlorperazine, megestrol, HCTZ, triamterene, metformin, amiloride, citalopram.
	Black box warning		TIKOSYN is available only to hospitals and prescribers who have received appropriate TIKOSYN dosing and treatment initiation education. To minimize the risk of induced arrhythmia, patients initiated or reinitiated on dofetilide should be placed for a minimum of three days in a facility that can provide cardiac resuscitation and continuous electrocardiographic monitoring.
Propafenone			
	12-lead ECG	Baseline, then every 6 mo	Consider dose decrease or discontinuation for second-degree or higher AV block or QRS >20% longer than baseline.
	Liver function tests	Baseline, then every 6 mo	If elevation seen in hepatic transaminases >3xULN, consider discontinuation or dose reduction.
	Electrolytes	Baseline, then every 6 mo	Consider potassium supplementation for potassium level <4.0 mmol/L. Consider magnesium supplementation for magnesium level <2.0 mg/dL and potassium level <4.0 mmol/L. Consider magnesium supplementation if level <1.5 mg/dL regardless of potassium level.
	CBC	Baseline, then every 6 mo	Consider dose decrease or discontinuation for agranulocytosis.
	Heart rate	Every visit	Consider intervention or closer monitoring at heart rate <50 bpm or >100 (risk of VT).
	Drug interaction screening	Every visit	Ritonavir, phenobarbital, rifampin, rifabutin, phenytoin.
	Interview or physical examination	Baseline, then every 6 mo	For rash, arthralgia, consider drawing antinuclear antibody. For severe taste disturbance or bronchospasm, consider dose reduction or discontinuation.
	Structural heart disease evaluation	Baseline, then at physician discretion	If myocardial ischemia seen, consider discontinuation.

TABLE 33-1 Example Clinical Protocols for Monitoring Long-Term Antiarrhythmic Therapy[3,4,5]

Drug	Monitoring Parameter	Frequency	Management
	Black box warning		An increased rate of death was seen in patients treated with encainide or flecainide compared with that seen in patients assigned to placebo; therefore, it is prudent to consider any IC antiarrhythmic to have a significant risk of provoking proarrhythmic events in patients with structural heart disease.
			Given the lack of any evidence that these drugs improve survival, antiarrhythmic agents should generally be avoided in patients with non–life-threatening ventricular arrhythmias, even if the patients are experiencing unpleasant, but not life-threatening, symptoms or signs.
Flecainide			
	12-lead ECG	Baseline, then every 6 mo	Consider dose decrease or discontinuation for second-degree or higher AV block or QRS >20% longer than baseline.
	Liver function tests	Baseline, then every 6 mo	If elevation seen in hepatic transaminases >3xULN, consider drawing flecainide trough.
	Renal function tests	Baseline, then every 6 mo	For renal impairment, consider dose reduction or monitoring flecainide trough.
	Electrolytes	Baseline, then every 6 mo	Consider potassium supplementation for potassium level <4.0 mmol/L.
			Consider magnesium supplementation for magnesium level <2.0 mg/dL and potassium level <4.0 mmol/L.
			Consider magnesium supplementation if level <1.5 mg/dL regardless of potassium level.
	Heart rate	Every visit	Consider intervention or closer monitoring at heart rate <50 or >100 bpm (risk of VT).
	Drug interaction screening	Every visit	Disopyramide, verapamil, amiodarone, urine alkalinizer, digoxin, cimetidine, phenytoin, carbamazepine, phenobarbital.
	Interview or physical examination	Baseline, then every 6 mo	If dizziness, nausea, blurred vision, photopsia, chest pain, or tremors occur, consider dose reduction or discontinuation.
	Structural heart disease evaluation	Baseline, then at physician discretion	If myocardial ischemia seen, consider discontinuation.
	Black box warning		An increased rate of death was seen in patients treated with encainide or flecainide compared with that seen in patients assigned to placebo, therefore it is prudent to consider any IC antiarrhythmic to have a significant risk of provoking proarrhythmic events in patients with structural heart disease.
			Given the lack of any evidence that these drugs improve survival, antiarrhythmic agents should generally be avoided in patients with non–life-threatening ventricular arrhythmias, even if the patients are experiencing unpleasant, but not life-threatening, symptoms or signs.

LONG TERM MONITORING OF ANTIARRHYTHMIC
DRUG THERAPY

SECTION V
ANTIARRHYTHMIC MEDICAL THERAPY
FOR ATRIAL FIBRILLATION

225

TABLE 33-1 Example Clinical Protocols for Monitoring Long-Term Antiarrhythmic Therapy[3,4,5] (*Continued*)

Drug	Monitoring Parameter	Frequency	Management
Mexiletine			
	12-lead ECG	Baseline, then every 6 mo	Consider dose decrease or discontinuation for second-degree or higher AV block, or QRS >20% longer than baseline.
	Liver function tests	Baseline, then every 6 mo	If elevation seen in hepatic transaminases >3xULN, consider discontinuation or dose reduction.
	CBC	Baseline, then every 6 mo	Consider dose decrease or discontinuation for agranulocytosis, leucopenia, or thrombocytopenia.
	Renal function test	Baseline, then every 6 mo	If severe impairment, consider dose reduction or discontinuation.
	Heart rate	Every visit	Consider intervention or closer monitoring at heart rate <50 bpm.
	Drug interaction screening	Every visit	CYP3A4 inducers, rasagiline, theophylline, tizanidine, fluvoxamine.
	Interview or physical examination	Baseline, then every 6 mo	For rash, arthralgia, consider drawing antinuclear antibody. For severe ataxia, dizziness, tremor, blurred vision, nausea, or taste disturbance, consider dose reduction or discontinuation.
	Black box warning		Considering the known proarrhythmic properties of MEXITIL (mexiletine hcl) and the lack of evidence of improved survival for any antiarrhythmic drug in patients without life-threatening arrhythmias, the use of MEXITIL (mexiletine hcl) as well as other antiarrhythmic agents should be reserved for patients with life-threatening ventricular arrhythmia.
Disopyramide			
	12-lead ECG	Baseline, then every 6 mo	Consider dose decrease or discontinuation for second-degree or higher AV block or QRS >20% longer than baseline, or QT/QTc >500 ms.
	Liver function tests	Baseline, then every 6 mo	If elevation seen in hepatic transaminases >3xULN, consider discontinuation or dose reduction.
	CBC	Baseline, then every 6 mo	Consider dose decrease or discontinuation for agranulocytosis.
	Renal function tests	Baseline, then every 6 mo	For renal impairment, adjust dose according to prescribing information.
	Heart rate	Every visit	Consider intervention or closer monitoring at heart rate <50 bpm.
	Drug interaction screening	Every visit	Many interactions present including QT prolonging drugs, sulfonylureas, lidocaine, phenytoin, ritonavir, propranolol, nivirapine, warfarin, atenolol, digoxin, rifampin, insulin, CYP3A4 inhibitors.
	Interview or physical examination	Baseline, then every 6 mo	For rash, arthralgia, consider drawing antinuclear antibody. For severe anticholinergic effects (urinary retention, glaucoma), consider dose reduction or discontinuation.
	Black box warning		Considering the known proarrhythmic properties of disopyramide phosphate and the lack of evidence of improved survival for any antiarrhythmic drug in patients without life-threatening arrhythmias, the use of disopyramide phosphate as well as other antiarrhythmic agents should be reserved for patients with life-threatening ventricular arrhythmias.

TABLE 33-1 Example Clinical Protocols for Monitoring Long-Term Antiarrhythmic Therapy[3,4,5]

Drug	Monitoring Parameter	Frequency	Management
Quinidine			
	12-lead ECG	Baseline, then every 6 mo	Consider dose decrease or discontinuation for second-degree or higher AV block or QRS >20% longer than baseline, or QT/QTc >500 ms.
	Liver function tests	Baseline, then every 6 mo	If elevation seen in hepatic transaminases >3xULN, consider discontinuation or dose reduction.
	Electrolytes	Baseline, then every 6 mo	Consider potassium supplementation for potassium level <4.0 mmol/L. Consider magnesium supplementation for magnesium level <2.0 mg/dL and potassium level <4.0 mmol/L. Consider magnesium supplementation if level <1.5 mg/dL regardless of potassium level.
	Renal function tests	Baseline, then every 6 mo	For renal impairment, consider adjustment due to variable renal elimination.
	CBC	Baseline, then every 6 mo	Consider dose decrease or discontinuation for blood dyscrasias.
	Heart rate	Every visit	Consider intervention or closer monitoring at heart rate <50 bpm.
	Drug interaction screening	Every visit	Great potential for interactions due to quinidine being a 3A4 substrate, strong 2D6 inhibitor, less strong 3A4 inhibitor, and Pgp inhibitor. Caution with azole antifungals, protease inhibitors, clarithromycin, diltiazem, verapamil, dabigatran, rivaroxaban, rifampin, anticonvulsants, digoxin, warfarin, and dronedarone.
	Interview or physical examination	Baseline, then every 6 mo	For severe anticholinergic effects, rash, or recurring sore throats, consider dose reduction or discontinuation.
	Black box warning		In the case of quinidine used to prevent or defer recurrence of atrial flutter/fibrillation, in a meta-analysis, the mortality associated with the use of quinidine was more than three times as great as the mortality associated with the use of placebo. Another meta-analysis showed that in patients with various non–life-threatening ventricular arrhythmias, the mortality associated with the use of quinidine was consistently greater than that associated with the use of any of a variety of alternative antiarrhythmics.

Abbreviations: ALT, alanine aminotransferase; AST, aspartate aminotransferase; AV, atrioventricular; BPM, beats per minute; CBC, complete blood count; CrCl, creatinine clearance rate; CXR, chest x-ray or chest radiograph; CYP, cytochrome P450; DLCO, diffusing capacity; ECG, electrocardiography; fT4, free thyroxine; GI, gastrointestinal; ms, milliseconds; PFT, pulmonary function tests; SCr, serum creatinine; TSH, thyroid stimulating hormone; ULN, upper limit of normal; UV, ultraviolet; VT, ventricular tachycardia.

LONG TERM MONITORING OF ANTIARRHYTHMIC
DRUG THERAPY

SECTION V
ANTIARRHYTHMIC MEDICAL THERAPY
FOR ATRIAL FIBRILLATION

227

TABLE 33-2 Example Alternate Structure of Clinical Protocols for Monitoring Long-Term Antiarrhythmic Therapy[3,4,5]

Drug	Adverse Drug Effects	Potential Drug Interactions	Monitoring Frequency for Antiarrhythmic Drug-Related Side Effects	Threshold For Considering Intervention
Amiodarone	Pulmonary fibrosis Hepatotoxicity Thyroid function abnormalities Optic neuritis Skin photosensitivity or discoloration	Simvastatin, lovastatin, digoxin, warfarin	ECG every 6 mo TFT every 6 mo LFT every 6 mo CXR and PFTs (diffusing capacity) every 12 mo, or for symptoms Ophthalmologic examination every 12 mo. Vitals every visit	QT or QTc >600 ms Abnormal TFT LFT >3xULN Findings indicative of pulmonary fibrosis Visual changes HR <45 bpm
Tikosyn	Torsades de pointes	QTc-prolonging drugs, cimetidine, verapamil, ketoconazole, trimethoprim, itraconazole, ketoconazole, prochlorperazine, megestrol, HCTZ, triamterene, metformin, amiloride, citalopram	ECG every 3 mo Renal function every 3 mo. Electrolytes every 3 mo Vitals every visit	QT or QTc >500 ms or HR <50 bpm Reduced CrCl Potassium <4.0 mmol/L or mg <2.0 mg/dL
Sotalol	Torsades de pointes bradycardia heart block fatigue dyspnea	QTc-prolonging drugs, diltiazem, verapamil, β-blockers, citalopram	ECG every 6 mo Renal function every 6 mo Electrolytes every 6 mo Vitals every visit	QT or QTc >500 ms or HR <50 bpm Reduced CrCl Potassium <4.0 mmol/L or mg <2.0 mg/dL

Abbreviations: BPM, beats per minute; CrCl, creatinine clearance rate; CXR, chest x-ray or chest radiograph; ECG, electrocardiography; LFT, liver function tests; ms, milliseconds; PFT, pulmonary function tests; TFT, thyroid function tests; ULN, upper limit of normal.

TABLE 33-3 Factors That Increase the QT or QT-U Interval[6]

- Bradycardia
- Hypokalemia
- Elderly
- Female
- Hypomagnesemia
- Hypocalcemia
- Use of drugs that block IKr potassium channels or prolong QT interval (class III or Ia antiarrhythmics, antibiotics, antidepressants, antiemetics, antihistamines, and antipsychotics are common classes containing QT prolonging medications)

- Therefore, consideration may be given to the development of a pharmacist-run, physician-supervised antiarrhythmic medications monitoring clinic.

- Development of such a service may involve:
  - Developing clinical protocols in conjunction with referring electrophysiologists.
  - Establishing thresholds for pharmacists to notify supervising or referring physician.
  - Reviewing clinical protocols regularly.
  - Forming scheduling templates, that is, 15 minutes for return, 30 minutes for new patients.
  - Designing billing structure, that is, incident-to, hospital facility fees, or fee-for-service.
  - Utilizing consult agreements, which in some states allow pharmacists to participate independently in direct patient care activities, that is, independently evaluating patients, performing medication reconciliation, interviewing patients, ordering testing per protocol, performing patient education, and communicating with physician at regular intervals.

CONCLUSION

- Risk versus benefit analysis should be considered for each unique patient case to truly individualize care.

- Operational considerations are essential for ensuring consistent and quality care at any institution prescribing antiarrhythmic medication monitoring.

REFERENCES

1. Steinberg BA, Holmes DN, Ezekowitz MD, et al. Rate versus rhythm control for management of atrial fibrillation in clinical practice: results from the Outcomes Registry for Better Informed Treatment of Atrial Fibrillation (ORBIT-AF) registry. *Am Heart J.* 2013;165(4):622-9.

2. Chinitz JS, Halperin JL, Reddy VY, et al. Rate or rhythm control for atrial fibrillation: update and controversies. *The American Journal of Medicine.* 2012;125(11):1049-1056.

3. Thomson Reuters Healthcare. Micromedex web site. http://www.micromedex.com. Accessed July 19, 2013.

4. Sanoski CA. Arrhythmia management: an evidence-based update. In Cheng JWM, Jaso T, Moser L, eds.: *Pharmacotherapy Self-Assessment Program,* 6th ed. Lenexa, KY: American College of Clinical Pharmacy; 2006:179-204.

5. Snider M, Kalbfleisch S, Carnes CA. Initial experience with antiarrhythmic medication monitoring by clinical pharmacists in an outpatient setting: a retrospective review. *Clin Ther.* 2009;31(6):1209-1218.

6. Ayad RF, Assar MD, Simpson L, et al. Causes and management of drug-induced long QT syndrome. *Proc (Bayl Univ Med Cent).* 2010;23(3):250-255.

7. Woosley RL. QT Drug Lists by Risk Groups. Tucson, AZ: Arizona Center for Research and Education on Therapeutics, 2009. Available at http://www.azcert.org/medical-pros/drug-lists/drug-lists.cfm. Accessed July 19, 2013.

8. Snider M, Carnes C, Grover J, et al. Cost-benefit and cost-savings analyses of antiarrhythmic medication monitoring. *Am J Health Syst Pharm.* 2012;69(18):1569-1573.

CATHETER ABLATION TECHNIQUES FOR MANAGING ATRIAL FIBRILLATION AND ATRIAL FLUTTER

34 PULMONARY VEIN INITIATION AND TACHYCARDIA

Han S. Lim, MBBS, PhD, Benjamin Berte, MD, Michel Haïssaguerre, MD, Pierre Jaïs, MD

INITIATION OF ATRIAL FIBRILLATION FROM THE PULMONARY VEINS

The seminal work of Haissaguerre and colleagues demonstrated spontaneous initiation of atrial fibrillation (AF) triggered by ectopic beats from the pulmonary veins (PVs).[1] Paroxysms of AF were induced by sudden bursts of local rapid depolarizations within the PVs. The arrhythmogenicity of PVs is contributed by complex fiber orientation within the myocardial sleeves at the LA-PV junction, with zones of activation delay correlating with abrupt changes in myofiber orientation, and distinctive electrophysiological properties in the PVs.[2-5] These foci were shown to respond to ablation,[1] and currently PV isolation remains the cornerstone of catheter ablation for AF.

P-WAVE MORPHOLOGY OF PULMONARY VEIN TACHYCARDIAS

The P-wave morphology of tachycardias arising from the PVs is associated with distinctive characteristics and can be used as a means to identify the source of a particular tachycardia. Furthermore, knowledge of the potential source of tachycardia aids in preprocedural planning of the ablation strategy.[6,7] Left-sided PV tachycardias typically give rise to a P wave that is broad and notched in lead II and V_1, and isoelectric in lead I.[6,8,9] Right-sided PV tachycardias produce a narrower P wave in accordance with its more septal origin. P waves tend to be positive in lead I and aVL, and have a shorter duration of positive phase in lead V_1.[6,8,9] Both superior PVs and inferior PVs typically produce a positive P wave in the inferior leads, although the P-wave amplitude in the inferior leads tends to be larger from the superior PVs ($\geq$100 μV in lead II).[6]

PULMONARY VEIN TACHYCARDIAS

The PVs play a dominant role in the initiation of AF and are also important sites of origins for tachycardias. Rapidly firing focal sources of activity have been identified originating from the PVs, resulting in an AF pattern or atrial tachycardia (AT) on surface ECG.[10] These discrete foci tend to originate from the ostia of the right and left PVs and respond to focal ablation.[10,11] Although patients with AF commonly have multiple PV foci and concurrent AT, for patients with sole AT originating from the PV successful focal ablation has been associated with good acute and long-term freedom from AT and AF.[10,11]

In patients with prior catheter ablation and PV isolation, the commonest form of recurrent AT is reconnection of the PV.[12,13] Delayed conduction between the LA and PV and specific conduction gaps in the prior PV isolation ablation line give rise to these tachycardias. These tachycardias could arise from a local gap in the prior ablation line, localized reentry or focal activity at the PV ostia, macroreentry around the entire PV orifice, or gap-to-gap reentry from multiple gaps in the prior line of isolation.[8,14,15] In patients with prior PV isolation and recurrent AT, the first diagnosis to rule out should be reconnection of the PVs as a cause of the AT. A systematic approach for mapping LA tachycardias following AF ablation can be undertaken by assessing for PV reconnection and mapping around the PV ostia, examining tachycardia cycle length regularity, excluding macroreentry by activation and entrainment mapping, and mapping of focal tachycardias.[16]

ISOLATION OF THE PULMONARY VEINS

Pulmonary vein isolation stands as the cornerstone of most AF ablation procedures with the goal of electrical isolation. The initial approach of segmental isolation of the PVs targeted specific earliest connections between the LA and PV at the PV ostia.[17] However, the recognition of PV stenosis as a complication when ablating distally within the PV has led to a shift in ablation strategy toward wider antral circumferential ablation, which is more commonly practiced nowadays. In a randomized study, a larger circumferential area of isolation targeting the atrial myocardium surrounding the PVs was shown to produce better outcomes than a smaller area of isolation.[18] The resumption of PV-LA conduction and the extent of atrial to PV conduction delay have been demonstrated to correlate directly with arrhythmia recurrence following ablation.[19]

PULMONARY VEIN INITIATION AND TACHYCARDIA

SECTION VI
CATHETER ABLATION TECHNIQUES
FOR MANAGING ATRIAL FIBRILLATION
AND ATRIAL FLUTTER

231

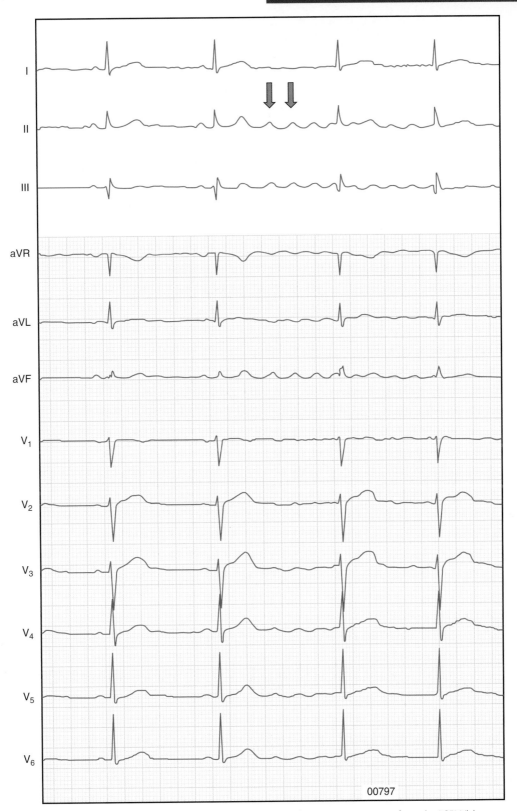

FIGURE 34-1 Pulmonary vein ectopic foci. Twelve-lead ECG of a patient in SR with intermittent ectopy from the LSPV (blue arrows).

232

SECTION VI
CATHETER ABLATION TECHNIQUES
FOR MANAGING ATRIAL FIBRILLATION
AND ATRIAL FLUTTER

CHAPTER 34

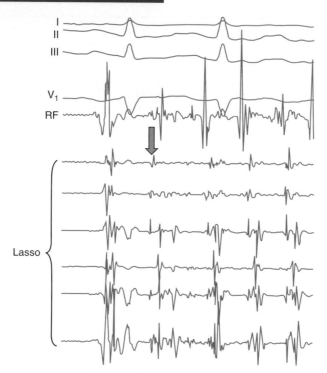

FIGURE 34-2 Pulmonary vein foci initiating AF. After the first beat of SR, a firing PV ectopic focus is observed in the Lasso catheter (blue arrow). This PV signal is early compared to the other intracardiac signals, and subsequently initiates AF. The PVs in patients with AF have distinctive electrophysiological properties such as short effective refractory periods, with decremental and slow conduction properties compared with the LA and patients without AF, which explain their arrhythmogenic role in AF.[2]

PULMONARY VEIN INITIATION AND TACHYCARDIA

SECTION VI
CATHETER ABLATION TECHNIQUES
FOR MANAGING ATRIAL FIBRILLATION
AND ATRIAL FLUTTER

233

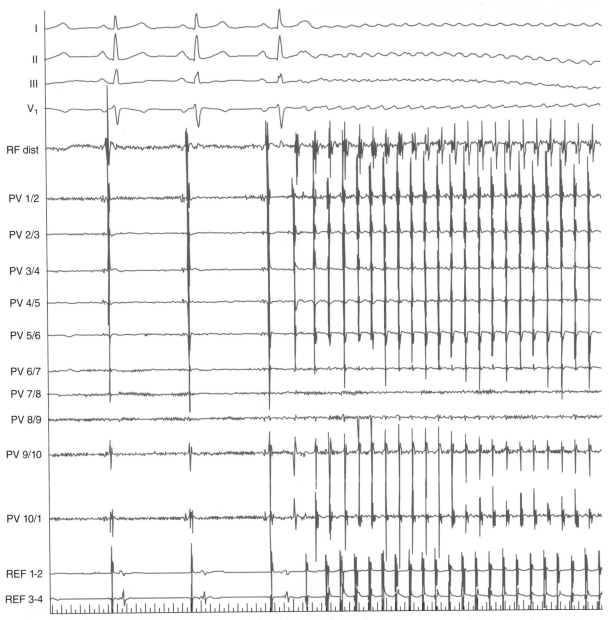

FIGURE 34-3 PV foci initiating AF in a patient with previous incomplete PV isolation. In the first three beats of SR, large and sharp PV potentials are seen following the smaller and blunt atrial signals in the PV catheter and P wave, indicative of persisting LA and PV connection. Immediately after the third sinus beat, a continuous burst of PV activity is observed, revealing it as the source of tachycardia and initiation of AF. The earliest signal during ectopic activity is seen in the PV catheter, followed by the RF distal electrode and coronary sinus catheter. Abbreviations: REF, reference (coronary sinus), speed 25 mm/s.

234

SECTION VI
CATHETER ABLATION TECHNIQUES
FOR MANAGING ATRIAL FIBRILLATION
AND ATRIAL FLUTTER

CHAPTER 34

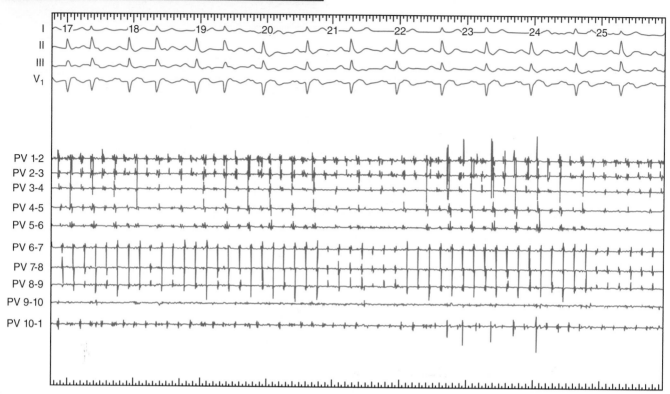

FIGURE 34-4 PV tachycardia from the LSPV. Note the broad and notched P-wave morphology in V₁.[6] The Lasso catheter positioned in the LSPV recorded PV ectopic activity at a much faster rate compared to the surface ECG. Ablation and isolation of the LSPV led to conversion of the tachycardia to SR (speed 25 mm/s).

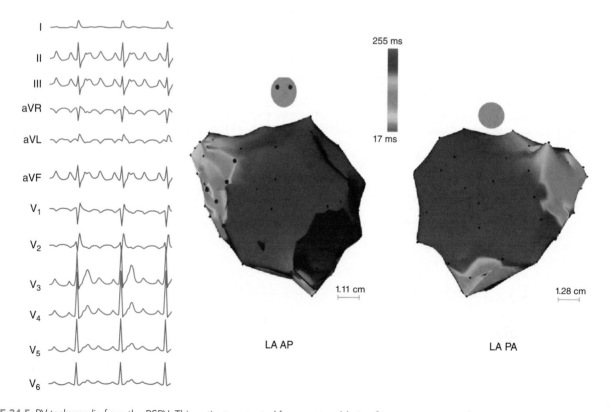

FIGURE 34-5 PV tachycardia from the RSPV. This patient presented for a repeat ablation for recurrent AT. (Left) Twelve-lead ECG of the tachycardia demonstrates tall and narrow P waves in leads II, III, and aVF without any notching in lead II, an amplitude ratio in lead III<II, and a short duration of positive phase in V₁, consistent with a tachycardia originating from the RSPV. (Right) A focal source with centrifugal activation was detected from CARTO 3-dimensional electroanatomical mapping (Biosense Webster, Diamond Bar, CA), emanating from the RSPV, which had reconnected despite previous isolation.

PULMONARY VEIN INITIATION AND TACHYCARDIA

SECTION VI
CATHETER ABLATION TECHNIQUES
FOR MANAGING ATRIAL FIBRILLATION
AND ATRIAL FLUTTER

235

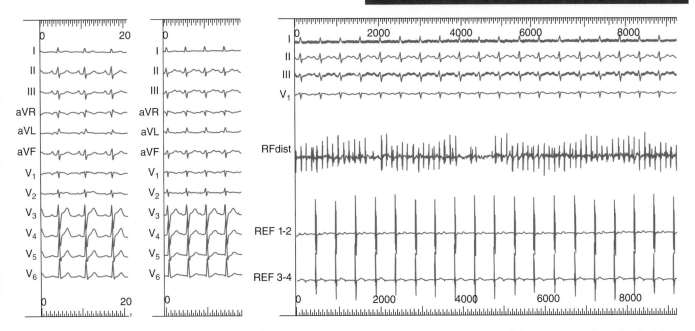

FIGURE 34-6 Pseudosinus rhythm. (Left) Twelve-lead ECG of the patient in SR. (Middle) Twelve-lead ECG of the patient in tachycardia. (Right) "Pseudosinus rhythm" on surface ECG due to underlying PV tachycardia originating from the RSPV. Rapid activity is observed in the RF distal electrode positioned in the RSPV, with delayed conduction to the LA (REF = reference, coronary sinus), giving the appearance of a regular rhythm. The P-wave morphology of tachycardias arising from the RSPV can be similar to that in SR or from the crista terminalis (however, most RSPV tachycardias change in configuration from a biphasic P wave in SR to positive in tachycardia);[9] hence these tachycardias could potentially masquerade as SR. Speed 25 mm/s for all figures.

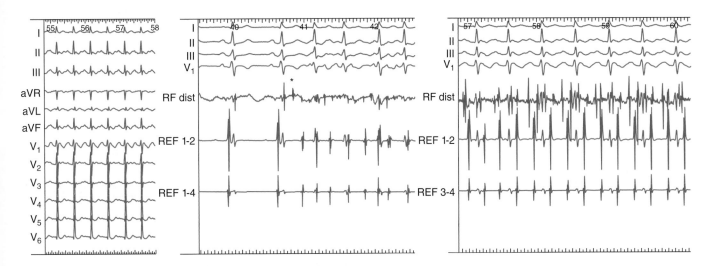

FIGURE 34-7 PV tachycardia from the LSPV. (Left) Twelve-lead ECG of the LSPV tachycardia. Note the P waves are upright in leads II, III, and aVF, negative in aVL, and are broad and notched in lead II, speed 25 mm/s. (Middle) Burst of rapid ectopic activity in the LSPV initiating tachyarrhythmia (black asterisk), speed 50 mm/s. (Right) Intracardiac recordings of the PV tachycardia with rapid activity seen in the distal RF catheter positioned in the LSPV. Delayed and regular activity is seen in the reference catheter (REF = reference, coronary sinus) and surface ECG recordings, speed 50 mm/s.

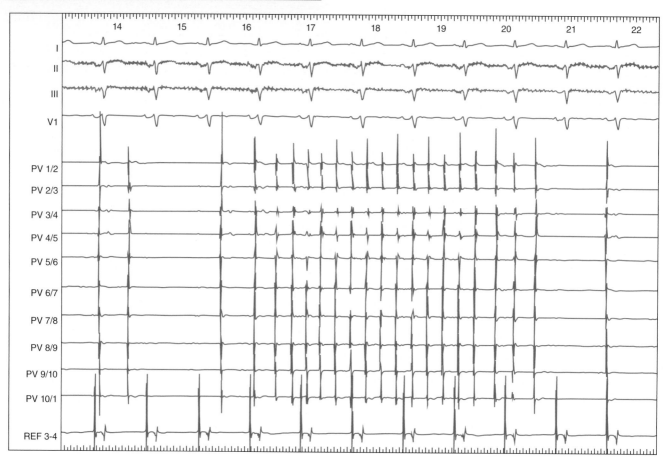

FIGURE 34-8 RIPV tachycardia. Following isolation of the RIPV in this patient with PV tachycardia, a burst of activity is seen within the RIPV, but does not conduct to the LA. Dissociated PV potentials are also observed, speed 25 mm/s.

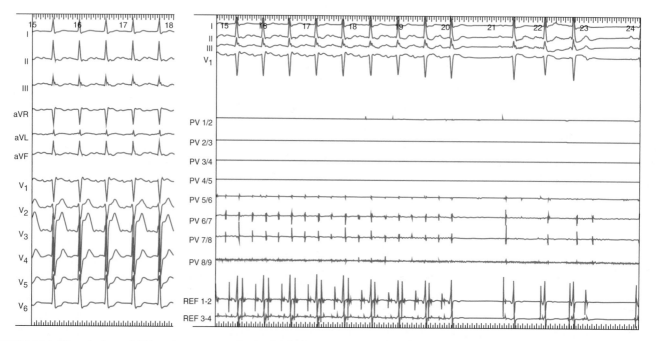

FIGURE 34-9 "Pseudo-flutter." This patient presented with AT following previous AF ablation with extensive defragmentation in both atria and linear ablation in the roof, mitral isthmus, and cavotricuspid isthmus. (Left) Twelve-lead ECG of the "pseudo-flutter." Upright P waves are seen inferiorly and are biphasic in V₁. (Right) A rapid signal is detected in electrodes PV 5-6. Ablation of the RSPV terminated the tachycardia, speed 25 mm/s. This case illustrates the importance of identifying and targeting the initiating foci and complete isolation of the PVs.

PULMONARY VEIN INITIATION AND TACHYCARDIA

SECTION VI
CATHETER ABLATION TECHNIQUES
FOR MANAGING ATRIAL FIBRILLATION
AND ATRIAL FLUTTER

237

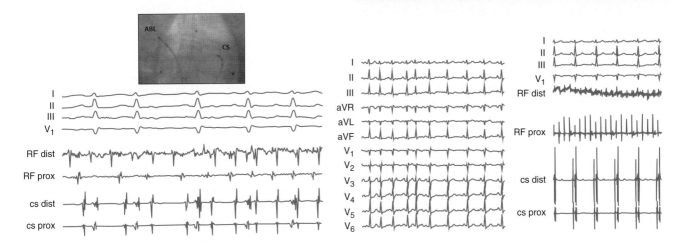

FIGURE 34-10 Focal source of AF. AF due to focal sources such as the PVs, right atrium and coronary sinus ostium have been described.[10] In this patient, the AF pattern on the surface ECG was due to focal activity from the RSPV. (Left) The distal electrode of the ablation (ABL) catheter placed in the RSPV demonstrates an early and rapid signal compared with the proximal electrode and the rest of the atrium (coronary sinus electrodes), speed 100 mm/s. The P-wave morphology is positive in the inferior leads, positive in lead I, and biphasic in V_1. (Middle) Ablation at this focal source restored SR (speed 25 mm/s). (Right) Following ablation the PV tachycardia continues within the isolated RSPV (RF distal and proximal electrodes), while the rest of the atrium remains in SR (coronary sinus electrodes and surface ECG), speed 25 mm/s. The fluoroscopy image is in the anteroposterior view.

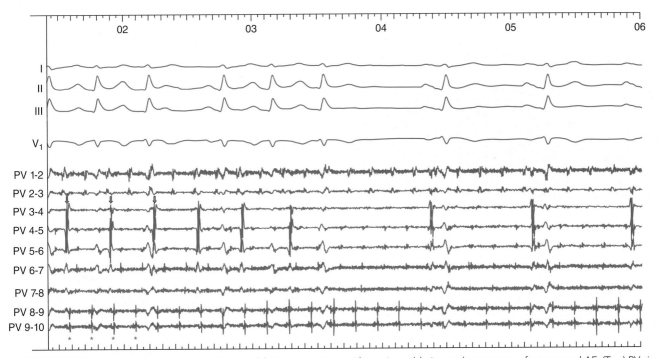

FIGURE 34-11 Pulmonary vein reconnection. Repeat ablation in a patient with previous ablation and recurrence of paroxysmal AF. (Top) PV signals within the LIPV (red asterisk) are seen at twice or three times the frequency compared with the far-field atrial signal (blue arrows). Note that the appearance of the PV potentials can be altered following prior to ablation. PV activity continues despite SR in the atria (Top right), and eventually terminates (Bottom, blue arrow), speed 50 mm/s.

238

SECTION VI
CATHETER ABLATION TECHNIQUES
FOR MANAGING ATRIAL FIBRILLATION
AND ATRIAL FLUTTER

CHAPTER 34

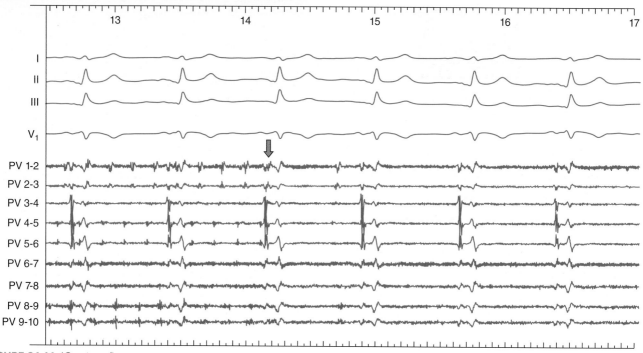

FIGURE 34-11 (*Continued*)

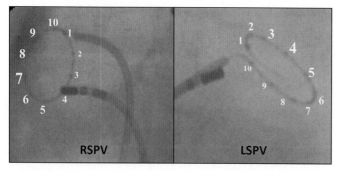

FIGURE 34-12 Orientation of the Lasso catheter electrodes. The electrodes in the Lasso catheter are arranged in the pattern of a clock face, such that when it is viewed end-on internally from the LA cavity towards the PV ostium, the electrodes are always displayed in a clockwise fashion from 1 to 10 around the perimeter of the PV ostium. Hence when the shaft of the catheter is positioned at the superior aspect of the PV, on the left-sided PVs, electrodes 1 to 5 would face anteriorly, and electrodes 6 to 10 would face posteriorly (Right, LSPV). Conversely, on the right-sided PVs with the shaft positioned at the roof of the PV, electrodes 1 to 5 would face posteriorly, and electrodes 6 to 10 would face anteriorly (Left, RSPV). Fluoroscopy images are provided in anteroposterior view.

PULMONARY VEIN INITIATION AND TACHYCARDIA

SECTION VI
CATHETER ABLATION TECHNIQUES
FOR MANAGING ATRIAL FIBRILLATION
AND ATRIAL FLUTTER

239

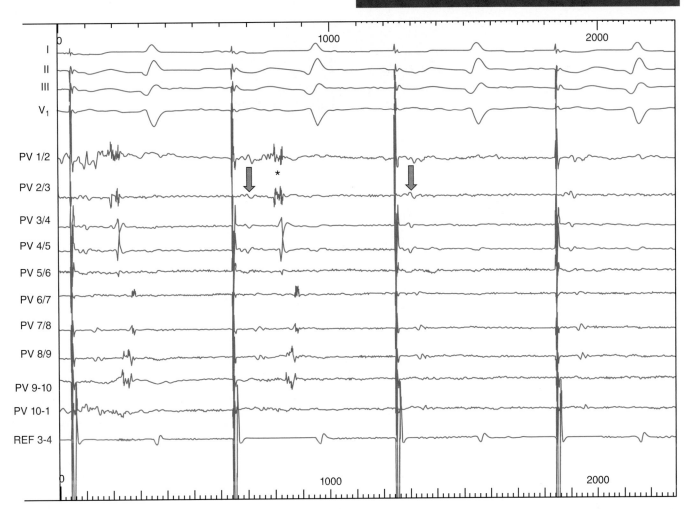

FIGURE 34-13 Isolation of the PV. Pacing from the coronary sinus (REF) is used to differentiate far-field atrial signals (arrow) from the PV potentials (second set of signals). A long LA to PV conduction time is observed from prior to ablation. The earliest activity is noted at PV electrodes 1 to 2 and 2 to 3 compared with the rest of the PV potentials. Furthermore, bipolar electrogram reversal of polarity is seen between PV 1 and 2 (predominantly positive deflection) and PV 2 and 3 (predominantly negative deflection), indicative of the earliest site of breakthrough and subsequent opposing excitation wavefronts.[20] Ablation at the site of earliest breakthrough (PV 1 to 2 and PV 2 to 3) (asterisk) results in complete isolation of the PV.

240

SECTION VI
CATHETER ABLATION TECHNIQUES
FOR MANAGING ATRIAL FIBRILLATION
AND ATRIAL FLUTTER

CHAPTER 34

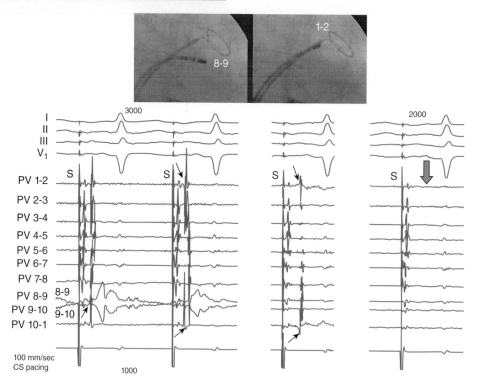

FIGURE 34-14 Segmental PV isolation. The first site of breakthrough is at the junction of the posterior LA wall and carina, nearest to electrodes PV 8- to 9 and PV 9 to 10 (black arrow, first beat). Ablation at this site (ablation artefact observed) delays the local signal, bringing about a change in the pattern of the PV potential on the Lasso catheter. The second earliest site of breakthrough is now at the superior section of the PV close to the roof, nearest to electrodes PV 1 to 2 and PV 10 to 1 (blue arrows, second beat). With ablation, progressive prolongation of LA to PV signals is seen between the second and third illustrated beats. Further ablation at the site of breakthrough (third illustrated beat) results in complete isolation of the LSPV (fourth illustrated beat and disappearance of PV potentials). S indicates stimulus pacing from the coronary sinus to separate the PV signals from far-field potentials.

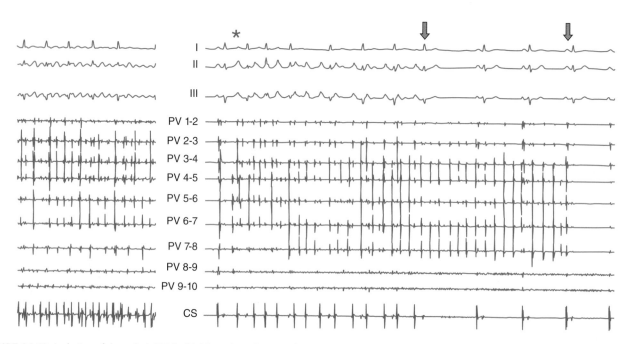

FIGURE 34-15 Isolation of the culprit PV. (Left) AF resulting from PV foci seen within the Lasso catheter (electrodes 1-10). (Right) Initiating bursts from the culprit PV is observed (red asterisk) in the Lasso PV catheter (labelled from electrodes 1-10), following the first sinus beat. Isolation of the PV with ablation leads to termination of the arrhythmia (first blue arrow). The PV ectopic activity continues briefly with no further conduction to the LA before disappearing (second blue arrow).

PULMONARY VEIN INITIATION AND TACHYCARDIA

SECTION VI
CATHETER ABLATION TECHNIQUES
FOR MANAGING ATRIAL FIBRILLATION
AND ATRIAL FLUTTER

241

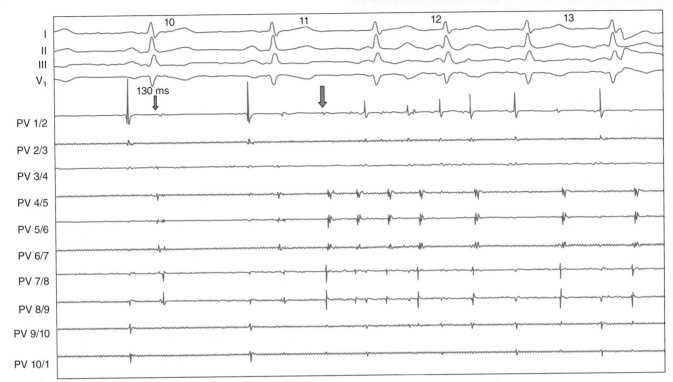

FIGURE 34-16 Delayed LA-PV conduction. LA-PV conduction delay is demonstrated in this patient during a repeat procedure (130 ms between the LA signals seen in the PV catheter and the PV potentials, indicated by the blue arrow). The resumption of LA-PV conduction and extent of LA-PV conduction delay has been shown to be directly related to AF recurrences following catheter ablation.[19] Despite the delay in LA-PV conduction in this patient, PV ectopy (red arrow) were still being conducted to the LA, resulting in AF.

242

SECTION VI
CATHETER ABLATION TECHNIQUES
FOR MANAGING ATRIAL FIBRILLATION
AND ATRIAL FLUTTER

CHAPTER 34

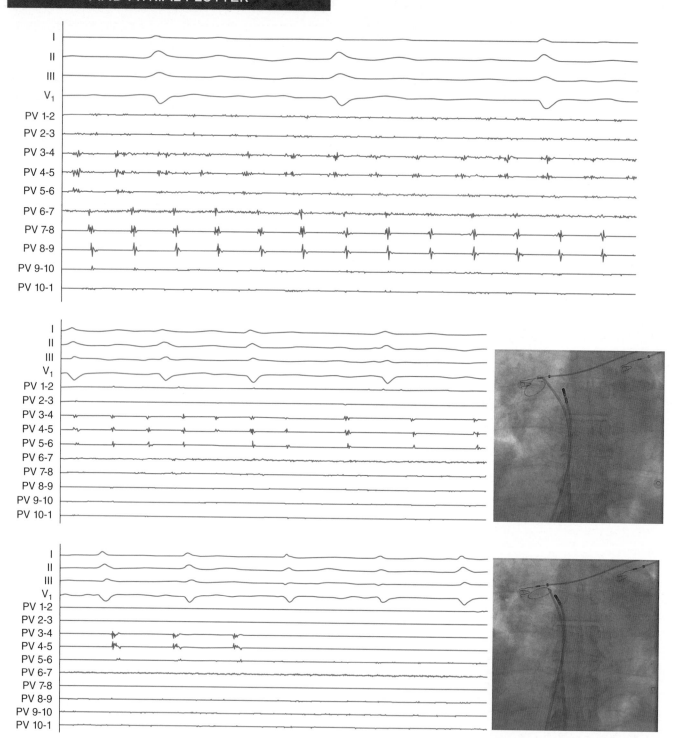

FIGURE 34-17 Isolation of the RSPV. Repeat procedure in a patient with prior PV isolation, electrogram-based and linear ablation for persistent AF who represented with recurrent paroxysmal AF. (Top) Reconnection in the RSPV is noted. (Middle) During reisolation of the RSPV, progressive cycle length slowing is recorded. (Bottom) Further ablation results in complete isolation of the PV. Fluoroscopy images are provided in anteroposterior view. Note that the Lasso catheter in the vein is quite distant from the ablation catheter and that antral isolation is possible while monitoring PV potentials in the vein.

PULMONARY VEIN INITIATION AND TACHYCARDIA

SECTION VI
CATHETER ABLATION TECHNIQUES
FOR MANAGING ATRIAL FIBRILLATION
AND ATRIAL FLUTTER

243

REFERENCES

1. Haissaguerre M, Jais P, Shah DC, et al. Spontaneous initiation of atrial fibrillation by ectopic beats originating in the pulmonary veins. *N Engl J Med*. 1998;339(10):659-666.

2. Jais P, Hocini M, Macle L, et al. Distinctive electrophysiological properties of pulmonary veins in patients with atrial fibrillation. *Circulation*. 2002;106:2479-2485.

3. Hocini M, Ho SY, Kawara T, et al. Electrical conduction in canine pulmonary veins: electrophysiological and anatomic correlation. *Circulation*. 2002;105:2442-2448.

4. Ho SY, Sanchez-Quintana D, Cabrera JA, et al. Anatomy of the left atrium: implications for radiofrequency ablation of atrial fibrillation. *J Cardiovasc Electrophysiol*. 1999;10:1525-1533.

5. Ho SY, Cabrera JA, Tran VH, et al. Architecture of the pulmonary veins: relevance to radiofrequency ablation. *Heart*. 2001;86:265-270.

6. Yamane T, Shah DC, Peng JT, et al. Morphological characteristics of P waves during selective pulmonary vein pacing. *J Am Coll Cardiol*. 2001;38:1505-1510.

7. Tang CW, Scheinman MM, Van Hare GF, et al. Use of P wave configuration during atrial tachycardia to predict site of origin. *J Am Coll Cardiol*. 1995;26:1315-1324.

8. Gerstenfeld EP, Marchlinski FE. Mapping and ablation of left atrial tachycardias occurring after atrial fibrillation ablation. *Heart Rhythm*. 2007;4:S65-72.

9. Kistler PM, Roberts-Thomson KC, Haqqani HM, et al. P-wave morphology in focal atrial tachycardia: development of an algorithm to predict the anatomic site of origin. *J Am Coll Cardiol*. 2006;48:1010-1017.

10. Jais P, Haissaguerre M, Shah DC, et al. A focal source of atrial fibrillation treated by discrete radiofrequency ablation. *Circulation*. 1997;95:572-576.

11. Kistler PM, Sanders P, Fynn SP, et al. Electrophysiological and electrocardiographic characteristics of focal atrial tachycardia originating from the pulmonary veins: acute and long-term outcomes of radiofrequency ablation. *Circulation*. 2003;108:1968-1975.

12. Gerstenfeld EP, Callans DJ, Dixit S, et al. Mechanisms of organized left atrial tachycardias occurring after pulmonary vein isolation. *Circulation*. 2004;110:1351-1357.

13. Ouyang F, Antz M, Ernst S, et al. Recovered pulmonary vein conduction as a dominant factor for recurrent atrial tachyarrhythmias after complete circular isolation of the pulmonary veins: lessons from double lasso technique. *Circulation*. 2005;111: 127-135.

14. Satomi K, Bansch D, Tilz R, et al. Left atrial and pulmonary vein macroreentrant tachycardia associated with double conduction gaps: a novel type of man-made tachycardia after circumferential pulmonary vein isolation. *Heart Rhythm*. 2008;5:43-51.

15. Ouyang F, Ernst S, Vogtmann T, et al. Characterization of reentrant circuits in left atrial macroreentrant tachycardia: critical isthmus block can prevent atrial tachycardia recurrence. *Circulation*. 2002;105:1934-1942.

16. Jais P, Matsuo S, Knecht S, et al. A deductive mapping strategy for atrial tachycardia following atrial fibrillation ablation: importance of localized reentry. *J Cardiovasc Electrophysiol*. 2009;20:480-491.

17. Haissaguerre M, Shah DC, Jais P, et al. Electrophysiological breakthroughs from the left atrium to the pulmonary veins. *Circulation*. 2000;102:2463-2465.

18. Arentz T, Weber R, Burkle G, et al. Small or large isolation areas around the pulmonary veins for the treatment of atrial fibrillation? Results from a prospective randomized study. *Circulation*. 2007;115:3057-3063.

19. Verma A, Kilicaslan F, Pisano E, et al. Response of atrial fibrillation to pulmonary vein antrum isolation is directly related to resumption and delay of pulmonary vein conduction. *Circulation*. 2005;112:627-635.

20. Yamane T, Shah DC, Jais P, et al. Electrogram polarity reversal as an additional indicator of breakthroughs from the left atrium to the pulmonary veins. *J Am Coll Cardiol*. 2002;39:1337-1344.

35 ANTRAL PULMONARY VEIN ISOLATION FOR ATRIAL FIBRILLATION

Mohamad C.N. Sinno, MD, and Hakan Oral, MD

CASE PRESENTATION

A 56-year-old woman presented for evaluation and management of recurrent paroxysmal palpitations over several years who remained symptomatic despite atrioventricular nodal blockade. Physical examination and laboratory studies were all normal. A transthoracic echocardiogram showed a normal left ventricular function with mild enlargement of the left atrium (LA diameter = 43 mm). Ambulatory monitoring revealed that the palpitations correlated with atrial fibrillation. Addition of class IC antiarrhythmic medication to her drug regimen was initially effective in suppressing her palpitations. Over the past few months, she noticed increased palpitations despite full adherence to medications. The patient was referred to for consideration of catheter ablation.

INTRODUCTION

Atrial fibrillation (AF) affects 1% to 2% of the general population and is the most prevalent cardiac arrhythmia. The incidence of AF increases with age and structural heart disease.[1] AF is often symptomatic and impairs quality of life. Affected patients are at 1.5- to 1.9-fold increased risk for mortality as reported in the Framingham study.[2] AF is a leading cause of stroke both due to loss of atrial systole and associated prothrombotic state often observed in patients with AF. AF with uncontrolled ventricular response is also responsible for tachycardia-mediated cardiomyopathy or acute systolic and diastolic heart failure exacerbations. In the AFFIRM trial, except for anticoagulation which is known to reduce stroke risk, there was no difference in mortality among patients randomized to a rate or rhythm control strategy.[3] However, it has been suggested that potential beneficial effects of sinus rhythm maintenance may have been negated by the proarrhythmic effects of antiarrhythmic drugs, which were exclusively used for rhythm control and were effective in maintaining sinus rhythm in only 30% of the patients in the AFFIRM trial. A subsequent post hoc analysis of the AFFIRM trial demonstrated a survival benefit in patients who remained in sinus rhythm. Catheter ablation of AF has been demonstrated to have a superior efficacy over antiarrhythmic drug therapy in patients with AF and has been associated with an improvement in quality of life, left atrial size, and left ventricular ejection fraction. Whether maintenance of sinus rhythm with catheter ablation is also associated with an improvement in survival remains to be determined in large and prospective randomized studies. However, early observations from single center case registries suggest a positive association.

PATHOGENESIS OF PAROXYSMAL ATRIAL FIBRILLATION

Initiators of atrial fibrillation are harbored inside the pulmonary veins (PVs) in >90% of the cases, and repetitive high frequency discharges from these PVs often trigger AF[5] (Figure 35-1). Ectopy can arise from different sites within the same PV or from different PVs in the same patient. Besides being triggers, PVs are also responsible for perpetuation of AF. Intermittent PV tachycardias have been demonstrated to play a critical role in initiation and perpetuation of AF.[6] In a prior study, isolation of PVs in patients with paroxysmal AF was associated with a progressive increase in AF cycle length and subsequent termination of AF in 75% of patients, rendered AF noninducible in 57%, and prevented recurrence in 74%.[7]

ELECTROPHYSIOLOGICAL PROPERTIES OF PULMONARY VEINS

Experimental evidence from isolated, blood-perfused dog hearts support triggered activity, reentry, and automaticity as the mechanisms of arrhythmogenesis in PVs.[8] Nonhomogenous muscle fiber orientation at the ostia of PVs correlates with zones of delayed conduction and fractionated signals facilitating reentry within the PVs. These electrophysiological properties of PVs were confirmed with optical mapping in atrial preparations of dog hearts demonstrating delayed conduction, heterogeneous depolarization, conduction block, and reentry in 60% of preparations. Besides, sustained focal discharges localized near the PV ostia were also demonstrated with isoproterenol infusion.[9]

In clinical studies, the effective refractory period (ERP) of the four PVs was shorter than the LA ERP in patients with AF. In the same study, the opposite was true for patients without AF. Decremental conduction between the PV and LA and the slow conduction within the PVs was also noted to be more prevalent in patients with AF suggesting a pivotal role for reentry within PV musculature in AF perpetuation.[10] Furthermore, pace-termination and entrainment of PV-induced arrhythmias provide indirect evidence supportive of reentry as a mechanism for AF.

There is also evidence that automaticity and triggered activity may play a role in the genesis of AF. Discrete ectopic discharges and adenosine sensitive focal tachycardias have been demonstrated using high-density mapping within PVs, and there was no evidence of reentry in some reports. Besides, early reports in animal models have identified pacemaker regions in the distal parts of the muscular sleeves within the pulmonary vein where it joins the smooth muscle. Those PV sites were referred to as subsidiary pacemakers in the 1980s and are capable of developing oscillatory after-potentials, large enough to reach threshold and cause extrasystoles.[11] Digitalis treated atrial preparations were shown to develop oscillatory after-potentials and act as ectopic foci.

PULMONARY VEIN ANATOMY

Embryologically, the PVs arise from the posterior LA without distinct boundaries separating the ostium, antrum, and LA (Figure 35-2). Nonuniform sleeves of myocardium extending from the LA into PVs constitute the arrhythmogenic substrate for paroxysmal AF. These myocardial sleeves are more developed in the upper than the lower PVs, extend between 2 and 25 mm distally into the vein, and are thickest at the LA-PV junction. Sleeves tend to be thicker in the "carina" region separating the inferior from the superior veins with fibrous tissue filling gaps between those sleeves at the LA-PV junction and within the PVs. Sleeves most commonly wrap around the LA-PV

ANTRAL PULMONARY VEIN ISOLATION
FOR ATRIAL FIBRILLATION

SECTION VI
CATHETER ABLATION TECHNIQUES FOR
MANAGING ATRIAL FIBRILLATION AND
ATRIAL FLUTTER

245

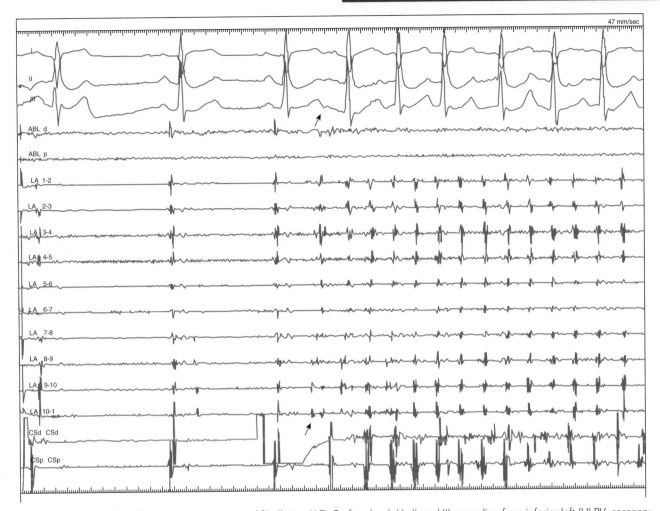

FIGURE 35-1 Pulmonary vein (PV) ectopy initiating atrial fibrillation (AF). Surface leads V₁, II, and III, recording from inferior left (LI) PV, coronary sinus (CS), and ablation catheter (ABL). A premature beat (arrow) arising from the LIPV, earliest LA 10-1, precedes atrial activity on the surface ECG (arrow on surface ECG), conducts to the left atrium (LA) and initiates AF.

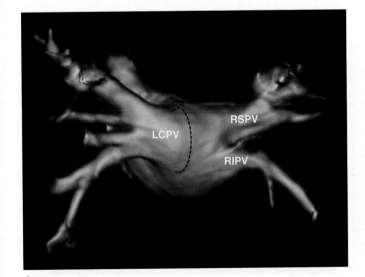

A

FIGURE 35-2A Magnetic resonance imaging reconstruction of the atrial and pulmonary vein anatomy. (A) Three-dimensional reconstruction of the left atrium and pulmonary veins, view from a posterior perspective. Note the left common ostium (LCPV) of the left pulmonary veins and the separate ostia of the right inferior pulmonary vein (RIPV) and right superior pulmonary vein (RSPV).

SECTION VI
CATHETER ABLATION TECHNIQUES FOR
MANAGING ATRIAL FIBRILLATION AND
ATRIAL FLUTTER

246

CHAPTER 35

junction in a circumferential manner, but some are oriented in a longitudinal or oblique fashion. Therefore, the anisotropic arrangement of these muscle fibers may provide a substrate for reentry.

CATHETER ABLATION OF ATRIAL FIBRILLATION

According to current guidelines, catheter ablation for symptomatic AF is considered a second-line treatment after failure of antiarrhythmic medications. Expert consensus acknowledges the pivotal role of PVs in AF and recommends complete electrical isolation of PVs.[12] Electrical isolation requires demonstration of entrance block into the vein. PV isolation is often sufficient in patients with paroxysmal AF. However, in patients with persistent AF who may have electroanatomical remodeling, modification of the atrial substrate beyond PVs may often be necessary.[13]

Initial efforts targeted arrhythmogenic foci within the PVs by focal applications of radiofrequency energy often within the PV or one of its branches.[5] However, this approach was associated with a high recurrence rate both from the same PV and also other PVs and with a high incidence of PV stenosis.[14] Since the electrical connection between the PVs and the left atrium occur via insulated, discrete myocardial fibers, referred to as PV fascicles, complete isolation of PVs by segmental ostial ablation followed.[5,15] Subsequently, left atrial circumferential ablation or wide area circumferential ablation (Figure 35-3) that included most if not all of the antrum was shown to be superior to isolation of PVs at the ostial level.[15]

The PV antrum that includes most of the posterior left atrium shares similar histoembryological origin to the tubular portion of the PV and appears to have a similar arrhythmogenic potential as the PVs. As a matter of fact a majority of the non-PV foci that initiate AF arise from the posterior left atrium and PV antrum. Later ablation strategies evolved as antral PV isolation that aims to isolate the PVs by antral ablation specifically targeting antral potentials (that have similar characteristics to the PV potentials such as high frequency activation) and by confirming complete isolation of PVs.[12] The mechanisms of

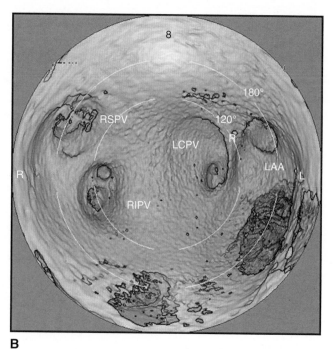

B

FIGURE 35-2B Computed tomography reconstruction of the atrial and pulmonary vein (PV) anatomy. Intra-atrial reconstructed views of the posterior LA. Note the "saddles" between adjacent PVs. The complex, funnel-shaped approaches to the veins are apparent. In this case, there is a common ostium for the left-sided veins (LCPV). Also demonstrated is the narrow ridge that separates the left PVs from the left atrial appendage (LAA). Abbreviations: R, ridge between LAA and PVs; RIPV, right inferior pulmonary vein; RSPV, right superior pulmonary vein.

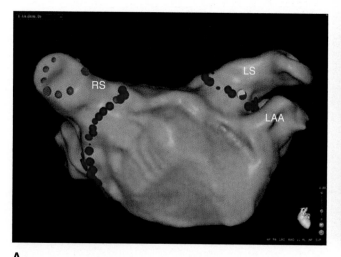

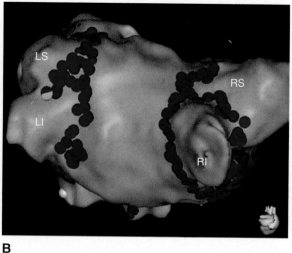

A   **B**

FIGURE 35-3 Three-dimensional reconstruction of the left atrium using the Biosense CARTO 3 mapping system. (A) Anteroposterior (AP) view of the left atrium (LA) and pulmonary veins (PVs) with circumferential ablation (red dots) around the antrum. (B) Posteroanterior (PA) view with a rightward tilt of the left atrium (LA) and pulmonary veins (PVs) with circumferential ablation (red dots) around the antra of individual PVs. Abbreviations: LAA, left atrial appendage; LI, left inferior pulmonary vein; LS, left superior pulmonary vein; RI, right inferior pulmonary vein; RS, right superior pulmonary vein.

ANTRAL PULMONARY VEIN ISOLATION
FOR ATRIAL FIBRILLATION

SECTION VI
CATHETER ABLATION TECHNIQUES FOR
MANAGING ATRIAL FIBRILLATION AND
ATRIAL FLUTTER

247

superior efficacy of antral PV isolation may include: (1) elimination of PV arrhythmogenicity; (2) elimination of drivers of AF such as rotors that often have anchor points in the antrum of PVs; (3) elimination of non-PV triggers that may originate within the PV antrum; (4) debulking of the left atrium; and (5) ablation of ganglionated plexi that often are located on the epicardial aspect of the PV antrum.

Technique

Access to the left atrium is established by transseptal puncture under fluoroscopic guidance with or without intracardiac echocardiography (ICE) (Figure 35-4). Once LA access is achieved, anticoagulation with unfractionated heparin is recommended with a target-activated clotting time between 300 and 350 seconds. Continuing anticoagulant therapy with warfarin or dabigatran throughout the ablation procedure has been associated with a lower incidence of thromboembolic complications without an increase in bleeding or pericardial tamponade.[16,17]

A circular mapping catheter along with the ablation catheter are advanced across the transseptal access site for mapping and ablation. Catheter navigation and ablation guidance inside the LA could be facilitated with fluoroscopy, ICE, and three-dimensional mapping systems. Electrical isolation of the pulmonary veins is typically performed at antral locations (Figure 35-5). It has been suggested to use a rowing circular catheter to precisely map the antral potentials in some studies. However, this often can be achieved with a typical ablation catheter. Mapping around the circumference of the vein allows recording of PV potentials that are often merged with LA signals. The PV potentials are sharp, high frequency signals that are <50 ms in duration and follow the left atrial electrograms during normal sinus rhythm. Pacing from within the coronary sinus advances the left atrial electrograms while delaying conduction into the left-sided PVs separating the two signals (Figure 35-6).

Visualization of the course of the esophagus along the posterior wall of the left atrium is helpful to avoid inadvertent applications of radiofrequency energy in the immediate proximity of the esophagus. Strategies to minimize the risk of esophageal injury include visual assessment of esophagus position relative to intended ablation targets, avoidance of ablation near the esophagus, titration of RF energy, and

duration and monitoring of intraluminal esophageal temperatures. However, the safest approach to avoid esophageal injury remains to be determined.

Real-time visualization of the esophagus could be achieved by fluoroscopic imaging of the esophageal lumen containing barium or another radio-opaque marker, or with real time intracardiac ultrasound from the right or left atrium.

Avoidance of ablation anterior to the esophagus is achieved by modifying the lesion sets either closer to the PVs or away from the antrum. A potential pitfall of creating a wider lesion set is the difficulty in achieving persistent and complete electrical isolation of the pulmonary veins.

RF energy titration is often used to minimize the risk of esophageal injury during catheter ablation of critical targets close to the esophagus. Observational studies reveal that esophageal heating can happen during RF applications along the posterior LA wall. Rapid heat transfer in the order of 0.05 to 0.1 degrees per second to the esophagus may predict potential thermal injury instances.[18] Besides, there is evidence that the esophagus cools slowly, and closely coupled RF applications at the same site can result in a greater degree of mural esophageal heating.[18] However, there are limited data on the safety thresholds for the maximum power, temperature, and duration during applications of energy. A commonly used approach is to limit the power to 15 to 20 watts and to not deliver energy for more than 10 to 15 seconds a time. However, it remains unclear whether this approach offers sufficient safety. Cryoablation can also lead to esophageal injury; therefore, caution should also be exercised with this modality.

After entrance block is confirmed within the PV (Figure 35-7), isoproterenol and/or adenosine can be administered to assess residual arrhythmogenic foci and dormant PV conduction[19] (Figure 35-8). Additional ablation after PV isolation targeting reconnected PV fascicles or sustained atrial ectopy after administration of adenosine or isoproterenol has been shown to predict improved clinical outcomes.[19]

COMPLICATIONS

Based on the results of world-wide registry, the overall complication rate for AF ablation procedures is estimated as 6%, may including

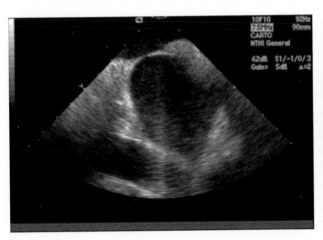

A

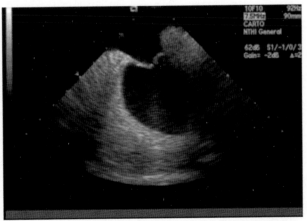

B

FIGURE 35-4 (A) Utilization of phased-array intracardiac echocardiography for visualizing the thin portion of the interatrial septum. (B) Tenting of the fossa ovalis by the dilator and BRK needle assembly. Note that the assembly is pointing toward the left atrial midcavity.

248

SECTION VI
CATHETER ABLATION TECHNIQUES FOR
MANAGING ATRIAL FIBRILLATION AND
ATRIAL FLUTTER

CHAPTER 35

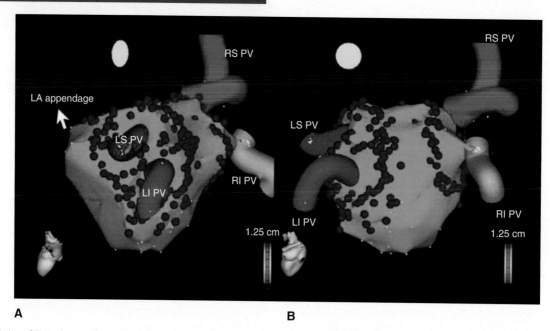

A   **B**

FIGURE 35-5 Antral PV isolation. Shown are left lateral (A) and posteroanterior (B) projections of a 3-dimensional electroanatomic depiction of the left atrium (LA). Red tags indicate ablation sites. Abbreviations: LI, left inferior; LS, left superior; PV, pulmonary vein; RI, right inferior; RS, right superior. Reproduced with permission from Oral H, Chugh A, Yoshida K, et al. A randomized assessment of the incremental role of ablation of complex fractionated atrial electrograms after antral pulmonary vein isolation for long-lasting persistent atrial fibrillation. *J Am Coll Cardiol.* 2009;53(9):782-789. Copyright Elsevier.

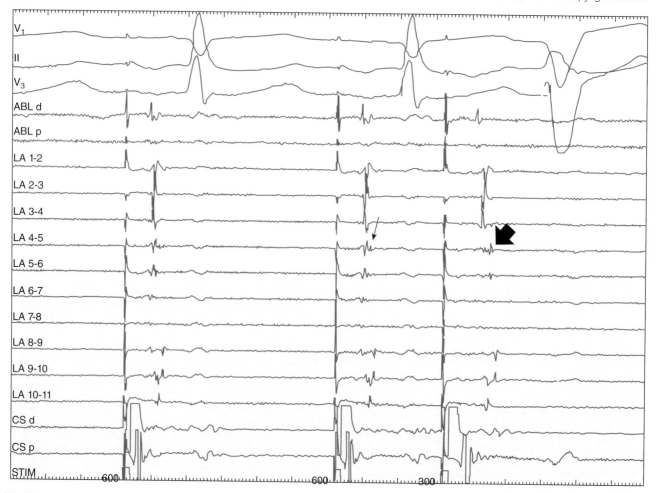

FIGURE 35-6 CS pacing at a drive cycle length of 600 ms and a single extrastimulus delivered at 300 ms after circumferential ablation around the left inferior pulmonary vein. The pulmonary vein potential on the circular mapping catheter during CS pacing at 600 ms is fused with the left atrial far field potential (arrow). There is decremental conduction into the pulmonary vein with the delivery of a single extrastimulus at 300 ms showing the earliest site of PV activation on LA 4-5 (arrow head). Targeted ablation at the antrum close to LA 4-5 electrically isolated this vein.

ANTRAL PULMONARY VEIN ISOLATION
FOR ATRIAL FIBRILLATION

SECTION VI
CATHETER ABLATION TECHNIQUES FOR
MANAGING ATRIAL FIBRILLATION AND
ATRIAL FLUTTER

249

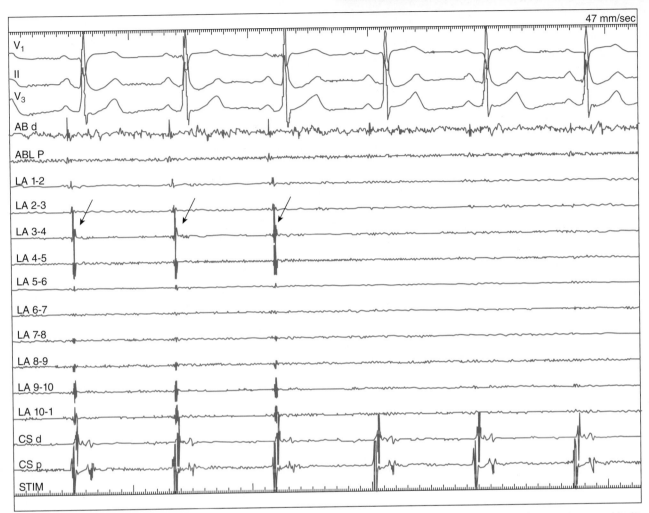

FIGURE 35-7 Ablation at the right superior pulmonary vein antrum results in electrical isolation of this PV from the left atrium (entrance block). Arrows highlight the sharp and narrow pulmonary vein potentials. Abbreviations: LA, circular mapping catheter; ABL, ablation; CS, coronary sinus.

a 0.2% risk of procedural death, 1.2% risk of tamponade, 1% for cerebrovascular accident, and <2% for PV stenosis. Atrioesophageal fistula is one of the most feared complications of catheter ablation and is often fatal. The incidence is about 0.01%. Vascular access related complications can also occur. Phrenic nerve injury may occur in 0.1% of patients using conventional RF catheters and up to 7% during cryoballoon ablation.

PATIENT MANAGEMENT AND FOLLOW-UP

Patients referred to for catheter ablation are started on oral anticoagulation prior to the procedure. Uninterrupted anticoagulation using warfarin at a target INR 2-3 in the periprocedural period has been demonstrated to be associated with a lower risk of thromboembolic events without an increase in hemorrhagic complications compared to interrupted anticoagulation and bridging with low molecular weight heparin.[16] LMWH has been shown to increase vascular access site complications. In a recent study, dabigatran was also found to be safe and as effective as uninterrupted warfarin, when discontinued 24 hours prior to the procedure and resumed 4 hours after vascular hemostasis is achieved. Similarly, rivaroxaban, with the dose held on the day of the procedure, appears to be equally safe and effective

when compared with uninterrupted coumadin.[20] Data is still lacking behind apixaban use in patients presenting for left atrial ablation procedures. The utility of newer anticoagulants, including apixaban, and optimal dosing regimens need to be confirmed in large-scale prospective studies.

Early recurrences of AF within the first 2 to 3 months can be transient most likely due to an inflammatory response to ablation. Although early recurrence of AF carries an independent risk of treatment failure, its occurrence should not prompt immediate reablation attempts, as 20% to 57% of patients may not have any further arrhythmias during long-term follow-up. Since the mechanism of AF postablation may be different from that of the patient's clinical arrhythmia and may resolve completely upon resolution of the inflammatory process, some operators choose to treat all patients with suppressive antiarrhythmic agents for the first 1 to 3 months following ablation (blanking period). Repeat ablation procedures should be delayed for at least 3 months following the initial procedure if the patient's symptoms can be controlled with medical therapy.

The HRS Consensus Statement suggests that follow-up should begin within 3 months after the ablation procedure and continue at 6-month intervals for at least 2 years.

250

SECTION VI
CATHETER ABLATION TECHNIQUES FOR
MANAGING ATRIAL FIBRILLATION AND
ATRIAL FLUTTER

CHAPTER 35

CONCLUSION

Pulmonary vein arrhythmogenicity plays an important role in initiation and perpetuation of AF. Antral pulmonary vein isolation remains as a key step in targeting AF and is often sufficient to eliminate paroxysmal AF. PV antrum is often as arrhythmogenic as the tubular portion of the PVs and should be included as an ablation target. Whether accurate identification and elimination of drivers of AF beyond the PVs and their antrum will improve the outcomes of antral PV isolation or even eliminate the need for it, remains to be determined in future studies.

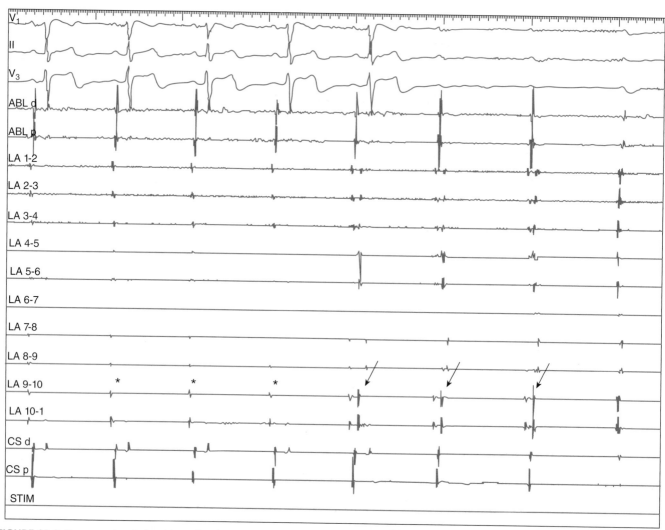

FIGURE 35-8 Dormant electrical activity within the right superior pulmonary vein. There are atrial far-field signals recorded on the circular mapping catheter (LA) positioned antrally (asterix). With administration of 12 mg of adenosine, AV nodal block occurs with evidence of pulmonary vein activity (arrows). Abbreviations: ABL, ablation; CS, coronary sinus.

REFERENCES

1. Kannel WB, Abbott RD, Savage DD, McNamara PM. Epidemiologic features of chronic atrial fibrillation: the Framingham study. *N Engl J Med.* 1982;306(17):1018-1022.

2. Benjamin EJ, Wolf PA, D'Agostino RB, Silbershatz H, Kannel WB, Levy D. Impact of atrial fibrillation on the risk of death: the Framingham Heart Study. *Circulation.* 1998;98(10):946-952.

3. Wyse DG, Waldo AL, DiMarco JP, et al. A comparison of rate control and rhythm control in patients with atrial fibrillation. *N Engl J Med.* 2002;347(23):1825-1833.

4. Corley SD, Epstein AE, DiMarco JP, et al. Relationships between sinus rhythm, treatment, and survival in the Atrial Fibrillation Follow-Up Investigation of Rhythm Management (AFFIRM) Study. *Circulation.* 2004;109(12):1509-1513.

5. Haissaguerre M, Jais P, Shah DC, et al. Spontaneous initiation of atrial fibrillation by ectopic beats originating in the pulmonary veins. *N Engl J Med.* 1998;339(10):659-666.

6. Oral H, Ozaydin M, Tada H, et al. Mechanistic significance of intermittent pulmonary vein tachycardia in patients with atrial fibrillation. *J Cardiovasc Electrophysiol.* 2002;13(7):645-650.

ANTRAL PULMONARY VEIN ISOLATION
FOR ATRIAL FIBRILLATION

SECTION VI
CATHETER ABLATION TECHNIQUES FOR
MANAGING ATRIAL FIBRILLATION AND
ATRIAL FLUTTER

251

7. Haissaguerre M, Sanders P, Hocini M, et al. Changes in atrial fibrillation cycle length and inducibility during catheter ablation and their relation to outcome. *Circulation.* 2004;109(24):3007-3013.

8. Hocini M, Ho SY, Kawara T, et al. Electrical conduction in canine pulmonary veins: electrophysiological and anatomic correlation. *Circulation.* 2002;105(20):2442-2448.

9. Arora R, Verheule S, Scott L, et al. Arrhythmogenic substrate of the pulmonary veins assessed by high-resolution optical mapping. *Circulation.* 2003;107(13):1816-1821.

10. Jais P, Hocini M, Macle L, et al. Distinctive electrophysiological properties of pulmonary veins in patients with atrial fibrillation. *Circulation.* 2002;106(19):2479-2485.

11. Cheung DW. Pulmonary vein as an ectopic focus in digitalis-induced arrhythmia. *Nature.* 1981;294(5841):582-584.

12. Calkins H, Brugada J, Packer DL, et al. HRS/EHRA/ECAS expert Consensus Statement on catheter and surgical ablation of atrial fibrillation: recommendations for personnel, policy, procedures and follow-up. A report of the Heart Rhythm Society (HRS) Task Force on catheter and surgical ablation of atrial fibrillation. *Heart Rhythm.* 2007;4(6):816-861.

13. Ouyang F, Bansch D, Ernst S, et al. Complete isolation of left atrium surrounding the pulmonary veins: new insights from the double-Lasso technique in paroxysmal atrial fibrillation. *Circulation.* 2004;110(15):2090-2096.

14. Yu WC, Hsu TL, Tai CT, et al. Acquired pulmonary vein stenosis after radiofrequency catheter ablation of paroxysmal atrial fibrillation. *J Cardiovasc Electrophysiol.* 2001;12(8):887-892.

15. Oral H, Knight BP, Tada H, et al. Pulmonary vein isolation for paroxysmal and persistent atrial fibrillation. *Circulation.* 2002;105(9):1077-1081.

16. Latchamsetty R, Gautam S, Bhakta D, et al. Management and outcomes of cardiac tamponade during atrial fibrillation ablation in the presence of therapeutic anticoagulation with warfarin. *Heart Rhythm.* 2011;8(6):805-808.

17. Lakkireddy D, Reddy YM, Di Biase L, et al. Feasibility and safety of dabigatran versus warfarin for periprocedural anticoagulation in patients undergoing radiofrequency ablation for atrial fibrillation: results from a multicenter prospective registry. *J Am Coll Cardiol.* 2012;59(13):1168-1174.

18. Perzanowski C, Teplitsky L, Hranitzky PM, Bahnson TD. Real-time monitoring of luminal esophageal temperature during left atrial radiofrequency catheter ablation for atrial fibrillation: observations about esophageal heating during ablation at the pulmonary vein ostia and posterior left atrium. *J Cardiovasc Electrophysiol.* 2006;17(2):166-170.

19. Crawford T, Chugh A, Good E, et al. Clinical value of noninducibility by high-dose isoproterenol versus rapid atrial pacing after catheter ablation of paroxysmal atrial fibrillation. *J Cardiovasc Electrophysiol.* 2010;21(1):13-20.

20. Varuna K, Gadiyaram M, Isabel Boero BA, et al. Rivaroxaban has similar safety and efficacy as warfarin for peri-procedural anticoagulation for atrial fibrillation ablation. Program and abstracts of the 34th Annual Scientific Sessions of the Heart Rhythm Society; May 8-11, 2013; Denver, Colorado.

SECTION VI
CATHETER ABLATION TECHNIQUES FOR
MANAGING ATRIAL FIBRILLATION AND
ATRIAL FLUTTER

252

CHAPTER 36

36 APPROACHES TO ABLATION OF ATRIAL FIBRILLATION: FRACTIONATED ELECTROGRAMS

Koonlawee Nademanee, MD

CASE PRESENTATION

A 74-year-old man with a history of hypertension and a transient ischemic attack has paroxysmal atrial fibrillation (AF) for 42 months. He has failed propafenone, sotalol, and dronedarone. His ejection fraction (EF) was 70%, and his left atrial (LA) diameter was 44 mm. AF was induced in the EP lab by isoproterenol infusion (Figure 36-1A) which precipitated spontaneous AF initiated by a premature atrial capture emanating from the right superior pulmonary vein (RSPV). Figure 36-1B shows the LA complex fractionated atrial electrogram (CFAE) map in PA and AP views on the electroanatomic map. The colors display the areas according to the cycle lengths of the CFAEs.

The map shows the CFAEs area localized around the left inferior pulmonary vein (LIPV), antrum of the RSPV, and septum as shown in the red color. The rest of the LA was relatively organized and being activated with a relatively much longer cycle length. In this case, the RSPV has the shortest cycle length of CFAEs (<100 ms) and serve as the prime target for ablation (Figure 36-1C). Note that there were also distinct differences between the cycle lengths of the electrograms recorded from RIPV antrum than those recorded from coronary sinus. Ablations at these sites progressively lengthened tachycardia cycle length and eventually reverted AF to sinus rhythm (SR) (Figure 36-1D). After ablation, both a high dose of isoproterenol infusion and rapid burst pacing could not induce any atrial tachyarrhythmias (Figure 36-1E). His procedure lasted only 86 minutes, and fluoroscopic time lasted only 4 minutes and 6 seconds. The patient remained symptom- and arrhythmia-free during the long-term follow-up.

ABLATION THERAPY FOR ATRIAL FIBRILLATION

The watershed observation by Haissguerre et al that PVs are an important source of triggering foci for paroxysmal AF has drawn electrophysiologists' attention to the PVs as important target sites for AF ablation[1]. Although the initial approach was to focally ablate the culprit PV that was identified as the triggering site initiating AF,[1,2] this approach quickly was out of vogue because numerous limitations:

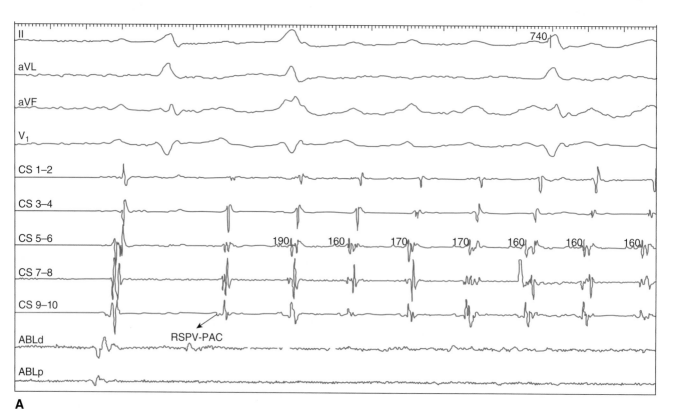

A

FIGURE 36-1 (A) PAC from the right superior pulmonary vein (RSPV) that triggered AF. Once AF was sustained, a CFAE map was performed as shown in B. The LA map was created during AF. The map displays CFAE areas with respect to the shortest cycle length of the fractionated electrogram. Red areas have the shortest cycle length, and in this patient the RSPV, septum, and antrum of the left inferior pulmonary vein (LIPV) had the shortest cycle length (<100 ms). (C) The electrograms recorded from the LIPV as shown in the inset (arrow); note the much shorter cycle length at this site compared to the electrograms recorded from the coronary sinus. The red dots are the RF application points. Ablations were performed in these areas and rendered AF termination (D) and noninducible tachyarrhythmias with a high dose isoproterenol infusion (20 μg/min E).

APPROACHES TO ABLATION OF ATRIAL
FIBRILLATION: FRACTIONATED ELECTROGRAMS

SECTION VI
CATHETER ABLATION TECHNIQUES FOR
MANAGING ATRIAL FIBRILLATION AND
ATRIAL FLUTTER

253

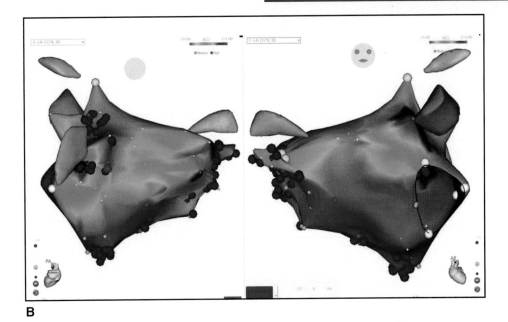

B

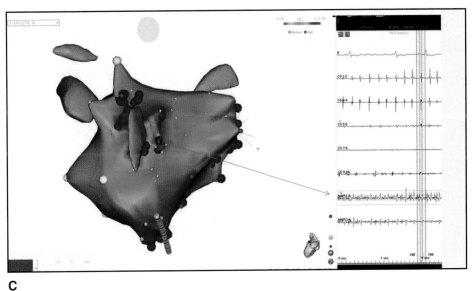

C

FIGURE 36-1 *(Continued)*

(1) difficulty of mapping the triggering focus due to a paucity of spontaneous AF coupling and time consuming because inducing the triggering arrhythmia often required multiple provocation and was quite inconsistent; (2) a daunting task of mapping multiple triggering foci; (3) multiple cardioversions were often needed for those whose AF became persistent. The strategy then changed to attempt to isolate the electrical connections of all four veins from the LA muscle.[3-5] Various techniques were utilized to achieve electrical isolation of PVs: segmental isolation introduced by Haissaguerre and his colleagues,[3] PV isolation at the antrum at the atrium-venous junction,[4] or electroanatomical mapping and circumferential PV ablation.[5]

However, a total isolation of all four PVs poses a risk of PV stenosis. Furthermore, this strategy assumes that PVs are virtually the primary source of triggers or the perpetuator of AF, and thus all AF patients

were essentially treated the same way—guided by anatomical scheme rather than electrophysiological mapping. As a result, electrical isolation of PVs has a variable rate of success in treating patients with all types of AF.[6,7]

We have utilized a different approach in ablating AF by using electroanatomical mapping of a substrate that perpetuates AF through identification of areas that have CFAEs during AF.

CHARACTERISTICS OF ATRIAL ELECTROGRAMS DURING ATRIAL FIBRILLATION

When one maps both atria during AF, one finds that there are three types of atrial electrogram characteristics[8-10] (Figure 36-2). Atrial electrograms during sustained AF have three distinct patterns: single potential, double potential, and complex fractionated potential (CFAE).

254

SECTION VI
CATHETER ABLATION TECHNIQUES FOR
MANAGING ATRIAL FIBRILLATION AND
ATRIAL FLUTTER

CHAPTER 36

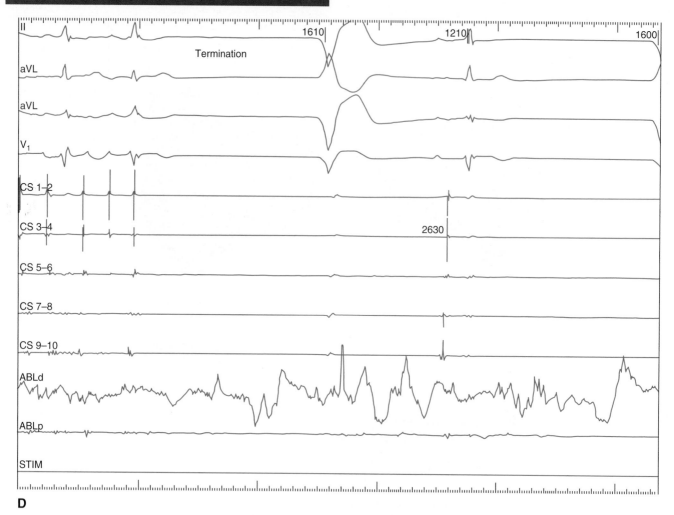

D

FIGURE 36-1 (*Continued*)

There are significant differences in these atrial electrograms during AF with respect to their cycle lengths and patterns and their regional distribution. Interestingly, areas that harbor CFAE with a very short cycle length have proclivity to localize and cluster in specific areas of the atria and do not meander; in other words, these atrial electrograms exhibit surprisingly remarkable temporal and spatial stability. These CFAE areas represent the AF substrate sites and become important target sites for AF ablation. By ablating such areas that have persistent CFAEs recording, one eliminates AF and usually renders AF noninducible. With this observation, CFAE mapping has become a novel approach for guiding a successful ablation of AF substrate with excellent long-term outcomes.

CFAEs are usually low voltage multiple potential signals between 0.05 and 0.15 mV. CFAEs are defined as follows: (1) atrial electrograms that have fractionated electrograms composed of two deflections or more, and/or have a perturbation of the baseline with continuous deflection of a prolonged activation complex (Figure36- 2). (2) Atrial electrograms with a very short cycle length (<120 ms) with or without multiple potential; however, when compared to the rest of the atria, this site has the shortest cycle length (Figure 36-3) that drives the rest of the atria. These CFAEs, as shown in Figure 36-3, are also important targets for ablations.

ELECTROPHYSIOLOGIC MECHANISMS UNDERLYING CFAEs

The elegant study by Konings et al showed that the complex, multiple component fractionated electrical potentials observed during intra-operative mapping of human AF were found mostly in the areas of slow conduction and/or pivot points where the wavelets turn around the end of the arch of the functional block.[8,9] Thus, such areas of fractionated electrical recordings during AF represent either continuous reentry of the fibrillatory waves into the same area or the overlap between different wavelets entering the same area at different times.

Kalifa et al[12] identified a key relationship between areas of dominant frequency and areas of fractionation in sheep. The investigators were able to localize areas with regular, fast, spatio-temporally organized activity and map the regions around them. Waves propagating from these areas were found to break and change direction recurrently at a boundary zone and demonstrate fractionation of local electrograms. Their findings suggested that one of the possible electrophysiologic mechanisms for AF relating to the hypothesis that high-frequency reentry at the boundary zones is responsible for the fractionation.

APPROACHES TO ABLATION OF ATRIAL
FIBRILLATION: FRACTIONATED ELECTROGRAMS

SECTION VI
CATHETER ABLATION TECHNIQUES FOR
MANAGING ATRIAL FIBRILLATION AND
ATRIAL FLUTTER

255

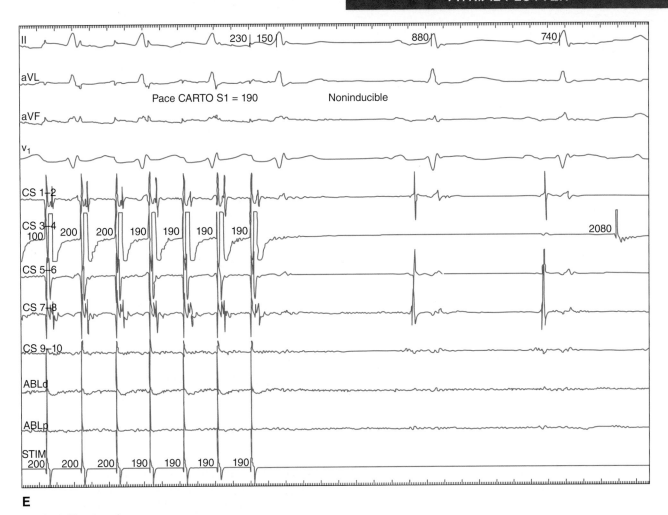

E

FIGURE 36-1 (*Continued*)

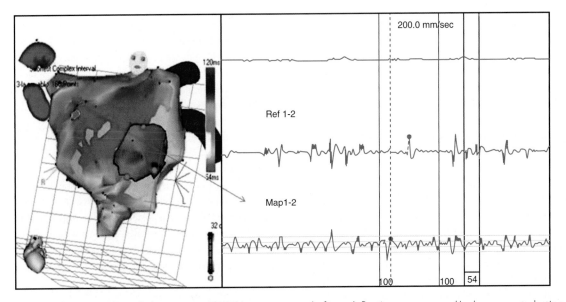

FIGURE 36-2 Complex fractionated atrial electrograms (CFAEs) are composed of two deflections or more and/or have a perturbation of the baseline with continuous deflections from a prolonged activation complex with a very short cycle length. This figure shows an electroanatomical map of the LA in the LAO-oblique view, displaying the shortest cycle length of the recording sites in the span of 2.5 seconds ranging from 50 to 120 ms. The site from anterior aspect of the LA around the antrum of right superior pulmonary veins (arrow) had continuous low voltage fractionated atrial electrograms with the shortest cycle length of 54 ms (Map 1-2). In contrast, electrograms recorded from the coronary sinus (Ref 1-2) showing varying three types of electrograms in the same short time span; note that CFAE of this site are fleeting, sandwiching between a double potential electrogram and a single potential; note also that the cycle length of this recording site is much longer than that of the Map 1-2 recording site. CFAE recorded from Map 1-2 is an ideal target for ablation.

256

SECTION VI
CATHETER ABLATION TECHNIQUES FOR
MANAGING ATRIAL FIBRILLATION AND
ATRIAL FLUTTER

CHAPTER 36

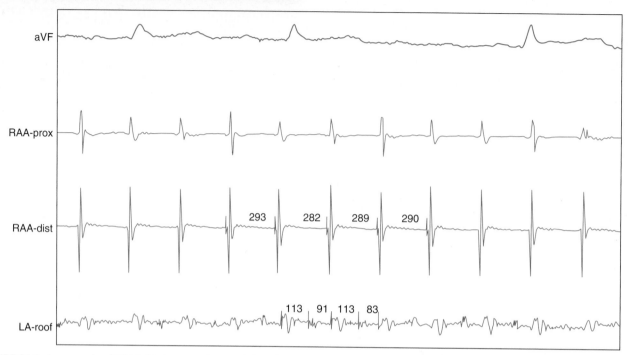

FIGURE 36-3 An example of CFAE that has very short cycle length. It is much shorter than those recorded from the rest of atria, despite having no multiple prolonged potentials.

The most prominent theory underlying the occurrence of CFAE involves the complex interplay of the intrinsic cardiac nervous system on atrial tissues. The cardiac ganglionic plexi (GP) are a collection of autonomic nervous tissues with afferent and efferent sympathetic and parasympathetic fibers.[13,14] Six major GPs that may exert influence on the atria are the superior LA, the posterolateral LA, the posteromedial LA, the anterior descending LA, the posterior right atrium (RA), and the superior RA. In animal models, the stimulation of parasympathetic fibers within the GP has been shown to decrease atrial effective refractory periods and allow AF to perpetuate. Quan KJ et al[13] showed that electrical stimulation of cardiac ganglia near the PV orifices significantly shortened the atrial refractoriness close to the site of the stimulation and that the effects diminished at >2 cm away from this site. This raises the possibility that neurotransmitter release ie, acetylcholine, at preganglionic, and/or postganglionic terminal may contribute to the genesis of CFAEs and may play role in the differences of CFAEs regional distribution in the atria during AF. Indeed, Scherlag et al[14] have demonstrated quite convincingly that in the areas of the LA where the GPs are identified by high frequency stimulation, CFAEs were almost always recorded after the high frequency stimulation initiated AF. They suggest that a marked shortening of action potential duration and formation of early repolarization caused ectopic beats, initiating AF that was sustained by the marked shortening of the refractory period. Ongoing research has identified a close relationship between the location of CFAE and the GP in animal models.[15-18] CFAE-targeted ablation may provide a surrogate for modification of the GP if this relationship can be confirmed in humans. Certainly, ablation in areas that have resulted in a vagal response has shown excellent results in the treatment of AF.

It is possible that all of the above electrophysiologic changes are the underlying causes of CFAE. However, regardless of the mechanism underlying CFAEs, it is very likely that CFAE areas represent substrate areas that perpetuate AF.

REGIONAL DISTRIBUTION OF CFAE

The regions that harbor CFAE are not symmetrically located within the atria, and the distribution of CFAE in the right and left atria is vastly different from one area to another but can be predictably sought in certain places during mapping.[10,11] CFAE are surprisingly stationary and exhibit relative spatial and temporal stability; thus, one can perform point-to-point mapping of these CFAE areas and associate them into an electroanatomical map. The following key areas have demonstrated a predominance of CFAE within our cohort: the proximal coronary sinus; the superior vena cava-RA junction; the septal wall anterior to the right superior and inferior PVs; the anterior wall medial to the LA appendage; the area between the LA appendage and left superior PV; and the posterosuperior wall medial to the left superior PV (Figure 36-3). Typically, patients with persistent or long-lasting AF have greater numbers and locations of sites with CFAE than those with paroxysmal AF.[10]

CFAE MAPPING TO GUIDE SUBSTRATE ABLATION

Mapping is always performed during AF by point-to-point mapping, although detailed mapping of the LA, coronary sinus, and, occasionally, RA is required. The spatial and temporal stability of CFAE allows the precise localization of these electrograms. A map with a minimum of 100 data points is usually created, especially in high-density areas commonly known to have CFAE. Additionally, we usually create a

APPROACHES TO ABLATION OF ATRIAL
FIBRILLATION: FRACTIONATED ELECTROGRAMS

SECTION VI
CATHETER ABLATION TECHNIQUES FOR
MANAGING ATRIAL FIBRILLATION AND
ATRIAL FLUTTER

257

detailed map of the proximal coronary sinus, and occasionally the RA. We identify locations with stable electrograms, and these are "tagged" to create targets for ablation. Areas with fleeting CFAE are not sought as primary targets. A highly reliable map allows for minimal use of fluoroscopy. We routinely use less than 10 minutes of fluoroscopic time during average procedure duration of approximately 120 minutes.

A customized software package to assist in the process of mapping (CFAE software module, CARTO, Biosense-Webster, Diamond Bar, CA, United States) was produced.[19] The software analyzes data on atrial electrograms collected from the ablation catheter over a 2.5-second recording window and interprets it according to two variables: (1) shortest complex interval (SCL) in milliseconds, out of all intervals identified between consecutive CFAE complexes over the span of 2.5 ms; and (2) interval confidence level, the number of intervals identified between consecutive complexes identified as CFAE. The assumption is that the more complex intervals recorded during the signal recording time (2.5 ms), that is, the more repetitions in a given time duration, the more confident the categorization of CFAE. Information from these variables is projected on a three-dimensional electroanatomical shell according to a color-coded scale. This allows targeting and retargeting of areas of significant CFAE.

PROCEDURAL DETAILS

A decapolar catheter is placed in the coronary sinus for reference and pacing. A single transseptal puncture under hemodynamic and fluoroscopic guidance is used to access the LA. Patients who are not in AF at the onset of the procedure undergo an aggressive induction protocol utilizing intravenous isoproterenol up to 20 µg/min and adenosine injection at the dose of 24 mg. If AF was not initiated, then burst pacing is performed in the coronary sinus and atria at a lower limit of 1:1 capture or the shortest cycle length of 180 msec. AF is considered stable for mapping if it can be sustained for greater than 30 seconds.

We use an open-irrigation 3.5-mm tip ablation catheter with a large or extra-large curve (Thermacool F or J, Biosense-Webster) irrigating at 30 mL/min during lesion creation. Power settings are 35 to 50 watts throughout the atria except for the posterior wall (25-35 watts) and coronary sinus (10-30 watts). Careful power titration is required during radiofrequency (RF) to ensure complete lesion creation. RF duration is usually 10 to 60 seconds and is halted because of patient discomfort or elimination of CFAE. Because of occasional noise on the ablation catheter during RF, multiple short (15-30 seconds) applications may be used.

One of the most important aspects of CFAE ablation (and one of the most common challenges early in the learning curve of this technique) is to revisit areas that were initially ablated to ensure that there has been no recovery of electrical activity. If the patient remains in AF despite elimination of all visible CFAE, intravenous ibutilide (1 mg over 10 minutes; may repeat once to a maximum of 2 mg) is used to increase the cycle length of the arrhythmia in "nondriver" atrial tissue and highlight the remaining areas of greatest significance (eg, CFAE associated with perpetuating AF). Often during CFAE-targeted AF ablation, the arrhythmia evolves into an atrial tachyarrhythmia (AT). Using the CS catheter as a reference, the AT is subsequently mapped and ablated. Most often the sites of origin of the AT are at the same locations as the CFAE, which were targeted during the initial part of the procedure. The end points employed are either termination of AF to SR (and if the presenting rhythm was paroxysmal AF, it must not be reinducible). or elimination of all CFAE. Occasionally, a patient will remain in AF or AT after an extensive ablation eliminating all CFAE, despite the use of ibutilide. In this small group of patients, an external cardioversion is required.

It is important to emphasize that the tachycardia cycle length is almost always progressively lengthening before the termination. If there is no change in the tachycardia cycle length, the ablation may not be effective, and one must reevaluate to determine if the RF power is delivered adequately or if remapping of the CFAEs is warranted.

CLINICAL OUTCOMES

The effectiveness of CFAE ablation for treatment of AF is highlighted in our study of high-risk patients with AF.[20] Our study involved screening 2356 high-risk AF patients similar to those in the Atrial Fibrillation Follow-up Investigation of Rhythm Management (AFFIRM) trial population. Patients were at least 65 years old or had at least one or more risk factors for stroke, including hypertension, diabetes, structural heart diseases (coronary artery disease, valvular disease, cardiomyopathy, etc), a prior history of stroke or transient ischemic attack, congestive heart failure, or a left ventricular ejection fraction of <40%. We excluded patients with chronic alcoholism, recent myocardial infarction within one month of the study, significant debilitating diseases or terminal disease, and those with documented LA thrombus. After the screening of these patients for catheter ablation, we enrolled 771 patients with symptomatic refractory AF who had a high risk for stroke and, similar to those patients studied in the AFFIRM trial, were candidates for ablation.

Of the 771 patients, 674 underwent catheter ablations for AF; 39 were lost to follow-up within the three-month period after the ablation and were excluded from the study. Of the 97 patients who were not treated, 27 were excluded due to a LA thrombus and the other 70 patients declined the procedure. A total of 1065 ablations were performed on our 635 patients. There were 329 patients (52%) who underwent one procedure, 204 patients (32%) who required two procedures, 80 patients (12.6%) who required the procedure three times, and only 22 patients (3%) who required four procedures.

MAINTAINING SINUS RHYTHM AFTER CATHETER ABLATION

After a mean follow-up period of 836 ± 605 days, 517 were in SR (81.4%). AF ablations are significantly more effective in maintaining SR in patients with paroxysmal AF (226 of 254 patients [90%]) and persistent AF (124 of 146 patients [86%]) compared with those with permanent AF (167 of 235 patients [70%]). Of the 517 patients who remained in SR, only 68 patients (13%) required antiarrhythmic agents to maintain SR (48 amiodarone, 19 sotalol, and 1 dofetilide).

MORTALITY REDUCTION AFTER MAINTAINING SINUS RHYTHM FOLLOWING ABLATION

Interestingly, maintaining SR was associated with improved survival rate compared to those whose AF ablation failed to restore SR (P <0.0001). Over the follow-up period, there were 29 deaths: 15 patients who remained in SR and 14 who remained in AF died. Patients whose AF ablation was effective in maintaining SR had a much lower 5-year mortality rate (8%) than those with recurrent

258

SECTION VI
CATHETER ABLATION TECHNIQUES FOR
MANAGING ATRIAL FIBRILLATION AND
ATRIAL FLUTTER

CHAPTER 36

AF after the ablation (36%; $P < 0.0001$) (Figure 36-4). It is possible that patients whose AF ablation failed to restore SR had more advanced heart disease or unrecognized risk factors that prevented them from maintaining SR and unfavorably influenced their overall survival. However, with the exception of the LA size and duration of AF, which were greater in patients who did not respond to AF ablation, there were no differences in terms of baseline patient characteristics, including EF. Multivariate analysis and Cox regression analysis convincingly show SR to be an independent predictor of a favorable prognosis, whereas EF, hypertension, and female gender had little effect. Sinus rhythm is an independent predictor of increased survival. Patients who maintained SR regardless of baseline EF had a lower mortality rate than their counterparts on the same corresponding EF stratum (Figure 36-5).

The reason that patients who had a lower EF (<40%) but maintained SR fared better is probably the significant recovery of their ventricular function after restoring SR. The average EF increased from a mean of 31% prior to ablation to 41% following successful ablation ($P < 0.001$). In contrast, patients who had recurrent AF after ablation had no change in their EF (Figure 36-6). Our data dovetail nicely with the findings of Hsu et al[21] and Gentlesk et al[22] that many AF patients with a depressed baseline EF show improvement in their EF after SR has been restored with a successful AF ablation.

RELATION BETWEEN DISCONTINUATION OF ANTICOAGULATION THERAPY AND BLEEDING, STROKE, AND EMBOLIC INCIDENCE

Warfarin therapy was discontinued in 434 patients (72.7%) whose AF was maintained after catheter ablation. Eleven patients experienced a major stroke or TIA. In the patients who discontinued warfarin, three patients developed a major stroke and two patients had a TIA compared with six patients in the group who required ongoing anticoagulation (five ischemic strokes and one fatal intracranial hemorrhage).

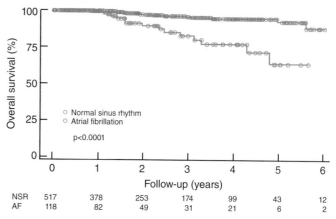

NSR	517	378	253	174	99	43	12
AF	118	82	49	31	21	6	2

FIGURE 36-4 Kaplan-Meir curve demonstrating improved survival in patients who remained in sinus rhythm from all-cause mortality compared to patients who remained in AF.

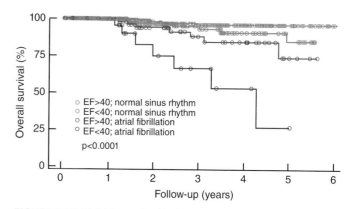

FIGURE 36-5 Multiple overlay Kaplan-Meir survival curves among four strata of patients: (1) patients with an EF >40% and NSR (orange circle); (2) patients with an EF ≤40% and NSR (green circle); (3) patients with an EF >40% and AF (magenta circle); and (4) patients with an EF ≤40% and AF (blue circle).

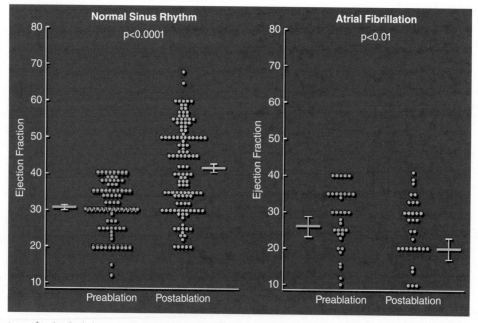

FIGURE 36-6 Comparison of individual changes of EF before and after ablation: Normal sinus rhythm (NSR) patients after ablation VS. AF patients after ablation: Pre = preablation and Post = 6-12 months postablation.

APPROACHES TO ABLATION OF ATRIAL
FIBRILLATION: FRACTIONATED ELECTROGRAMS

SECTION VI
CATHETER ABLATION TECHNIQUES FOR
MANAGING ATRIAL FIBRILLATION AND
ATRIAL FLUTTER

259

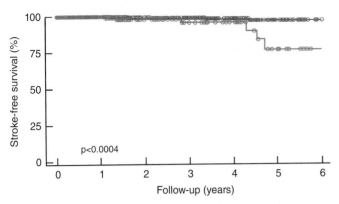

FIGURE 36-7 Comparison of stroke-free survival between the two groups of patients: those who were on Coumadin (green) and those who were not (red).

The Kaplan-Meier curves for stroke rate are shown in Figure 35-7. The 5-year stroke rate was 3% in the group of patients who were off warfarin compared with 23% in the group of patients who remained in AF and continued taking warfarin ($P = 0.004$).

PROCEDURE COMPLICATIONS

Five patients (0.9%) suffered from cerebrovascular accident (CVA). Incidentally, two of the five CVAs occurred 24 to 48 hours after the procedure. Hemopericardium occurred in seven patients (1.4%); one of these seven patients required cardiovascular surgical repair of the perforation of the LA at the ablation site, while the remaining six patients were treated successfully with pericardiocentesis. Nine patients developed major vascular complications at the groin sites (seven pseudoanerysm and two atrioventricular fistulas). Two patients developed atrioventricular block and required permanent pacemaker implantation. Three patients had a transient pulmonary edema after the procedure.

OTHER STUDIES AND CONTROVERSY

Our introduction of CFAE mapping to guide AF ablation, as an alternative to anatomical approach of PVI, spurred other investigators to follow our approach. However, our results were not fully reproduced by others.[23-25] While it is unclear what exactly the factors are underlying the differences in both acute and long-term outcomes between our studies and others, it seems likely that one or more of the following key variables may help explain the differences between these studies[26]:

• RA ablation. Other investigators often did not map and ablate the RA. We found that 15% of our patients required RA ablation; the common sites are right postero-septum, cavotricuspid isthmus, tricuspid annulus, and, rarely, posterior wall of the RA and SVC-RA junction.

• Power and duration of RF energy applications. Our power of RF applications is significantly higher than those of others. We use RF power up to 50 watts over the anterior and septal wall and 30 to 40 watts in the posterior wall that is not close to the esophagus but titrates down to about 20 to 30 watts in the areas close to the esophagus.

• Ablation endpoint. Perhaps this variable is the most significant factor influencing the differences among these studies. CFAE are low

voltage atrial signals usually ranging from 0.05 to 0.25 mV, and the areas with the very low voltage signals (between 0.05 and 0.1 mV) are often the most desirable. By contrast, other investigators defined successful lesion creation as a voltage reduction to <0.1 mV or decreased by <80%. This single factor may explain why the investigators did not have a high success rate of acute termination. In our experience, the ablation sites where AF terminated are often the sites that we had applied RF before, and often the voltage of atrial signals at these successful sites were in the range of 0.5 to 0.8 mV.

• Procedure endpoint. The procedure endpoint in our study is SR and/or complete elimination of CFAE target sites. We deliberately attempt to ablate all "new" arrhythmias including pleomorphic forms of atrial tachyarrhythmias whereas others often did not and elected to merely perform cardioversion to convert the arrhythmias to SR.

• Comprehensive mapping. Lastly, the electroanatomic map for CFAE should have high density of evenly spaced mapping points. It was unclear whether other investigators committed to detailed mapping of the CFAE; but there is no question that the key to the success of AF ablation guided by CFAE must have all areas of the atria and coronary sinus explored.

CONCLUSIONS

The above discussion and data of AF ablation guided by CFAE mapping are in contrast with previous studies in AF ablation that included largely young patients with paroxysmal AF population and show that our ablation techniques have greater benefit for the elderly and high risk populations with structural heart disease. Clearly, one must wait for more studies before recommending catheter ablation as the first line therapy for all high-risk AF patients. In the meantime, it is safe to say that catheter-based ablative approach is a promising modality for many symptomatic AF patients and that it has great potential to become the mainstay of AF treatment.

Finally, one must recognize that AF ablation, regardless of the technique, is a challenging task that requires operator skills in manipulating catheters in the atrial chambers, in understanding all facets of clinical electrophysiology, and in early recognition and treating procedure-related complications. Many of these skills could be achieved by proper training and hands-on experience after exposure to an adequate number of procedures. Advances in technology and development of new tools such as robotic navigation of catheters are being introduced at an impressive pace and will undoubtedly help electrophysiologists become more proficient in these tasks. Similarly, it is imperative that AF ablation procedures be done in centers that are well resourced with an advanced electrophysiology mapping system and ancillary equipment along with an experienced team to ensure the best possible outcome for patients.

REFERENCES

1. Haissaguerre M, Jais P, Shah DC, et al. Spontaneous initiation of atrial fibrillation by ectopic beats originating in the pulmonary veins. *N Engl J Med.* 1998;339(10):659-666.

2. Chen SA, Hsieh MH, Tai CT, et al. Initiation of atrial fibrillation by ectopic beats originating from the pulmonary veins: electrophysiological characteristics, pharmacological responses, and

260

SECTION VI
CATHETER ABLATION TECHNIQUES FOR
MANAGING ATRIAL FIBRILLATION AND
ATRIAL FLUTTER

CHAPTER 36

effects of radiofrequency ablation. *Circulation.* 1999;100: 1879-1886.

3. Haïssaguerre M, Shah DC, Jaïs P, et al. Electrophysiological breakthroughs from the left atrium to the pulmonary veins. *Circulation.* 2000;102:2463-2465.

4. Marrouch NF, Dresing T, Cole C, et al. Circular mapping and ablation of the pulmonary vein for treatment of atrial fibrillation. *J Am Coll Cardiol.* 2002;40:464-474.

5. Pappone C, Oreto G, Lamberti F, et al. Catheter ablation of paroxysmal atrial fibrillation using a 3D mapping system. *Circulation.* 1999;100:1203-1208.

6. Calkins H, Kuck KH, Cappato R, et al. 2012 HRS/EHRA/ECAS expert consensus statement on catheter and surgical ablation of atrial fibrillation: recommendations for patient selection, procedural techniques, patient management and follow-up, definitions, endpoints, and research trial design: a report of the Heart Rhythm Society (HRS) Task Force on Catheter and Surgical Ablation of Atrial Fibrillation. *Heart Rhythm.* 2012;9:632-696.

7. Cappato R, Calkins H, Chen S, et al. Worldwide survey on the methods, efficacy, and safety of catheter ablation for human atrial fibrillation. *Circulation.* 2005;111:1100-1105.

8. Konings KTS, Kirchhof CJHJ, Smeets JRLM, et al. High-density mapping of electrically induced atrial fibrillation in humans. *Circulation.* 1994;89:1665-1680.

9. Konings KTS, Smeets JLRM, Penn OC, et al. Configuration of unipolar atrial electrograms during electrically induced atrial fibrillation in humans. *Circulation.* 1997;95:1231-1241.

10. Nademanee K, McKenzie J, Kosar E, et al. A new approach for catheter ablation of atrial fibrillation: mapping of electrophysiologic substrate. *J Am Coll Cardiol.* 2004;43:2044-2053.

11. Jaïs P, Haïssaguerre M, Shah DC, et al. Regional disparities of endocardial atrial activation in paroxysmal atrial fibrillation. *Pacing Clin Electrophysiol.* 1996;19(pt 2):1998-2003.

12. Kalifa J, Tanaka K, Zaitsev AV, et al. Mechanisms of wave fractionation at boundaries of high-frequency excitation in the posterior left atrium of the isolated sheep heart during atrial fibrillation. *Circulation.* 2006;113:626-633.

13. Quan KJ, Lee JH, Van Hare GF, Biblo LA, Mackall, JA Carlson MD. Identification and characterization of atrioventricular parasympathetic innervation in humans. *J Cardiovasc Electrophysiol.* 2002;13:735-739.

14. Scherlag BJ, Nakagawa H, Jackman WM, et al. Electrical stimulation to identify neural elements on the heart: their role in atrial fibrillation. *J Interv Card Electrophysiol.* 2005:13:37-42.

15. Armour JA, Murphy DA, Yuan BX, et al. Gross and microscopic anatomy of the human intrinsic cardiac nervous system. *Anat Rec.* 1997;247:289-298.

16. Pauza DH, Skripka V, Pauziene N, Stropus R. Morphology, distribution, and variability of the epicardial neural ganglionated subplexuses in the human heart. *Anat Rec.* 2000;259:353-382.

17. Scherlag BJ, Yamanashi W, Patel U, et al. Autonomically induced conversion of pulmonary vein focal firing into atrial fibrillation. *J Am Coll Cardiol.* 2005;45:1878-1886.

18. Patterson E, Po SS, Scherlag BJ, et al. Triggered firing in pulmonary veins initiated by in vitro autonomic nerve stimulation. *Heart Rhythm.* 2005;2:624-631.

19. Nademanee K, Schwab M, Porath J, Abbo R. How to perform electrogram guided atrial fibrillation ablation. *Heart Rhythm.* 2006;3:981-984.

20. Nademanee K, Schwab MC, Kosar EM, et al. Clinical outcomes of catheter substrate ablation for high-risk patients with atrial fibrillation. *J Am Coll Cardiol.* 2008;51:843-849.

21. Hsu LF, Jais P. Sanders P, et al. Catheter ablation for atrial fibrillation in congestive heart failure. *N Engl J Med.* 2004;351:2373-2383.

22. Gentlesk PJ, Sauer WH, Gerstenfeld EP, et al. Reversal of the left ventricular dysfunction following ablation of atrial fibrillation. *J Cardiovasc Electrophysiol.* 2007; 18:9-14.

23. Oral H, Chugh A, Good E, et al. Radiofrequency catheter ablation of chronic atrial fibrillation guided by complex electrograms. *Circulation.* 2007;115:2606-2612.

24. Schmitt C, Estner H, Hecher B, et al. Radiofrequency ablation of complex fractionated atrial electrograms (CFAE): preferential sites of acute termination and regularization in paroxysmal and persistent atrial fibrillation. *J Cardiovasc Electrophysiol.* 2007;18:1039-1046.

25. Verma A, Sanders P, Champagne J, et al. Selective complex fractionated atrial electrograms targeting for atrial fibrillation study (SELECT AF) a multicenter, randomized trial. *Circ Arrhythm Electrophysiol.* 2014;7(1):55-56.

26. Nademanee K. Trials and travails of electrogram-guided ablation of chronic atrial fibrillation. *Circulation.* 2007;115:2592-2594.

37 APPROACHES TO ATRIAL FIBRILLATION: CRYOABLATION

Justin Ng, MBBS, Chirag Barbhaiya, MD, Gregory Michaud, MD

CASE PRESENTATION

The patient is a 58-year-old man with a long-standing history of paroxysmal atrial fibrillation and flutter. On sotalol he developed atrial flutter and underwent a right-sided cavotricuspid isthmus flutter ablation. He was switched to dofetilide, but continued to have breakthrough episodes of symptomatic atrial fibrillation (AF). A decision was made to proceed with pulmonary vein isolation.

A preprocedural MRI was performed confirming suitable anatomy for pulmonary vein isolation with cryoballoon ablation. Isolation of the left pulmonary veins resulted in termination of AF. Pacing of the phrenic nerve was performed from the SVC during ablation of the right-sided veins. Two minutes into the first cryoapplication to the right superior pulmonary vein (RSPV), phrenic nerve capture diminished, indicating injury to the phrenic nerve. Despite immediate termination of the freeze, phrenic nerve capture was lost completely, and by case end the phrenic nerve had not recovered.

The patient continued to have persistent elevation of the right hemidiaphragm until about 1 year postablation (Figure 37-1), after which he became asymptomatic.

EXPERT OPINION

This case highlights the risk of phrenic nerve palsy associated with cryoballoon ablation and the importance of early recognition of injury to the phrenic nerve. The course of the phrenic nerve typically traverses anterior to the right-sided pulmonary veins and may be injured during cryoapplication, particularly in the RSPV. A pacing catheter is usually inserted in a superior part of the superior vena cava to pace the phrenic nerve continuously during ablation. The simplest method of determining phrenic nerve capture is direct palpation of the abdomen to confirm contraction of the right hemidiaphragm. Phrenic injury during cryoapplication is often first recognized by reduced strength of diaphragmatic capture. Many other methods to determine phrenic capture have been developed, including direct measurement of diaphragmatic potentials via surface electrodes, and other means to detect the contraction, such as visualization with intracardiac ultrasound, auditory surveillance with Doppler ultrasound, and others. The earlier phrenic nerve injury is detected, the faster the recovery of diaphragmatic function, which often occurs by the end of the procedure.

Despite taking all these precautions, phrenic nerve paralysis will still occur, and often the patient is very symptomatic, with a recovery period of up to a year or more.

INTRODUCTION

The mainstay of an ablative approach to paroxysmal AF is pulmonary vein isolation using a single-tip radiofrequency catheter. In an attempt

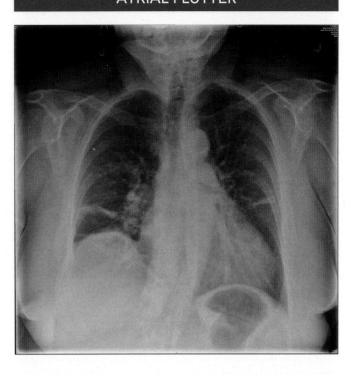

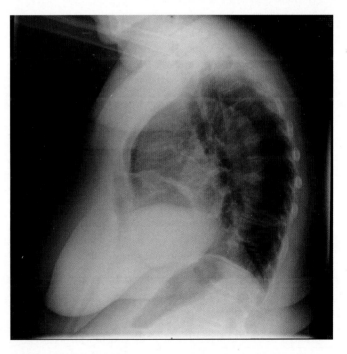

FIGURE 37-1A AND 37-1B PA (A) and lateral (B) chest radiograph demonstrating elevated right hemidiaphragm due to phrenic nerve injury following cryoablation.

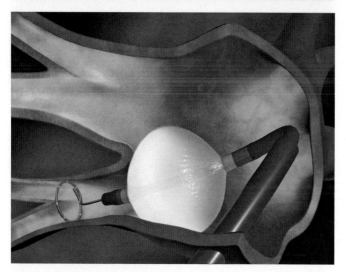

FIGURE 37-2 Illustration of the Medtronic Arctic Front cryoballoon catheter within a steerable sheath, with the Achieve spiral mapping catheter within the central lumen of the catheter. (Reproduced with permission of Medtronic, Inc.)

to eliminate the need for point-by-point ablation, balloon-based ablation systems have been developed to produce circumferential lesions.

The most commonly used system is the Medtronic Arctic Front over-the-wire cryoballoon catheter. The catheter is introduced into the left atrium through a 12-Fr steerable sheath. The shaft of the cryoballoon catheter has a central lumen that can accommodate a wire or allow the passage of a spiral catheter for real time mapping and is used for injection of saline or contrast (Figure 37-2).

The inner balloon of the cryoballoon catheter is cooled to a temperature of $-112°F$ ($-80°C$) with nitrous oxide.[1] The cold outer skin of the balloon adheres to the underlying tissue (much like a tongue on a frozen metal pole), and a large thermal gradient removes heat causing irreversible cellular injury below $23°F$ ($0°C$). Cryothermal energy produces progressive necrosis but does not result in significant alteration of tissue structure at thaw.[2] The cryothermal lesion formation can be divided in three sequential stages: the freeze/thaw phase, the hemorrhagic inflammatory phase, and the replacement fibrosis phase stage.[2] Theoretically, the absence of endothelial disruption with cryoablation is thought to result in less thrombogenicity.[2]

PATIENT SELECTION

- Cryoablation is reserved for patients with drug-refractory symptomatic paroxysmal AF for which pulmonary vein isolation is the mainstay of therapy. It is not ideal for the patient with persistent or chronic AF where additional lesion sets are generally required, since additional ablation catheters are often necessary.

- We strongly recommend the use of imaging prior to the procedure with either a CT pulmonary venogram or an MRI to assess the suitability of the pulmonary venous anatomy for the balloon and to assist with sizing of the cryoballoon.

ADVANTAGES

- Shorter time to proficiency than point-by-point radiofrequency catheter ablation.

- Less dependent on operator dexterity.

- Potentially shorter procedural and fluoroscopy times in nonrandomized trials.[3]

DISADVANTAGES

- Not cost-effective if additional ablation is required to treat non-PV sources of arrhythmia, as is commonly encountered in patients with persistent AF, or if PV isolation cannot be achieved a high percentage of the time with cryoablation.

- Certain venous anatomy less compatible with cryoballoon ablation such as a large common left pulmonary vein trunk (Figure 37-3).

- Higher incidence of phrenic nerve paralysis.[4]

KEY PROCEDURAL STEPS

- Access: Given that most patients do not interrupt anticoagulation for the PVI procedure, safe vascular access is essential. We recommend micropuncture kits (21 gauge needle and 4 French dilator) for initial venous access prior to exchanging for larger sheaths. A minimum of two venous sheaths are required; one is exchanged for the steerable 12 Fr sheath after transseptal puncture and another as a conduit for a catheter to pace the phrenic nerve, which can be as small as 4 Fr. In our lab, we typically place a third venous sheath for the placement of a coronary sinus catheter and a fourth for placement of an intracardiac echocardiogram (ICE) probe (Figures 37-4 and 37-5).

- Transeptal puncture: At our institution, the transeptal puncture is initially performed with a fixed curve sheath, such as the 8.5-Fr SL-1, with the 12-Fr steerable cryoballoon sheath exchanged over an 0.035" relatively stiff J-tip guide wire.

- Anticoagulation: Prior to transeptal access, a bolus of 80 to 120 units/kg of unfractionated heparin is administered, depending on the patient's INR, followed by boluses every 20 to 30 minutes to maintain the ACT >350s.

- The only commercially available cryoballoon in the United States is the Medtronic Arctic Front CryoAblation Catheter. It comes in 23 mm and 28 mm balloon sizes. We rarely choose a 23-mm balloon, unless the largest PV size is 15 mm or less. The central lumen accommodates a spiral catheter (Achieve) for mapping and confirming isolation, which we use in place of a guide wire.

- Documentation of pulmonary vein electrical activity is performed with the mapping catheter prior to any ablation.

- Positioning the cryoballoon:

  1. The guidewire or mapping catheter is advanced into the target vein, which we visualize using ICE (Figure 37-6A).

  2. The cryoballoon is inflated in the body of the atrium as visualized on ICE or fluoroscopy (Figure 37-6B).

  3. The inflated cryoballoon is advanced into the antrum of the vein using ICE and fluoroscopy (Figure 37-6C).

  4. Cryoapplication begins only after occlusion of the vein is confirmed.

  5. Firm pressure should be applied during the first 60 to 90 seconds until freezing occurs and the balloon adheres.

  6. Two to three applications of 4 minutes duration is recommended, although shorter periods are being investigated using the newest

APPROACHES TO ATRIAL
FIBRILLATION:
CRYOABLATION

SECTION VI
CATHETER ABLATION TECHNIQUES FOR
MANAGING ATRIAL FIBRILLATION AND
ATRIAL FLUTTER

263

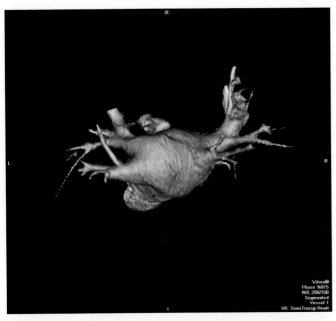

FIGURE 37-3 CT venogram of the left atrium showing a large common left pulmonary vein trunk, which is usually not suitable for cryoablation.

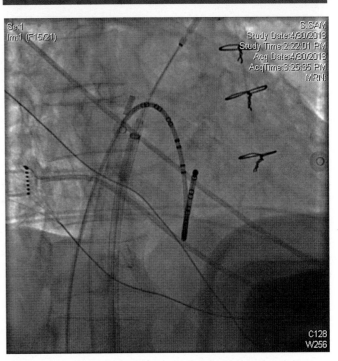

FIGURE 37-5 RAO view of the set-up in Figure 37-4.

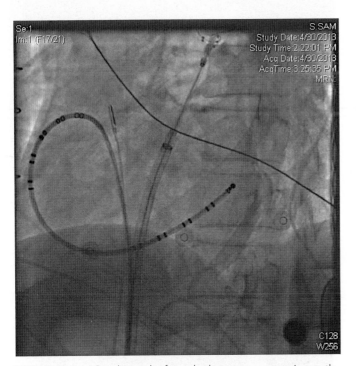

FIGURE 37-4 LAO radiograph of standard set up: coronary sinus catheter, ablation catheter in SVC for phrenic nerve pacing, cryoballoon at antrum of left upper pulmonary vein, ICE catheter imaging from the right atrium at the level of the fossa.

generation of the cryoballoon, the Arctic Front Advance, which has more uniform cooling patterns on the outer surface and may require less application time and perhaps fewer applications.

• Assessing adequacy of venous occlusion: Complete occlusion of the pulmonary vein is necessary for successful isolation. Any leakage of blood around the balloon will limit the fall in temperature required for effective ablation.

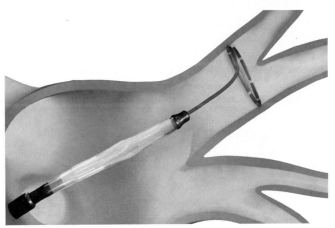

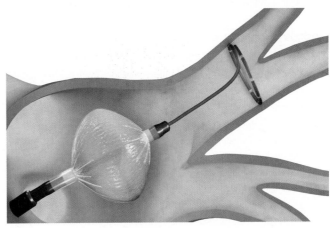

FIGURE 37-6 Steps in positioning the cryoballoon: (A) mapping catheter advanced into the target vein; (B) cryoballoon is inflated in the body of the atrium; (C) inflated cryoballoon is advanced into the antrum of the target vein. (Reproduced with permission of Medtronic, Inc.)

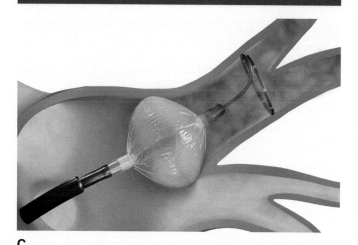

C

FIGURE 37-6 (Continued)

1. The traditional method for confirming total occlusion of the vein is the injection of contrast though the balloon's tip lumen under fluoroscopy, while observing accumulation of contrast in the PV without flow back the left atrium.

2. At our institution, ICE with color flow Doppler is used as an alternative to assess for leaks (Figures 37-7 and 37-8).

- A surrogate for PV occlusion is the rate of drop in temperature measured in the balloon and the ultimate temperature achieved. Studies have shown that cryoballoon temperature achieved predicts acute pulmonary vein isolation; however, no cutoff value is practical because of the wide spread in temperatures associated with occlusion[5] (Figure 37-9).

- Another surrogate is the time it takes to achieve PV isolation as observed on the circular mapping catheter. Most occluded PVs will be electrically isolated by 30 to 60 seconds after the application has begun (Figure 37-10).

- Confirming isolation: The circular mapping catheter is used to confirm pulmonary vein isolation. Typically, the inferior surface of the right inferior vein is difficult to isolate and may require reangulation of the balloon, rewiring other branches of the same PV to provide a different angle of approach and other techniques.

TROUBLESHOOTING THE DIFFICULT CASE

- Techniques to achieve venous occlusion:

1. Positioning the guidewire in different venous branches may aid in changing the balloon orientation in the antrum to achieve venous occlusion.

2. The "pull down" technique can be useful when a gap is present in the inferior border of the vein. Freezing is commenced despite the presence of the gap. At 60 to 90 seconds into the freeze, the balloon and the sheath are both gently pulled down in order to close the gap in the inferior portion of the vein. With the new generation cryoballoon, this technique is rarely necessary, since small gaps will often seal during the cryoapplication.

AVOIDING COMPLICATIONS

- Avoiding phrenic nerve paralysis: During freezing of the right pulmonary veins, the phrenic nerve may be damaged, especially when

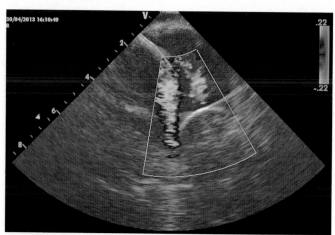

FIGURE 37-7 ICE catheter image of the cryoballoon in the left inferior pulmonary vein with a large leak demonstrated by color flow Doppler.

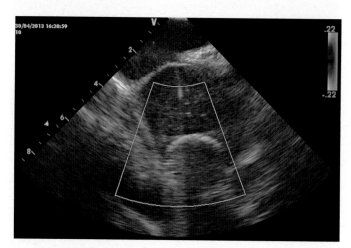

FIGURE 37-8 Adjustment of the cryoballoon in the left inferior pulmonary vein results in occlusion of the vein and closure of the leak.

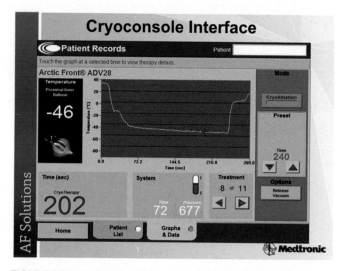

FIGURE 37-9 The Medtronic Cryoconsole Interface demonstrating an appropriate fall in balloon temperature with appropriate venous occlusion. (Reproduced with permission of Medtronic, Inc.)

APPROACHES TO ATRIAL
FIBRILLATION:
CRYOABLATION

SECTION VI
CATHETER ABLATION TECHNIQUES FOR
MANAGING ATRIAL FIBRILLATION AND
ATRIAL FLUTTER   265

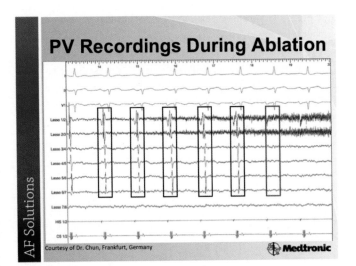

FIGURE 37-10 Isolation of pulmonary vein during cryoapplication. (Reproduced with permission of Medtronic, Inc.)

ablating the right superior PV. A number of techniques can be used to minimize the risk of this complication.

1. Pacing the phrenic nerve during ablation on the right: A catheter is placed in the SVC in a position to capture the phrenic nerve and freezing is performed during pacing of the right phrenic nerve. Loss of capture should prompt immediate termination of the freeze. It is important to capture the phrenic nerve proximal to where the potential injury will occur, and in the case of general anesthesia, also to remind the anesthetist to avoid paralytic agents.

2. Use of the larger 28 mm balloon: Use of the larger 28 mm balloon results in a more antral lesion, which theoretically will reduce the risk of phrenic nerve palsy (PNP).[1]

CLINICAL STUDIES AND OUTCOMES

- In the largest prospective study, 346 patients in 3 centers with drug refractory paroxysmal AF (n = 293) or persistent AF (n = 53) underwent cryoablation. At 12 months follow-up, 74% of the PAF group and 42% of the persistent group remained in sinus rhythm.[6]

- In a recent meta-analysis of cryoballoon ablation studies reporting a 3-month blanking period (time frame during which transient arrhythmias were not considered recurrences), at 1-year follow-up, 72.8% were free from recurrent AF.[4]

- The STOP-AF trial, randomized patients with PAF in a 2:1 fashion to either PV isolation with cryoballoon or antiarrhythmic drug (AAD). Balloon-only isolation of PVs was achieved in 90.8%. The success rate at 12-month follow-up was 69.9%, that is, patients free of symptomatic AF off AAD (60.1% with a single procedure).[7]

- Nonrandomized controlled trials have showed similar short-term efficacy compared with RF ablation along with slightly shorter procedural and fluoroscopic times.[3] The Freeze AF trial is a randomized controlled trial currently underway to compare cryoballoon catheter ablation with open-irrigated RF ablation.

- Procedural times: In the STOP AF trial the mean procedural duration was 371 minutes (range 200-650) with 62.8 (8-229) minutes fluoroscopy time.[7] In the subanalysis of operator experience presented at the 2011 Boston AF symposium, experience with the cryoballoon reduced procedure time by 15% and fluoroscopy time by 24% compared to first-time users.[8]

COMPLICATIONS

- Phrenic nerve palsy (PNP): The most common complication of cryoballoon ablation is PNP with an incidence of 6.38% in a recent meta-analysis. In the STOP AF study, PNP was reported in 29 out of 259 procedures (11.2%). Of these, only 4 patients (13.8%) had persistent PNP at 12 months and 1 had symptoms.[7]

- Pulmonary vein stenosis: STOP AF demonstrated 3.1% risk of PV stenosis in its study population defined as a >75% narrowing.[7]

- Atrial-esophageal fistula: There have been case reports of this catastrophic complication, but a true incidence is unknown. The incidence of Atrial-esophageal fistula using cryoablation appears less commonly then with RF ablation.

- Comparable with RF ablation, the incidence of thromboembolic complications including periprocedural stroke, TIA, or MI was 0.57%, and pericardial effusion or tamponade occurred in 1.46% of cases.[4]

- The incidence of secondary left atrial tachycardia following cryoablation is low.

CONCLUSION

The cryoballoon provides a comparable alternative to point-by-point RF ablation in patients with drug refractory paroxysmal atrial fibrillation where complete isolation of the pulmonary veins is the mainstay of therapy. Imaging is useful to select the appropriate patient for this therapy, and knowledge of the potential complications and the techniques used to minimize these are essential for a safe and successful procedure.

REFERENCES

1. Kühne M, Sticherling C. Cryoballoon ablation for pulmonary vein isolation of atrial fibrillation: a better way to complete the circle? *Innovations (Phila)*. 2011;2:264-270.

2. Lustgarten DL, Keane D, Ruskin J. Cryothermal ablation: mechanism of tissue injury and current experience in the treatment of tacharrhythmias. *Prog Cardiovasc Dis*. 1999;41(6):481-498.

3. Kojodjojo P, O'Neill MD, Lim PB, et al. Pulmonary venous isolation by antral ablation with a large cryoballoon for treatment of paroxysmal and persistent atrial fibrillation: medium-term outcomes and non-randomised comparison with pulmonary venous isolation by radiofrequency ablation. *Heart*. 2010:96,(17):1379-1384.

4. Andrade JG, Khairy P, Guerra PG, et al. Efficacy and safety of cryoballoon ablation for atrial fibrillation—a systematic review of published studies. *Heart Rhythm*. 2011;8(9):1828.

5. Fürnkranz A, Koster I, Chun KR, et al. Cryoballoon temperature predicts acute pulmonary vein isolation. *Heart Rhythm*. 2011;8(6):821-9.

6. Neumann T, Vogt J, Schumacher B, et al. Circumferential pulmonary vein isolation with the cryoballoon technique results from a

SECTION VI
CATHETER ABLATION TECHNIQUES FOR
MANAGING ATRIAL FIBRILLATION AND
ATRIAL FLUTTER

266

CHAPTER 37

prospective 3-center study. *J Am Coll Cardiol.* 2008;52(4): 273-278.

7. Packer D, Irwin JM, Champagne J, et al. Cryoballoon ablation of pulmonary veins for paroxysmal atrial fibrillation: first results of the North American Arctic Front STOP- AF pivotal trial. *J Am Coll Cardiol.* 2010;55:E3015-3016.

8. T Bunch. Cryoballoon ablation for atrial fibrillation. Is it the right choice for my practice? *Innovations (Phila).* 2011;2:272-273.

9. Van Belle Y, Janse P, Theuns D, Szili-Torok T, Jordaens L. One year follow-up after cryoballoon isolation of the pulmonary veins in patients with paroxysmal atrial fibrillation. *Europace.* 2008;10(11):1271-1276.

TECHNOLOGIES
FOR ABLATION OF ATRIAL FIBRILLATION:
DUTY-CYCLE ABLATION

SECTION VI
CATHETER ABLATION TECHNIQUES FOR
MANAGING ATRIAL FIBRILLATION AND
ATRIAL FLUTTER

267

38 TECHNOLOGIES FOR ABLATION OF ATRIAL FIBRILLATION: DUTY-CYCLE ABLATION

John D. Hummel, MD

CASE PRESENTATION

A 67-year-old man presented with a 3-year history of atrial fibrillation (AF) that was symptomatic with dyspnea on exertion. He underwent echocardiography as well as treadmill nuclear stress testing revealing a left ventricular ejection fraction of 40% without evidence of significant valve or coronary artery disease. The left ventricle was diffusely hypokinetic. Holter monitoring revealed rate-controlled atrial fibrillation. He was initially treated with sotalol and spontaneously converted to and maintained NSR for approximately 14 months with resolution of his cardiomyopathy. His symptomatic AF then recurred, and the patient required two cardioversions with early recurrence of AF, which remained persistent. He presented with dyspnea on moderate exertion and complaints of mild swelling in his lower extremities. His left ventricular ejection fraction was globally depressed with an ejection fraction of 40%. The patient was referred for ablation of his AF and was enrolled in the TTOP-AF trial (a randomized, prospective trial of antiarrhythmic medical therapy versus phased-RF ablation therapy).[1] He was randomized to curative ablation, utilizing three specially designed catheters (Figure 38-1). The patient underwent percutaneous catheter placement in the left atrium with pulmonary vein isolation using the PVAC catheter (Figures 38-2 and 38-3). Pulmonary vein isolation was followed by septal ablation with the MASC catheter (Figure 38-4). Subsequent ablation of complex fractionated atrial electrograms using the MAAC catheter completed the procedure (Figure 38-5).

EPIDEMIOLOGY

AF and heart failure (HF) are two of the most pervasive cardiovascular diseases, costing millions of people loss of quality of life and a decrease in survival. AF affects over 2 million Americans, and the lifetime risk of developing AF for adults aged >40 is 25%, while the AF population carries an elevated risk of developing heart failure in the range of 20%.[2-4]

ETIOLOGY AND PATHOPHYSIOLOGY

The causes of AF are myriad, and AF and HF represent a deadly intersection with AF promoting HF and HF promoting AF as AF is present in 5% of NYHA class I patients and up to 50% of NYHA class IV patients.[5] AF can promote HF through rapid ventricular rates, poor

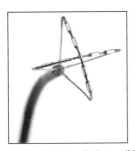

A) Multi Array Ablation Catheter (MAAC)

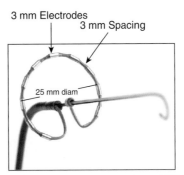

B) Pulmonary Vein Ablation Catheter (PVAC)

3 mm Electrodes
3 mm Spacing
25 mm diam

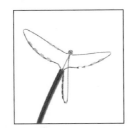

C) Multi Array Septal Catheter (MASC)

FIGURE 38-1 The three primary catheters for phased radiofrequency energy delivery are (A) the MAAC used for targeting regions of complex fractionated electrograms or creating areas of ablation in the body of the left atrium such as the LA roof and mitral isthmus; (B) the PVAC placed in the pulmonary veins over a guidewire and rotated between RF applications to allow electrical isolation of the pulmonary veins; (C) the MASC delivered through the transseptal sheath, pulled back against the septum and rotated between RF applications to eliminate septal electrical activity.

atrial transport, or the irregularity of ventricular contraction. Resolution of AF can result in reverse remodeling and restoration of atrial and ventricular cellular and mechanical function as evidenced by trials comparing AF ablation versus atrioventricular nodal ablation with cardiac resynchronization pacing or medical therapy.[6,7]

MANAGEMENT

Patients with persistent AF have lower success rates than those with paroxysmal AF, and the use of phased RF in the persistent AF population was examined in the TTOP-AF trial as an initial step in assessing efficacy of a different form of RF ablation in this challenging population. Although no benefit has been demonstrated for attempted medical rhythm control over rate control, several studies of AF and CHF suggest clear benefit with restoration of NSR via AF ablation.[7] This may indicate that the deleterious effects of medication offset the beneficial effects of restoration of NSR in previous studies. This patient was enrolled in the TTOP-AF trial. Patients who had failed at least one antiarrhythmic drug were randomized to phased-RF ablation or antiarrhythmic drug. The primary endpoints of TTOP-AF included chronic effectiveness and safety at 6 months and acute safety within 7 days of the ablation.

At 6 months, a greater proportion of ablation patients achieved effectiveness (77/138; 55.8%) compared with medically managed patients (19/72; 26.4%) ($p < 0.0001$). Acutely, 92.8% of procedures were successful, while 12.3% experienced a serious procedure and/or device-related adverse event. The predefined acute safety end point was not met. This trial demonstrated superiority of phased-RF AF ablation over medical therapy but with a higher than expected risk of clinical stroke. Thus, the phased RF system

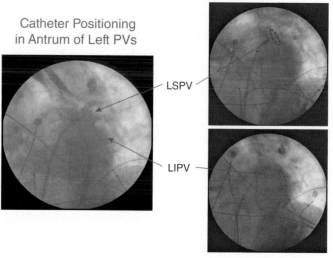

Catheter Positioning in Antrum of Left PVs

LSPV

LIPV

FIGURE 38-2 Fluoroscopic image of the PVAC deployed in the left superior and inferior veins to allow energy delivery.

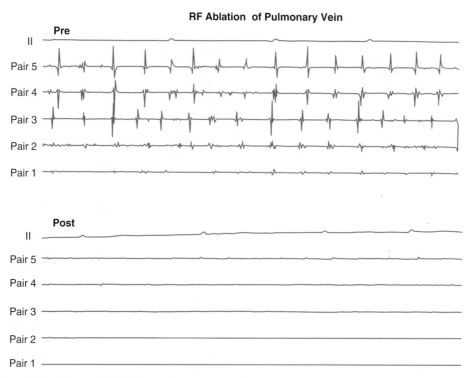

FIGURE 38-3 Elimination of PV activity in the left inferior pulmonary vein after RF delivery.

TECHNOLOGIES
FOR ABLATION OF ATRIAL FIBRILLATION:
DUTY-CYCLE ABLATION

SECTION VI
CATHETER ABLATION TECHNIQUES FOR MANAGING ATRIAL FIBRILLATION AND ATRIAL FLUTTER

269

was approved as efficacious by the FDA panel, but rejected for use in the United States due to safety concerns, which are now being addressed after catheter and protocol modifications embodied in the Victory AF trial.

THE TECHNOLOGY

The Phased RF system (Medtronic Ablation Frontiers, Carlsbad, CA, United States) employs three multielectrode catheters to deliver duty-cycled, phased energy via a multichannel RF generator to targeted left atrial regions (Figure 38-1). Phase-shifted energy delivery between adjacent catheter electrodes (bipolar) and return electrodes (unipolar) allows creation of long, contiguous lesions. Modulating unipolar-to-bipolar RF ratios controls lesion depth (Figures 38-6 and 38-7). RF is delivered in temperature-controlled and power-limited fashion (140°F [60°C], 8 or 10 watts) with typical duration of 60 seconds, with the lower power limits being all that is needed due to increased current density on the small electrodes.

PATIENT OUTCOME

The phased-RF procedure was uncomplicated and successful in maintaining sinus rhythm off antiarrhythmic therapy. Three months postablation the patient's echocardiogram demonstrated recovery of normal left ventricular function.

3 Spline Catheter – Septal Positioning

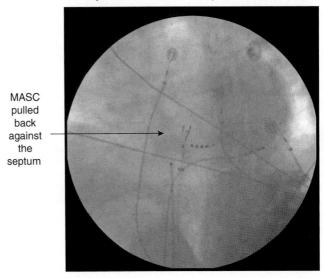

MASC pulled back against the septum →

FIGURE 38-4 Position of the MASC against the septum on fluoroscopy.

LA Roof and Floor Ablation Sites

MAAC at roof line

MAAC at mitral annulus

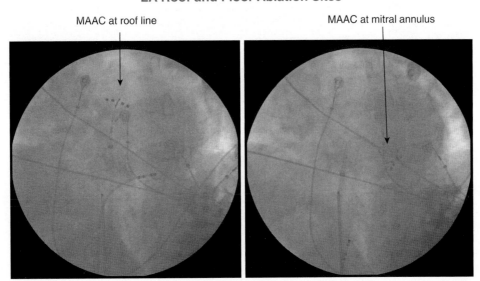

FIGURE 38-5 Position of the MAAC catheter on flouroscopy along the left atrial roof line and between the left inferior pulmonary vein and the mitral isthmus.

Radiofrequency Energy Modes

- Five different selectable energy modes:

  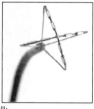

  – Unipolar only
  – 1:1 (50% bipolar, 50% unipolar)
  – 2:1 (66% bipolar, 33% unipolar)
  – 4:1 (80% bipolar, 20% unipolar)
  – Bipolar only

- Modes allow user to control lesion depth and fill:

Depth				
Unipolar only	1:1	2:1	4:1	Bipolar only
Fill				

FIGURE 38-6 Schematic diagram of decreasing lesion depth and increasing lesion fill between electrodes as phasing of RF energy transitions from primarily unipolar to primarily bipolar.

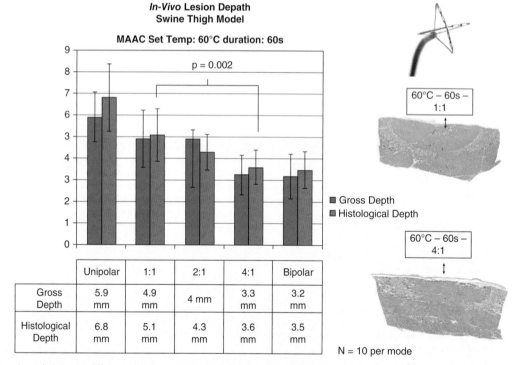

In-Vivo Lesion Depath
Swine Thigh Model

MAAC Set Temp: 60°C duration: 60s

p = 0.002

■ Gross Depth
■ Histological Depth

	Unipolar	1:1	2:1	4:1	Bipolar
Gross Depth	5.9 mm	4.9 mm	4 mm	3.3 mm	3.2 mm
Histological Depth	6.8 mm	5.1 mm	4.3 mm	3.6 mm	3.5 mm

60°C – 60s – 1:1

60°C – 60s – 4:1

N = 10 per mode

FIGURE 38-7 Preclinical data on differing degrees of lesion depth based on differing ratios of unipolar to bipolar phasing of the RF energy delivery to swine thigh muscle in a perfused tissue bath.

TECHNOLOGIES
FOR ABLATION OF ATRIAL FIBRILLATION:
DUTY-CYCLE ABLATION

SECTION VI
CATHETER ABLATION TECHNIQUES FOR
MANAGING ATRIAL FIBRILLATION AND
ATRIAL FLUTTER

271

REFERENCES

1. Hummel J, Michaud G, Hoyt R, et al. Phased RF ablation of persistent atrial fibrillation. *Heart Rhythm*. 2014;11(2): 202-209.

2. Lloyd-Jones DM, Larson MG, Leip EP, et al. Lifetime risk for developing congestive heart failure: the Framingham Heart Study. *Circulation*. 2002;106(24):3068-3072.

3. Roger VL, Go AS, Lloyd-Jones DM, et al. Heart disease and stroke statistics—2011 update: a report from the American Heart Association. *Circulation*. 2011;123:e18-e209.

4. Lloyd-Jones DM, Wang TJ, Leip EP, et al. Lifetime risk for development of atrial fibrillation: the Framingham Heart Study. *Circulation*. 2004;110:1042-1046.

5. Maisel WH, Stevenson LW. Atrial fibrillation in heart failure: epidemiology, pathophysiology, and rationale for therapy. *Am J Cardiol*. 2003;91:2D-8D.

6. Carson PE, Johnson GR, Dunkman WB, Fletcher RD, Farrell L, Cohn JN. The influence of atrial fibrillation on prognosis in mild to moderate heart failure: theV-HeFT Studies. *Circulation*. 1993;87(6 Suppl):VI102-110.

7. Khan MN, Jaïs P, Cummings J, et al. Pulmonary-vein isolation for atrial fibrillation in patients with heart failure. *N Engl J Med*. 2008;359:1778-1785.

8. Dagres N, Varounis C, Gaspar T, et al. Catheter ablation for atrial fibrillation in patients with left ventricular systolic dysfunction. A systematic review and meta-analysis. *J Card Fail*. 2011;17:964-970.

272

SECTION VI
CATHETER ABLATION TECHNIQUES FOR
MANAGING ATRIAL FIBRILLATION AND
ATRIAL FLUTTER

CHAPTER 39

39 TECHNOLOGIES FOR ABLATION OF ATRIAL FIBRILLATION: ROTOR MAPPING

Ismail Hamam, MD, and John D. Hummel, MD

CASE PRESENTATION

A 61-year-old woman was brought to the electrophysiology (EP) laboratory for catheter-based atrial fibrillation (AF) ablation. She was diagnosed with AF 3 years ago and has history of stroke and hypertension. She failed AF ablation 6 months ago, and despite treatment with drondedarone and sotalol, she continues to have recurrent symptomatic episodes of AF. An implantable loop recorder was placed for AF monitoring.

After discontinuation of the sotalol for 3 days and exclusion of left atrial (LA) thrombus by tranesophageal echocardiography, the patient was brought to the EP lab, and 3 venous sheaths were introduced into the right femoral vein and 2 venous sheaths into the left femoral vein. The patient presented in normal sinus rhythm, and AF was induced by isoproterenol infusion and rapid atrial pacing.

Initially, the circular mapping catheter was advanced to the right atrium (RA) and the SVC, and an electroanatomic RA shell was created using a 3-D mapping system. Under intracardiac echo guidance, the first transseptal puncture was performed with advancement of the circular mapping catheter into the LA. The circular mapping catheter was used to create an electroanatomic LA shell including the pulmonary veins using a 3-D electroanatomic mapping system. Through an 8.5-F steerable sheath, a 64-pole basket catheter was carefully advanced to the RA body and then to the LA body, and the position of each basket spline was correlated to the electroanatomic shell (Figures 39-1 to 39-3).

In each atria, after basket insertion and careful positioning, meticulous computer-based AF signal analysis was performed using specialized software (Topera, San Diego, CA, United States). After localizing these rotors in relation to the basket electrodes, radiofrequency (RF) ablation of these sites was applied in both atria (Figures 39-4 to 39-7). After matching the signal location in relation to the basket electrodes and confirming the signals with repeat recordings, several RF applications were applied to the site, which resulted in slowing and organization of the AF (see Figure 39-6). In the LA there was another rotor signal recorded on the posterior wall. Applying several RF applications resulted in acute termination of the AF to normal sinus rhythm (see Figure 39-7). The rotor ablation was complemented by conventional pulmonary vein isolation. On follow-up after 3 months, the patient was free of symptoms, and loop recorder interrogation showed no evidence of AF.

EPIDEMIOLOGY AND PATHOPHYSIOLOGY

AF is the most common human arrhythmia and is characterized by chaotic contraction of the atrium. Mechanisms of AF can be divided into the mechanisms of initiation and mechanisms of perpetuation of arrhythmia. There are three widely held theories on the mechanisms of AF perpetuation: multiple random propagating wavelets, focal electrical discharges, and localized reentrant activity with fibrillatory conduction.

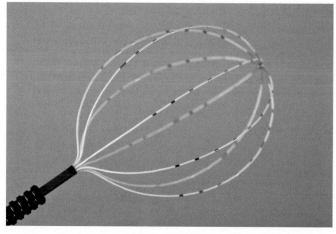

FIGURE 39-1 The 64-pole Constellation basket mapping catheter is shown. It consists of eight splies, and each spline has eight electrodes.

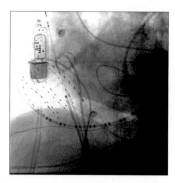

FIGURE 39-2 The 64-pole Constellation basket mapping catheter deployed in the right atrium. An implantable loop recorder, 20-pole steerable catheter, and circular mapping catheter are also seen in the fluoroscopic image.

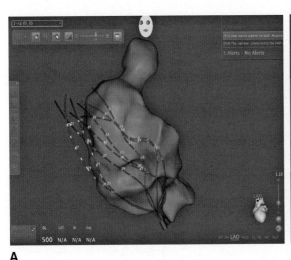
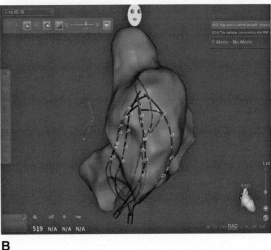

A   **B**

FIGURE 39-3 (A) An LAO image of a 3-dimensional shell of the right atrium derived from an intracardiac roving mapping catheter with the 64-pole basket catheter overlaid. The basket catheter clearly lies outside the shell of the atrium revealing a lack of complete reconstruction of the atrium with the roving catheter. (B) An RAO image of a 3-dimensional shell of the right atrium derived from an intracardiac roving mapping catheter with the 64-pole basket catheter overlaid.

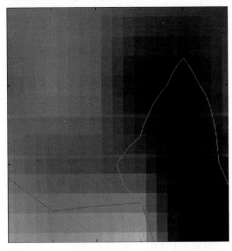
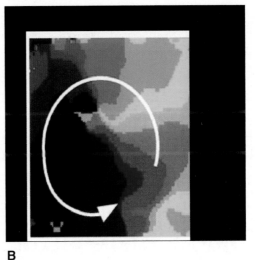

A   **B**

FIGURE 39-4 (A) The image is a still frame of a movie depicting the rotation of the rotor around the central core depicted by the red spot. This movie was created from the electrograms recorded from the basket electrode during AF. The signals are then processed to identify a rotor. (B) The right image is a map of the wavefront of activation of the rotor around its core.

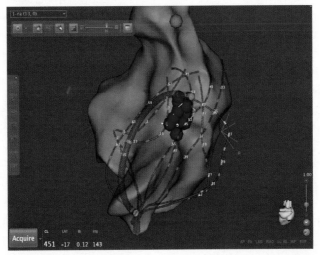

FIGURE 39-5 This is an electroanatomic map displaying the 64-pole basket catheter deployed in the left atrium. The green shell represents the left atrium anatomy. The sites of delivery of RF current are marked by the red dots and are delivered at the region of rotor activation. The ablation catheter tip is highlighted in green.

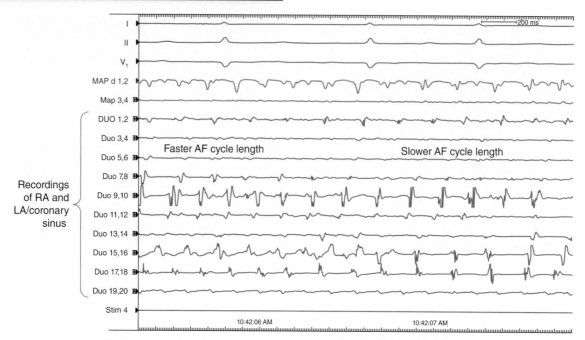

FIGURE 39-6 More rapid atrial fibrillation cycle length (on left side of electrogram tracing) slows (longer cycle length and more organized AF tracing on right side of electrogram tracing) during RF ablation of a left atrial rotor.

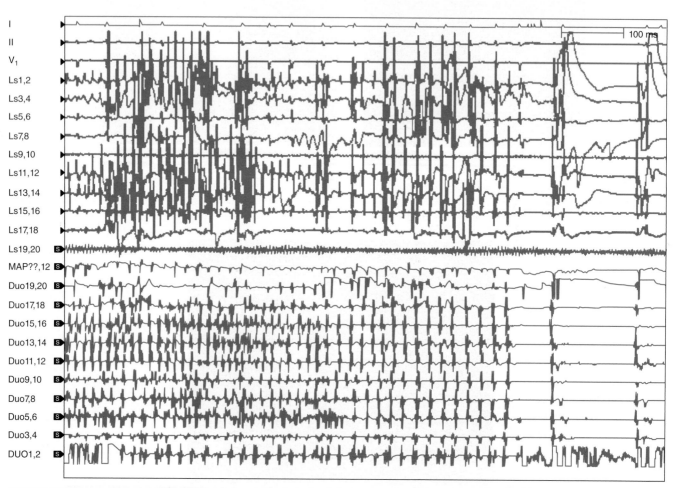

FIGURE 39-7 Termination of atrial fibrillation during application of radiofrequency energy at a rotor site identified by processing of AF electrograms recorded from the 64-basket electrode.

TECHNOLOGIES FOR ABLATION OF ATRIAL
FIBRILLATION: ROTOR MAPPING

SECTION VI
CATHETER ABLATION TECHNIQUES FOR
MANAGING ATRIAL FIBRILLATION AND
ATRIAL FLUTTER

275

Multiple Wavelet Hypothesis

In 1959, Moe and Abildskov proposed the multiple wavelet hypothesis.[1,2] This theory was experimentally confirmed in 1985 by the work of Allessie and colleagues.[3] According to this hypothesis, AF results from the presence of multiple independent wavelets occurring simultaneously and propagating randomly throughout the LA and RA. This model suggests that the number of wavelets at any point in time depends on the atrial conduction velocity, refractory period, and excitable mass. The perpetuation of AF appears to require at least four to six coexisting wavelets and is favored by slowed conduction, shortened refractory periods, and increased atrial mass. One of the practical implications of this hypothesis was the fact that chronic AF could be cured in some patients by the placement of multiple surgical lesions (maze procedure) to compartmentalize the atria into regions presumably unable to sustain multiple wavelet reentry.[5]

Despite the fact that this theory was widely accepted, this hypothesis failed to answer many questions, such as why AF exhibits consistent spatial nonuniformities in rate and activation vectors, how ablation may terminate AF relatively early, in some cases before compartmentalization of meandering wavelets, or why extensive ablation often has little acute impact.[6-8]

Focal Triggers

In clinical practice, the concept of focal triggers as a cause of AF was verified to the greatest extent by Haissaguerre and colleagues who found that ectopic beats from the pulmonary veins initiated AF and that a localized catheter ablation procedure to eliminate these triggers could cure AF in some patients.[9-11] This important finding made the pulmonary veins and the posterior wall of the LA the primary targets to cure AF.

Mother Rotors

Based on animal models, some authors have proposed that in the presence of an appropriately heterogeneous AF substrate a focal trigger can result in sustained high-frequency reentrant AF drivers (rotors).[12-15] The waves that emerge from the rotors undergo spatially distributed fragmentation and give rise to fibrillatory conduction. In the early 1990s, Schuessler and colleagues demonstrated in an isolated canine RA that with increasing concentrations of acetylcholine, activation patterns characterized by multiple reentrant circuits converted to a single, relatively stable, high-frequency reentrant circuit that resulted in fibrillatory conduction.[15]

In humans, multiple studies have used spectral analysis and dominant frequency mapping as a surrogate for localized AF sources, with ablation at these sites resulting in prolongation of the AF cycle length and termination of paroxysmal AF, indicating their role in the maintenance of AF.[16,17] Recent human studies have directly demonstrated, for the first time, that a majority of AF patients exhibit rotors and focal impulses where targeted ablation alone can acutely eliminate AF.[18,19]

Identifying and Ablating AF Rotors

During the EP study, a 64-pole basket catheter (see Figure 39-1) is introduced through an 8.5-F steerable sheath to the RA and then to the LA after transseptal puncture. The basket catheter has a unique, flexible basket design that conforms to atrial anatomy to aid in accurate placement and to save repositioning time. The 64 electrodes provide comprehensive, real-time 3-D information in a single beat. The average interelectrode spacing of 4 to 8 mm is sufficient to detect small reentry circuits in human atria. Care should be taken to optimize the contact between the atrial wall and the catheter's electrodes by using fluoroscopy, electrogram analysis, and intracardiac echocardiography. An ACT of more than 300 seconds should be maintained throughout the procedure to prevent thromboembolic complications. After appropriate positioning of the basket catheter and placement of a unipolar catheter as a reference, AF is induced in patients who present in normal sinus rhythm by decremental atrial pacing or with a high dose of isoproterenol.

Computational AF maps are generated intraprocedurally using a novel software system, where electrograms from the basket electrodes are acquired and then analyzed. This software preprocesses electrograms to remove QRS signals and improve signal-to-noise ratio, and then it analyzes AF cycles at each electrode using reported human atrial tissue electrophysiology from previous studies to reconstruct propagation movies of electrogram amplitude at each electrode over successive time points, projected onto a grid.[20-22]

These maps often reveal electrical rotors defined as sequential clockwise or counterclockwise activation contours (isochrones) around a center of rotation emanating outward to control local AF activation, or focal impulses defined by centrifugal activation contours (isochrones) from an origin (see Figure 39-4). Rotors and focal impulses should be considered AF sources only if consistent in multiple recordings over a period of time (usually 10 minutes). The location of these AF sources can be defined in relation to the basket electrodes and then correlated to the electroanatomical map in order to apply RF ablation at these anatomic sites.

In a study of 80 consecutive AF patients, it was concluded that rotors and focal sources are common in AF.[23] It was found that rotors exist in 96% of the patients. Study patients often demonstrated more than one coexisting electrical rotor or repetitive focal beat, for an average of 1.8 ± 0.9 for both atria. In the initial study, the authors showed that rotational centers and focal beat origins in fibrillation were unexpectedly stable and can last for at least several hours.

In the Conventional Ablation for Atrial Fibrillation With or Without Focal Impulse and Rotor Modulation (CONFIRM) trial, electrical rotors and focal impulses were present in 98 of 101 cases with sustained AF (97%). Each subject demonstrated 2.1 ± 1.0 sources of which 70% were rotors and 30% focal impulses.[19] Also, the authors concluded that when sources were present, their number was higher for persistent than for paroxysmal AF and for spontaneous versus induced AF, and was unrelated to age, historical duration of AF, or whether subjects were undergoing first ablation or had had prior conventional ablation.

In another series of 14 patients, localized sources were demonstrated in all mapped patients for an average of 1.9 ± 0.8 sources per patient. Of 23 AF sources in this series (21 rotors, 2 focal sources), 18 were found in LA and 5 in the RA. All sources were stable for at least 20 to 30 minutes during mapping and remapping.[24]

MANAGEMENT

Localizing the critical sites in human AF yields a promising opportunity to eliminate AF by targeting these sources with radiofrequency energy. The CONFIRM trial was the first prospective study to test the hypothesis that by eliminating the rotors or focal impulses, the outcome after AF ablation will improve.[19] The authors in this trial concluded that the acute endpoint (AF termination or consistent slowing) was achieved in 86% of sites targeted ablation group versus in 20% of the conventional ablation therapy cohort, and resulted in higher

276

SECTION VI
CATHETER ABLATION TECHNIQUES FOR
MANAGING ATRIAL FIBRILLATION AND
ATRIAL FLUTTER

CHAPTER 39

freedom from AF during a median 273 days (interquartile range: 132 to 681 days) after a single procedure (82.4% versus 44.9%; $P = 0.001$). These conclusions were similar in other studies.[23,24]

The mechanism by which localized ablation terminates rotors is unclear but likely involves the elimination or alteration of functional or anatomical heterogeneities such as fiber anisotropy, fibrosis, scar, or other factors central to maintaining AF, leading to its termination.[23]

LIMITATIONS

Despite the high rate of acute AF termination and improved success rate over the long term, there are many limitations and complications that have been reported. The technical connectivity, basket availability, and limitation of basket size in patients with large atria are the most important limitations. The distance between the electrodes in the basket catheter may produce suboptimal resolution for a small focal origin or rotor core, so there is a possibility that many rotors that originate between the electrodes will not be detected. There is also the possibility that additional sources will not be mapped (septal LA) due to the suboptimal contact between the atrial surface and the basket splines.

REFERENCES

1. Moe GK, Abildskov JA. Atrial fibrillation as a self-sustaining arrhythmia independent of focal discharge. *Am Heart J.* 1959;58(1): 59-70.

2. Moe GK, Rheinboldt WC, Abildskov JA. A computer model of atrial fibrillation. *Am Heart J.* 1964;67:200-220.

3. Allessie MA, Lammers WJEP, Bonke FIM, Hollen J. Experimental evaluation of Moe's multiple wavelet hypothesis of atrial fibrillation. In: Zipes DP, Jalife J, eds. *Cardiac Electrophysiology and Arrhythmias.* Orlando, FL: Grune and Straton, Inc; 1985: 265-275.

4. Jalife J, Berenfeld O, Mansour M. Mother rotors and fibrillatory conduction: a mechanism of atrial fibrillation. *Cardiovasc Res.* 2002;54:204-216.

5. Cox JL, Canavan TE, Schuessler RB, et al. The surgical treatment of atrial fibrillation. II. Intraoperative electrophysiologic mapping and description of the electrophysiologic basis of atrial flutter and atrial fibrillation. *J Thorac Cardiovasc Surg.* 1991;101(3):406-426.

6. Gerstenfeld E, Sahakian A, Swiryn S. Evidence for transient linking of atrial excitation during atrial fibrillation in humans. *Circulation.* 1992;86:375-382.

7. Lazar S, Dixit S, Marchlinski FE, Callans DJ, Gerstenfeld EP. Presence of left-to-right atrial frequency gradient in paroxysmal but not persistent atrial fibrillation in humans. *Circulation.* 2004;110:3181-3186.

8. Sahadevan J, Ryu K, Peltz L, et al. Epicardial mapping of chronic atrial fibrillation in patients: preliminary observations. *Circulation.* 2004;110:3293-3299.

9. Haissaguerre M, Marcus FI, Fischer B, Clementy J. Radiofrequency catheter ablation in unusual mechanisms of atrial fibrillation: report of three cases. *J Cardiovasc Electrophysiol.* 1994;5(9):743-751.

10. Jais P, Haissaguerre M, Shah DC, et al. A focal source of atrial fibrillation treated by discrete radiofrequency ablation. *Circulation.* 1997;95(3):572-576.

11. Haissaguerre M, Jais P, Shah DC, et al. Spontaneous initiation of atrial fibrillation by ectopic beats originating in the pulmonary veins. *N Engl J Med.* 1998;339(10):659-666.

12. Berenfeld O, Mandapati R, Dixit S, et al. Spatially distributed dominant excitation frequencies reveal hidden organization in atrial fibrillation in the Langendorff perfused sheep heart. *J Cardiovasc Electrophysiol.* 2000;11(8):869-879.

13. Mandapati R, Skanes A, Chen J, Berenfeld O, Jalife J. Stable microreentrant sources as a mechanism of atrial fibrillation in the isolated sheep heart. *Circulation.* 2000;101(2):194-199.

14. Skanes AC, Mandapati R, Berenfeld O, Davidenko JM, Jalife J. Spatiotemporal periodicity during atrial fibrillation in the isolated sheep heart. *Circulation.* 1998;98(12):1236-1248.

15. Schuessler RB, Grayson TM, Bromberg BI, Cox JL, Boineau JP. Cholinergically mediated tachyarrhythmias induced by a single extrastimulus in the isolated canine right atrium. *Circ Res.* 1992;71:1254-1267.

16. Atienza F, Almendral J, Jalife J, et al. Real-time dominant frequency mapping and ablation of dominant frequency sites in atrial fibrillation with left-to-right frequency gradients predicts long-term maintenance of sinus rhythm. *Heart Rhythm.* 2009;6:33-40.

17. Sanders P, Berenfeld O, Hocini M, et al. Spectral analysis identifies sites of high frequency activity maintaining atrial fibrillation in humans. *Circulation.* 2005;112:789-797.

18. Narayan SM, Krummen DE, Rappel WJ. Clinical mapping approach to diagnose electrical rotors and focal impulse sources for human atrial fibrillation. *J Cardiovasc Electrophysiol.* 2012;23:447-454.

19. Narayan SM, Krummen DE, Shivkumar K, Clopton P, Rappel WJ, Miller JM. Treatment of atrial fibrillation by the ablation of localized sources: CONFIRM (Conventional Ablation for Atrial Fibrillation With or Without Focal Impulse and Rotor Modulation) trial. *J Am Coll Cardiol.* 2012;60:628-636.

20. Narayan SM, Kazi D, Krummen DE, Rappel WJ. Repolarization and activation restitution near human pulmonary veins and atrial fibrillation initiation: a mechanism for the initiation of atrial fibrillation by premature beats. *J Am Coll Cardiol.* 2008;52: 1222-1230.

21. Narayan SM, Franz MR, Clopton P, Pruvot EJ, Krummen DE. Repolarization alternans reveals vulnerability to human atrial fibrillation. *Circulation.* 2011;123:2922-2930.

22. Lalani G, Gibson M, Schricker A, Rostamanian A, Krummen DE, Narayan SM. Slowing of atrial conduction prior to the initiation of human atrial fibrillation: a bi-atrial contact mapping study of transitions to atrial fibrillation. *J Am Coll Cardiol.* 2012;59:595-606.

23. Narayan SM, Krummen DE, Enyeart MW, Rappel WJ. Computational mapping identifies localized mechanisms for ablation of atrial fibrillation. *PLoS One.* 2012;7(9):e46034. doi: 10.1371/journal.pone.0046034. Epub 2012 Sep 26.

24. Shivkumar K, Ellenbogen KA, Hummel JD, Miller JM, Steinberg JS. Acute termination of human atrial fibrillation by identification and catheter ablation of localized rotors and sources: first multicenter experience of Focal Impulse and Rotor Modulation (FIRM) ablation. *J Cardiovasc Electrophysiol.* 2012;23(12):1277-1285.

TECHNOLOGIES FOR ABLATION OF ATRIAL
FIBRILLATION: MRI ANALYSIS OF ATRIAL TISSUE
REMODELING AND SCARRING

SECTION VI
CATHETER ABLATION TECHNIQUES FOR
MANAGING ATRIAL FIBRILLATION AND
ATRIAL FLUTTER

277

40 TECHNOLOGIES FOR ABLATION OF ATRIAL FIBRILLATION: MRI ANALYSIS OF ATRIAL TISSUE REMODELING AND SCARRING

Matthias Koopmann, MD, Nazem Akoum, MD, MS,
Nassir Marrouche, MD

CASE PRESENTATION

CASE 1

A 75-year-old woman with paroxysmal atrial fibrillation (AF) presented to our clinic for evaluation. The patient had been having AF for a few years. During AF episodes, she has palpitations and an irregular heart beat. Recently, the frequency of her episodes increased, and antiarrhythmic drug therapy with sotalol and flecainide failed to satisfactorily improve her symptoms, so she presents to discuss further treatment options. No significant comorbidities were apparent. A CHADS$_2$ score of 1 (age) and a transthoracic echocardiogram showed normal left ventricular systolic function. Late gadolinium enhancement magnetic resonance imaging (LGE-MRI) demonstrated 12% LA tissue fibrosis, consistent with Utah stage II (Figure 40-1). After careful consideration and because of severe symptoms associated with AF, the patient elected to undergo an AF ablation. Given an early disease stage, the ablation procedure was limited to pulmonary vein antrum isolation (PVAI) only. Repeat LGE-MRI 10 months postablation demonstrated 12.5% LA scar formation (see Figure 40-1). After follow-up of 15 months, the patient remains free of AF.

CASE 2

A 68-year-old man presents who was first diagnosed with paroxysmal AF at the age of 52. Initially, episodes lasted 2 to 3 days and were associated with palpitations. Over the following 15 years, the frequency, duration, and severity of symptoms of AF episodes increased, some lasting for weeks. While initially he only felt palpitations, with time he increasingly had shortness of breath, with a sensation of not getting enough oxygen, and lightheadedness. He always, however, converted spontaneously to sinus rhythm. During those episodes

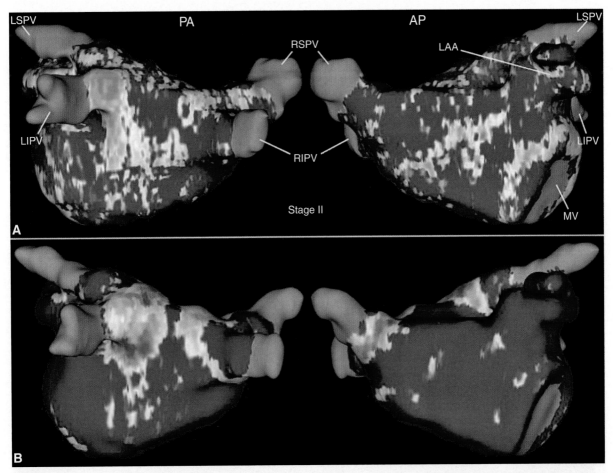

FIGURE 40-1 Three-dimensional LA reconstruction showing LASRM (A) and chronic LA Scar (B) after PVAI. (A) LASRM estimated at 12% (stage II). (B) LGE-MRI was obtained 10 months post-AF ablation, exhibiting 12.5% LA scar. Blue, healthy myocardium; green, LASRM; red, scarred tissue. Dark green/red indicates transmurality; white indicates nontransmurality. Wall contours are smoothened.

278

SECTION VI
CATHETER ABLATION TECHNIQUES FOR
MANAGING ATRIAL FIBRILLATION AND
ATRIAL FLUTTER

CHAPTER 40

his quality of life was significantly impacted. Antiarrhythmic drug therapy with flecainide failed after a short period of success in suppressing AF. Four years ago he experienced a stroke, which occurred 1 day after a liposuction procedure. Fortunately he does not exhibit any residual effects. No other significant cardiovascular risk factors were apparent, thus having a CHADS$_2$ score of 2. Due to increased symptoms, he elected to undergo AF ablation. Cardiac LGE-MRI was performed, and postimage acquisition processing revealed 22% atrial tissue fibrosis (Figure 40-2), fitting with stage III disease as depicted in Figure 40-3, which illustrates the Utah classification. Based on this individual's extent of fibrosis, he was deemed eligible for ablation with an approach tailored to pulmonary vein antrum isolation (PVAI) and fibrotic area debulking. Immediate postablation, MRI demonstrated acute tissue lesions with regions of "no-reflow" at the posterior and septal wall (Figure 40-4), a predictor of appropriate scarring or lesion formation on MRI. Three months later MRI was repeated to assess chronic atrial scarring, which showed a scar burden of 19% of the LA volume (see Figure 40-2). Figure 40-5 illustrates 3 consecutive MRIs at preablation, immediate postablation, and 3 months postablation. At follow-up of 12 months the patient remains free of AF.

CASE 3

A 29-year-old man was referred to our electrophysiology clinic for paroxysmal AF. He reported having episodes of fast heart rates for several years, occurring at a frequency of 1 to 3 times per months, each lasting about 2 to 3 days. He had a remarkable family history with many family members with sudden cardiac death (SCD), cardiomyopathy, and early onset AF. A thorough workup including cardiac MRI was performed given his significant family history of SCD. MRI showed normal left ventricular function, no signs of ventricular delayed enhancement, myocardial infarction, or scar. Postimage acquisition processing revealed 24% left atrial fibrosis (Utah stage III; Figure 40-6). Hence the patient was eligible for catheter ablation for AF with a tailored approach of pulmonary vein antrum isolation (PVAI) and posterior wall debulking. Acute postablation MRIs were performed within 24 hours and uncovered extensive posterior wall and esophageal enhancement. A day following ablation the patient complained of symptoms of heartburn and some pain with swallowing. Endoscopy was performed showing esophageal injury at the level of the left atrium (maximum diameter 11 mm) with no bleeding 30 to 31 cm from the incisors (Figure 40-7). LGE-MRI was repeated at 48 and 96 hours following AF ablation. Three-dimensional segmentations of the preablation MRI in this patient demonstrated the close topographic anatomical relationship between the left atrium and the posteriorly located esophagus (Figure 40-8). Figure 40-9 shows the temporal evolvement of the esophageal lesions. Proton pump inhibitors were initially given intravenously, sucralfate suspension (1 gram per mouth 4 times a day for 5 weeks), and mechanically soft

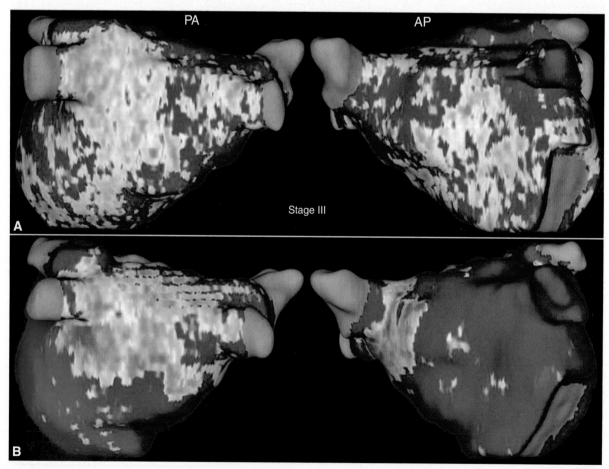

FIGURE 40-2 Three-dimensional LA reconstruction showing LASRM (A) and chronic LA scar (B) after PVAI and PWD. (A) LASRM estimated at 22% (stage III). (B) LGE-MRI 3 months post-AF ablation, exhibiting 19.1% LA scar.

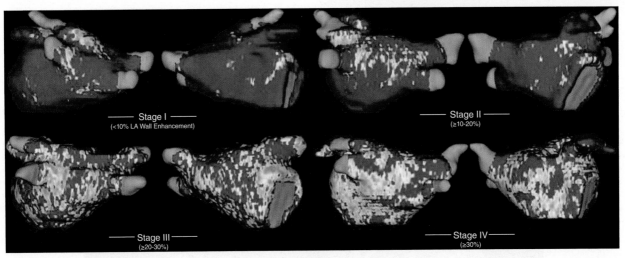

FIGURE 40-3 Utah classification of LASRM, a quantitative LGE-MRI based clinical staging system reflecting disease progression of atrial fibrillation. Utah stage I (minimal) as <10% LASRM, stage II (mild) as ≥10% and <20%, stage III (moderate) as ≥20% and <30%, and stage IV (extensive) as ≥30%.

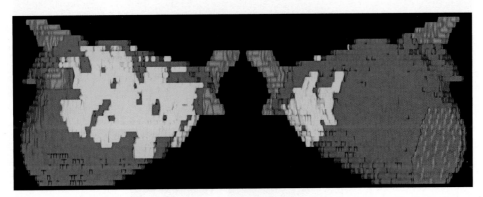

FIGURE 40-4 Three-dimensional LA reconstruction showing areas of no-reflow (yellow) indicating regions of catheter-induced tissue injury, immediately after AF ablation. Regions of no-reflow later enhance on 3 months postablation LGE-MRI, predicting permanent scar formation. Yellow, regions of no-reflow; blue, normal myocardium.

diet was instituted for 5 weeks. Repeat endoscopies over the next days showed progressive healing of the esophageal ulcerations. After a clinical follow-up of more than 12 months, the patient remains free of AF, without any gastrointestinal symptoms.

MRI TECHNOLOGY FOR IMAGING ATRIAL TISSUE

Late gadolinium enhancement magnetic resonance imaging has emerged as a key noninvasive modality in the armory of heart imaging in modern cardiology. The well established ability to assess precisely myocardial viability and accurately depict anatomy and function has lead to its widespread clinical use. Left atrial and pulmonary vein anatomy (including anatomic variability) and major thoracic structures such as the esophagus have been thoroughly investigated using MRI.[1,2] Recently, the utility of LGE-MRI has been significantly expanded with the demonstration of its ability to assess atrial tissue changes that contribute to the arrhythmic substrate, as well as acute and chronic postablation tissue lesions. In this chapter, we illustrate these MRI-based approaches and emphasize how the clinical application of these modalities are instrumental in tailoring treatment by selecting appropriate ablation candidates and the adequate ablation strategy, and predicting individual ablation outcome.

ASSESSMENT OF ATRIAL STRUCTURAL REMODELING

Atrial fibrillation is associated with atrial electrical, contractile, and structural remodeling. As AF perpetuates, apoptosis of atrial myocytes and fibrotic replacement occurs. Conversely, an increase in fibrosis within atrial tissue contributes to the arrhythmic substrate for AF. While for a long time the evaluation of tissue relied on invasive means either through surgical or postmortem histological specimens, MRI is now the noninvasive gold standard for tissue characterization, especially for the ventricular myocardium. Imaging of the atrial myocardium is more challenging, particularly due to the much thinner and nonuniform atrial wall, ranging from 1 to 7 mm. LGE-MRI relies on the differences in washout kinetics of gadolinium, an extracellular contrast agent, to differentiate between healthy myocardium and diseased tissue. Unlike in normal tissue where intracellular myocyte space forms the vast volume, in chronic diseased tissue the extracellular space is increased due to fibrous tissue replacement. This eventually leads to increase of gadolinium concentration and therefore delayed washout and subsequent enhancement. Figure 40-10 illustrates workflows which are used to generate different LA images. The detection and quantification of fibrous tissue in the LA wall using

280

SECTION VI
CATHETER ABLATION TECHNIQUES FOR
MANAGING ATRIAL FIBRILLATION AND
ATRIAL FLUTTER

CHAPTER 40

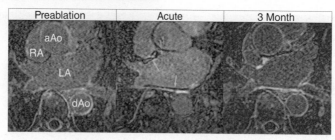

FIGURE 40-5 LGE-MRIs prior to ablation with LASRM, immediate postablation with dark regions of no-reflow at the posterior and septal wall (yellow arrows), and their transformation into areas that enhance on LGE-MRI, indicating permanent atrial scarring (red arrows) 3 months postablation.

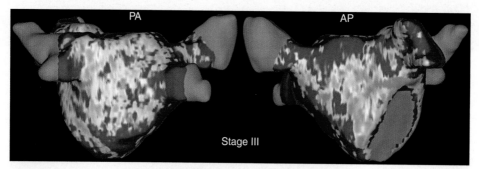

FIGURE 40-6 Three-dimensional LA reconstruction showing preablation LASRM of 24% fibrosis (stage III). Note the extensive fibrosis in this young patient (aged 29 years) with a CHADS$_2$ score of 0.

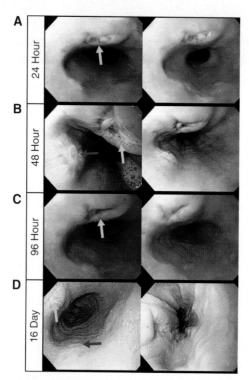

FIGURE 40-7 Repeat upper gastrointestinal endoscopies at (A) 24 hours, (B) 48 hours, (C) 96 hours, and (D) 16 days post-AF ablation. Spatial and temporal development of two distinct esophageal lesions (lesion 1, yellow arrows; lesion 2, blue arrows).

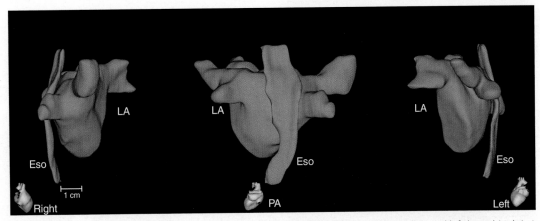

FIGURE 40-8 Three-dimensional reconstruction of the LA and esophagus in right-lateral (left), PA (middle), and left-lateral (right) views. Note the close spatial anatomical proximity between the anterior-located LA to the posterior-located esophagus. The distance between these structures varies among individuals and is about 3 to 13 mm away from the LA endocardium (frequently around 5 mm).

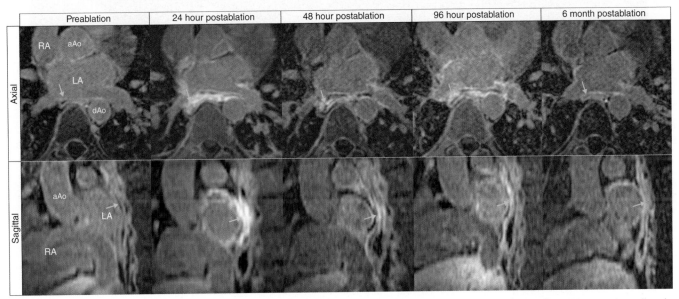

FIGURE 40-9 Consecutive 2-D LGE-MRI slices in axial (top) and sagital (bottom) views. Catheter ablation caused significant LA posterior wall and esophageal wall (yellow arrows) enhancement, indicating remarkable thermal tissue injury. Note the spatial extention and temporal behavior of the thermal eosphageal injuries.

LGE-MRI was first introduced by our group at the University of Utah. We demonstrated that low-voltage areas derived by electroanatomical mapping during AF ablation correlated well with areas showing enhancement on LGE. Further, AF recurrence following ablation was best predicted by the degree of fibrosis[3] (Figure 40-11). Using this approach assessment of distribution, amount, and transmurality of diseased fibrotic tissue was feasible. LA fibrosis seems to have no significant association with clinical congestive heart failure, coronary artery disease, arterial hypertension, or diabetes mellitus. However, an association was found with left ventricular hypertrophy[4] and left ventricular dysfunction[5] in AF patients. Paroxysmal AF is more prevalent in Utah I while persistent AF is more in Utah IV. Nevertheless, all 4 Utah stages include a heterogeneous mix of both AF phenotypes.

Subsequent work of our group investigated the value of guiding treatment of AF patients based on their individual degree and distribution of LASRM.[6] Patients with more advanced AF tend to have more LA tissue involved with fibrosis, and our data support

extending the ablation strategy from pulmonary vein antrum isolation (PVAI) to posterior and septal wall debulking to improve ablation outcome.[7,8] Patients in Utah stages I and II receive PVAI alone, while Utah IV patients are counseled to receive medical therapy rather than ablation. An inverse relationship of complex fractionated atrial electrograms (CFAEs) to atrial fibrosis has also been defined using LGE-MRI. Almost 90% of CFAE sites were found to occur at nonfibrotic and patchy fibrosis locations in the LA.[9] Further, as sinus node dysfunction (SND) is a frequent phenomenon in AF patients, significant atrial fibrosis assessed by LGE-MRI is associated with clinically significant SND requiring pacemaker implantation, while fibrosis affects the left atrium more than the right.[10]

Ischemic stroke is an imminent threat in AF patients. Current schemes to predict stroke risk, such as the widely used CHADS$_2$ score, do not include any assessment of individual LA structural remodeling. We showed that AF patients who experienced an ischemic stroke exhibit significantly higher levels of LA fibrosis as

282

SECTION VI
CATHETER ABLATION TECHNIQUES FOR
MANAGING ATRIAL FIBRILLATION AND
ATRIAL FLUTTER

CHAPTER 40

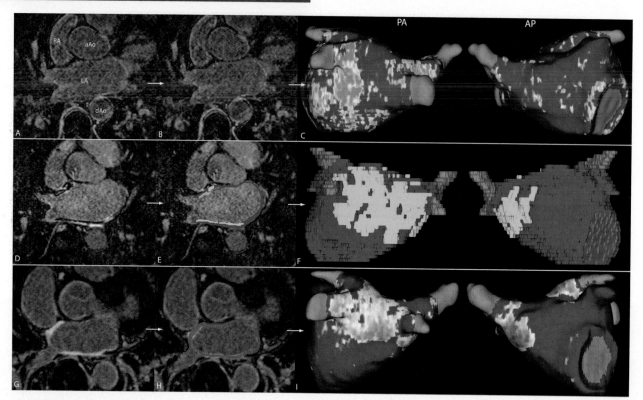

FIGURE 40-10 Workflows from LGE-MRI image acquisition to quantification/detection of LASRM (top), acute atrial lesions after ablation of AF with regions of no-reflow (middle), and chronic atrial scarring postablation (bottom). Figures A, D, and G show 2-D image slices; B, E, and H show endo- and epicardial LA wall contours; and C, F, and I show 3-D reconstructions.

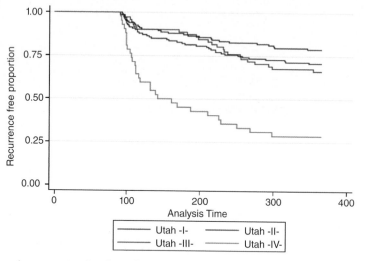

FIGURE 40-11 Kaplan-Meier curve demonstrating freedom of arrhythmia recurrence in days following a single AF ablation procedure based on the Utah classification (mean follow-up 746 ± 428 days). Note the strong correlation between recurrence arrhythmias to higher LASRM (unpublished data).

quantified by LGE-MRI.[11] LGE-MRI has also uncovered an association of higher levels of fibrosis in the left atrial appendage, a common site of thrombus formation in AF, to echocardiographic findings of LAA thrombi and spontaneous echocardiographic contrast (SEC).[12] Knowledge of individual LA fibrosis degrees in conjunction with the CHADS$_2$ score may help clinicians improve stroke risk stratification and weigh risk and benefits for anticoagulation regimens.

ASSESSMENT OF ACUTE ATRIAL LESIONS AFTER CATHETER ABLATION

Significant heterogeneity is seen in the LA wall on acute LGE-MRI following AF ablation, and those changes occur and dissolve quickly within the first 24 hours. Delivery of radiofrequency energy to the myocardial tissue creates remarkable edema with hyperenhancement, as well as nonenhancing regions showing characteristics similar to the no-reflow phenomenon. Unlike chronic myocardial remodeling, the mechanism of gadolinium enhancement in the setting of acute LGE-MRI is based on cell membrane rupture, allowing Gadolinium to diffuse into what was previously intracellular space, causing an increase in gadolinium concentration and therefore LGE. The proposed mechanism for the no-reflow phenomenon is based on intracapillary red blood cell stasis in the central necrotic region caused by capillary plugging. Those vascular changes induced either by an infarction or via catheter induced tissue injury result in tissue hypoperfusion, thus regions or no-reflow will appear dark on LGE-MRI. Nonenhancing or regions of no-reflow are more likely to transform into permanent scar on repeat LGE-MRI than hyperenhancing regions representing edema.[13] Interestingly, edema is not only seen in regions directly subjected to RF energy but also in distant nonablated regions, such as parts of the anterior LA wall. It is worth noting that those regions do not predict final scar formation, even though they correlate with low-voltage areas during the procedure. The optimal timing of imaging postablation is crucial to visualize no-reflow phenomena. Those observations shed important light on the importance of early scar detection following ablation. However, with the expansion of knowledge regarding early lesion formation, the ultimate goal remains to titrate and monitor lesion formation in real time during the procedure.

ASSESSMENT OF CHRONIC ATRIAL SCARRING AFTER CATHETER ABLATION

Time periods ranging from weeks to months after ablation have been thoroughly investigated using LGE-MRI to assess chronic atrial ablation induced scarring. Tissue edema and regions of no-reflow observed acutely result in a heterogeneous mix of recovered and permanently scarred tissue in different subjects. Early studies demonstrated that subjects undergoing AF ablation exhibit LGE in the LA and around the PV ostia 1 to 3 months postablation.[14] Subsequently, this finding was confirmed using a novel imaging approach and processing methods,[15] also showing that catheter-induced scarring on MRI predicted procedural outcome. Later studies proposed a time period of approximately 3 months postablation to permanently reflect chronic atrial scar formation.[13] The amount of LA scar and the number of scarred pulmonary vein antra is associated with better ablation outcome; however, attaining complete PV encirclement as defined by LGE-MRI is difficult to achieve.[15,16] Specifically higher procedure success was seen in those individuals exhibiting >23% LA scar, with lower success rates in those with <23% LA scar. The mechanism is likely multifactorial, but is at least in part due to the fact that certain tissue changes seen acutely (especially edema) will resolve over time, thus not being detectable on repeat MRI at 3 months. Catheter ablation of AF has also been associated with a decrease of LA size and systolic function, with a correlation to the total LA scar volume.[17] LGE-MRI enables further to accurately define atrial scarring after AF ablation, and to identify gaps in PV lesion sets, which can be specifically targeted during a repeat ablation procedure.[18] Of note, achieving complete circumferential isolation of all four PVs is a difficult task to achieve, and is likely less frequently achieved than previously assumed. It is important to mention that patients who remained in sinus rhythm exhibited incomplete PV scarring. This observation suggests the involvement of other mechanisms influencing AF recurrence after ablation. Since AF ablation procedures are guided by

electroanatomic mapping systems, another study compared intended radiofrequency ablation sites using CARTO with postablation LA scar location detected by LGE-MRI and reported good qualitative and quantitative agreement between CARTO representations of ablation sites and LA scar by LGE-MRI.[19] Both early and chronic atrial scar imaging is of significant clinical interest. While the presence of no-reflow phenomena likely predicts permanent scarring, lesion breaks on chronic scar imaging helps to individually plan redo procedures in patients who failed previous ablation.

FUTURE USE OF MRI

MRI is an extremely valuable tool in planning, performing, and follow-up of catheter-based ablation procedures in EP. Consequently, there is a growing interest in cardiac MRI in EP, and the past 7 years have witnessed major strides in this field. Specifically, imaging of remodeled atrial tissue, acute and chronic ablation-induced tissue lesions, and scarring have seen improved accuracy, reliability, and reproducibility. The proposed modalities, however, allow clinicians to better select appropriate ablation candidates, plan the ablation strategy prior to the procedure, individually predict stroke risk and ablation outcome, and plan redo procedures as necessary. Moreover, MRI precisely elaborates left atrial, pulmonary vein anatomy, and the anatomical relationship to critical adjacent mediastinal structures, which is of particular interest for planning an invasive procedure. Further, LGE-MRI is instrumental for the detection and management of ablation-related complications, such as in our case of thermal esophageal injury.

To further improve arrhythmia management, future work will focus on intraprocedural real-time visualization of tissue lesions, giving the operator immediate feedback during energy delivery. Real-time MRI would further allow monitoring of critical adjacent anatomical structures, such as the esophagus, pericardial space, and PVs, thereby improving both efficacy and safety of ablation procedures. Safely navigating catheters in the heart, pacing maneuvers, recording intracardiac ECGs, transseptal punctures, and exploring all four cardiac chambers under real-time MRI is feasible. While major steps have already been accomplished, hurdles remain, including MRI-compatible EP catheters and equipment. Accomplishments of those steps will serve to expand further the utility of MRI in modern cardiac electrophysiology, increase curative rates for AF and other arrhythmias, while simultaneously decreasing procedural-associated complications.

REFERENCES

1. Hauser TH, Peters DC, Wylie JV, Manning WJ. Evaluating the left atrium by magnetic resonance imaging. *Europace.* 2008;10(Suppl 3):iii22-27.

2. Mansour M, Holmvang G, Sosnovik D, et al. Assessment of pulmonary vein anatomic variability by magnetic resonance imaging: implications for catheter ablation techniques for atrial fibrillation. *J Cardiovasc Electrophysiol.* 2004;15(4):387-393.

3. Oakes RS, Badger TJ, Kholmovski EG, et al. Detection and quantification of left atrial structural remodeling with delayed-enhancement magnetic resonance imaging in patients with atrial fibrillation. *Circulation.* 2009;119(113):1758-1767.

4. Akkaya M, Higuchi K, Koopmann M, et al. Relationship between left atrial tissue structural remodelling detected using late gadolinium enhancement MRI and left ventricular hypertrophy in patients with atrial fibrillation. *Europace.* 2013;15(12):1725-1732.

5. Akkaya M, Higuchi K, Koopmann M, et al. Higher degree of left atrial structural remodeling in patients with atrial fibrillation and left ventricular systolic dysfunction. *J Cardiovasc Electrophysiol.* 2013;24(5):485-491.

6. Akoum N, Daccarett M, McGann C, et al. Atrial fibrosis helps select the appropriate patient and strategy in catheter ablation of atrial fibrillation: a DE-MRI guided approach. *J Cardiovasc Electrophysiol.* 2011;22(1):16-22.

7. Segerson NM, Daccarett M, Badger TJ, et al. Magnetic resonance imaging-confirmed ablative debulking of the left atrial posterior wall and septum for treatment of persistent atrial fibrillation: rationale and initial experience. *J Cardiovasc Electrophysiol.* 2010;21(2):126-132.

8. Daccarett M, McGann CJ, Akoum NW, MacLeod RS, Marrouche NF. MRI of the left atrium: predicting clinical outcomes in patients with atrial fibrillation. *Expert Rev Cardiovasc Ther.* 2011;9(1):105-111.

9. Jadidi AS, Cochet H, Shah AJ, et al. Inverse relationship between fractionated electrograms and atrial fibrosis in persistent atrial fibrillation: combined magnetic resonance imaging and high-density mapping. *J Am Coll Cardiol.* 2013;62(9):802-812.

10. Akoum N, McGann C, Vergara G, et al. Atrial fibrosis quantified using late gadolinium enhancement MRI is associated with sinus node dysfunction requiring pacemaker implant. *J Cardiovasc Electrophysiol.* 2012;23(1):44-50.

11. Daccarett M, Badger TJ, Akoum N, et al. Association of left atrial fibrosis detected by delayed-enhancement magnetic resonance imaging and the risk of stroke in patients with atrial fibrillation. *J Am Coll Cardiol.* 2011;57(7):831-838.

12. Akoum N, Fernandez G, Wilson B, McGann C, Kholmovski E, Marrouche N. Association of atrial fibrosis quantified using LGE-MRI with atrial appendage thrombus and spontaneous contrast on transesophageal echocardiography in patients with atrial fibrillation. [Epub ahead of print]. *J Cardiovasc Electrophysiol.* 2013. doi:10(10) 1104-1109.1111/jce.12199.

13. McGann C, Kholmovski E, Blauer J, et al. Dark regions of no-reflow on late gadolinium enhancement magnetic resonance imaging result in scar formation after atrial fibrillation ablation. *J Am Coll Cardiol.* 2011;58(2):177-185.

14. Peters DC, Wylie JV, Hauser TH, et al. Detection of pulmonary vein and left atrial scar after catheter ablation with three-dimensional navigator-gated delayed enhancement mr imaging: initial experience. *Radiology.* 2007;243(3):690-695.

15. McGann CJ, Kholmovski EG, Oakes RS, et al. New magnetic resonance imaging-based method for defining the extent of left atrial wall injury after the ablation of atrial fibrillation. *J Am Coll Cardiol.* 2008;52(15):1263-1271.

16. Peters DC, Wylie JV, Hauser TH, et al. Recurrence of atrial fibrillation correlates with the extent of postprocedural late gadolinium enhancement: a pilot study. *JACC Cardiovasc Imaging.* 2009;2(3):308-316.

17. Wylie JV Jr, Peters DC, Essebag V, Manning WJ, Josephson ME, Hauser TH. Left atrial function and scar after catheter ablation of atrial fibrillation. *Heart Rhythm.* 2008;5(5):656-662.

18. Badger TJ, Daccarett M, Akoum NW, et al. Evaluation of left atrial lesions after initial and repeat atrial fibrillation ablation: lessons learned from delayed-enhancement MRI in repeat ablation procedures. *Circ Arrhythm Electrophysiol.* 2010;3(3):249-259.

19. Taclas JE, Nezafat R, Wylie JV, et al. Relationship between intended sites of RF ablation and post-procedural scar in AF patients, using late gadolinium enhancement cardiovascular magnetic resonance. *Heart Rhythm.* 2010;7(4):489-496.

ATRIAL TACHYCARDIA OCCURRING
AFTER ABLATION OF ATRIAL
FIBRILLATION

SECTION VI
CATHETER ABLATION TECHNIQUES FOR
MANAGING ATRIAL FIBRILLATION AND
ATRIAL FLUTTER

285

41 ATRIAL TACHYCARDIA OCCURRING AFTER ABLATION OF ATRIAL FIBRILLATION

Aman Chugh, MD

CASE PRESENTATION

A 76-year-old man was referred to for catheter ablation of atrial tachycardia (AT) that occurred after an ablation procedure of atrial fibrillation (AF) performed 9 months ago. Four years ago, he underwent mitral and aortic valve replacement (both porcine) for rheumatic heart disease (ejection fraction, 45%; left atrial [LA] diameter, 6.1 cm). He developed postoperative AF for which he was prescribed amiodarone. He remained free of AF for approximately 18 months at which time he developed symptomatic-persistent AF. He was pretreated with amiodarone and underwent transthoracic cardioversion. However, sinus rhythm only lasted for 2 weeks. He then underwent catheter ablation of persistent AF, which consisted of antral pulmonary vein (PV) isolation, ablation of complex fractionated electrograms, and linear ablation at the left atrial (LA) roof.

The electrocardiogram (ECG) during AT showed that the initial portion of the flutter wave in the inferior leads was slightly negative, followed by notching (Figure 41-1). In addition, apart from lead V₁, the remaining precordial leads were isoelectric. This pattern

is consistent with an LA origin. Insertion of a multipolar catheter into the coronary sinus (CS) revealed distal-to-proximal activation, verifying LA origin. The cycle length of the tachycardia was 265 ms. A high-density activation map of the LA using more than 500 points confirmed macroreentry around the mitral valve in a clockwise fashion (Figure 41-2). The mechanism was confirmed by entrainment mapping around the mitral valve (Figure 41-3). Linear ablation was commenced from the lateral annulus to the left-sided PVs. Radiofrequency (RF) energy slowed and terminated the tachycardia to sinus rhythm. Pacing from anterior to the ablation line showed a proximal-to-distal activation of the CS, consistent with bidirectional block. Programmed atrial stimulation and rapid atrial pacing during isoproterenol infusion failed to reveal any arrhythmias. Eighteen months after the ablation procedure, there is not evidence of recurrent arrhythmia on long-term ambulatory monitoring. His symptoms of dyspnea and fatigue, along with the ejection fraction, have also improved.

EPIDEMIOLOGY

Patients undergoing catheter ablation of atrial fibrillation (AF) may develop atrial tachycardia (AT) during follow-up.[1,2] The incidence of postablation AT depends on a number of factors, including the underlying atrial substrate, the ablation approach, and possibly treatment with antiarrhythmic medications. In patients undergoing only pulmonary vein isolation, the incidence of postablation AT is low.[3] Patients who undergo empiric linear ablation, the incidence is about 33%,[2] with about one-fourth of the patients requiring a repeat ablation procedure for AT. AT is quite common when a step-wise approach is utilized in an attempt to acutely terminate AF during radiofrequency ablation. In fact, about 40% to 50% of such patients require a repeat ablation for AT.[4]

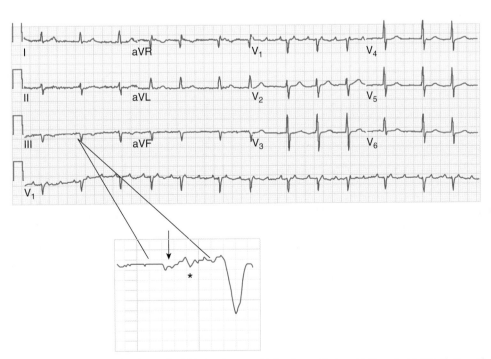

FIGURE 41-1 Electrocardiogram during atrial tachycardia (AT) that occurred following catheter ablation of atrial fibrillation. The lack of a "sawtooth" morphology of the P waves in the inferior leads and the presence of isoelectric P waves in the lateral precordial leads point to a left atrial (LA) origin. Also, note the notching (∗) after the initial negative deflection (arrow).

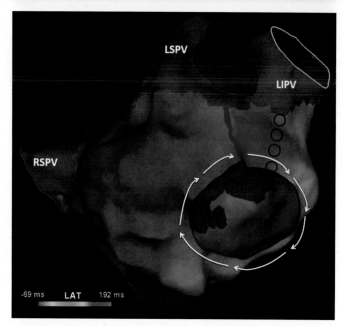

FIGURE 41-2 Activation map of the LA constructed using more than 500 points suggests that the mechanism of the AT (cycle length = 265 ms) is macroreentry around the mitral valve in a clockwise direction. The color spectrum (261 ms) shows that mapping accounted for almost the entire cycle length of the tachycardia, confirming a macroreentrant mechanism. The appendage (LAA) has been removed for clarity. Abbreviations: LI, left inferior; LS, left superior; PV, pulmonary vein; RS, right superior.

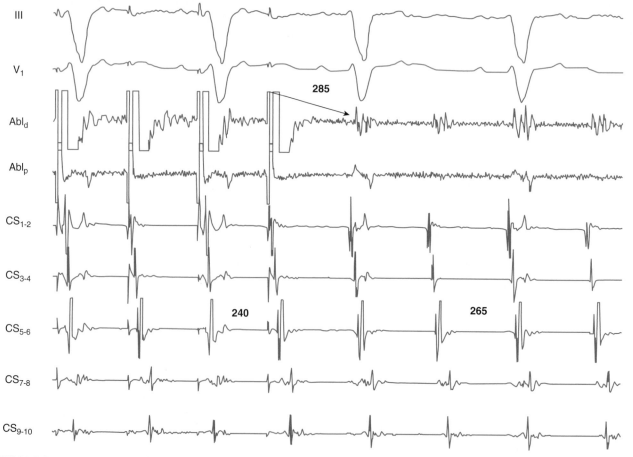

FIGURE 41-3 Entrainment mapping from the mitral isthmus (region between the lateral mitral annulus and the left inferior PV). The tachycardia is accelerated to the pacing rate, and the postpacing interval upon cessation of pacing approximates the cycle length of the tachycardia, confirming the findings on activation mapping shown in Figure 41-2. Abbreviations: Abl, ablation; CS, coronary sinus.

ATRIAL TACHYCARDIA OCCURRING
AFTER ABLATION OF ATRIAL
FIBRILLATION

SECTION VI
CATHETER ABLATION TECHNIQUES FOR
MANAGING ATRIAL FIBRILLATION AND
ATRIAL FLUTTER

287

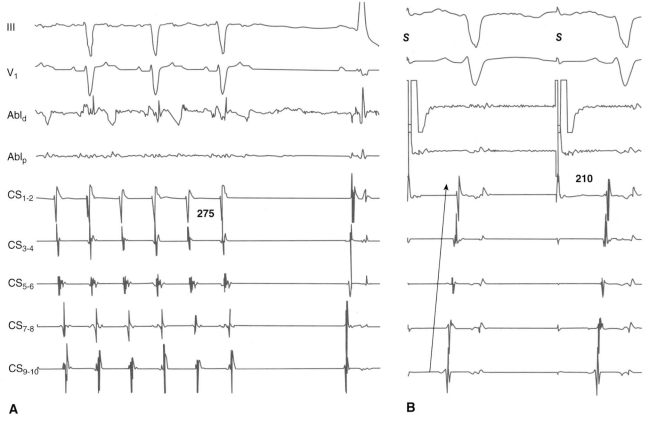

FIGURE 41-4 (A) Termination of mitral isthmus-dependent flutter during radiofrequency energy delivery along the line (black circles in Figure 41-2). (B) Pacing anterior to the line (from the region of the LAA) results in a proximal-to-distal activation of the coronary sinus, confirming the presence of linear block at the mitral isthmus. Abbreviation: S, stimulus.

ETIOLOGY AND PATHOPHYSIOLOGY

Broadly speaking, there are two main hypotheses that help explain the emergence of AT after catheter ablation of AF.[5] It is possible that postablation AT represents an underlying "driver" that is only unmasked after eliminating AF or more precisely, fibrillatory conduction. A prior study using spectral analysis showed that the frequency (ie, activation rate) of the resultant AT after elimination of AF matched the frequency of a spectral component that was present during the initial periodogram during AF.[6] This finding suggests that the substrate for AT—macroreentrant in the majority—is already present during AF and that the AT is destined to be encountered at some point. Although this hypothesis is certainly plausible, it may not be applicable to all patients. The other hypothesis posits that postablation AT is a result of the ablation approach, that is, a proarrhythmic complication of the initial AF procedure. There is a wealth of data that supports this contention. First, it is well known that both antral PVI and circumferential PV ablation (ie, circular lesions around the PVs, along with linear lesions at the mitral isthmus and the posterior wall/roof) are very effective in eliminating AF in patients with paroxysmal AF.[7] However, the former does so without intervening macroreentrant AT, which is quite common with the latter approach. So if patients were destined to develop macroreentrant AT, why should they only do so with one technique and not both? In fact, one could argue that they should be less likely to develop macroreentrant AT with an approach that involves linear lesions than with one that

does not. Second, a recent study showed that the area of slowest conduction velocity, requisite for the development of macroreentry, during either roof or perimitral flutter was found at the precise location where ablation was performed during the initial AF procedure.[8] In other words, the area of slowest velocity during a roof- or mitral-isthmus-dependent AT was identified at the most cranial aspect of the roof, and the lateral mitral annulus, respectively. If macroreentrant AT were due to the underlying substrate, why would the area of slowest conduction be confined to the site that was ablated, and not other sites along the reentrant path? When sources of AF are mapped, as opposed to an empiric lesion set for all patients, ablation of AF often yields sinus rhythm without an intervening atrial tachycardia.[9] Lastly, a prior study showed that >95% reentrant AT following circumferential PV ablation arose from the prior ablation targets/lines for AF.[10] Therefore, AT in most patients is likely related to a proarrhythmic effect of ablation.

DIAGNOSIS

Establishing a diagnosis of postablation AT is straightforward. The diagnosis can be made on the ECG or ambulatory monitoring, or by analysis of stored electrograms in the patient with an implantable device. The ECG shows evidence of organized atrial activity, and that the P or flutter waves are identical with a consistent cycle length. This may require careful analysis of the ECG to distinguish between organized AF and AT. If the P waves are even slightly dissimilar in

SECTION VI
CATHETER ABLATION TECHNIQUES FOR
MANAGING ATRIAL FIBRILLATION AND
ATRIAL FLUTTER

288

CHAPTER 41

rate or appearance, the rhythm is likely AF and not AT. Not infrequently, the P waves may not be apparent due to low amplitude or are obscured by the QRS or T waves during rapid ventricular rates. An ECG during postablation AT is sometimes misdiagnosed as sinus tachycardia. A closer inspection of the ECG usually shows a P wave that is obscured by the QRS/T wave. Resting sinus tachycardia, in the absence of a coexisting illness in these patients—recall that patients with persistent AF have evidence of structural and sinus node remodeling—is uncommon.

The ECG may also be helpful in elucidating the mechanism of the atrial tachycardia. The P-wave duration during macroreentrant tachycardias (ie, "atrial flutter") is longer owing to continuous atrial activation. A recent study suggested that a cut-off value >185 ms is consistent with macroreentry.[8] During focal tachycardias or in situations in which reentry is confined to a small region of the atrium (ie, localized reentry or small reentrant circuits), the activation time is shorter, and the diastolic interval is longer as compared to large circuits. These features result in a shorter P-wave duration and a presence of an isoelectric interval between successive P waves. It should be stressed that in atria with multiple areas of conduction block or extensive scarring, these observations may not be applicable.

MANAGEMENT

Preprocedure Preparation

Not all patients with post-AF atrial tachycardia need to undergo a repeat ablation procedure. It is not unreasonable to perform transthoracic cardioversion (for persistent AT) or recommend antiarrhythmic medications (for paroxysmal AT) in the acute phase (within the first 3 months) following the AF procedure. In some of these patients, AT may not recur during long-term follow-up.[2] For AT that occurs after 3 months of the AF procedure, our practice is to recommend catheter ablation. Note that most of these patients were referred to for the initial AF procedure after failure or intolerance of antiarrhythmic medications. Thus, to prescribe antiarrhythmic medications on an indefinite basis is not an attractive option.

We prefer to perform the repeat procedure for AT during the arrhythmia, as opposed to sinus rhythm, as some clinical ATs may not be readily inducible in the electrophysiology laboratory. If the clinical arrhythmia is not inducible, the patient may experience recurrence, despite elimination of possible triggers (eg, reisolation of connected PVs) or empiric linear ablation at the major isthmi. Patients with paroxysmal tachycardia while taking antiarrhythmic medications are instructed to discontinue rhythm-controlling drugs a few weeks prior to the scheduled procedure. If the arrhythmia fails to recur, the procedure is postponed. Amiodarone should be discontinued at least 2 months prior to the ablation procedure given its long half-life. Another reason to discontinue antiarrhythmic medications prior to the ablation procedure is the possibility that the drug may be masking AF. The ablation procedure may eliminate AT, but underlying drivers may not be manifest and hence cannot be mapped and ablated.

One should be aware of the rapid atrioventricular (AV) nodal conduction that may occur in patients with AT as compared to patients with AF. As patients are asked to discontinue rate-controlling (and of course, rhythm-controlling) medications in preparation for the procedure, unchecked AV nodal conduction may result in tachycardia.

Occasionally, 1:1 AV nodal conduction may occur leading to hemodynamic collapse and syncope, and may require urgent transthoracic cardioversion. In such patients, our practice is to admit them to the hospital a day prior to the procedure allowing for drug washout and initiation of intravenous rate-controlling medications as needed.

Our preference is to perform the procedure on therapeutic oral anticoagulation to prevent not only thromboembolism but also access site complications, which are more likely related to intravenous or subcutaneous heparin. We ask patients who are taking one of the novel oral anticoagulants (dabigatran, rivaroxaban, or apixaban) to discontinue the drug 36 hours prior to the procedure. All patients who present to the electrophysiology laboratory in AT undergo transesophageal echocardiography to rule out LA thrombus prior to the procedure.

Mapping and Ablation of AT

A question often arises whether to map the right atrium first prior to performing transseptal catheterization or whether LA mapping may be obviated in some patients altogether. From a practical standpoint, all patients who have previously undergone LA ablation of AF deserve LA mapping at the repeat session to ensure that the PVs remain disconnected and that any linear lesions that were deployed previously are complete. Nonetheless, there are some clues on the ECG that suggest a right atrial source. Although cavotricuspid isthmus dependent flutter is not uncommonly seen after AF ablation, its ECG signature is frequently obscured by the attendant LA ablation. The end result is that the ECG may not show the classic saw-tooth pattern of the flutter waves in the inferior leads.[11] Initial negativity of the flutter waves, especially in the absence of notching, is suggestive a right atrial source. Further, a transition of positive to negative in the precordial leads is also suggestive (but not diagnostic) of flutter from the right atrial isthmus. Isoelectric flutter waves across the precordium are also suggestive of an LA origin.

A minimum of two venous sheaths is required for mapping and ablation of post-AF atrial tachycardia. A multipolar catheter is placed into the coronary sinus (CS). A distal-to-proximal activation confirms the presence of a LA source, whereas a proximal-to-distal activation is not as informative. The latter could be consistent with a right atrial, septal, or even lateral left atrial origin. For example, during counterclockwise mitral isthmus dependent flutter (which, unlike typical flutter, is equally prevalent as the clockwise version) or even during AT from the lateral LA in a patient with prior mitral isthmus conduction block, the CS is activated in proximal-to-distal fashion.

After LA access, the operator has a choice to map the AT using activation mapping using a 3-dimensional mapping system or entrainment mapping. There are advantages and disadvantages with either approach. A criticism of activation mapping is that it is time consuming and needs to be repeated in case of multiple tachycardias, which is not uncommon. However, a high-density map using a multipolar catheter (either a ring catheter [Lasso]or Pentaray, Biosense Webster, Diamond Bar, CA) can be constructed within 10 to 15 minutes. Currently, however, the operator still needs to review each point to accurate annotation, which may be time consuming. Further refinements and other promising technologies should help reduce the need of user intervention in assigning timing to activation points.

ATRIAL TACHYCARDIA OCCURRING
AFTER ABLATION OF ATRIAL
FIBRILLATION

SECTION VI
CATHETER ABLATION TECHNIQUES FOR
MANAGING ATRIAL FIBRILLATION AND
ATRIAL FLUTTER

289

The advantage of entrainment mapping is that it quickly informs the operator if the site in question is involved in the reentry circuit. If the postpacing interval (PPI) is within 20 to 30 ms of the tachycardia cycle length (without a change in atrial activation), the site in question is part of the reentry circuit. A PPI that approximates the TCL but with a change in atrial activation during pacing or a long PPI identifies a site that is not critical to the reentry circuit. A single "good" return cycle is not enough to establish the diagnosis or mechanism of the tachycardia. For large circuits, one has to show good PPIs from the opposite walls of the LA (anterior and posterior or superior and inferior in the case of roof flutter, and analogously around the mitral valve for perimitral flutter). The major drawback of such an approach is that pacing may change or terminate the tachycardia, which may not be inducible. If the clinical tachycardia cannot be reinduced, it may recur during follow-up. Occasionally, the return cycle may be significantly longer than the TCL despite that the fact target site lies in the reentrant path. As has been shown for typical flutter, delayed conduction may result in a spuriously long PPI.[12] Another problem with entrainment mapping is that it presupposes that the mechanism of the AT is macroreentry. The other possible mechanisms, eg, small reentrant circuits (during which the reentrant activity is restricted to a small segment of the atrium) and focal tachycardias, are probably best targeted by identifying the diastolic or presystolic activity, respectively, on the ECG.

The prevalence of these various mechanisms probably depends on the ablation approach that was utilized during the AF procedure. If multiple linear lesions were deployed, macroreentry is a good bet. In general, a macroreentrant mechanism involving the mitral isthmus, LA roof, the cavotricuspid isthmus, and other, less common areas is found in the majority of patients. In about 20% to 30% of patients, small reentrant or focal sources are found. For large circuits, the operator strives to design an ablation line that connects nonconductive areas, such as the two upper veins in the case of roof reentry, and lateral mitral valve to the left-sided PVs for perimitral reentry. The critical site within small reentrant circuits is characterized by very fractioned electrograms[13] that cover about 50% of the TCL, and these sites are exquisitely responsive to radiofrequency (RF) energy or even pacing.[8] For focal arrhythmias, the site with the earliest activation with respect to the P wave is targeted.

The endocardial mitral isthmus is typically ablated using about 35 watts of irrigated RF energy. The majority of patients with perimitral flutter require RF energy delivery within the distal CS (at 20 watts) for either tachycardia termination[14] or creation of isthmus block or both. If a lateral approach is ineffective, an anterior approach (from the anterior annulus to the right-side PVs) or a superior approach (from the anterolateral annulus, along the left lateral ridge, to the left upper PV) usually results in tachycardia termination. After tachycardia termination, pacing from anterior to the line (usually from the LA appendage) is performed to determine whether linear block is present. With incomplete block, one observes the anticipated activation of the CS, that is, from distal-to-proximal. With block, the CS is activated from proximal-to-distal, with prolongation of the conduction time (Figure 41-5). Linear block at the mitral isthmus can be achieved in about 90% of patients. Recently, an alternative to CS ablation has been introduced in patients undergoing mitral isthmus ablation.[15] The vein of Marshall, an atrial branch that is identified on CS venography, is injected with ethanol, which may reduce the amount of RF energy required (especially within the CS) for linear block.

The left atrial roof is ablated using 25 to 30 watts of irrigated RF depending upon the degree of sheath support. If an initial line at the most cranial aspect of the roof is ineffective, a slightly anterior approach may be effective. If tachycardia or conduction persists, RF energy is delivered at the high posterior wall and even the low posterior wall at the level of the PV antra. With a more posterior approach, one has to be aware of the location of the esophagus, and the line may be altered as appropriate. Linear block is confirmed by observing ascending activation of the posterior LA during pacing from the appendage or sinus rhythm (Figure 41-6). Linear block at the roof may be demonstrated in about 95% of patients, but it may be difficult to distinguish from slow conduction.

Procedural End Points

After tachycardia termination and demonstration of linear block, the next step is to ensure that all PVs remain isolated. Then, we perform an induction protocol using programmed atrial stimulation and rapid atrial pacing during isoproterenol infusion (10-20 mcg/min). It is important to note that despite tachycardia termination, PV reisolation, and noninducibility, some patients still experience recurrence.[8] In roughly one-half of the patients, recurrence is due to resumption of conduction along previously ablated lesions, and in the other half, emergence of a new tachycardia substrate that was not apparent at the previous session. To minimize the prevalence of the latter, we perform rapid atrial pacing to atrial refractoriness (to cycle lengths as short as 160 ms) during isoproterenol infusion, which may be the only way to induce ATs that may manifest themselves clinically during follow-up. With such an aggressive induction protocol, AF may occasionally be encountered. At this point, isoproterenol is discontinued to see if AF gives way to AT, which is then mapped and ablated. The clinical import of inducible AF that persists in this setting is not clear, but it is probably not unreasonable to perform cardioversion if the patient has not demonstrated AF clinically. Empiric ablation of the cavotricuspid isthmus is also reasonable to prevent recurrent arrhythmias.

OUTCOMES

Clinical AT can be eliminated in >90% of patients. Reasons for an unsuccessful ablation procedure include multiloop ATs that involve multiple circuits/mechanisms, extensive atrial scar, and involvement of the septum (especially involving the atrioventricular junction). Linear block at the roof and the mitral isthmus may be demonstrable in roughly 90% of patients. Nonetheless, 20% develop recurrence necessitating a repeat procedure.[8] After multiple procedures, long-term freedom from AT/AF can be achieved in about 80% of patients without antiarrhythmic medications.[8] The risk of a serious complication including vascular site issues that require transfusion or surgery, tamponade, or thromboembolism is about 1%. Anticoagulation is discontinued in most patients (except those with a prior stroke) in whom long-term ambulatory monitoring fails to show atrial arrhythmias. In case of procedural failure, other options include medical therapy (with either rhythm or rate-controlling medications) or AV junction ablation with a permanent pacemaker if the ventricular rates cannot be adequately managed. In the latter case, a pacemaker with

290

SECTION VI
CATHETER ABLATION TECHNIQUES FOR
MANAGING ATRIAL FIBRILLATION AND
ATRIAL FLUTTER

CHAPTER 41

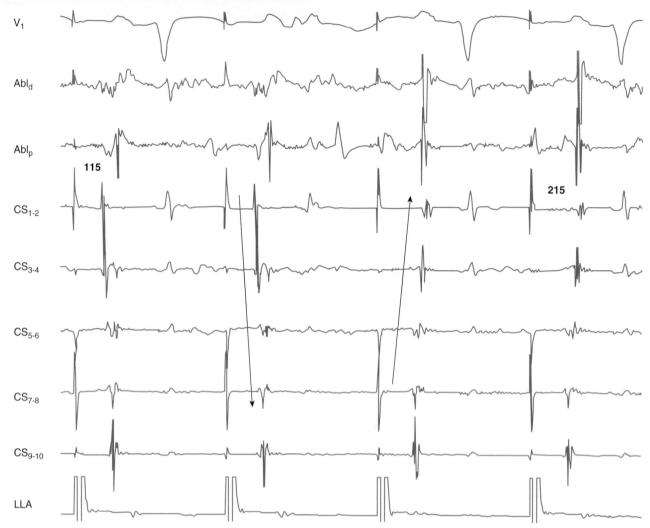

FIGURE 41-5 Linear block at the mitral isthmus usually requires radiofrequency ablation within the CS, as shown in this tracing from another patient. Note that during LAA pacing, the activation of the CS abruptly changes from the expected (distal-to-proximal) to the unexpected (proximal-to-distal), heralding conduction block at the mitral isthmus. Concomitantly, there is a sudden increase in the mitral isthmus conduction time from 115 to 215 ms.

ATRIAL TACHYCARDIA OCCURRING
AFTER ABLATION OF ATRIAL
FIBRILLATION

SECTION VI
CATHETER ABLATION TECHNIQUES FOR
MANAGING ATRIAL FIBRILLATION AND
ATRIAL FLUTTER

291

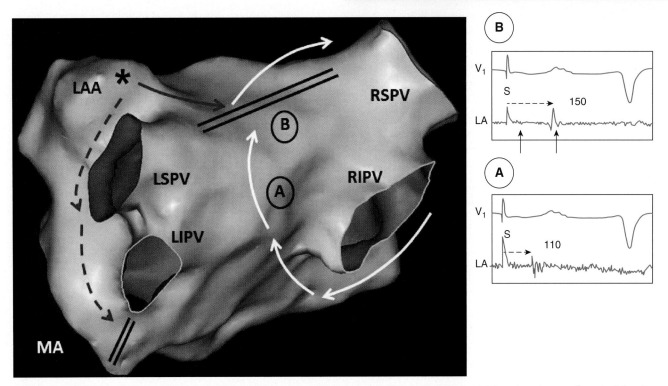

FIGURE 41-6 Confirmation of linear block at the LA roof from the same patient as in Figure 41-5. During LAA pacing, the wavefront (solid red arrow) blocks at the roof, and then descends the anterior wall (solid, white, downward pointing arrow). The latter wavefront then *ascends* the posterior wall, confirming conduction block at the roof. With persistent conduction across the roofline, one would expect to see *descending* activation of the posterior wall. Also shown are representative electrograms from the mid posterior LA (A) and high posterior LA, near the roofline (B). The increase in conduction time from A → B (110 to 150 ms) is consistent with ascending activation of the posterior wall and linear block at the roof. Also, note the presence of widely split double potentials (solid arrows on top electrogram) recorded on the line. In this patient, there was also block at the mitral isthmus (dashed arrows) LA.

atrial antitachycardia pacing is recommended as pacing is much more efficacious in terminating organized tachycardia as opposed to AF.

PATIENT EDUCATION

Some patients may not be able to distinguish symptoms during AT versus AF. However, others are particularly bothered by the higher heart rates that are present during AT as opposed to AF despite AV nodal medications. Some patients with facile AV nodal conduction may experience extremely fast heart rates during AT leading to syncope and may require urgent cardioversion. For these reasons and the fact that recurrences are common (even after an acutely successful procedure), patients with postablation AT require an experienced and dedicated team of outpatient clinical care coordinators, inpatient nurses and midlevel providers, and physicians to ensure optimal outcomes.

REFERENCES

1. Mesas CE, Pappone C, Lang CC, et al. Left atrial tachycardia after circumferential pulmonary vein ablation for atrial fibrillation: electroanatomic characterization and treatment. *J Am Coll Cardiol.* 2004;44(5):1071-1079.

2. Chugh A, Oral H, Lemola K, et al. Prevalence, mechanisms, and clinical significance of macroreentrant atrial tachycardia during and following left atrial ablation for atrial fibrillation. *Heart Rhythm.* 2005;2:464-471.

3. Gerstenfeld EP, Callans DJ, Dixit S, et al. Mechanisms of organized left atrial tachycardias occurring after pulmonary vein isolation. *Circulation.* 2004;110:1351-1357.

4. O'Neill MD, Wright M, Knecht S, et al. Long-term follow-up of persistent atrial fibrillation ablation using termination as a procedural endpoint. *Eur Heart J.* 2009;30:1105-1112.

5. Chugh A. Atrial tachycardia after ablation of persistent atrial fibrillation: is it us or them? *Circ Arrhythm Electrophysiol.* 2013;6:1047-1049.

6. Yoshida K, Chugh A, Ulfarsson M, et al. Relationship between the spectral characteristics of atrial fibrillation and atrial tachycardias that occur after catheter ablation of atrial fibrillation. *Heart Rhythm.* 2009;6:11-17.

7. Oral H, Scharf C, Chugh A, et al. Catheter ablation for paroxysmal atrial fibrillation: segmental pulmonary vein ostial ablation versus left atrial ablation. *Circulation.* 2003;108:2355-2360.

8. Yokokawa M, Latchamsetty R, Ghanbari H, et al. Characteristics of atrial tachycardia due to small vs large reentrant circuits after ablation of persistent atrial fibrillation. *Heart Rhythm.* 2013;10:469-476.

9. Narayan SM, Krummen DE, Shivkumar K, Clopton P, Rappel WJ, Miller JM. Treatment of atrial fibrillation by the ablation of localized sources: CONFIRM (Conventional Ablation for Atrial

Fibrillation With or Without Focal Impulse and Rotor Modulation) trial. *J Am Coll Cardiol.* 2012;60:628-636.

10. Chae S, Oral H, Good E, et al. Atrial tachycardia after circumferential pulmonary vein ablation of atrial fibrillation: mechanistic insights, results of catheter ablation, and risk factors for recurrence. *J Am Coll Cardiol.* 2007;50:1781-1787.

11. Chugh A, Latchamsetty R, Oral H, et al. Characteristics of cavotricuspid isthmus-dependent atrial flutter after left atrial ablation of atrial fibrillation. *Circulation.* 2006;113:609-615.

12. Vollmann D, Stevenson WG, Luthje L, et al. Misleading long post-pacing interval after entrainment of typical atrial flutter from the cavotricuspid isthmus. *J Am Coll Cardiol.* 2012;59:819-824.

13. Jais P, Matsuo S, Knecht S, et al. A deductive mapping strategy for atrial tachycardia following atrial fibrillation ablation: importance of localized reentry. *J Cardiovasc Electrophysiol.* 2009;20:480-491.

14. Chugh A, Oral H, Good E, et al. Catheter ablation of atypical atrial flutter and atrial tachycardia within the coronary sinus after left atrial ablation for atrial fibrillation. *J Am Coll Cardiol.* 2005;46:83-91.

15. Baez-Escudero JL, Morales PF, Dave AS, et al. Ethanol infusion in the vein of Marshall facilitates mitral isthmus ablation. *Heart Rhythm.* 2012;9:1207-1215.

PULMONARY VEIN STENOSIS

SECTION VI
CATHETER ABLATION TECHNIQUES FOR
MANAGING ATRIAL FIBRILLATION AND
ATRIAL FLUTTER

293

42 PULMONARY VEIN STENOSIS

Farbod Raiszadeh, MD, PhD, Luigi Di Biase, MD, PhD, FACC, FHRS, Pasquale Santangeli, MD, Rodney Horton, MD, Conor Barrett, MD, Stephan Danik, MD, Alessandro Paoletti Perini, MD, Francesco Santoro, MD, Sanghamitra Mohanty, MD, Rong Bai, MD, Javier E. Sanchez, MD, J. Joseph Gallinghouse, MD, J. David Burkhardt, MD, Andrea Natale, MD, FACC, FHRS, FESC

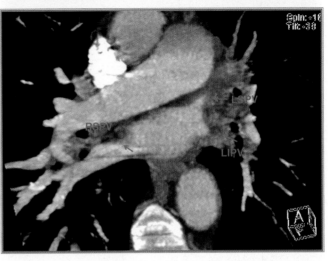

FIGURE 42-1 A 2-D CT scan image showing complete occlusion of the left inferior pulmonary veins (LIPVs) and severe stenosis of both left and right superior pulmonary veins (RSPVs).

CASE PRESENTATION

A 66-year-old man with hypertension and a history of bilateral hernia surgery was referred to our institution with persistent shortness of breath after two pulmonary vein isolations (PVIs) performed at another institution. At admission, he denied any chest discomfort, palpitations, syncope, or dizziness. The patient's arrhythmia history started in 2003 when he first developed symptomatic episodes of atrial fibrillation (AF). After determination of normal left ventricular function on echocardiogram, the arrhythmia was initially treated both with propafenone and flecainide at the appropriate doses, but this was ineffective. The patient's AF became more persistent, and he underwent several cardioversions. In 2006, he underwent his first PVI procedure with no complications. A CT scan performed 3 months after PVI showed no evidence of pulmonary vein (PV) stenosis. Five months after ablation, the patient developed atrial flutter, which required cardioversion. In 2008, the patient underwent a redo PVI procedure.

One month after the redo procedure, the patient started to experience progressively worsening dyspnea on exertion with daily activities such as walking on a flat surface. At admission, the results of blood screening tests and physical examination were normal. To establish the diagnosis, the patient had a CT scan and an echocardiogram 11 months after the redo procedure. The echocardiogram confirmed a normal LV EF but showed an enlarged pulmonary artery with increased pulmonic valve velocities consistent with pulmonary hypertension. There was also evidence of mild right ventricular hypertrophy and mild tricuspid regurgitation.

A transesophageal echocardiogram was performed to better assess the cardiac structures, but this was technically difficult and had suboptimal echocardiographic images. No thrombus was seen in the left atrium or the left atrial appendage. EF was estimated at 60%, and other cardiac structures were poorly visualized. Only the left superior PV was properly visualized and showed increased velocities on its distal portion on Doppler echocardiogram consistent with a significant stenosis. A CT scan was performed showing complete occlusion of the left inferior pulmonary veins (LIPVs) and severe stenosis of both left and RSPV. An enlarged pulmonary artery was also noted (Figures 42-1 and 42-2). Due to the presence of significant dyspnea and pulmonary hypertension related to PV stenosis of three PVs, the decision was made to recommend balloon angioplasty and possible stenting of the stenotic PVs. On angiography, the left superior, left inferior, and RSPVs were found severely stenosed (>90%) and were

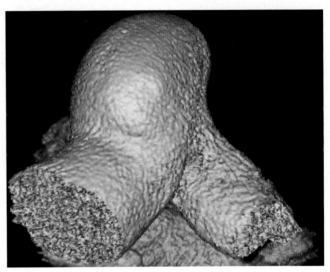

FIGURE 42-2 A 3-D CT scan image of the same patient (Figure 42-1) showing an enlarged pulmonary artery due to severe stenosis in three out of the four pulmonary veins.

294

SECTION VI
CATHETER ABLATION TECHNIQUES FOR
MANAGING ATRIAL FIBRILLATION AND
ATRIAL FLUTTER

CHAPTER 42

dilated with balloon angioplasty. There was no significant gradient across the stenotic segments following the dilation.

EPIDEMIOLOGY

Pulmonary vein stenosis/occlusion is defined as >70% narrowing of a PV and affects 3.4% of patients following catheter ablation of atrial fibrillation. The incidence of PV stenosis is partly explained by the method of ablation and partly by the experience of the operator and the volume of cases performed.[1-3] The incidence rate of PV stenosis is decreasing due to advances in intraprocedural imaging modalities and in improved ablation methods that limit the burning in the antrum of the PV,[2] but given the increasing and widespread use of catheter ablation as a treatment modality for atrial fibrillation, the overall incidence of this complication may rise.

ETIOLOGY AND PATHOPHYSIOLOGY

Pulmonary vein stenosis is a clinical condition caused by delivery of radiofrequency energy within or at the orifice of the PVs. The exact etiology and pathophysiology of PV stenosis after catheter ablation of atrial fibrillation is not completely understood. Application of radiofrequency lesions within the PVs or close to the ostium of PVs is the culprit. Animal models of PV stenosis suggest periadventitial inflammation and collagen deposition as the likely mechanisms leading to stenosis formation.[4] This is supported by imaging findings of fibrosis in perihilar PV tissues and presence of inflammatory protein precursors in involved PV areas.[5-7] Extensive ablation of PVs in dogs was shown to result in necrotic atrial myocardium interspersed with macrophages and red cells after 2 weeks and replacement of necrotic myocardium by collagen and appearance of organized thrombus by 4 weeks. Occlusion of PVs accompanied by cartilaginous metaplasia happens around 6 to 8 weeks, followed by replacement of necrotic atrial muscle with collagenous matrix and neovascularization in about 10 to 14 weeks after ablation.[6] The series of steps that lead from the application of radiofrequency energy around or inside the PV ostia to the stenosis of PVs can be summarized as:

- Metaplasia
- Proliferation of the elastic lamina/intima
- Hyperplasia
- Neovascularization
- Fibrosis and endovascular contraction
- Thrombosis

Clinical presentation of PV stenosis is widely variable in patients.[1-4] Severe stenosis of a single PV can be asymptomatic in a large number of cases. In symptomatic patients, the clinical presentation of PV stenosis can include any of the following symptoms:

- Chest pain
- Dyspnea
- Decreased exercise tolerance
- Cough
- Hemoptysis
- Fever

- Recurrent lung infection
- Pulmonary hypertension (is rare and requires severe stenosis of multiple PVs)

The severity of clinical symptoms is related to the number of involved PVs, the severity and length of stenosis, and the time course of stenosis formation.[4,8]

DIAGNOSIS

The diagnosis of PV stenosis after catheter ablation of atrial fibrillation relies on a high index of suspicion and obtaining appropriate imaging studies. Misdiagnosis is very common in patients with PV stenosis (pulmonary embolism, lung cancer, pneumonia, and new onset of asthma are most commonly misdiagnosed) because symptoms may occur far from the procedural time.[1-3] This is why timely imaging following catheter ablation is crucial even in asymptomatic patients. Indeed, most of the cases with PV stenosis are asymptomatic and may progress insidiously. Those who are symptomatic demonstrate a myriad of nonspecific symptoms.

Chest x-ray is usually not helpful in diagnosing PV stenosis. As demonstrated in the case history above, transesophageal echocardiogram (TEE) does not always provide clear images of the PVs in order to rule out PV stenosis. CT scan with contrast and MRI with contrast are the main imaging modalities used in diagnosis of PV stenosis[9,10] (Figure 42-3). Many groups recommend assessment of PV diameter using CT scan or MRI 3 months after PVI together with comparison of preablation measurements to ensure best identification of PV stenosis after ablation because the caliber remains relatively stable beyond 3 months after an ablation[11] (Figure 42-4). However, late progressions from a mild stenosis to a more severe stenosis have been described, and repeat imaging study is required in any patient who develops new symptoms suggestive of PV stenosis.[2]

In patients with moderate to severe stenosis, a ventilation/perfusion (V/Q) scan may be useful because it provides a reliable measure of the functional impact of the stenosis. Usually, more than 70% narrowing is required to have an abnormal (V/Q) scan.

The CSI (cumulative stenosis index = sum of percent stenosis of the unilateral veins divided by the total number ipsilateral veins) has been proposed with a cutoff value of 75% to identify patients at greatest risk of severe symptoms and lung disease.[2,11] Other diagnostic modalities include TTE, nuclear perfusion scans, and intracardiac echocardiograms (ICEs) employed during repeat catheter ablation procedures. Each of these modalities has its advantages and disadvantages (Table 42-1).

DIFFERENTIAL DIAGNOSIS

- Bronchopneumonia
- Interstitial lung disease
- Lung infection
- Pulmonary embolism
- Asthma
- Heart failure, diastolic
- Lung consolidation (cancer)

PULMONARY VEIN STENOSIS

SECTION VI
CATHETER ABLATION TECHNIQUES FOR
MANAGING ATRIAL FIBRILLATION AND
ATRIAL FLUTTER

295

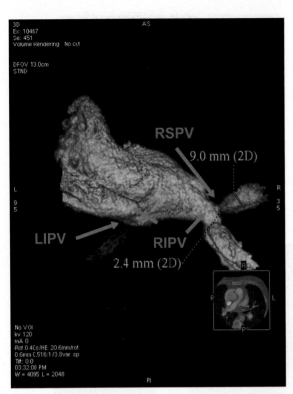

FIGURE 42-3 A 3-D CT scan of the same patient (Figures 42-1 and 42-2) showing complete occlusion of the left inferior pulmonary veins (LIPVs) and severe stenosis of both right superior PV (RSPV) and left superior PV (LSPV).

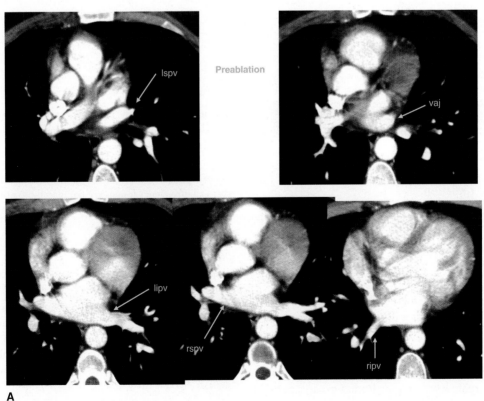

FIGURE 42-4 Preablation (A) and postablation (B). (A) A 2-D CT scan with contrast shows normal pulmonary venous anatomy and (B) thickening and narrowing of the venoatrial junction at the left superior pulmonary vein from 16 to 5 mm (arrow) with associated occlusion of a left tributary vein of the anterior apical left upper lobe. Minimal narrowing of the right and left inferior pulmonary veins. (Reproduced with permission from Feld GK, Srivatsa U, Hoppe B. Ablation of isthmus dependent atrial flutters. In: Huang SS, Wood MA, editors. Catheter ablation of cardiac arrhythmias. Philadelphia: Elsevier; 2011)

296

SECTION VI
CATHETER ABLATION TECHNIQUES FOR
MANAGING ATRIAL FIBRILLATION AND
ATRIAL FLUTTER

CHAPTER 42

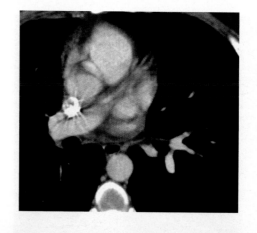

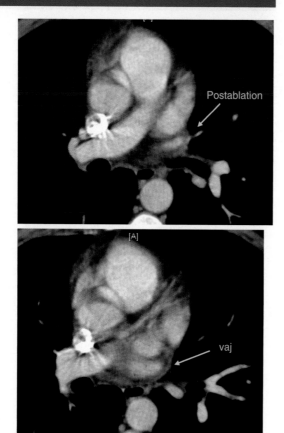

Postablation

vaj

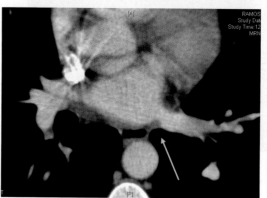

B

FIGURE 42-4 (Continued)

TABLE 42-1 Diagnostic Modalities Used in Diagnosis of PV Stenosis After Catheter Ablation of Atrial Fibrillation

Imaging Modalities	Advantages	Disadvantages
CT	Readily available.	Radiation exposure. Contrast exposure.
MRI	No radiation.	
TEE	Real-time reading and rapid interpretation. Doppler flow information.	Difficulty visualizing inferior veins.
Nuclear perfusion scan	Physiologic information on significance of observed stenosis.	Radiation exposure. In some cases may mimic pulmonary embolism.
PV angiography	Combined with treatment procedure.	Invasive procedure. Radiation and contrast exposure.
ICE	Real-time information during repeat ablation.	Invasive procedure.

MANAGEMENT

The best approach to the management of PV stenosis is prevention. Antral and segmental ablation approaches are preferred over focal and linear approaches as the risk of PV stenosis is lower with the latter. The cornerstone of prevention of PV stenosis for patients undergoing catheter ablation of atrial fibrillation is ensuring that radiofrequency lesions are not placed too distally into the PV veins.[13] Use of 3-D imaging and ICE can be useful in visualizing the location of the ablation catheter during ablation.[2,4] Multiple methods have been proposed to reduce the risk of PV stenosis during ablation (Table 42-2).

In patients who develop PV stenosis and who have abnormal CSI values, early and, when required, repeated PV intervention should be considered for restoration of pulmonary blood flow and prevention of associated lung disease.[2] Late opening of a stenotic vein, though feasible, may not provide the same benefit in reducing a patient's symptoms and restoring lung functionality. There is no consensus on the best approach to asymptomatic patients with PV stenosis. In these cases, CSI can be used to identify patients at higher risk for lung dysfunction and progressive disease.

For symptomatic patients with PV stenosis, angioplasty and stenting of the stenotic vein should be considered depending on the patients' symptoms and severity of the stenotic vein. Timely intervention after diagnosis of symptomatic PV stenosis is important

PULMONARY VEIN STENOSIS

SECTION VI
CATHETER ABLATION TECHNIQUES FOR
MANAGING ATRIAL FIBRILLATION AND
ATRIAL FLUTTER

297

TABLE 42-2 Procedural Methods to Prevent Development of Future PV Stenosis after Catheter Ablation of Atrial Fibrillation

Avoiding energy delivery inside the PV

Minimizing delivered power/energy

Avoiding high temperature readings

Use of intracardiac echo

Use of cryo as power source

Use of 3-D mapping systems

Increased operator experience

because later intervention, even when venous patency is restored, is not associated with significant improvement in lung perfusion and therefore does not result in symptom relief.[11]

Balloon angioplasty with or without stenting has been shown to achieve satisfactory results, although restenosis requiring repeat interventions is necessary in about 45% to 50% of patients[2,12] (Figure 42-5). Stent size of above 10 mm is associated with higher long-term patency rate; therefore, early intervention and using larger stents (if possible) is recommended.[4,14]

PATIENT EDUCATION

Patients undergoing catheter ablation of atrial fibrillation should be alerted to the possibility of PV stenosis and be educated about its symptoms so they can seek medical care in case any of the nonspecific symptoms of PV stenosis develop within weeks or months after their ablation procedure.

Patients who undergo treatment procedures for PV stenosis should be regularly followed up and undergo noninvasive diagnostic imaging to determine the response to therapy and recurrence of stenosis as a

significant number of patients will develop restenosis after angioplasty and stenting procedures and could potentially benefit from a repeat procedure.

CASE CONCLUSION

In the previously described case, the patient did not undergo an imaging study after the second ablation. As we explained, imaging is very important in the timely detection of PV stenosis even in asymptomatic patients. The dyspnea reported by the patients was underestimated and not investigated for nearly a year. This resulted in severe pulmonary hypertension and pulmonary artery dilatation (as seen on CT scan). In such a case, late dilation of the occluded PVs is angiographically possible but very likely will not solve the patient's symptoms. Indeed, this patient, despite a successful dilatation and stenting, died of severe pulmonary hypertension 2 years after the diagnosis.

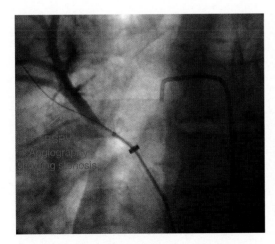
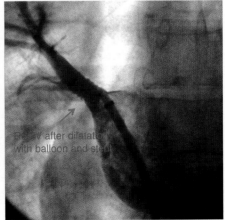

FIGURE 42-5 Pulmonary vein angiography demonstrating significant stenosis of RSPV (left) and acute resolution of stenosis after dilatation with balloon angioplasty and placement of a stent (right).

REFERENCES

1. Saad EB, Marrouche NF, Saad CP, et al. Pulmonary vein stenosis after catheter ablation of atrial fibrillation: emergence of a new clinical syndrome. *Ann Intern Med.* 2003;138(8):634-638.

2. Di Biase L, Fahmy TS, Wazni OM, et al. Pulmonary vein total occlusion following catheter ablation for atrial fibrillation: clinical implications after long-term follow-up. *J Am Coll Cardiol.* 2006;48(12):2493-2499.

3. Saad EB, Rossillo A, Saad CP, et al. Pulmonary vein stenosis after radiofrequency ablation of atrial fibrillation: functional characterization, evolution, and influence of the ablation strategy. *Circulation.* 2003;108(25):3102-3107.

4. Holmes DR Jr, Monahan KH, Packer D. Pulmonary vein stenosis complicating ablation for atrial fibrillation: clinical spectrum and interventional considerations. *JACC Cardiovasc Interv.* 2009;2(4):267-276.

5. Milton MA, Peterson TE, Johnson SB, et al. Marked cellular proliferation in pulmonary vein stenosis—a potential target of cell cycle inhibiting agents. *Pacing Clin Electrophysiol.* 2003;26(4p2):1054.

6. Taylor GW, Kay GN, Zheng X, Bishop S, Ideker RE. Pathological effects of extensive radiofrequency energy applications in the pulmonary veins in dogs. *Circulation.* 2000;101(14):1736-1742.

7. Li S, Li H, Mingyan E, Yu B. Expression of TGFbeta1 in pulmonary vein stenosis after radiofrequency ablation in chronic atrial fibrillation of dogs. *Mol Biol Rep.* 2009;36(2):221-225.

8. Tsao HM, Chen SA. Evaluation of pulmonary vein stenosis after catheter ablation of atrial fibrillation. *Card Electrophysiol Rev.* 2002;6(4):397-400.

9. Packer DL, Keelan P, Munger TM, et al. Clinical presentation, investigation, and management of pulmonary vein stenosis complicating ablation for atrial fibrillation. *Circulation.* 2005;111(5):546-554.

10. Neumann T, Sperzel J, Dill T, et al. Percutaneous pulmonary vein stenting for the treatment of severe stenosis after pulmonary vein isolation. *J Cardiovasc Electrophysiol.* 2005;16(11):1180-1188.

11. Barrett CD, Di Biase L, Natale A. How to identify and treat patient with pulmonary vein stenosis post atrial fibrillation ablation. *Curr Opin Cardiol.* 2009;24(1):42-49.

12. Qureshi AM, Prieto LR, Latson LA, et al. Transcatheter angioplasty for acquired pulmonary vein stenosis after radiofrequency ablation. *Circulation.* 2003;108(11):1336-1342.

13. Pürerfellner H, Martinek M. Pulmonary vein stenosis following catheter ablation of atrial fibrillation. *Curr Opin Cardiol.* 2005;20(6):484-490.

14. Prieto LR, Schoenhagen P, Arruda MJ, Natale A, Worley SE. Comparison of stent versus balloon angioplasty for pulmonary vein stenosis complicating pulmonary vein isolation. *J Cardiovasc Electrophysiol.* 2008;19(7):673-678.

ISTHMUS-DEPENDENT ATRIAL FLUTTER

SECTION VI
CATHETER ABLATION TECHNIQUES
FOR MANAGING ATRIAL FIBRILLATION
AND ATRIAL FLUTTER

299

43 ISTHMUS-DEPENDENT ATRIAL FLUTTER

Thomas McGarry, MD, and Gregory K. Feld, MD

CASE PRESENTATION

The patient, a 65-year-old retired physician, presented to our institution for evaluation of recurrent palpitations. The patient had a history of typical atrial flutter (AFL) documented by electrocardiogram (ECG) on several previous occasions (Figure 43-1A), including several emergency department visits during which he had undergone cardioversion. After failure of antiarrhythmic therapy, the patient underwent electrophysiology study (EPS) and cavotricuspid isthmus (CTI) ablation at another institution, in an attempt to cure the atrial flutter. The initial EPS confirmed the mechanism of typical AFL, but attempted ablation of the CTI was unsuccessful in producing bidirectional CTI conduction block. The patient continued to have recurrent palpitations and presented to our institution for further evaluation with an ECG showing a slightly modified flutter pattern suggesting an atypical AFL (Figure 43-2A). Repeat EPS with three-dimensional (3-D) electroanatomical mapping in this case demonstrated incomplete

CTI ablation with a large area of low voltage (ie, <0.5 mV) due to scarring in the CTI from prior ablation, but with persistent CTI conduction along a rim of viable myocardium near the tricuspid valve annulus, resulting in reinducibility of typical AFL (Figure 43-2B). Additional ablation of the CTI near the tricuspid valve annulus terminated AFL (Figure 43-3), and eliminated further clinical recurrences in this patient.

ELECTROPHYSIOLOGIC MECHANISMS OF ISTHMUS-DEPENDENT (TYPICAL AND REVERSE TYPICAL) ATRIAL FLUTTER

Electrophysiologic studies have shown typical and reverse typical AFL to be due to counterclockwise (typical) or clockwise (reverse typical) macroreentry around the tricuspid valve annulus (Figure 43-4, left and right), with an area of slow conduction in the CTI accounting for one-third to one-half of the AFL cycle length.[1-10] The CTI is bounded by the inferior vena cava and Eustachian ridge posteriorly and the tricuspid valve annulus (TVA) anteriorly (see Figure 43-4, left and right), forming barriers delineating a protected zone in the reentry circuit.[5,11-13] Lines of block, including the Eustachian ridge and the crista terminalis, along which double potentials are typically recorded during AFL (Figure 43-5A and B), are necessary to establish an adequate path-length for reentry to be sustained and to prevent short circuiting of the reentrant circuit.[12-14]

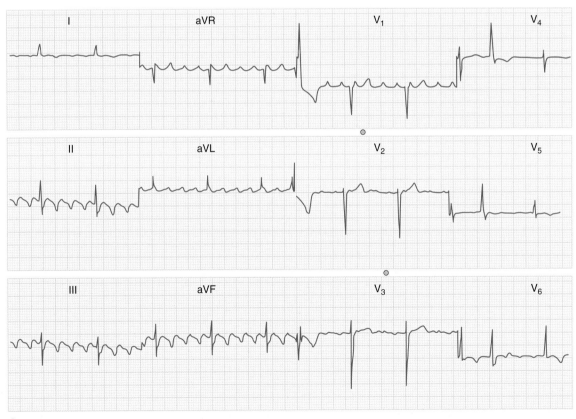

A

FIGURE 43-1 (A) A 12-lead ECG recorded during typical AFL, with typical saw-toothed pattern of inverted F waves in the inferior leads II, III, and aVF. (B) A 12-lead ECG recorded during reverse typical AFL, with atypical F wave pattern in the inferior leads. (Reproduced with permission from Feld GK, Srivatsa U, Hoppe B. Ablation of isthmus-dependent atrial flutters. In: Huang SS, Wood MA, eds. *Catheter Ablation of Cardiac Arrhythmias*. Philadelphia, PA: Elsevier; 2011.)

300

SECTION VI
CATHETER ABLATION TECHNIQUES
FOR MANAGING ATRIAL FIBRILLATION
AND ATRIAL FLUTTER

CHAPTER 43

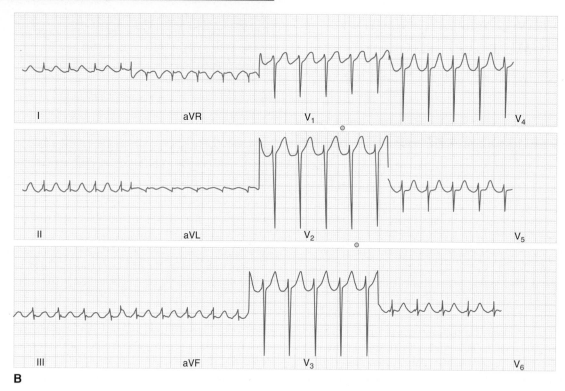

B

FIGURE 43-1 *(Continued)*

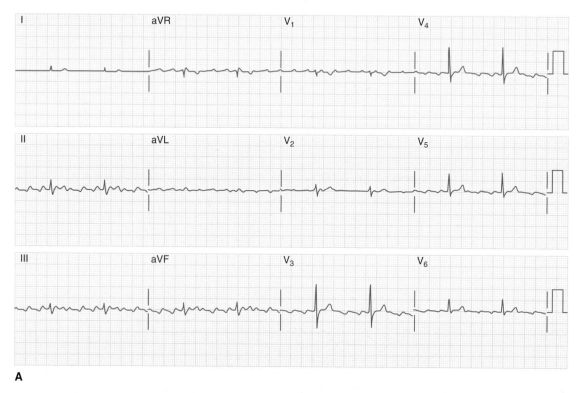

A

FIGURE 43-2 (A) A 12-lead ECG recorded during AFL following initial CTI ablation attempt. Note the biphasic F waves in the inferior leads II, III, and aVF, an atypical AFL pattern suggesting possible non–isthmus-dependent AFL. (B) During EPS a CARTO map of induced atrial flutter demonstrates an area of scarring (grey area) throughout the CTI near the Eustachian ridge, but continued activation of the CTI near the tricuspid valve annulus in a counterclockwise direction producing typical AFL. Color red = earliest activation, color purple = latest activation, reference coronary sinus electrogram. [(B) Reproduced with permission from Feld GK, Birgersdotter-Green U, Narayan S. Diagnosis and ablation of typical and reverse typical (type 1) atrial flutter. In: Wilber D, Packer D, Stevenson W, eds. *Catheter Ablation of Cardiac Arrhythmias: Basic Concepts and Clinical Applications.* 3rd ed. Oxford, England: Blackwell Publishing; 2007:173-192.]

ISTHMUS-DEPENDENT ATRIAL FLUTTER

SECTION VI
CATHETER ABLATION TECHNIQUES
FOR MANAGING ATRIAL FIBRILLATION
AND ATRIAL FLUTTER

301

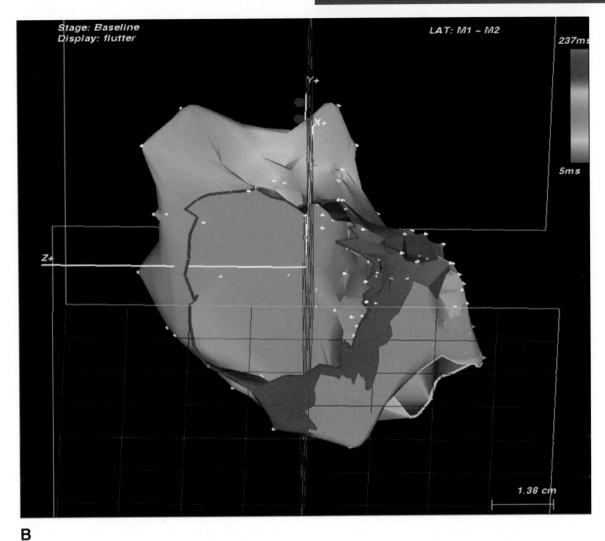

B

FIGURE 43-2 (*Continued*)

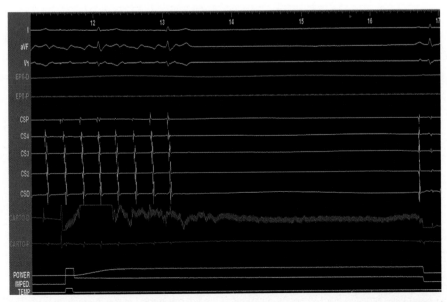

FIGURE 43-3 Surface ECG leads I, aVF, and V$_1$ and endocardial electrograms from the coronary sinus catheter (CSP-D), the ablation catheter (CARTO P&D), and power, impedance, and temperature readouts, show termination of AFL and restoration of sinus rhythm immediately after initiating ablation near the tricuspid valve annulus.

302

SECTION VI
CATHETER ABLATION TECHNIQUES
FOR MANAGING ATRIAL FIBRILLATION
AND ATRIAL FLUTTER

CHAPTER 43

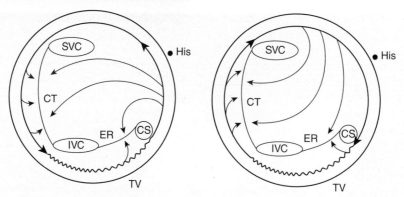

FIGURE 43-4 Schematic diagrams demonstrating right atrial activation patterns in typical (left) and reverse typical (right) forms of CTI-dependent AFL. In typical AFL, reentry occurs in a counterclockwise direction around the tricuspid valve annulus (TVA), whereas in reverse typical AFL reentry is clockwise. The Eustachian ridge (ER) and crista terminalis (CT) form lines of block, and an area of slow conduction (wavy line) is present in the CTI between the inferior vena cava (IVC) and Eustachian ridge and the tricuspid valve annulus. Abbreviations: CS, coronary sinus ostium; His, His bundle, SVC, superior vena cava. (Reproduced with permission from Feld GK, Srivatsa U, Hoppe B. Ablation of isthmus dependent atrial flutters. In: Huang SS, Wood MA, eds. *Catheter Ablation of Cardiac Arrhythmias.* Philadelphia: Elsevier; 2011.)

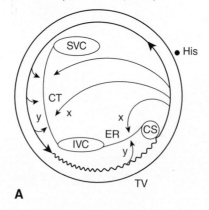

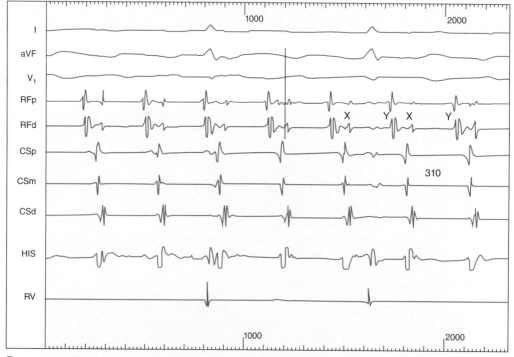

FIGURE 43-5 (A) Schematic diagram demonstrating where double potentials (x, y) are recorded during typical AFL along the Eustachian ridge and crista terminalis. (B) Double potentials recorded from an ablation catheter (RFp&d) positioned at the Eustachian ridge during typical AFL. Abbreviations: I, aVF, V₁, surface ECG leads; RFp&d, proximal and distal bipolar recordings from the ablation catheter; CSp-d, proximal to distal CS electrogram recordings; RV, right ventricular electrogram recording. (Reproduced with permission from Feld GK, Srivatsa U, Hoppe B. Ablation of isthmus dependent atrial flutters. In: Huang SS, Wood MA, eds. *Catheter Ablation of Cardiac Arrhythmias.* Philadelphia: Elsevier; 2011.)

ISTHMUS-DEPENDENT ATRIAL FLUTTER

SECTION VI
CATHETER ABLATION TECHNIQUES
FOR MANAGING ATRIAL FIBRILLATION
AND ATRIAL FLUTTER

303

Slow conduction in the CTI may be caused by anisotropic fiber orientation, predisposing it to development of unidirectional block during rapid activation.[2,8-10,15-19] The predominate clinical presentation of isthmus-dependent AFL is typical AFL, likely triggered by premature atrial contractions originating from the left atrium (LA) or nonsustained atrial fibrillation (AF),[20] both of which result in clockwise unidirectional block in the CTI and initiation of counterclockwise macroreentry.

ECG PATTERNS OF TYPICAL (AND REVERSE TYPICAL) ATRIAL FLUTTER

In typical AFL, there is a characteristic inverted saw-tooth F wave pattern in the inferior leads II, III, and aVF. In reverse typical AFL, in contrast, the F wave pattern on the 12-lead ECG is less specific, often with a sine wave pattern in the inferior ECG leads (Figure 43-1A and B). The F wave pattern on ECG is dependent in part on the activation sequence of the LA, with inverted F waves in the inferior leads in typical AFL the result of activation of the left atrium initially near the coronary sinus (CS), and upright F waves in the inferior leads in reverse typical AFL resulting from activation of the LA near Bachman bundle.[21,22] However, following LA ablation, and even right atrial ablation as in this case, the ECG presentation of isthmus-dependent AFL may be significantly different from the characteristic patterns described above.[23]

STANDARD CATHETER MAPPING OF ISTHMUS-DEPENDENT ATRIAL FLUTTER

Despite the characteristic 12-lead ECG pattern, electrophysiologic mapping and entrainment must be performed prior to radiofrequency catheter ablation of AFL. For standard catheter mapping, multielectrode catheters are typically positioned in the right atrium (RA), His bundle region, CS, and around the TVA (Figure 43-6). Recordings obtained during AFL (ie, spontaneous or induced) are then analyzed

to determine the RA activation sequence. Typical or reverse typical AFL is confirmed by observing a counterclockwise or clockwise activation pattern in the RA around the TVA, respectively, (Figures 43-7A and B) and demonstration of concealed entrainment during pacing from the CTI (Figures 43-8 A and B).[5]

RADIOFREQUENCY CATHETER ABLATION OF TYPICAL ATRIAL FLUTTER

Radiofrequency catheter ablation (RFCA) of isthmus-dependent AFL is performed with a steerable mapping/ablation catheter positioned across the CTI via a femoral vein.[3,5-7,24-26] Catheters with either saline-irrigated ablation electrodes (Thermocool Classic or SF, Biosense Webster, Inc, Diamond Bar, CA, or Chili, Boston Scientific, Inc., Natick, MA), or large distal ablation electrodes (ie, 8-10 mm Blazer, Boston Scientific, Inc, Natick, MA) are preferred for CTI ablation.[27,29,30-33]

The preferred target for isthmus-dependent AFL ablation is the CTI (Figure 43-9A).[3,5-7,24-30, 32,33] The ablation catheter is positioned across the CTI (Figure 43-6) with the ablation electrode near the TVA, midway between the septum and RA free wall, in order to record an atrial-to-ventricular electrogram amplitude ratio of 1:2 to 1:4 (Figure 43-6). The ablation catheter is then withdrawn a few millimeters at a time, pausing for 30 to 60 seconds at each location during a continuous or interrupted RF energy application. The catheter should be withdrawn until the ablation electrode records no atrial electrogram or until it is noted to abruptly slip off the Eustachian ridge. Radiofrequency energy application should be immediately interrupted when the catheter reaches the inferior vena cava, since ablation in venous structures may cause significant pain.

PROCEDURE END POINTS FOR RADIOFREQUENCY CATHETER ABLATION OF TYPICAL ATRIAL FLUTTER

Ablation may be performed during AFL or sinus rhythm. If performed during AFL, the first end point is its termination (Figure 43-9B).

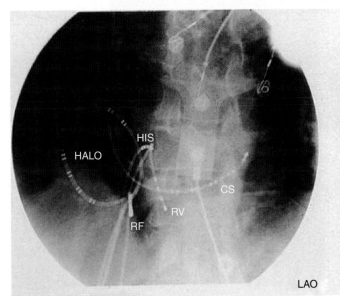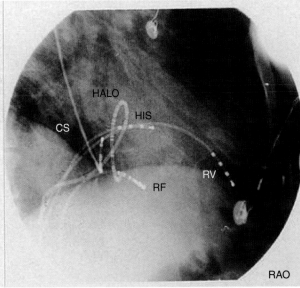

FIGURE 43-6 Left anterior oblique (LAO) and right anterior oblique (RAO) fluoroscopic projections showing common intracardiac positions of the right ventricular (RV), His bundle (HIS), coronary sinus (CS), Halo (HALO), and mapping/ablation catheters (RF). (Reproduced with permission from Feld GK, Srivatsa U, Hoppe B. Ablation of isthmus dependent atrial flutters. In: Huang SS, Wood MA, eds. *Catheter Ablation of Cardiac Arrhythmias.* Philadelphia: Elsevier; 2006:195-218.)

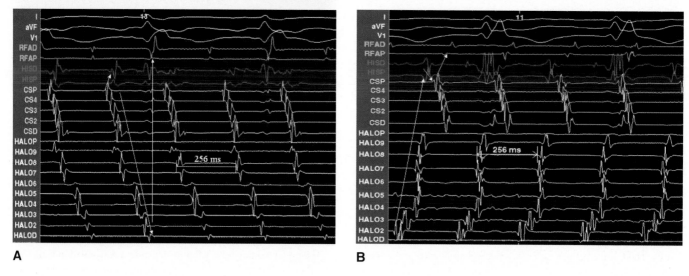

FIGURE 43-7 Endocardial electrograms from the mapping/ablation, Halo, CS, and His bundle catheters, and surface ECG leads I and aVF, during typical AFL (A) and reverse typical AFL (B). The atrial cycle length was 256 ms for both, and the arrows demonstrate the activation sequence. Abbreviations: CSP, electrograms recorded from the CS ostium; HISP, electrograms recorded at the proximal His bundle; RF, electrograms recorded from the mapping/ablation catheter in the CTI. (Reproduced with permission from Feld GK, Srivatsa U, Hoppe B. Ablation of isthmus dependent atrial flutters. In: Huang SS, Wood MA, editors. Catheter ablation of cardiac arrhythmias. Philadelphia: Elsevier; 2011.)

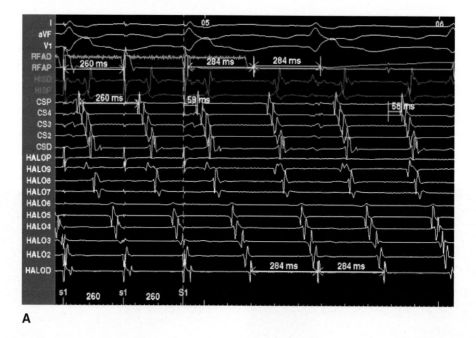

FIGURE 43-8 Endocardial electrograms from the RF, Halo, CS, and His bundle catheters, and surface ECG leads I, aVF, and V₁, demonstrating concealed entrainment during pacing at the CTI in typical AFL (A) and reverse typical AFL (B). Abbreviations: Halo D-Halo P, bipolar electrograms from the distal to proximal poles of the Halo catheter around the TVA; CSP-D, bipolar electrograms recorded from the proximal to distal CS catheter electrode pairs; HISP&D, bipolar electrograms recorded from the proximal and distal His bundle catheter; RFAP&D, bipolar electrograms recorded from the proximal and distal electrode pairs of the mapping/ablation catheter at the CTI. (Reproduced with permission from Feld GK, Srivatsa U, Hoppe B. Ablation of isthmus dependent atrial flutters. In: Huang SS, Wood MA, editors. Catheter ablation of cardiac arrhythmias. Philadelphia: Elsevier; 2011.)

After CTI ablation, electrophysiologic testing is required to ensure the presence of bidirectional conduction block (Figures 43-10A and B and 43-11A and B), which is confirmed by demonstrating a strictly cranial-to-caudal activation sequence in the contralateral RA, and widely spaced double potentials (ie, usually ≥120 ms apart) along the ablation line, during pacing from the low lateral right atrium and CS ostium, respectively (Figure 43-12).[34-38] Electrophysiologic testing should be repeated up to 30 to 60 minutes after ablation to ensure that bidirectional CTI block persists, and that AFL cannot be reinduced, in order to significantly lower the risk of recurrent AFL during long-term follow-up.[3,5-7,24-28,30-36,39-40]

OUTCOMES AND COMPLICATIONS OF CTI ABLATION FOR ISTHMUS-DEPENDENT ATRIAL FLUTTER

Although early reports of RFCA for AFL revealed recurrence rates up to 20% to 45%, subsequent studies have demonstrated acute and chronic efficacy in excess of 95% (Table 43-1), although patients with complex CTI anatomy may have higher recurrence rates in long-term follow-up.[41] Randomized comparisons of internally cooled, externally cooled, and large-tip ablation catheters, suggest a slightly better acute and chronic success rate with externally cooled ablation catheters, compared to internally cooled or large-tip ablation catheters.[27,28,30,33,40,42]

Radiofrequency catheter ablation for typical AFL is relatively safe, but serious complications can occur, including AV block, cardiac perforation, pericardial tamponade, and thromboembolic events, including pulmonary embolism and stroke. In recent large-scale studies, including those using large-tip ablation catheters and high power generators, major complications have been observed in only 2.5% to 3.0% of patients.[32,33,40]

ALTERNATIVE ENERGY SOURCES FOR ABLATION OF TYPICAL ATRIAL FLUTTER

Alternate energy sources for CTI ablation are being studied due to the disadvantages of RFCA, including pain, risk of coagulum formation and embolization, tissue charring, and subendocardial steam pops resulting in perforation. Several studies have been published on cryoablation and microwave ablation of AFL.[43-46] Cryoablation of isthmus-dependent AFL can achieve results similar to RFCA.[43,44] Cryoablation produces less pain during ablation and does not cause tissue charring or coagulum formation, or steam pops.[43,44] In addition, the CTI may be ablated with microwave energy (Medwaves, Inc., San Diego, CA) using a catheter-mounted antennae with lengths up to 4 cm.[45,46] Microwave ablation might reduce procedure time considering the length of the electrodes that can effectively ablate tissue.[45,46]

COMPUTERIZED 3-D MAPPING AND INTRACARDIAC ECHOCARDIOGRAPHY (ICE) GUIDANCE FOR CTI ABLATION

Three-dimensional (3-D) electroanatomical activation mapping systems (CARTO, BioSense-Webster, Diamond Bar, CA, and ESI NavX, St. Jude, Inc., St. Paul, MN) and noncontact balloon (Ensite, St. Jude, Inc., St. Paul, MN), although not required for isthmus-dependent AFL ablation, are now widely used. Although it is not

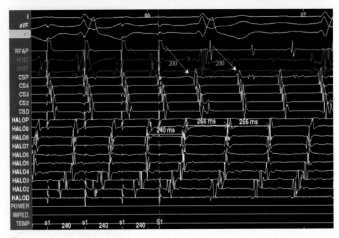

B

FIGURE 43-8 (Continued)

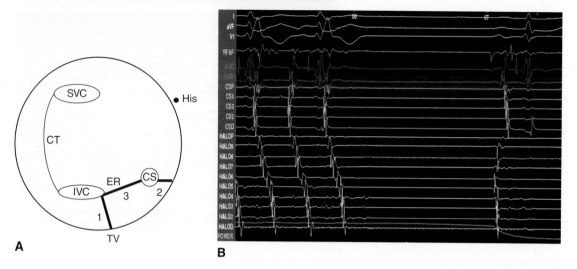

FIGURE 43-9 (A) A schematic diagram of the right atrium demonstrating the potential targets for ablation of CTI-dependent AFL. The preferred target for ablation is the CTI. (B) Surface ECG and endocardial electrogram recordings during ablation of the CTI showing termination of AFL. Abbreviations: I, aVF, V₁, surface ECG leads; RFAP, proximal ablation electrogram; Hisp&d, proximal and distal His bundle electrograms; CSd-p, distal to proximal CS electrograms; Halo d-p, distal to proximal Halo catheter electrograms (Reproduced with permission from Feld GK, Srivatsa U, Hoppe B. Ablation of isthmus dependent atrial flutters. In: Huang SS, Wood MA, editors. Catheter ablation of cardiac arrhythmias. Philadelphia: Elsevier; 2011.)

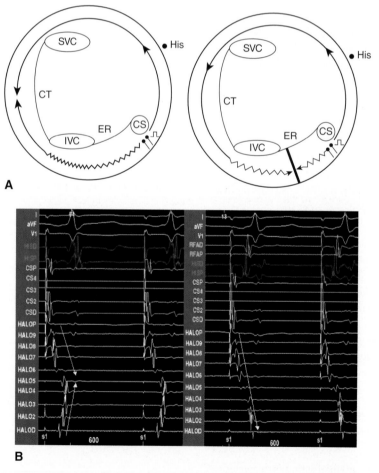

FIGURE 43-10 (A) A schematic diagram of the expected right atrial activation sequence during pacing in sinus rhythm from the CS ostium before (left) and after (right) ablation of the CTI. Abbreviations: CT, crista terminalis; ER, Eustachian ridge; His, His bundle; IVC, inferior vena cava; SVC, superior vena cava. (B) Surface ECG and right atrial endocardial electrograms recorded during pacing in sinus rhythm from the CS ostium before (left) and after (right) CTI ablation. (Reproduced with permission from Feld GK, Srivatsa U, Hoppe B. Ablation of isthmus dependent atrial flutters. In: Huang SS, Wood MA, editors. Catheter ablation of cardiac arrhythmias. Philadelphia: Elsevier; 2011.)

ISTHMUS-DEPENDENT ATRIAL FLUTTER

SECTION VI
CATHETER ABLATION TECHNIQUES
FOR MANAGING ATRIAL FIBRILLATION
AND ATRIAL FLUTTER

307

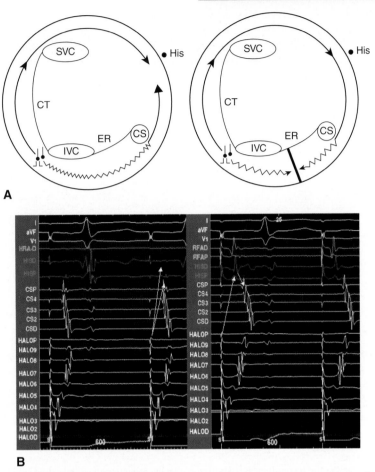

FIGURE 43-11 (A) A schematic diagram of the expected right atrial activation sequence during pacing in sinus rhythm from the low lateral right atrium before (left) and after (right) ablation of the CTI. Abbreviations: CT, crista terminalis; ER, Eustachian ridge; His, His bundle; SVC, superior vena cava; IVC, inferior vena cava. (B) Surface ECG and right atrial endocardial electrograms recorded during pacing in sinus rhythm from the low lateral right atrium before (left) and after (right) ablation of the CTI. (Reproduced with permission from Feld GK, Srivatsa U, Hoppe B. Ablation of isthmus dependent atrial flutters. In: Huang SS, Wood MA, editors. Catheter ablation of cardiac arrhythmias. Philadelphia: Elsevier; 2011.)

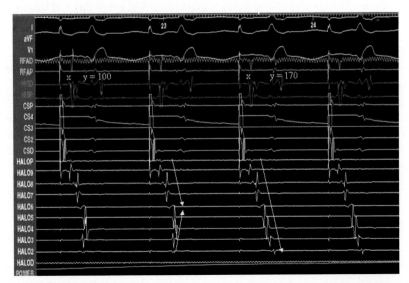

FIGURE 43-12 Surface ECG leads I, aVF, and V$_1$, and endocardial electrograms from the CS sinus, His bundle, Halo, mapping/ablation (RF), and right ventricular (RV) catheters during ablation of the CTI while pacing from the CS ostium. Note the change in activation sequence in the lateral right atrium on the Halo catheter from bidirectional to unidirectional, indicating development of clockwise block in the CTI. This was associated with development of widely spaced (170 ms) double potentials (x and y) on the RF catheter along the ablation line, confirming medial to lateral conduction block. All abbreviations are the same as in previous figures. (Reproduced with permission from Feld GK, Srivatsa U, Hoppe B. Ablation of isthmus dependent atrial flutters. In: Huang SS, Wood MA, editors. Catheter ablation of cardiac arrhythmias. Philadelphia: Elsevier; 2011.)

308

SECTION VI
CATHETER ABLATION TECHNIQUES
FOR MANAGING ATRIAL FIBRILLATION
AND ATRIAL FLUTTER

CHAPTER 43

TABLE 43-1 Success Rates for Radiofrequency Catheter Ablation of Atrial Flutter

Author	Year (ref)	N	Electrode Length	% Acute Success	Follow-Up (Months)	% Chronic Success
Feld	1992[5]	16	4	100	4±2	83
Cosio	1993[6]	9	4	100	2–18	56
Kirkorian	1994[25]	22	4	86	8±13	84
Fischer	1995[24]	80	4	73	20±8	81
Poty	1995[35]	12	6/8	100	9±3	92
Schwartzman	1996[36]	35	8	100	1-21	92
Chauchemez	1996[39]	20	4	100	8±2	80
Tsai	1999[31]	50	8	92	10±5	100
Atiga	2002[30]	59	4 versus cooled	88	13±4	93
Scavee	2004[28]	80	8 versus cooled	80	15	98
Feld	2004[32]	169	8 or 10	93	6	97
Calkins	2004[40]	150	8	88	6	87
Ventura	2004[33]	130	8 versus cooled	100	14±2	98

Abbreviations: N, number of patients studied; % acute success, termination of AFL during ablation and/or demonstration of bidirectional CTI block following ablation; % chronic success, percentage of patients in whom type 1 atrial flutter did not recur during follow-up. Acute and chronic success rates are reported as overall results in randomized or comparison studies.

within the scope of this chapter to describe the technological basis of these systems in detail, there are unique characteristics of each system that make them more or less suitable for mapping and ablation of atrial flutter.

A 3-D mapping system may be particularly useful in difficult cases such as those where prior ablation has failed, similar to the case described herein (Figure 43-2B), those with complex CTI anatomy, or those with surgically corrected congenital heart disease such as an atrial septal defect. Voltage mapping, alone or in combination with activation mapping, may also be helpful to identify areas of thinner muscle in the CTI that may be more easily ablated. Following CTI ablation, 3-D mapping may also be used to confirm CTI block, when pacing from the proximal CS catheter electrodes (Figure 43-13) or the low lateral right atrium. ICE may also be used to identify anatomical variations in the CTI, such as a wide or thickened CTI or deep pouches in the CTI that may make ablation difficult using standard techniques. Visualization of these anatomical variations with ICE may allow their avoidance or better catheter contact with the CTI, increasing the acute and long-term success rates of ablation (Figure 43-14).

ATYPICAL FORMS OF ISTHMUS-DEPENDENT ATRIAL FLUTTER

In lower loop reentrant AFL, the activation wave front spreads through the crista terminalis and around the inferior vena cava through the CTI (Figure 43-15A). This is in contrast to typical AFL, where the crista terminalis behaves as a line of block, albeit functional in most cases. The diagnosis of lower loop reentrant AFL is confirmed by the demonstration of concealed entrainment of the

tachycardia from not only the CTI but also the inferior-posterior right atrium.[47] In lower loop reentry, the posterior right atrium is part of the reentry circuit, and wave fronts collide in the lateral right atrium[47] (Figure 15B). Lower loop reentrant AFL may be slowed or terminated by ablation posteriorly along the crista terminalis from the superior vena cava to the inferior vena cava, but will usually convert to typical AFL and require CTI ablation for cure.

In partial isthmus-dependent AFL, the wave front bypasses the (CTI) to enter it laterally and medially in opposite directions, with collision of wave fronts near the middle of the CTI[48] (Figure 43-16). Partial isthmus-dependent AFL is confirmed by the demonstration of concealed entrainment from the lateral margin of the CTI but not from the medial portion near the tricuspid valve.[48] In addition, there is early activation of the CS ostium and evidence of collision with double potentials recorded within the medial CTI.[48] Cure of partial isthmus-dependent AFL can be achieved by ablation at the lateral CTI.

SIMPLIFIED APPROACH TO ABLATION OF TYPICAL (AND REVERSE TYPICAL) AFL

We have developed a simplified approach for CTI ablation in patients with isthmus-dependent AFL, using only two catheters. CTI ablation can be rapidly achieved with minimal fluoroscopy time using this approach. After percutaneous insertion via the right femoral vein, a steerable decapolar catheter is positioned in the CS with the proximal electrode pair at the ostium near the medial CTI, and an ablation catheter is flexed in the low lateral right atrium with the distal pair near the lateral CTI (Figure 43-17A). Pacing from the proximal CS

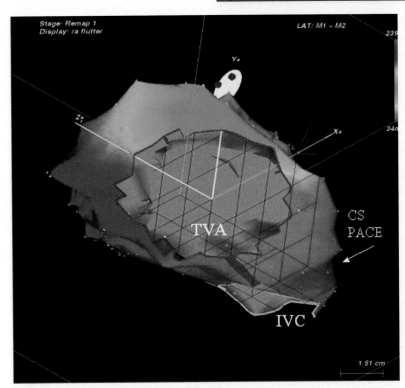

FIGURE 43-13 A 3-D electroanatomical (CARTO) map of the right atrium is shown in a patient with typical AFL after CTI ablation. Following ablation of the CTI, during pacing from the coronary sinus ostium, there is evidence of medial-to-lateral isthmus block as indicated by juxtaposition of orange and purple color in the CTI, indicating early and late activation, respectively. (Reproduced with permission from Feld GK, Birgersdotter-Green U, Narayan S. Diagnosis and Ablation of Typical and Reverse Typical (Type 1) Atrial Flutter. In: Catheter Ablation of Cardiac Arrhythmias: Basic Concepts and Clinical Applications, 3rd Edition, Wilber D, Packer D, Stevenson W, eds., Blackwell Publishing, Oxford, England, pp:173-192, 2007.)

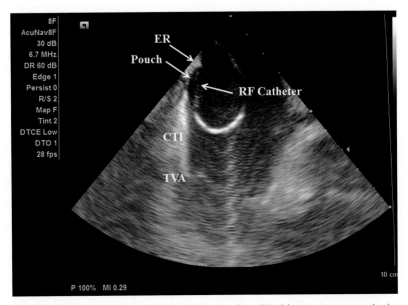

FIGURE 43-14 Intracardiac echo (ICE) image of a deep pouch preventing complete CTI ablation using a standard approach, due to difficulty in achieving adequate contact between the ablation catheter tip and the CTI in the pouch near the Eustachian ridge (ER). Positioning the ablation catheter in the CTI under ICE guidance, with a reverse curl from the inferior vena cava, such that the ablation electrode was just beneath the ER resulted in improved catheter-tissue contact with complete CTI ablation and bidirectional conduction block. Abbreviations: CTI, cavotricuspid isthmus; RF, radiofrequency; TVA, tricuspid valve annulus.

310

SECTION VI
CATHETER ABLATION TECHNIQUES
FOR MANAGING ATRIAL FIBRILLATION
AND ATRIAL FLUTTER

CHAPTER 43

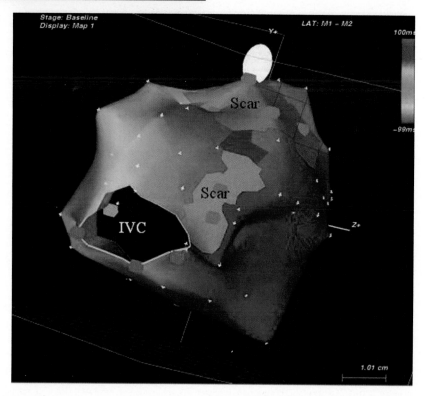

FIGURE 43-15 A CARTO 3-D activation sequence map (posterior caudal view) is shown in a patient with lower loop reentry. Note that the activation wave front spreads counterclockwise in the right atrium and horizontally across the crista terminalis between two (superior and inferior) areas of scarring in the posterior right atrial wall. Ablation between the scarred areas converted this atypical AFL into a typical AFL, which was ablated at the CTI. Abbreviation: IVC, inferior vena cava. (Reproduced with permission from Feld GK, Birgersdotter-Green U, Narayan S. Diagnosis and Ablation of Typical and Reverse Typical (Type 1) Atrial Flutter. In: Catheter Ablation of Cardiac Arrhythmias: Basic Concepts and Clinical Applications, 3rd Edition, Wilber D, Packer D, Stevenson W, eds., Blackwell Publishing, Oxford, England, pp:173-192, 2007)

ISTHMUS-DEPENDENT ATRIAL FLUTTER

SECTION VI
CATHETER ABLATION TECHNIQUES
FOR MANAGING ATRIAL FIBRILLATION
AND ATRIAL FLUTTER

311

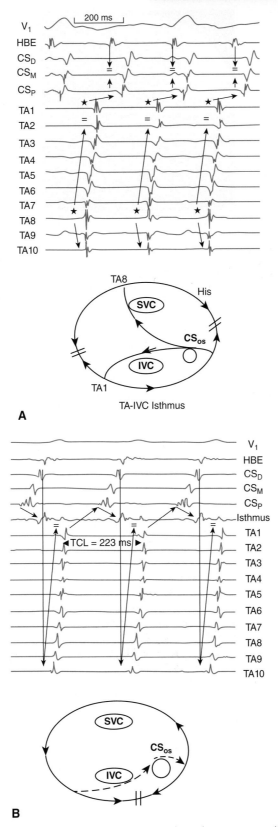

FIGURE 43-16 Electrograms and schematic representation of atrial activation in lower loop reentry and partial isthmus-dependent flutter. (A) In lower loop reentry, the posterior right atrium is part of the reentry circuit and wave fronts collide in the lateral right atrium. The electrograms show multiple collisions at TA1 and TA8 (stars). (B) In partial isthmus-dependent flutter, the wave front bypasses the cavotricuspid isthmus (CTI) to enter it laterally and medially. The coronary sinus (CS) ostium is activated prematurely, and the tachycardia is not entrained from the CTI itself. Abbreviations: IVC, inferior vena cava; SVC, superior vena cava; TA10, proximal recording electrodes on Halo catheter near upper septum; TA1, distal recording electrodes on Halo catheter near lateral aspect of the CTI. (Reproduced with permission from Yang Y, Cheng J, Bochoeyer A, et al. Atypical right atrial flutter patterns. Circulation 2001;Jun 26;103(25):3092-3098.)

312

SECTION VI
CATHETER ABLATION TECHNIQUES
FOR MANAGING ATRIAL FIBRILLATION
AND ATRIAL FLUTTER

CHAPTER 43

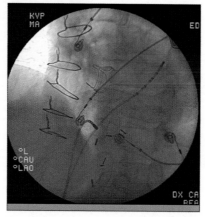

A

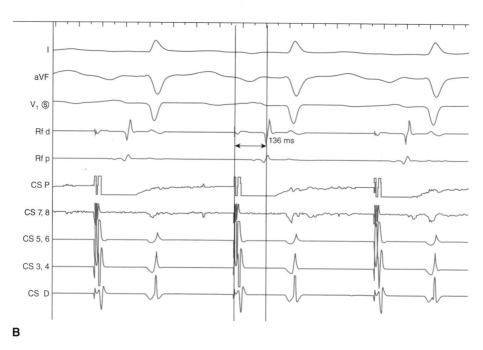

B

FIGURE 43-17 (A) Left anterior oblique fluoroscopic projection showing the positions of the CS and ablation catheter after CTI ablation to demonstrate conduction block. The proximal CS catheter electrode is positioned near the CS ostium, and the ablation catheter is positioned at the lateral CTI. (B) Surface ECG and endocardial electrogram recordings during pacing from the proximal CS demonstrating a proximal to distal (high to low) activation sequence on the ablation catheter with a conduction time of 136 ms confirming medial to lateral CTI conduction block. Abbreviations: I, aVF, V_1, surface ECG leads; RFd&p, distal and proximal ablation catheter electrograms; CSd-p, distal to proximal CS electrograms. (C) Surface ECG and endocardial electrogram recordings during pacing from the ablation catheter at the low lateral right atrium demonstrating a conduction time to the proximal CS of 138 ms, similar to the medial to lateral conduction time, confirming lateral to medial CTI conduction block. Abbreviations same as in Figure 43-16B. (D) Surface ECG and endocardial electrogram recordings during pacing from the proximal CS demonstrating widely spaced (130 ms) double potentials (x and y) at the ablation line, confirming medial to lateral conduction block. Abbreviations same as in previous figures. (Reproduced with permission from Sawhney NS, Wayne Whitwam W, Feld GK. Mapping of Human Atrial Flutter and Its Variants, In: Cardiac Mapping, 4th Edition, Shenasa M, Hindricks G, Borggrefe M, Briethardt G, eds., Wiley-Blackwell, Hoboken, NJ, 2012, pp: 191-212.)

ISTHMUS-DEPENDENT ATRIAL FLUTTER

SECTION VI
CATHETER ABLATION TECHNIQUES
FOR MANAGING ATRIAL FIBRILLATION
AND ATRIAL FLUTTER

313

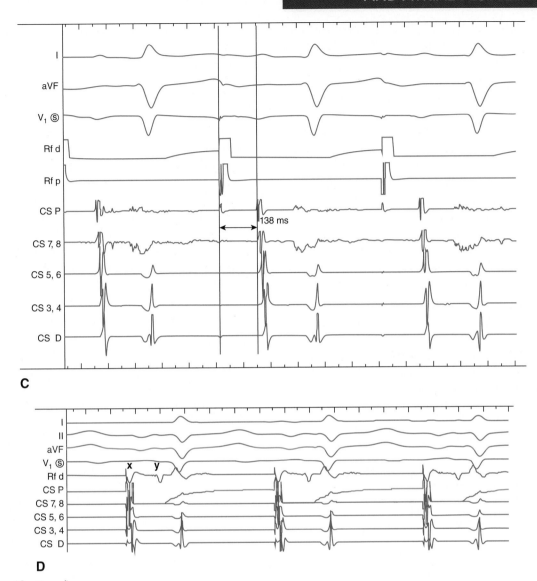

FIGURE 43-17 *(Continued)*

and the ablation catheter demonstrates bidirectional CTI conduction before and block after CTI ablation (Figure 43-17B and C). Using this simplified catheter approach, medial to lateral CTI conduction block is defined by both the presence of a high to low (ie, proximal to distal) activation sequence on the ablation catheter during pacing from the proximal CS, and by equal conduction times (ie, >130 ms) from medial to lateral and from lateral to medial, during pacing from the proximal CS and low lateral RA, respectively. In addition, pacing from the proximal CS with the ablation catheter positioned on the ablation line will demonstrate widely spaced double potentials (Figure 43-17D).

SUMMARY

Mapping of isthmus-dependent AFL can be performed using standard catheter techniques, allowing one to make an accurate diagnosis that will result in successful ablation. Computerized 3-D activation mapping is an adjunctive method, which, while not mandatory, may have significant advantages in some cases resulting in improved success

rates overall. Radiofrequency catheter ablation has become a first-line treatment for AFL with nearly uniform acute and chronic success and low complication rates. Currently, the use of large-tip or irrigated ablation catheters is recommended for optimal success. Alternate energy sources including cryoablation and microwave ablation are under investigation with the hope of further improving procedure times and success rates and potentially reducing the risk of complications during AFL ablation.

REFERENCES

1. Saoudi N, Cosio F, Waldo A, et al. Classification of atrial flutter and regular atrial tachycardia according to electrophysiologic mechanism and anatomic bases: a statement from a joint expert group from the Working Group of Arrhythmias of the European Society of Cardiology and the North American Society of Pacing and Electrophysiology. *J Cardiovasc Electrophysiol*. 2001;12: 852-866.

2. Olshansky B, Okumura K, Hess PG, Waldo AL. Demonstration of an area of slow conduction in human atrial flutter. *J Am Coll Cardiol.* 1990;16:1639-1648.

3. Lesh MD, Van Hare GF, Epstein LM, et al. Radiofrequency catheter ablation of atrial arrhythmias. Results and mechanisms. *Circulation.* 1994;89:1074-1089.

4. Cosio FG, Goicolea A, Lopez-Gil M, Arribas F, Barroso JL, Chicote R. Atrial endocardial mapping in the rare form of atrial flutter. *Am J Cardiol.* 1990;66:715-720.

5. Feld GK, Fleck RP, Chen PS, et al. Radiofrequency catheter ablation for the treatment of human type 1 atrial flutter. Identification of a critical zone in the reentrant circuit by endocardial mapping techniques. *Circulation.* 1992;86:1233-1240.

6. Cosio FG, Lopez-Gil M, Goicolea A, Arribas F, Barroso JL. Radiofrequency ablation of the inferior vena cava-tricuspid valve isthmus in common atrial flutter. *Am J Cardiol.* 1993;71:705-709.

7. Tai CT, Chen SA, Chiang CE, et al. Electrophysiologic characteristics and radiofrequency catheter ablation in patients with clockwise atrial flutter. *J Cardiovasc Electrophysiol.* 1997;8:24-34.

8. Feld GK, Mollerus M, Birgersdotter-Green U, et al. Conduction velocity in the tricuspid valve-inferior vena cava isthmus is slower in patients with type I atrial flutter compared to those without a history of atrial flutter. *J Cardiovasc Electrophysiol.* 1997;8:1338-1348.

9. Kinder C, Kall J, Kopp D, Rubenstein D, Burke M, Wilber D. Conduction properties of the inferior vena cava-tricuspid annular isthmus in patients with typical atrial flutter. *J Cardiovasc Electrophysiol.* 1997;8:727-737.

10. Da Costa A, Mourot S, Romeyer-Bouchard C, et al. Anatomic and electrophysiological differences between chronic and paroxysmal forms of common atrial flutter and comparison with controls. *Pacing Clin Electrophysiol.* 2004;27:1202-1211.

11. Kalman JM, Olgin JE, Saxon LA, Fisher WG, Lee RJ, Lesh MD. Activation and entrainment mapping defines the tricuspid annulus as the anterior barrier in typical atrial flutter. *Circulation.* 1996;94:398-406.

12. Olgin JE, Kalman JM, Lesh MD. Conduction barriers in human atrial flutter: correlation of electrophysiology and anatomy. *J Cardiovasc Electrophysiol.* 1996;7:1112-1126.

13. Olgin JE, Kalman JM, Fitzpatrick AP, Lesh MD. Role of right atrial endocardial structures as barriers to conduction during human type I atrial flutter. Activation and entrainment mapping guided by intracardiac echocardiography. *Circulation.* 1995;92:1839-1848.

14. Tai CT, Huang JL, Lee PC, Ding YA, Chang MS, Chen SA. High-resolution mapping around the crista terminalis during typical atrial flutter: new insights into mechanisms. *J Cardiovasc Electrophysiol.* 2004;15:406-414.

15. Spach MS, Dolber PC, Heidlage JF. Influence of the passive anisotropic properties on directional differences in propagation following modification of the sodium conductance in human atrial muscle. A model of reentry based on anisotropic discontinuous propagation. *Circ Res.* 1988;62:811-832.

16. Spach MS, Miller WT 3rd, Dolber PC, Kootsey JM, Sommer JR, Mosher CE Jr. The functional role of structural complexities in the propagation of depolarization in the atrium of the dog. Cardiac conduction disturbances due to discontinuities of effective axial resistivity. *Circ Res.* 1982;50:175-191.

17. Olgin JE, Kalman JM, Saxon LA, Lee RJ, Lesh MD. Mechanism of initiation of atrial flutter in humans: site of unidirectional block and direction of rotation. *J Am Coll Cardiol.* 1997;29:376-384.

18. Suzuki F, Toshida N, Nawata H, et al. Coronary sinus pacing initiates counterclockwise atrial flutter while pacing from the low lateral right atrium initiates clockwise atrial flutter. Analysis of episodes of direct initiation of atrial flutter. *J Electrocardiol.* 1998;31:345-361.

19. Feld GK, Shahandeh-Rad F. Activation patterns in experimental canine atrial flutter produced by right atrial crush injury. *J Am Coll Cardiol.* 1992;20:441-451.

20. Haissaguerre M, Sanders P, Hocini M, Jais P, Clementy J. Pulmonary veins in the substrate for atrial fibrillation: the "venous wave" hypothesis. *J Am Coll Cardiol.* 2004;43:2290-2292.

21. Oshikawa N, Watanabe I, Masaki R, et al. Relationship between polarity of the flutter wave in the surface ECG and endocardial atrial activation sequence in patients with typical counterclockwise and clockwise atrial flutter. *J Interv Card Electrophysiol.* 2002;7:215-223.

22. Okumura K, Plumb VJ, Page PL, Waldo AL. Atrial activation sequence during atrial flutter in the canine pericarditis model and its effects on the polarity of the flutter wave in the electrocardiogram. *J Am Coll Cardiol.* 1991;17:509-518.

23. Chugh A, Latchamsetty R, Oral H, et al. Characteristics of cavotricuspid isthmus-dependent atrial flutter after left atrial ablation of atrial fibrillation. *Circulation.* 2006;113:609-615.

24. Fischer B, Haissaguerre M, Garrigues S, et al. Radiofrequency catheter ablation of common atrial flutter in 80 patients. *J Am Coll Cardiol.* 1995;25:1365-1372.

25. Kirkorian G, Moncada E, Chevalier P, et al.. Radiofrequency ablation of atrial flutter. Efficacy of an anatomically guided approach. *Circulation.* 1994;90:2804-2814.

26. Calkins H, Leon AR, Deam AG, Kalbfleisch SJ, Langberg JJ, Morady F. Catheter ablation of atrial flutter using radiofrequency energy. *Am J Cardiol.* 1994;73:353-356.

27. Jais P, Haissaguerre M, Shah DC, et al. Successful irrigated-tip catheter ablation of atrial flutter resistant to conventional radiofrequency ablation. *Circulation.* 1998;98:835-838.

28. Scavee C, Jais P, Hsu LF, et al. Prospective randomised comparison of irrigated-tip and large-tip catheter ablation of cavotricuspid isthmus-dependent atrial flutter. *Eur Heart J.* 2004;25:963-969.

29. Calkins H. Catheter ablation of atrial flutter: do outcomes of catheter ablation with "large-tip" versus "cooled-tip" catheters really differ? *J Cardiovasc Electrophysiol.* 2004;15:1131-1132.

30. Atiga WL, Worley SJ, Hummel J, et al. Prospective randomized comparison of cooled radiofrequency versus standard radiofrequency energy for ablation of typical atrial flutter. *Pacing Clin Electrophysiol.* 2002;25:1172-1178.

ISTHMUS-DEPENDENT ATRIAL FLUTTER

SECTION VI
CATHETER ABLATION TECHNIQUES
FOR MANAGING ATRIAL FIBRILLATION
AND ATRIAL FLUTTER

315

31. Tsai CF, Tai CT, Yu WC, et al. Is 8-mm more effective than 4-mm tip electrode catheter for ablation of typical atrial flutter? *Circulation.* 1999;100:768-771.

32. Feld G, Wharton M, Plumb V, Daoud E, Friehling T, Epstein L. Radiofrequency catheter ablation of type 1 atrial flutter using large-tip 8- or 10-mm electrode catheters and a high-output radiofrequency energy generator: results of a multicenter safety and efficacy study. *J Am Coll Cardiol.* 2004;43:1466-1472.

33. Ventura R, Klemm H, Lutomsky B, et al. Pattern of isthmus conduction recovery using open cooled and solid large-tip catheters for radiofrequency ablation of typical atrial flutter. *J Cardiovasc Electrophysiol.* 2004;15:1126-1130.

34. Mangat I, Tschopp DR Jr, Yang Y, Cheng J, Keung EC, Scheinman MM. Optimizing the detection of bidirectional block across the flutter isthmus for patients with typical isthmus-dependent atrial flutter. *Am J Cardiol.* 2003;91:559-564.

35. Poty H, Saoudi N, Abdel Aziz A, Nair M, Letac B. Radiofrequency catheter ablation of type 1 atrial flutter. Prediction of late success by electrophysiological criteria. *Circulation.* 1995;92:1389-1392.

36. Schwartzman D, Callans DJ, Gottlieb CD, Dillon SM, Movsowitz C, Marchlinski FE. Conduction block in the inferior vena caval-tricuspid valve isthmus: association with outcome of radiofrequency ablation of type I atrial flutter. *J Am Coll Cardiol.* 1996;28:1519-1531.

37. Tada H, Oral H, Sticherling C, et al. Double potentials along the ablation line as a guide to radiofrequency ablation of typical atrial flutter. *J Am Coll Cardiol.* 2001;38:750-755.

38. Tai CT, Haque A, Lin YK, et al. Double potential interval and transisthmus conduction time for prediction of cavotricuspid isthmus block after ablation of typical atrial flutter. *J Interv Card Electrophysiol.* 2002;7:77-82.

39. Cauchemez B, Haissaguerre M, Fischer B, Thomas O, Clementy J, Coumel P. Electrophysiological effects of catheter ablation of inferior vena cava-tricuspid annulus isthmus in common atrial flutter. *Circulation.* 1996;93:284-294.

40. Calkins H, Canby R, Weiss R, et al. Results of catheter ablation of typical atrial flutter. *Am J Cardiol.* 2004;94:437-442.

41. Lo LW, Tai CT, Lin YJ, et al. Characteristics of the cavotricuspid isthmus in predicting recurrent conduction in the long-term follow-up. *J Cardiovasc Electrophysiol.* 2009;20:39-43.

42. Ilg KJ, Kuhne M, Crawford T, et al. Randomized comparison of cavotricuspid isthmus ablation for atrial flutter using an open irrigation-tip versus a large-tip radiofrequency ablation catheter. *J Cardiovasc Electrophysiol.* 2011;22:1007-1012.

43. Timmermans C, Ayers GM, Crijns HJ, Rodriguez LM. Randomized study comparing radiofrequency ablation with cryoablation for the treatment of atrial flutter with emphasis on pain perception. *Circulation.* 2003;107:1250-1252.

44. Feld GK, Daubert JP, Weiss R, Miles WM, and Pelkey W; Cryoablation Atrial Flutter Efficacy Trial Investigators. Acute and long-term efficacy and safety of catheter cryoablation of the cavotricuspid isthmus for treatment of type 1 atrial flutter. *Heart Rhythm.* 2008;5:1009-1014.

45. Iwasa A, Storey J, Yao B, Liem LB, Feld GK. Efficacy of a microwave antenna for ablation of the tricuspid valve—inferior vena cava isthmus in dogs as a treatment for type 1 atrial flutter. *J Interv Card Electrophysiol.* 2004;10:191-198.

46. Chan JY, Fung JW, Yu CM, Feld GK. Preliminary results with percutaneous transcatheter microwave ablation of typical atrial flutter. *J Cardiovasc Electrophysiol.* 2007;18:286-289.

47. Yang Y, Cheng J, Bochoeyer A, et al. Atypical right atrial flutter patterns. *Circulation.* 2001;103:3092-3098.

48. Yang Y, Varma N, Badhwar N, et al. Prospective observations in the clinical and electrophysiological characteristics of intra-isthmus reentry. *J Cardiovasc Electrophysiol.* 2010;21:1099-106.

316

SECTION VI
CATHETER ABLATION TECHNIQUES
FOR MANAGING ATRIAL FIBRILLATION
AND ATRIAL FLUTTER

CHAPTER 44

44 INCISIONAL ATRIAL FLUTTER: INSIGHTS ON HOW TO MAP AND ABLATE NON–ISTHMUS-DEPENDENT ATRIAL FLUTTERS

Emile G. Daoud, MD, FACC, FHRS

CASE PRESENTATION

The patient is a 64-year-old man who underwent mitral valve repair 12 years earlier. He presents with fatigue and palpitations and is found to be in atrial flutter (AFlr). After a transesophageal echocardiogram excludes left atrial clot, he is referred to the electrophysiology laboratory for catheter ablation.

A 20-pole catheter is positioned in the right atrium (Figure 44-1). The flutter wave morphology suggests a non–isthmus-dependent, incisional AFlr. To confirm this diagnosis and to map and ablate the tachycardia, the strategy is to utilize the response to pacing to assess the postpacing interval, assess for concealed entrainment of the tachycardia, and identify low-amplitude/fractionated atrial electrograms and activation and voltage map information from the electroanatomic map.

MAPPING OF INCISIONAL, PATCH, AND SCAR-RELATED MACROREENTRANT ATRIAL FLUTTER

This case is an example of atrial reentry around an area of scar/incision, termed "incisional flutter." As is common with these tachycardias, the patient has undergone an atriotomy several years prior to onset of the tachycardia as part of valve surgery.[1] Incisional AFlr usually does not respond to antiarrhythmic medication and typically requires ablation.

In addition to understanding the anatomy based on prior operative procedure notes, there are four features that aid in mapping AFlr due to incision-related scar. These features are also equally applicable to mapping and ablating any form of macroreentrant AFlr (inclusive of isthmus-dependent AFlr, AFlr/atrial tachycardias following congenital heart surgery, and postatrial fibrillation ablation AFlr):

1. **Postpacing intervals.**[2] The differential diagnosis of the tachycardia mechanism for this case is clockwise rotation of an isthmus-dependent flutter or an incisional flutter. To diagnose the mechanism, the response to pacing is helpful. When the tachycardia is entrained by atrial pacing, the tip of the pacing catheter is in or near the reentrant circuit if the first return beat of the tachycardia recorded from the pacing catheter, after pacing is stopped, is within 30 ms of the tachycardia cycle length: post-pacing interval (PPI) measured from the pacing catheter minus the tachycardia cycle length (TCL) ≤ 30 ms.

2. **Atrial concealed entrainment.**[3,4] When an atrial tachycardia is entrained, there is often fusion between the wave of depolarization generated from the pacing catheter colliding with the wave of depolarization of the tachycardia. The resultant P wave is a fusion beat: a

P-wave morphology that is "fused" between the two sources. *Progressive* fusion, meaning that the P-wave morphology is changing during the first several beats of pacing, confirms that the pacing catheter is not in the reentrant circuit. However, when pacing from within the circuit, there is no fusion, and the P-wave morphology generated from the pacing catheter is identical to the P wave generated by the tachycardia. This is called "concealed entrainment" and implies that the pacing catheter is within the circuit. Although this technique is effective for mapping reentrant ventricular arrhythmias since changes in QRS morphology are obvious, change in the P-wave morphology using surface ECG analysis is subtle. Concealed entrainment, for any mechanism of macroreentrant AFlr, is therefore determined by the absence of change in the atrial activation sequence, amplitude, *and* morphology of intracardiac atrial recordings when pacing from within the reentrant circuit.

3. **Low amplitude/fractionated electrograms.**[4] An essential feature of ablating non–isthmus-dependent AFlr is to identify the zone of slow conduction that is critical to the reentrant arrhythmia. This slow zone of conduction is characterized by anisotropic conduction. Anisotropic conduction is slow conduction related to local disorganized atrial architecture, often at sites of atrial myocardium intertwined with atrial scar/fibrosis. Atrial electrograms at these sites have low amplitude and are highly fractionated. Identification of these electrograms coupled with response to pacing and atrial entrainment (listed previously), help to identify the zone of slow conduction and sites to target for ablation.

These three features of assessing a macroreentrant arrhythmia (postpacing intervals, atrial concealed entrainment, and low amplitude/fractionated electrograms) are demonstrated in Figures 44-2 to 44-6 for this case of incisional AFlr (see figure legend for further explanation).

The fourth feature that is quite valuable to map incisional AFlr (as well as other non–isthmus-dependent AFlr) is the activation and voltage map that is completed with an electroanatomic map.

4. **Activation and voltage map.**[5,6] An electroanatomic map allows creation of a voltage and an activation sequence map of the atrium during the tachycardia. Scar is identified by low amplitude or absent atrial electrograms, which can be the area for slow conduction/reentry and often the region for the patch/scar/incisional AFlr. Mapping of the endocardial activation sequence during the tachycardia allows creation of the reentrant circuit by identifying the sites of earliest and latest activation. Figures 44-7 and 44-8 demonstrate the activation maps (CARTO system) that were used in this case to identify the reentrant incisional AFlr and to guide the ablation lesion set (see figure legend for further explanation).

For incisional AFlr, successful ablation sites often have all four of these features, yet ablation is unlikely to be successful with a single application of radiofrequency energy. The zone of slow conduction is often broad and, similar to ablation of isthmus-dependent AFlr, a permanent elimination of a patch/scar/incision-related AFlr requires a line of ablation to another electrical inert region of the heart. In the current case example, a line of ablation was completed between the superior vena cava and the tricuspid valve annulus, thus transecting the critical zone of slow conduction.

The key to long-term freedom from AFlr is confirmation of bidirectional conduction block, not merely termination of the tachycardia.[7] The mechanism to confirm bidirectional conduction block

INCISIONAL ATRIAL FLUTTER: INSIGHTS
ON HOW TO MAP AND ABLATE
NON– ISTHMUS-DEPENDENT ATRIAL FLUTTERS

SECTION VI
CATHETER ABLATION TECHNIQUES
FOR MANAGING ATRIAL FIBRILLATION
AND ATRIAL FLUTTER

317

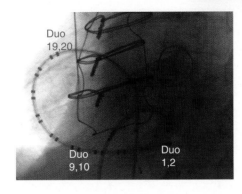

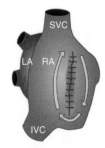

FIGURE 44-1. This is an LAO fluoroscopic image of a 20-pole catheter in the right atrium. Poles 1 and 2 (distal) are located in the proximal coronary sinus and poles 19 and 20 are in the high right atrium. The catheter lies across the cavotricuspid isthmus (poles 1-10) and then along the right atrial free wall (poles 11-20). The diagram in the lower right corner depicts a right atrial free wall atriotomy with a macroreentrant circuit rotating around the scar/incision (yellow arrows).

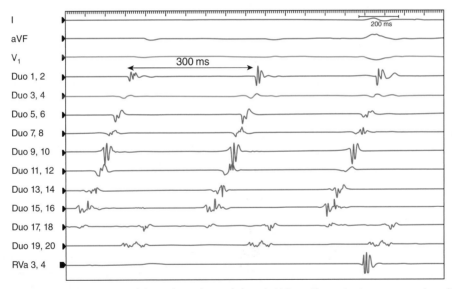

FIGURE 44-2. This is the initial intracardiac tracing of the tachycardia, cycle length 300 ms. The activation sequence is earliest at poles 17 and 18 and last at poles 1 and 2. The differential diagnosis is clockwise isthmus-dependent AFlr or incisional AFlr. The widely split electrograms on poles 17 and 18 and the late activation of poles 19 and 20 coupled with the history of a prior atriotomy suggest an incisional flutter, but response to pacing is required to confirm a diagnosis (see Figure 44-3). Abbreviations: aVF, V_1, surface ECG I; 20-pole recordings labeled as Duo 1-20; RVa, right ventricular apical recording.

318

SECTION VI
CATHETER ABLATION TECHNIQUES
FOR MANAGING ATRIAL FIBRILLATION
AND ATRIAL FLUTTER

CHAPTER 44

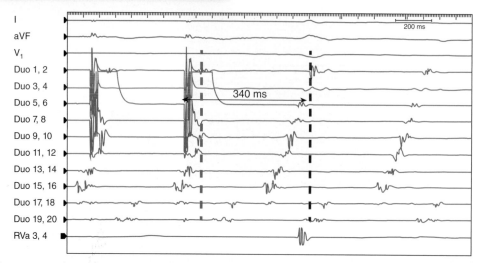

FIGURE 44-3 This demonstrates the response to pacing from poles 5 to 6. These poles are located within the cavotricuspid isthmus. If the tachycardia is an isthmus-dependent AFlr, the response to pacing should confirm this mechanism. However, pacing confirms that the mechanism is *not* isthmus-dependent. When pacing is stopped, the postpacing interval measured at poles 5 and 6 is 40 ms (340 ms − 300 ms = 45 ms), consistent with poles 5 and 6 not located within the AFlr circuit. Also, the atrial activation sequence during atrial pacing from poles 5 and 6 is *not* consistent with concealed entrainment of the AFlr. The activation sequence during pacing is not identical to the activation sequence during the tachycardia. Note that the electrogram recorded from poles 1 and 2 during pacing is nearly simultaneous with the electrogram on poles 9 and 10 (dashed green line); however, during the tachycardia, poles 1 and 2 are activated well after poles 9 and 10 (dashed blue line). Abbreviations same as Figure 44-2.

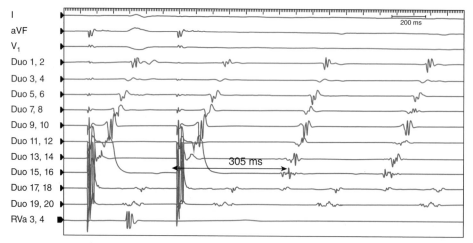

FIGURE 44-4. Since the original tracing (Figure 44-2) showed split potentials at poles 17 and 18 and an isthmus-dependent AFlr is excluded (Figure 44-3), response to pacing is then assessed by pacing at poles 15 and 16, presumably near the circuit. The postpacing interval is quite good, 305 ms (a difference of 5 ms), consistent with pacing from near/within the circuit. Furthermore, pacing from poles 15 and 16 results in an atrial activation sequence that is identical to the activation sequence during the tachycardia, but also note that the atrial electrogram features (amplitude and fractionation) are also nearly identical with pacing as compared to during tachycardia. This response to pacing confirms atrial concealed entrainment, another clue that poles 15 and 16 are within the AFlr circuit. Abbreviations same as Figure 44-2.

INCISIONAL ATRIAL FLUTTER: INSIGHTS
ON HOW TO MAP AND ABLATE
NON– ISTHMUS-DEPENDENT ATRIAL FLUTTERS

SECTION VI
CATHETER ABLATION TECHNIQUES
FOR MANAGING ATRIAL FIBRILLATION
AND ATRIAL FLUTTER

319

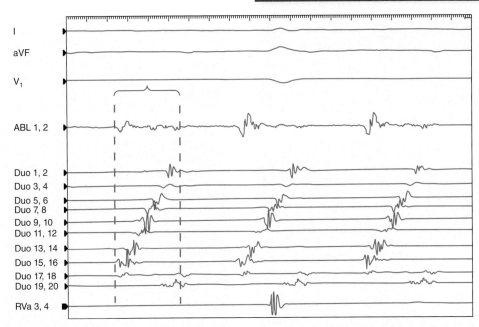

FIGURE 44-5. With pacing only at two sites, the mechanism and location of the AFlr is confirmed. The ablation catheter is then advanced into the right atrium and is directed to the region near poles 15 and 16. In this figure, note that the electrograms at the ablation catheter (ABL 1, 2) are low amplitude, fractionated, and split (at times into three components). Also, the electrograms recorded from the ABL 1, 2 span the electrograms on the 20-pole catheter (red dashed lines), indicating that ABL 1, 2 is in a region of slow activation and likely a turnaround point of the tachycardia as it rotates around the edge of the atriotomy incision. Abbreviations same as Figure 44-2.

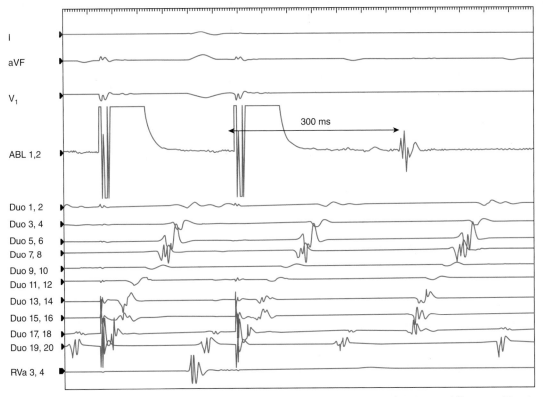

FIGURE 44-6 Response to pacing at ablation catheter (ABL 1, 2) shows excellent postpacing interval (300 ms, a difference of 0 ms) and atrial concealed entrainment (as explained in Figure 44-4). Abbreviations same as Figure 44-2.

320

SECTION VI
CATHETER ABLATION TECHNIQUES
FOR MANAGING ATRIAL FIBRILLATION
AND ATRIAL FLUTTER

CHAPTER 44

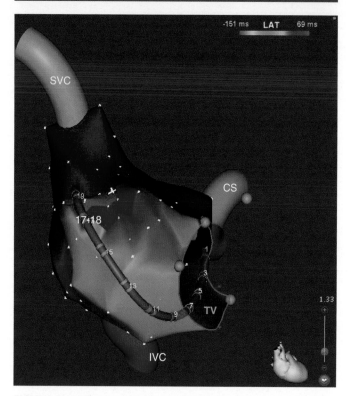

FIGURE 44-7. This is an RAO projection of the electroanatomic map of the right atrium during the incisional AFlr. This map was created by annotating electrograms recorded from the ablation catheter relative to a fixed electrode in the heart (in this patient, it was Duo 1, 2). The ablation catheter was moved throughout the atria, and signals that were "early," relative to the electrogram on Duo 1, 2, were annotated as red, and "late" signals were annotated as dark colors (latest = purple color). Also shown are the 20-pole electrodes, deployed along the cavotricuspid isthmus and the right atrial free wall. Poles 17 and 18 (noted to have a split electrogram on the first recording, see Figure 44-2) are highlighted in white. The electroanatomic map shows a region of "early meets late," a dark red zone, squeezed between the early red/yellow colored region and the late blue/purple colored region. The "early meets late" region suggests the turnaround point of the tachycardia. The tricuspid valve annulus is noted by light blue colored dots and ring. The single gold-colored dot represents the location of the His bundle. Abbreviations: CS, coronary sinus; IVC, inferior vena cava; SVC, superior vena cava; TV, tricuspid valve.

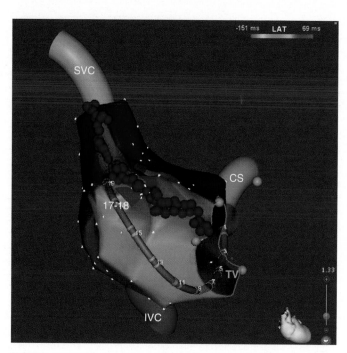

FIGURE 44-8 With the tachycardia mechanism confirmed and mapping completed, a line of ablation (red dots) is completed between the superior vena cava and the tricuspid valve annulus, resulting in termination of the tachycardia. During this line of ablation, careful attention was made not to ablate at sites near the phrenic nerve, identified by activation of the diaphragm with high-output pacing from the ablation catheter. Abbreviations same as Figure 44-7.

in this case is the same technique to confirm bidirectional block across any linear ablation lesion (eg, a cavotricuspid isthmus line for isthmus-dependent AFlr, or a roof line or mitral valve line created as part of ablation for atrial fibrillation). The concept is that two catheters are positioned on either side of the line of ablation. When pacing from one catheter, the time to the atrial signal recorded on the second catheter will be longer as the recording catheter is moved toward the line of block, compared to when the catheter is further from the line of ablation (but closer to the pacing source). In other words, if the line of ablation is complete, and there are no gaps, the wave of depolarization from the pacing catheter must travel in only one direction and hence activate the other side of the ablation line last (Figure 44-9).

Shown is the response to pacing from the HRAd catheter and the time to the local atrial signal recorded when the ablation catheter is first at the white dot and then located at the pink dot. With the ablation catheter located at the white dot, the time from the pacing stimulus from HRAd

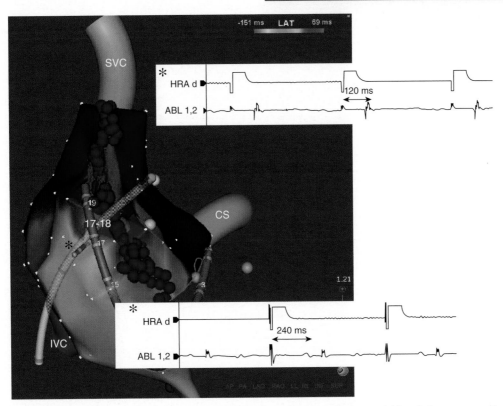

FIGURE 44-9 Confirmation of bidirectional conduction block. Figure 44-9 is an electroanatomic map (abbreviations same as Figure 44-7) after completion of the line of ablation and termination of the AFlr. The goal is to confirm bidirectional conduction block. Pacing will be completed from the tip of the catheter highlighted by the * and labeled as HRAd on the intracardiac tracings. HRA catheter is visualized on the electroanatomic map and is positioned just lateral to the line of ablation. The ablation catheter (ABL 1, 2) is located at the white dot, which is anatomically further away from the pacing tip compared to the pink dot. However, if there is complete block along the ablation line, then the pacing impulse must first travel past the white dot before reaching the area near the ablation line, noted by the pink dot.

to the atrial electrogram on the ablation catheter (ABL 1, 2) is 120 ms (upper electrogram tracing). When the ablation catheter is then moved to the pink dot, even though it is anatomically closer to the pacing catheter (*, HRA), because there is complete conduction block across the ablation line (ie, no gaps), the time from the HRAd to the ABL 1, 2 at the pink dot is longer (240 ms; lower electrogram tracing) compared to the time recorded at the white dot (120 ms). Bidirectional block is confirmed when the same maneuver is performed with pacing from the ablation catheter and recording from the HRA catheter (not shown).

REFERENCES

1. Pap R, Kohári M, Makai A, et al. Surgical technique and the mechanism of atrial tachycardia late after open heart surgery. *J Interv Card Electrophysiol.* 2012;35:127-135.

2. Santucci PA, Varma N, Cytron J, et al. Electroanatomic mapping of postpacing intervals clarifies the complete active circuit and variants in atrial flutter. *Heart Rhythm.* 2009;6:1586-1595.

3. Coffey JO, d'Avila A, Dukkipati S, et al. Catheter ablation of scar-related atypical atrial flutter. *Europace.* 2013;15:414-419.

4. Wu RC, Berger R, Calkins H. Catheter ablation of atrial flutter and macroreentrant atrial tachycardia. *Curr Opin Cardiol.* 2002;17:58-64.

5. Peichl P, Kautzner J, Cihák R, Vancura V, Bytesník J. Clinical application of electroanatomical mapping in the characterization of "incisional" atrial tachycardias. *Pacing Clin Electrophysiol.* 2003;26:420-425.

6. Reithmann C, Hoffmann E, Dorwarth U, Remp T, Steinbeck G. Electroanatomical mapping for visualization of atrial activation in patients with incisional atrial tachycardias. *Eur Heart J.* 2001;22:237-246.

7. Snowdon RL, Balasubramaniam R, Teh AW, et al. Linear ablation of right atrial free wall flutter: demonstration of bidirectional conduction block as an endpoint associated with long-term success. *J Cardiovasc Electrophysiol.* 2010;21:526-531.

SECTION VII

SYNCOPE

45 SYNCOPE: A MANAGEMENT STRATEGY

Venkata Krishna Puppala, MD, and David G. Benditt, MD

CASE PRESENTATION

A 67-year-old man came to the Syncope/Electrophysiology Clinic complaining of experiencing periodic "dizzy spells" and, more recently, two frank collapse events. The dizzy spells have become more frequent over the past year, and during these episodes he feels that his vision diminishes briefly then recovers. The two abrupt transient loss of consciousness spells were more severe. The first occurred as he was getting ready for bed, and he found himself on the bedroom floor. There were no warning symptoms. His wife indicated that his color seemed flushed, and his eyelids remained open. The second occurred while pushing a shopping cart but not otherwise exerting himself. There was no warning as far as he could recall; he held on to the cart in order to avoid injury as he collapsed. He recovered promptly and was not injured.

The patient's only cardiac history is hyperlipidemia for which he takes simvastatin. A recent echocardiogram showed modest left atrial enlargement (43 mm), mild concentric left ventricular hypertrophy (septal and free wall thickness approximately 12 mm), and a normal left ventricular ejection fraction (55%-60%). His 12-lead ECG was normal.

Given the infrequent nature of the frank syncope events in a patient without major structural heart disease (ie, presumably a low risk of a life-threatening cardiac cause for syncope) an ambulatory ECG monitoring strategy was chosen for subsequent evaluation; specifically, an implantable loop recorder (ILR) was selected since it would permit long-term monitoring to capture infrequent evens (Figure 45-1). Within a few days he reported an episode of his usual dizziness, accompanied by extreme fatigue and weakness. His ILR recording revealed sinus rhythm with ventricular bigeminy resulting in a slow effective heart rate (Figure 45-2). Given his weakness with this rhythm, the possibility was entertained that the bigeminy could be the basis for his dizziness and syncope, but it was decided to wait longer and continue monitoring.

Approximately 6 weeks later, the patient slumped to the floor while sweeping out his garage. His wife called 911, and he was brought to the emergency department. His ILR was interrogated, and a diagnosis of symptomatic bradycardia was established (Figure 45-3). Based on this finding a pacemaker was indicated. During the subsequent year he has not suffered any further syncope episodes. However, ablation of ventricular ectopy has been scheduled given his persistent ventricular bigeminy and "dizzy" spells.

EPIDEMIOLOGY

Syncope ("faint") is a brief, self-limited period (usually less than 1-2 minutes) in which loss of consciousness occurs a result of transient cerebral hypoperfusion. There are many possible causes. The percentage

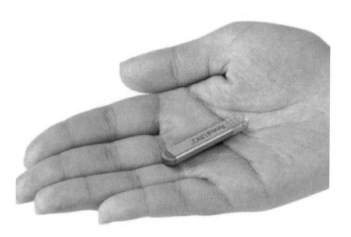

FIGURE 45-1 Picture of a typical implantable loop recorder. Note the size relative to the finger. (Image used with permission of Medtronic Inc., Minneapolis, Minnesota.)

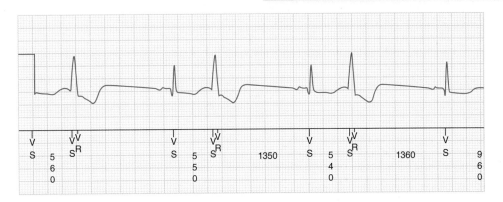

FIGURE 45-2 Ventricular bigeminy associated with "dizzy" spell, presumably due to a slow net heart rate.

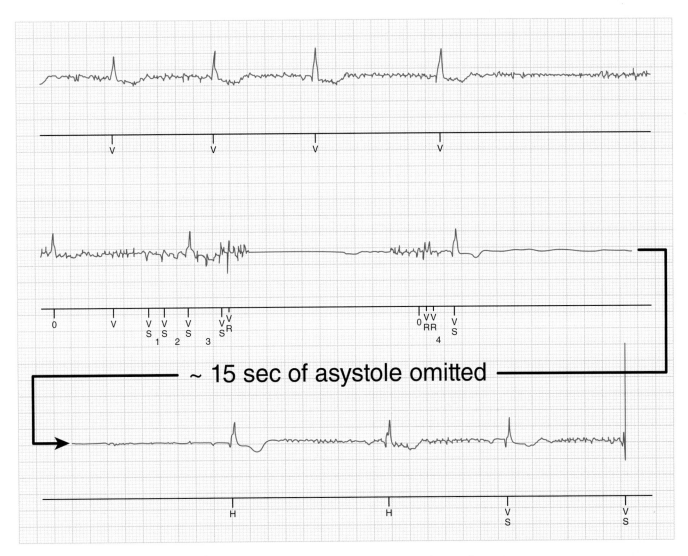

~ 15 sec of asystole omitted

FIGURE 45-3 Prolonged asystolic pause recorded by ILR in conjunction with the patient's abrupt collapse.

of patients who report having experienced a faint varies from 15% to 25% in Western countries.[1,2] Syncope accounts for 1% of all visits to emergency departments or urgent care clinics in Europe and around 1% to 6% of such visits in the United States.[1-3]

CAUSES

Vasovagal and orthostatic faints are the most common forms of syncope across all age groups.[1,4-6] In younger patients without any structural heart disease, neurally mediated reflex faints, particularly vasovagal syncope or situational faints (eg, postmicturition syncope, cough syncope), account for the vast majority. In older patients, carotid sinus syndrome (CSS) becomes of increasing importance and has been reported to account for up to 20% of syncope in this group.[1,4] Older patients are also more likely to experience orthostatic syncope.[4]

Cardiac causes of syncope include structural heart disease (ie, coronary artery disease, valvular disease, cardiomyopathies, consequences of hypertension) and arrhythmias. Increased mortality risk is a concern in these patients[1,5]; however, the primary mortality "driver" is the severity of the underlying heart disease rather than the syncope itself.[1] In the absence of overt structural disease, the possibility of a so-called channelopathy (eg, long QT syndrome, Brugada syndrome, catecholaminergic paroxysmal VT) should not be overlooked.[1] In addition, occasionally premature coronary artery disease may trigger an arrhythmia in individuals who are seemingly healthy.

ESTABLISHING THE BASIS FOR SYNCOPE AND RISK STRATIFICATION

The urgency of establishing the basis of syncope is determined by assessment of the patient's short-term and long-term potential morbidity and mortality risk. This "risk assessment" step has received considerable attention recently.[1-6,11] Its importance relates in part to potential for sudden unexpected death in such patients, but also (and perhaps more commonly) to susceptibility for syncope to recur in affected individuals and result in falls with injury and economic and life-style disruption. Table 45-1 provides a list of clinical findings (derived from multiple reports) that trigger concern regarding high risk of early (<1 month) syncope recurrence.

Longer-term risk of syncope recurrence (ie, <1 year) is more difficult to predict. However, a few studies have attempted to address this issue.[1,6] Table 45-1 summarizes a number of clinical observations that should raise concern regarding increased risk of syncope recurrence over the next year.

DIAGNOSTIC STRATEGY AND SPECIFIC CLINICAL CONSIDERATIONS

Figure 45-4 summarizes a basic strategy for the initial clinical evaluation and disposition of syncope/collapse patients. The initial evaluation requires a careful medical history (including accounts from witnesses) followed by risk assessment or risk stratification. The availability of a syncope clini or syncope management unit is of value in order to enhance efficiency of patient care by avoiding unnecessary hospitalizations and diminishing the number of "diagnostic" tests being ordered, while increasing diagnostic yield.

TABLE 45-1 Clinical Observations Suggesting Increased Risk in Syncope/Collapse Patients

Short-term increased risk	- Abnormal ECG (other than minor abnormalities) - Low blood pressure - Chest pain - Heart failure - Collapse while supine or in the midst of exertion -No warning
Long-term increased risk	- Older age (>65 years) - History of cardiac disease - Syncope during effort or supine - Ventricular arrhythmia present - No warning

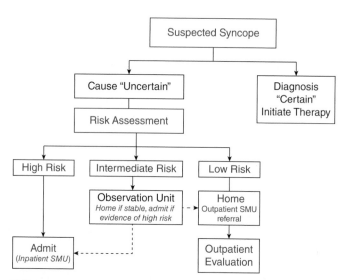

FIGURE 45-4 Management strategy for patients presenting to emergency departments or clinics with transient loss of consciousness and presumed syncope.

A preprepared history form may facilitate the recording of a complete story. The provider should try to obtain the answers for the following key questions as part of the history taking:

- Is loss of consciousness attributable to true syncope versus other causes of real or seemingly real loss of consciousness, including accidental falls?

- Is heart disease present?

- Are there important clinical features in the history that suggest the diagnosis? (eg, premonitory symptoms in vasovagal fainters)

- What were the circumstances of the collapse? (eg, emotional upset, fear, pain, during or after exertion, after cough, while supine or recumbent, after having recently stood up from a seated or supine position)

In regard to physical findings, most "presumed syncope" patients have fully recovered by the time they are first seen by a medical practitioner. Consequently, the relation between physical finding abnormalities (if any) and the cause of syncope is inferential in most cases. However, physical findings that may assist in uncovering a basis for syncope include marked drop in blood pressure when arising (ie, orthostatic blood pressure changes), important cardiac murmurs or bruits, evidence of heart failure or left ventricular disease, and an abnormal response to carotid sinus massage.

INVESTIGATIVE STUDIES

Pooled data from population-based studies indicate that the history and physical examination can identify a potential cause of syncope in approximately 50% of the patients.[1] An ECG should be obtained in all patients presenting with syncope. The ECG has been noted to be helpful in diagnosing a cardiac cause of syncope in approximately 6% of all patients with syncope and 50% of patients with a cardiac cause of syncope. On the other hand, routine blood tests rarely yield diagnostically useful information, and any such tests should be selected based on suspicion arising during the history taking. Very rarely such tests may yield other nonsyncope diagnoses such as hypoglycemia and intoxication. Similarly, head imaging (in the absence of head injury) and carotid Doppler imaging are to be avoided in most cases as they are highly unlikely to explain the faint.

DIAGNOSIS AND MANAGEMENT OF SPECIFIC CONDITIONS

Neurally Mediated Syncope

As noted earlier, "reflex" faints, and particularly vasovagal syncope (VVS), are the most common causes of syncope when one considers all age groups. VVS alone is reported to occur in 10% to 20% of the general population.

In the case of VVS and the closely related situational syncope (eg, syncope associated with swallowing, cough, and postmicturition), a good medical history is generally sufficient to establish the diagnosis.[1] Treatment of these forms of reflex syncope mainly consists of avoiding or ameliorating triggers when possible (ie, for situational faints), along with education and increased salt and volume intake if medically safe. Pharmacologic treatments have been proposed, but none have showed convincing benefit in placebo-controlled trials with the exception of midodrine.[12-17] The role of cardiac pacing for vasovagal syncope remains controversial. ISSUE 2

and the more recent ISSUE 3 trials suggest that cardiac pacing may be beneficial in older patients with a documented prolonged spontaneous asystole.[18,19]

Carotid sinus syndrome (CSS) occurs most often in older males. The conventional criteria for a diagnostic finding with carotid sinus massage (CSM) is a pause ≥3 sec with symptoms.[1] However, such a finding is only likely to occur if the CSM test is conducted with the patient in an upright posture, and even then the test has been criticized for not being sufficiently specific.[20] A recent consensus opinion suggests that the CSS diagnostic bar should be set higher[20]; specifically, CSM with a pause ≥6 sec with reproduction of syncope or near-syncope is almost certainly a more specific manner in which to establish a CSS diagnosis. Cardiac pacing is generally effective, although vasoconstrictors such as midodrine may also be needed if a prominent vasodepressor response is also present.

Orthostatic Syncope

Orthostatic syncope is diagnosed when there is documentation of posturally induced hypotension associated with syncope or near-syncope. Two forms are recognized: the "immediate" form that occurs promptly after movement to the upright posture and then disappears quickly, and the more troublesome "delayed" form, which consists of a drop in systolic blood pressure by ≥20 mm Hg within 3 to 5 minutes (sometimes longer) after assuming a standing posture.

Orthostatic syncope can be the result of either nonneurogenic reversible causes (eg, volume depletion, effect of medications) or primary neurologic conditions like Parkinson's disease or pure autonomic failure. When physical maneuvers and salt/volume repletion alone are not sufficient to suppress orthostatic symptoms, pharmacological interventions may be justified. Fludrocortisone and midodrine are probably the most commonly used drugs.[15,16]

Cardiac Arrhythmias

Syncope can be caused by both brady- and tachyarrhythmias. Bradyarrhythmias may be due to sinus node dysfunction (eg, severe sinoatrial bradycardia, sinus pauses, or occasionally asystolic pauses following termination of atrial tachyarrhythmias), chronic or paroxysmal atrioventricular (AV) block, or third-degree AV block. The severity of the bradycardia must be sufficient to account for abrupt cerebral hypoperfusion. In situations where the diagnosis is not certain, further testing with ambulatory event monitoring, electrophysiological assessment of AV conduction, and sometimes exercise testing to look for rate-dependent AV block. Pacemaker therapy is usually appropriate and effective in such cases. In our patient, despite absence of overt heart disease, intermittent sinus arrest was determined to be the cause of syncope, whereas his ventricular bigeminy was a less serious issue, but the apparent cause of his "dizzy" spells.

Tachyarrhythmias, of either supraventricular or ventricular origin, can cause syncope. Depending on the arrhythmia at fault, treatment options may include any combination of antiarrhythmic drugs (including β-blockers and calcium channel blockers) and radiofrequency catheter ablation (RFA). RFA is the treatment of choice for certain idiopathic monomorphic VTs (eg, right and left ventricular outflow tract VTs and the so-called fascicular VTs). Other, less common but important arrhythmic causes of syncope include torsades de pointes associated with long-QT syndromes (including drug-induced forms) or Brugada syndrome.

Structural Cardiac and Cardiopulmonary Causes of Syncope

In patients with structural cardiac or cardiopulmonary disease, syncope may be due to direct result of the structural disturbance or as a consequence of a neural-reflex disturbance triggered by the condition, or due to an arrhythmia (bradycardia or tachycardia). Important causes in this group include acute myocardial infarction, severe aortic stenosis, hypertrophic cardiomyopathy, and arrhythmogenic right ventricular cardiomyopathy.

Cerebrovascular Causes of Syncope

In general, cerebrovascular diseases are seldom the cause of true syncope; extensive neurologic testing such as head imaging or electroencephalography are rarely of value in the initial assessment of patients presenting with syncope. Head imaging may be occasionally necessary if there is a concern that the patient may have sustained an intracranial injury as a consequence of their collapse.

Conditions That Mimic Syncope

Certain conditions may cause a real or apparent loss of consciousness that might appear to be syncope, but is not true syncope.[17] Examples of such situations include seizures, pseudosyncope (pseudoseizures), concussions, or intoxication. Cataplexy and certain rare types of akinetic or minimally kinetic seizures may also be considered here.

CONCLUSION

Syncope is a syndrome that is a particularly frequent cause for emergency department and urgent care clinic visits. The physician's key tasks are to establish a confident causal diagnosis, assess prognostic implications, and then provide appropriate advice to prevent recurrences. To achieve these goals, it is important to develop an organized approach to assessment of the syncope patient. The initial patient evaluation, particularly a detailed medical history, is the key to identifying the most likely diagnosis and ascertaining the short-term mortality/morbidity risk. The latter allows one to determine whether urgent hospitalization is needed or whether the patient can be safely (and more economically) be evaluated as an outpatient. Based on findings from this initial step, subsequent carefully selected diagnostic tests can be chosen to confirm the diagnostic clinical suspicion, and thereby initiate effective preventive therapy.

REFERENCES

1. Moya A, Sutton R, Ammirati F, et al. Guidelines for the diagnosis and treatment of syncope (version 2009). *Eur Heart J.* 2009;30(21):2631-2671.

2. Van Dijk JG, Thijs RD, Benditt DG, Wieling W. A guide to disorders causing transient loss of consciousness: focus on syncope. *Nat Rev Neurol.* 2009;5:438-448.

3. Blanc JJ, L'Her C, Touiza A, Garo B, et al. Prospective evaluation and outcome of patients admitted for syncope over a 1 year period. *Eur Heart J.* 2002;23:815-820.

4. Newton JL, Marsh A, Frith J, Parry S. Experience of a rapid access blackout clinic for older people. *Age Ageing.* 2010;39:265-268.

5. Soteriades ES, Evans JC, Larson MG, et al. Incidence and prognosis of syncope. *N Engl J Med.* 2002;347:878-885.

6. Benditt DG. Syncope risk assessment in the emergency department and clinic. *Prog Cardiovasc Dis.* 2013;55:376-381.

7. Ammirati F, Colivicchi F, Minardi G, et al. The management of syncope in the hospital: the OESIL Study (Osservatorio Epidemiologico della Sincope nel Lazio). *G Ital Cardiol.* 1999;29:533-539.

8. Ammirati F, Colivicchi F, Santini M. Implementation of a simplified diagnostic algorithm in a multicentre prospective trial—the OESIL 2 Study (Osservatorio Epidemiologico della Sincope nel Lazio. *Eur Heart J.* 2000;21:935-940.

9. Shen W, Decker W, Smars P, et al. Syncope evaluation in the emergency department study (SEEDS). A multidisciplinary approach to syncope management. *Circulation.* 2004;110:3636-3645.

10. Quinn J, McDermott D, Stiell I, et al. Prospective validation of the San Francisco Syncope Rule to predict patients with serious outcomes. *Ann Emerg Med.* 2006;47:448-454.

11. Martin GJ, Adams SL, Martin HG, et al. Prospective evaluation of syncope. *Ann Emerg Med.* 1984;13:499-504.

12. Sumner GL, Rose MS, Koshman ML, Ritchie D, Sheldon RS; Prevention of Syncope Trial. Recent history of vasovagal syncope in a young, referral-based population is a stronger predictor of recurrent syncope than lifetime syncope burden. *J Cardiovasc Electrophysiol.* 2010;21:1375-1380.

13. Raj S, Coffin ST. Medical therapy and physical maneuvers in the treatment of vasovagal syncope and orthostatic hypotension. *Prog Cardiovasc Dis.* 2013;55:425-433.

14. Moya A, Rivas N, Perez-Rodon J. Overview of the contribution of recent trials to advancement of syncope management. *Prog Cardiovasc Dis.* 2013;55: 396-401.

15. Krediet CT, van Dijk N, Linzer M, et al. Management of vasovagal syncope: controlling or aborting faints by leg crossing and muscle tensing. *Circulation.* 2002;106:1684-1689.

16. Perez-Lugones A, Schweikert R, Pavia S, et al. Usefulness of midodrine in patients with severely symptomatic neurocardiogenic syncope: a randomized control study. *J Cardiovasc Electrophysiol.* 2001;12:935-938.

17. van Dijk G, Wieling W. Pathophysiological basis of syncope and neurological conditions that mimic syncope. *Prog Cardiovasc Dis.* 2013:55:345-356.

18. Brignole M, Sutton R, Menozzi C, et al; International Study on Syncope of Uncertain Etiology 2 (ISSUE 2) Group. Early application of an implantable loop recorder allows effective specific therapy in patients with recurrent Eur Heart J; 2006;27:1085-92.

19. Brignole M, Menozzi C, Moya A, et al. Pacemaker therapy in patients with neurally-mediated syncope and documented asystole. Third international study on syncope of uncertain etiology (ISSUE-3): a randomized trial. *Circulation.* 2012;125:2566-2571.

20. Krediet CDP, Parry SW, Jardine DL, Benditt DG, Brignole M, Wieling W. The history of diagnosing carotid sinus hypersensitivity: why are the current criteria too sensitive. *Europace.* 2011;13:14-22.

46 VASODEPRESSOR SYNCOPE

David G. Benditt, MD, Barry L.S. Detloff, BS, Oana Dickinson, MD

CASE PRESENTATION

A 39-year-old otherwise healthy active woman was seen in consultation at the Syncope/Arrhythmia Clinic at the University of Minnesota Medical Center complaining of multiple "faints" and numerous near-faints. The faints that she did experience were always similar in presentation; they tended to occur more often early in the day and developed within a few minutes after she stood up from a seated or lying position. Typically, within seconds of arising she experienced dull ache in her shoulder and arms, lightheadedness, and "blurry vision." These symptoms usually resolved promptly. However, from time-to-time 1 or 2 minutes later she would sense palpitations, sweatiness, cold skin, and occasional nausea. Observers noted marked pallor. In response, she had learned to lie down on the floor. However, even though lying down prevented complete loss of consciousness, she volunteered that afterward she felt "drained" and wanted to rest.

The patient does not recall fainting as a child, and there is no family history of transient loss of consciousness or premature death. She does not recollect ever having a faint triggered by prolonged standing, blood draws, emotional upset, or pain. Her only medications, apart from vitamin supplements, are occasional pain relievers and a vasoconstrictor for migraine control. Physical examination in the clinic was normal with a seated blood pressure of 104/69 mm Hg and a heart rate of 80 beats/min. Her ECG was normal, as was an echocardiogram.

ETIOLOGY AND PATHOPHYSIOLOGY

Faints occurring as the result of transient neural reflex-mediated systemic hypotension (so-called "neural-reflex syncope") are the most common form of syncope encountered in clinical practice (40%-50% of cases), with vasovagal syncope being the most frequent of all forms of neural-reflex syncope. Others include carotid sinus syndrome and situational faints (eg, cough syncope, postmicturition syncope) (Figure 46-1).

Neural reflex faints (particularly the vasovagal faint) not only comprise the vast majority of syncope events in younger, otherwise healthy patients but also remain a major contributing cause of syncope in older individuals (Figure 46-2).[3,4] However, due to a higher prevalence of heart and vascular disease in older individuals, establishing the diagnosis may be difficult. In any case, no matter the patient's age, it is the "reflex" nature of the faint, most often detected by the patient's symptoms documented during a carefully obtained medical history, that most effectively distinguishes neural-reflex faints from other causes of collapse.

NOMENCLATURE

In neurally mediated reflex syncope, systemic hypotension with consequent cerebral hypoperfusion may be caused by either vasodilation

Neurally Mediated Reflex Syncope: Most Common Forms

Vasovagal syncope (VVS)
Carotid sinus syndrome (CSS)
Situational faints

- Micturition syncope
- Cough syncope
- Defecation syncope
- Swallow syncope
- Trumpet blower's syncope
- Mess trick

FIGURE 46-1 Summary of the most common forms of neurally mediated reflex syncope. In each case the basis of the faint may be "vasodepressor" or "cardioinhibitory" or both ("mixed").

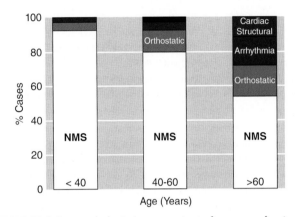

FIGURE 46-2 Bar graph depicting approximate frequency of various causes of syncope by age. Note that neurally mediated syncope (NMS, white) remains a common cause in all age groups. Orthostatic syncope increases with advancing age (light blue). (Modified with permission from Parry SW, Tan MP: An approach to the evaluation and management of syncope in adults, BMJ 2010 Feb 27;340(7744): 468-473.)

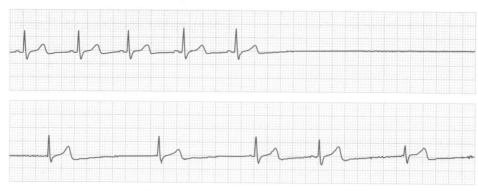

FIGURE 46-3 Sinus arrest suggestive of a cardioinhibitory syncope in a young patient with typical vasovagal symptoms. However, it should be recognized that a vasodepressor mechanism may also be present but cannot be confirmed in the absence of documenting the presence of hypotension during cardiac pacing to overcome the bradycardia.

or severe bradycardia acting alone, or as is more often the case, both working together.[1] When vasodilatation is the primary cause of symptomatic hypotension, the faint is termed "vasodepressor" and is the result of some degree of diminished arterial resistance, but an even greater component of increased venous capacitance (particularly in the splanchnic bed) with consequent diminished venous return to the heart. If bradycardia is the principal cause of hypotension, then the faint is termed "cardioinhibitory," and is due to the occurrence of a predominantly vagally-mediated slow heart rate (often prolonged asystolic pauses [Figure 46-3]) of sufficient severity to compromise cardiac output and cerebral blood flow. Most often both mechanisms are present, and the pathophysiology of the syncope is said to be "mixed."[1,2]

Given the pathophysiology described above, "vasodepressor" syncope is best considered a subset of the vasovagal reaction in which systemic hypotension is primarily due to vaso- and venodilatation; in the vasodepressor faint, cardioinhibition is either nonexistent or modest. The physiology of the "vasodepressor" faint was investigated in the classic study by Weissler et al in 1957.[5] These investigators pointed out that muscarinic blockade and correction of bradycardia (by atropine) had little impact on susceptibility to syncope. Thus a "vasodepressor" faint should be considered a physiologic unique entity (albeit often found in a "mixed" form with a cardioinhibitory feature) and should not be simply employed as another term for vasovagal syncope or "neural reflex faint." However, and rather unfortunately, the term "vasodepressor" often continues to be misused; this erroneous usage is confusing and should be abandoned.

CLINICAL EVALUATION

Initially, the medical history of the patient described here was interpreted to suggest that this patient was experiencing both "immediate" and subsequently the more classic "delayed" form of orthostatic hypotension. However, her age and absence of evident triggers (eg, drugs, neurologic disease) made orthostatic syncope unlikely. Furthermore, her symptom complex (ie, palpitations, sweating, feeling cold, pallor, and later, fatigue) were more compatible with a neurally mediated reflex vasovagal reaction triggered by abrupt movement to upright posture. Consequently, an autonomic study using noninvasive ECG and hemodynamic monitoring (Finometer, Finapres Medical Systems, Arnhem, The Netherlands) was undertaken. In brief, after a 10-minute period of being quietly seated in a chair, "active" standing resulted in evidence for immediate orthostatic hypotension (Figure 46-4A).

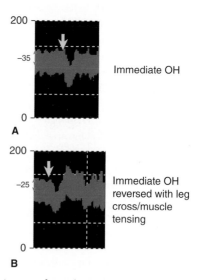

FIGURE 46-4 Impact of muscle tensing on immediate orthostatic hypotension (OH) response. Vertical blue arrows indicate time of movement from sitting to standing. The almost "immediate" fall of systemic pressure is apparent. PCM = physical counter maneuver. (A) Control test. Approximate drop in blood pressure is 35 mm Hg. (B) PCM test. Approximate drop of blood pressure is 25 mm Hg. Leg and buttock muscle tensing results in prompt normalization of pressure with slight overshoot evident.

The test was repeated in both the drug-free state and after sublingual nitroglycerin (0.4 mg) pretreatment; both resulted in her experiencing typical symptoms of "dizziness" and brief visual disturbance associated with an immediate but transient fall of systemic blood pressure but without substantial bradycardia. The observation strongly favored a predominantly "vasodepressor" response. The patient indicated that the sequence of events was typical of her spontaneous attacks.

DIAGNOSIS

The medical history is crucial to recognition of reflex syncope. Factors initiating the vasovagal form of neural reflex syncope, whether it be cardioinhibitory or vasodepressor in nature, are often elusive. Nevertheless, certain triggers are well recognized, including extreme emotion, relative dehydration, excessively warm confining environments, and acute pain. In addition, onset may be associated with prolonged periods of upright posture. However, the finding in the patient reported here, that abrupt postural change was to the best of our knowledge the only trigger, is uncommon. Nevertheless, it was the history that essentially excluded the primary contending diagnosis (ie, "delayed" form of orthostatic hypotension) and led to undertaking confirmatory laboratory testing.

Identifying vasodepressor hypotension is difficult in free-living individuals, as current ambulatory blood pressure recording technology is unsuitable to the task, and ambulatory ECG monitoring is not helpful. With regard to the latter, however, until newer ambulatory sensor systems able to detect blood pressure in a continuous manner become available,[6] indirect evidence may be used to implicate a vasodepressor response. Specifically, the recording of sinus tachycardia prior to a reported syncope in which the heart rate is now essentially "normal," suggests the possibility of a vasodepressor event. However, psychogenic pseudosyncope may exhibit a similar footprint. Consequently, findings during "active standing test" and/or head-up tilt table test may need to be relied upon even though they are at best surrogates for the spontaneous event.

Neurally mediated reflex faints, such as postural faints, are more likely to occur during periods of prolonged upright posture, especially if the affected individual is dehydrated or somewhat "volume down" (eg, in the morning after night-long fasting, or in the presence of excess diuretics or hot environments), or deconditioned.

The role of rapid postural change for triggering vasovagal reactions is difficult to assess using conventional tilt-table technique and is more amenable to evaluation by the "active standing test" or even more aggressively by the "squat-stand" test. In this regard, Rickards et al[7] compared the immediate cardiovascular effects of tilt-table testing to those of the squat-stand test in healthy subjects. In essence, squat-stand triggered a greater and more prolonged fall of systemic blood pressure (systolic and diastolic), with the principal driver being the dramatic impact on reduction of diastolic pressure (an indirect marker of a more severe diminution of arterial peripheral resistance). Others[8] have hypothesized that squatting impairs blood flow to the legs and increases local accumulation of vasodilator metabolites. Upon movement to upright posture, and despite otherwise normal neural (baroreceptor) reflex adaptation, there is more persistent reduction of peripheral resistance than would be observed with tilt. The impact may be more prolonged hypotension in certain susceptible patients (such as the individual described here) and the consequent triggering of a vasovagal response, and particularly a vasodepressor response.

TREATMENT RECOMMENDATIONS

In most cases of vasovagal syncope, whether predominantly cardioinhibitory or vasodepressor, patient education and advice regarding maintenance of hydration (with low calorie electrolyte solutions), along with warning regarding the potential for falls and injury are the foundations of treatment. Thereafter it may be useful to introduce physical countermaneuvers. Only infrequently are drugs such as midodrine and fludrocortisone required. Pacing therapy is used only on very rare occasions and generally in older patients in whom a marked cardioinhibitory form of vasovagal syncope has been confirmed by ambulatory monitoring (not by tilt table testing alone).

In the case of our patient, physical counter-maneuvers[9,10] were explained as part of the autonomic testing procedure; buttock and thigh muscle tensing clearly ameliorated the postural drop of blood pressure and eliminated near-syncope symptoms associated with abruptly moving to an upright posture (Figure 46-4B). Thereafter, a conventional head-up tilt table test was undertaken. A drug-free tilt-test was well tolerated for 20 minutes at which time sublingual nitroglycerin (0.4 mg) was administered (Figure 46-5). The patient experienced her usual near-syncope symptoms with an associated drop of blood pressure but only a modest reduction of heart rate (see Figure 46-5, top); however, the near-syncope symptoms were rapidly reversed by having her perform thigh and buttock muscle tensing as had been taught earlier in the study (see Figure 46-5).

Based on her history and the autonomic testing results, and in addition to general education regarding her condition, the patient was initiated on a treatment regimen comprised of increased dietary salt and volume (focusing on low-calorie electrolyte-containing "sport drinks") and physical counter-maneuvers (principally thigh and buttock muscle tensing) to minimize the "immediate orthostatic hypotensive" trigger. Follow-up at 8 months has been associated with absence of syncope and only infrequent near-syncope symptoms.

CONCLUSION

In conclusion, this case study highlights vasodepressor syncope as a unique entity and points out that this term is best considered a subset of the vasovagal reaction. Furthermore, the case illustrates the potential (albeit seemingly uncommon) for recurrent vasovagal reactions of the vasodepressor form to be triggered by immediate ("initial") orthostatic hypotension.

ACKNOWLEDGEMENT

The authors wish to thank Professor Wouter Wieling, University of Amsterdam, Amsterdam, The Netherlands, for his assistance with this manuscript and his invaluable teaching over many years.

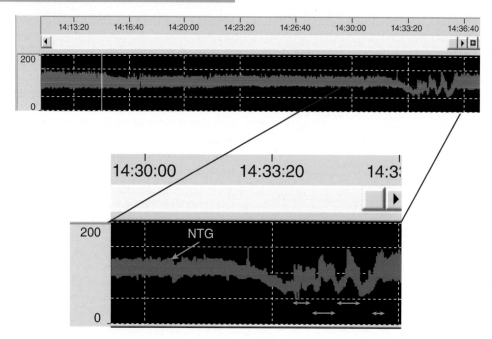

FIGURE 46-5 Recording depicting head-up tilt table findings. (Top) The white vertical bar at left indicates the time when the patient is tilted to 70 degrees. (Bottom) After approximately 15 minutes, the blood pressure was stable, and nitroglycerine (NTG) was administered sublingually. Within 2 to 3 minutes, marked hypotension and modest bradycardia (not shown) began to evolve. The patient developed typical vasovagal symptoms primarily on a vasodepressor basis. Thereafter a series of muscle tensing physical countermaneuvers (PCM) were initiated (noted by horizontal blue double arrows). Note the prompt increase in blood pressure with each intervention and subsequent blood pressure fall after each PCM termination, except for the last one. The patient's symptoms were ameliorated by the maneuvers, and these maneuvers could permit an affected individual to seek a safe gravitationally neutral location (ie, sitting, lying down) until the episode self-terminates. The tilt-test was concluded after the last PCM and accounts for normalization of pressure at that time.

REFERENCES

1. Moya, A, Sutton R, Ammirati F, et al. The Task Force for the Diagnosis and Management of Syncope of the European Society of Cardiology (ESC). Guidelines for the diagnosis and management of syncope (version 2009). European Heart J. 2009;30: 2631-2671.

2. Wieling W, Thijs RD, van Dijk N, Wilde AA, Benditt DG, van Dijk JG. Symptoms and signs of syncope: a review of the link between physiology and clinical clues. *Brain.* 2009;132:2630-2642.

3. Samniah N, Sakaguchi S, Ermis C, Lurie KG, Benditt DG. Transient modification of baroreceptor response during tilt-induced vasovagal syncope. *Europace.* 2004;6:48-54.

4. Parry SW, Tan MP. An approach to the evaluation and management of syncope in adults. *BMJ.* 2010;340:468-473.

5. Weissler AM, Warren JV, Estes EH Jr, McIntosh HD, Leonard JJ. Vaodepressor syncope: factors affecting cardiac output. *Circulation.* 1957;15:875-882.

6. Benditt DG, Sakaguchi S, van Dijk JG. Autonomic nervous system and cardiac arrhythmias. In: Saksena S, Camm AJ, Boyden PA, Dorian P, Goldschlager N, Vetter VL, Zareba W, eds.

Electrophysiology Disorders of the Heart, 2nd ed. Philadelphia, PA: Elsevier Saunders; 2012:61-71.

7. Venugopal D, Patterson R, Jhanjee R, et al. Subcutaneous bioimpedance recording: assessment of a method for hemodynamic monitoring by implanted devices. *J Cardiovasc Electrophysiol.* 2009;20:76-81.

8. Rickards CA, Newman DG. A comparative assessment of two techniques for investigating initial cardiovascular reflexes under acute orthostatic stress. *Eur J Appl Physiol.* 2003;90:449-457.

9. Convertino VA, Tripp LD, Ludwig DA, Duff J, Chelette TL. Female exposure to high G: chronic adaptations of cardiovascular functions. *Aviat Space Environ Med.* 1998;69:875-882.

9. Krediet CT, Go-Schon IK, Kim YS, Linzer M, Van Lieshout JJ, Wieling W. Management of initial orthostatic hypotension: lower body muscle tensing attenuates the transient arterial blood pressure decrease upon standing from squatting. *Clin Sci (Lond).* 2007;113:401-407.

10. van Dijk N, Quartieri F, Blanc JJ, et al; PC-Trial Investigators. Effectiveness of physical counterpressure maneuvers in preventing vasovagal syncope: the Physical Counterpressure Manoeuvres Trial (PC-Trial). *J Am Coll Cardiol.* 2006;48:1652-1657.

47 MEDICAL AND PACING THERAPIES FOR NEURO-CARDIOGENIC SYNCOPE

Blair P. Grubb, MD, FACC

CASE PRESENTATION

A 32-year-old woman presents after suffering a series of syncopal events. During one of these events she fractured her shoulder. Each of the episodes has occurred while she was standing, and in each case she experienced a sensation of light-headedness lasting 2 or 3 seconds followed by an abrupt loss of consciousness during which she would fall to the ground. The actual loss of consciousness was brief (less than 2-3 minutes) and was usually not associated with injury. After each syncopal event the patient was mildly confused for a brief period and was severely fatigued. Bystanders who have observed some of her events report that she suddenly becomes pale and often becomes "stiff and sometimes shakes." Physical examination is unremarkable. There are no orthostatic changes in heart rate or blood pressure. An electrocardiogram, echocardiogram, and electroencephalogram are all within normal limits. During head upright tilt table testing, at minute 15 of upright tilt she complains of light-headedness followed by an abrupt loss of consciousness. At the time of syncope her blood pressure fell from 120/80 mm Hg to 60/40 mm Hg and was associated with a 5-second period of asystole. She regained consciousness after being returned to the supine position. She reported that this episode felt identical to those she had experienced clinically. The patient was educated as to the nature of her condition, and therapeutic options were discussed.

ETIOLOGY AND PATHOPHYSIOLOGY

Syncope is defined as a loss of consciousness and postural tone with spontaneous recovery.[1] Both a symptom and sign, syncope may be the sole warning prior to an episode of sudden death.[2] Even when the cause is benign, recurrent syncope can result in injury and provoke a degree of functional and emotional impairment similar to that seen in other chronic debilitating disorders.[3] Neurocardiogenic (or vasovagal) syncope is the most common of a group of disorders known as reflex (or naturally mediated) syncopes. These are characterized by a sudden failure of the autonomic nervous system (ANS) to maintain blood pressure (and on occasion heart rate) at levels sufficient to maintain cerebral perfusion and consciousness. Other types of reflex syncopes include carotid sinus hypersensitivity and syncope brought on by activities such as coughing, swallowing, defecation, and urination.[4]

While the exact etiology is still uncertain, it is currently felt that neurocardiogenic syncope occurs in people who are predisposed to these events as a consequence of excessive peripheral venous pooling which results in a sudden decline in peripheral venous return to the heart. The lack of volume produces a "hypercontractile" state in the heart, which causes activation of cardiac mechanoreceptors that normally are stimulated only by stretch. This generates an abrupt increase in afferent neural input to the brain, which duplicates the situation normally seen in severe hypertension, resulting in a sudden withdrawal of sympathetic nerve activity. This action produces an apparent "paradoxical" reflex, causing bradycardia and a drop in peripheral vascular resistance and resulting in systemic hypotension which, if sufficiently profound, leads to cerebral hypoperfusion and syncope. In the susceptible individual, activation of other mechanoreceptor beds in the body (such as those found in the rectum, bladder, lungs, and esophagus) can produce similar responses.

Neurocardiogenic syncope can be brought on by being in a warm environment, prolonged standing, pain, fear, and emotional distress. Prodromal symptoms include light-headedness, sweating, headache, fatigue, visual disturbances, feeling cold or hot, and nausea. External signs may include paleness, dilation of the pupils, yawning, and unsteady gait. While most patients will experience some kind of prodrome a significant number (often older patients) will not, in which case syncope may result in a fall with the risk of subsequent physical trauma. The actual loss of consciousness is usually short, often between 30 seconds and several minutes, (however in older patients it maybe longer). Some patients may experience body rigidity and stiffness (or even tonic–clonic-like activity in some) during an episode. Recovery is usually fairly rapid, with only mild confusion afterward. Following an episode the patient may exhibit pallor and experience weakness, headache, and fatigue.

DIAGNOSIS

A comprehensive history and physical examination are vital to the diagnosis, which necessitates excluding cardiovascular or neurologic disease. Patients should be queried as to any family history of cardiac disease or sudden death. Information should be obtained as to the frequency of events and the conditions under which they occur. Bystander descriptions are also quite helpful. The finding of a cardiac murmur or focal neurologic sign requires further evaluation by echocardiography or magnetic resonance imaging (MRI). We routinely obtain a 12-lead electrocardiogram on all patients and echocardiography if there is any question that the heart is normal.

Tilt table testing is the sole medical test for diagnosing neurocardiogenic syncope that has undergone careful evaluation. A positive test is one that elicits a hypotensive response that duplicates the patient's clinical episodes. Several comprehensive resources have been published on the technical details of tilt table testing, established protocols, (including pharmacologic provocation), and the various patterns of hemodynamic response, to which the interested reader is directed.

Implantable loop recorders are also useful tools in determining whether severe bradycardia or asystole is associated with a syncopal event. The interested reader is directed to Chapter 49 The Implantable Loop Recorder in this book on the subject.

TREATMENT

In situations where syncope only occurs in particular circumstances, management principally centers around educating both the patient and their family as to the nature of the disorder and the situations to be avoided, for example, dehydration, extreme heat, prolonged standing, as well as agents that facilitate syncope such as vasodilators and alcohol.

In patients with an adequate prodrome, isometric contractions of the leg and arm muscles can sometimes abort episodes by virtue of activation

TABLE 47-1 Treatment Modalities for Neurocardiogenic Syncope

	Treatment	Use and Dosage	Drawbacks
Lifestyle-related	Physical maneuvers Fluid intake Salt intake	Leg crossing Isometric contractions Around 2 L/d ~120 mmol/d	Cannot use if prodrome absent Frequent urination Poor compliance Gastrointestinal upset, edema

Medications	β-Blockers
	Midodrine
	Fludrocortisone
	Selective serotonin
	  reuptake inhibitors
		Metoprolol 50 mg orally twice a day
		Nebivolol 5 mg/d
		2.5 to 10 mg three times a day
		0.1 to 0.2 mg/d
		Paroxetine 20 mg/d
		Sertraline 50 mg/d
			Bradycardia, fatigue, prolonged
			  syncope
			Hypertension
			Nausea
			Piloerection
			Fluid retention
			Edema
			Hypertension
			Nausea
			Insomnia
			Agitation

Devices	Permanent cardiac pacing	DDD mode with rate drop or CLS function	Expense, infection, thrombosis

of the skeletal muscle pump, which seems to augment venous return. Increasing fluid and salt intake may reduce the frequency of syncopal episodes. While a variety of pharmacotherapies are employed to treat neurocardiogenic syncope, only a small number have been prospectively evaluated, and no drug has been approved by the U.S. Food and Drug Administration for the treatment of neurocardiogenic syncope. A list of potential treatments can be found in Table 47-1.

Briefly, while β-blockers have been used to prevent neurocardiogenic syncope, some studies have cast doubt on their effectiveness. While most studies have used metoprolol, we prefer nebivolol due to is low side effect profile. Fludrocortisone is a synthetic mineral corticoid that promotes retention of sodium as well as the expansion of central blood volume and sensitization of α-receptors in the peripheral vasculature. Midodrine hydrochloride is a direct α-1 receptor agonist which exerts direct vasoconstrictive effects (methylphenidate may be an acceptable alternative agent). The selective serotonin reuptake inhibitors are sometimes helpful, presumably by their desensitization of central reflexes.

Other treatments undergoing evaluation for refractory patients include octreotide, desmopression, and erythropoietin.

Permanent cardiac pacemaker placement has been advocated as a treatment for medically refractory patients based on the finding that up to one-third of these patients may experience severe bradycardia or asystole during either tilt-induced or spontaneously occurring syncope. While initial controlled studies of pacing were disappointing, it was realized that when pacemakers were placed in patients in whom asystole or bradycardia was documented during syncope using an implantable loop recorder the success rate was much higher (see Chapter 49, The Implantable Loop Recorder).

The recent ISSUE-3 trial was a randomized, double-blind, placebo-controlled trial of pacing in syncope patients with periods of asystole or profound bradycardia documented by an implantable loop recorder.[10] Patients were randomized to pacing "on" or pacing "off." At the end of 2 years, the acute recurrence in the pacemaker "off" group was 57% while the recurrence rate in the pacemaker on group was 25%.

These studies were performed using standard pacing systems that sense heart rate only. However, in neurocardiogenic syncope blood pressure falls first followed by a decline in heart rate. Therefore, in this condition standard pacemakers can only detect an event after it is well underway, offering "too little too late." The recent development of pacemakers that have the ability to sense blood pressure have addressed this issue. Pacing systems using "closed loop stimulation" (CLS) have been show to be superior to standard pacing systems in preventing neurocardiogenic syncope.[11,12] Ongoing studies will help clarify this finding.

REFERENCES

1. Grubb BP. Neurocardiogenic syncope. In: Grubb BP, Olshansky B, eds. *Syncope: Mechanisms and Management*. Malden, MA: Blackwell/Futura Press; 2005:47-67.

2. Grubb BP. Clinical practice. Neurocardiogenic syncope. *N Engl J Med*. 2005;352(10):1004-1010.

3. Linzer M, Pontinen M, Gold GT, Divine GW, Felder A, Brooks WB. Impairment of physical and psychosocial function in recurrent syncope. *J Clin Epidemiol*. 1991;44:1037-1043.

4. Grubb BP. Neurocardiogenic syncope and related disorders of orthostatic intolerance. *Circulation*. 2005;111:2997-3006.

5. Moya A, Sutton R, Ammirati F, et al. Guidelines for the evaluation and management of syncope. *Eur Heart J*. 2009;30:2631-2671.

6. Grubb BP. Kosinski D. Tilt table testing: concepts and limitations. *Pacing Clin Electrophysiol*. 1997;20:760-776.

7. Brignole M. Tilt table testing. In: Grubb BP, Olshansky B, eds. *Syncope: Mechanisms and Management*. Malden, MA: Blackwell/ Futura Press; 2005:159-168.

8. Brignole M, Croci F, Menozzi C, et al. Isometric arm counter-pressure maneuvers to abort impending vasovagal syncope. *J Am Coll Cardiol*. 2002;40:2053-2059.

9. Bringole M. Randomized Clinical trials of neurally medicated syncope. *J Cardiovasc Electrophysiol*. 2003;14(S9):S64-S69.

10. Brignole M, Menozzi C, Moya A, et al. Pacemaker therapy in patients with neutrally medicated syncope and documented asystole: Third International Study on Syncope of Uncertain Etiology (ISSUE-3): a randomized trial. *Circulation*. 2012;125:2566-2571.

11. Kanjwal K, Karabin B, Kanjwal Y, Grubb BP. Preliminary observations on the use of closed-loop cardiac pacing in patients with refractory neurocardiogenic syncope. *J Interv Card Electrophysiol*. 2010;27:69-73.

12. Palmisano P, Zaccaria M, Luzzi G, Nacci F, Anacierio M, Favala S. Closed loop cardiac pacing vs. conventional dual chamber cardiac pacing with specialized sensing and pacing algorithms for syncope prevention in patients with refractory vasovagal syncope: results of a long term follow up. *Europace*. 2012:14(7):1038-1043.

48 SYNCOPE IN THE ATHLETE

Yousef Bader, MD, and Mark Estes, MD

CASE PRESENTATION

A 17-year-old woman presents for evaluation of recurrent episodes of abrupt loss of consciousness without a prodrome. She had been diagnosed as having epilepsy in infancy. In early life, she had been having seizures occurring both at rest and during exertion. She was seen by a pediatric neurologist, and despite multiple antiepileptic medications her seizures persisted. Four years prior to her presentation, her seizures began to occur exclusively with exercise. One of her seizures occurred while she was running at a picnic on a Sunday afternoon. A cardiologist who was present at the time witnessed this seizure and took her to the local emergency department to be evaluated. Her vitals were normal; her examination was benign except for a small scalp abrasion. Her complete blood count and basic metabolic panel were normal. An ECG was performed and is shown in Figure 48-1. She was sent home with a 24-hour Holter monitor. The following day she had yet another episode of loss of consciousness while rowing with her high school team. The Holter monitor demonstrated several minutes of torsades de pointes (Figure 48-2).

CASE EXPLANATION

Although this patient was diagnosed as having a seizure disorder, it is important to note that these episodes of altered consciousness have been refractory to antiepileptic medications. Recently they occurred during exercise, raising concerns for alternative diagnoses. A seizure can of course be the result of a primary neurologic problem. However, seizure-like activity, or convulsive syncope, can be the result of cerebral hypoperfusion. This can result from common neurocardiogenic syncope or even fatal cardiac arrhythmias. In this case, the typical prodromal features of vasovagal syncope did not precede the loss of consciousness, making that an unlikely diagnosis. Syncope occurring during exercise is a strong predictor that the underlying problem is likely cardiac in origin. The scalp abrasion our patient suffered also supports the diagnosis of a cardiac arrhythmia which would result in a sudden drop in blood pressure and therefore the inability of a patient to protect their head as they fall. (Table 48-1 demonstrates features of cardiac and noncardiac syncope.[1])

- Exertional syncope is a precursor of sudden cardiac death (SCD). When identified, an appropriate workup should be initiated quickly to achieve a diagnosis and begin managing the patient.

- The differential diagnosis of cardiac syncope in this setting is seen in Table 48-2.

- Our patient's ECG clearly demonstrates a prolonged QT with a broad based, notched T wave. In the absence of QT prolonging medications this is highly suggestive of an inherited long QT syndrome (LQT) type 1. Her Holter also confirmed that her syncope is secondary to torsades de pointes, which is defined as polymorphic ventricular tachycardia (VT) resulting from a prolonged QT.

EPIDEMIOLOGY

- Loss of consciousness in athletes, although rare, is devastating, and this is due to our growing understanding of SCD in athletes and its causes. Cardiac causes of syncope can be due to either

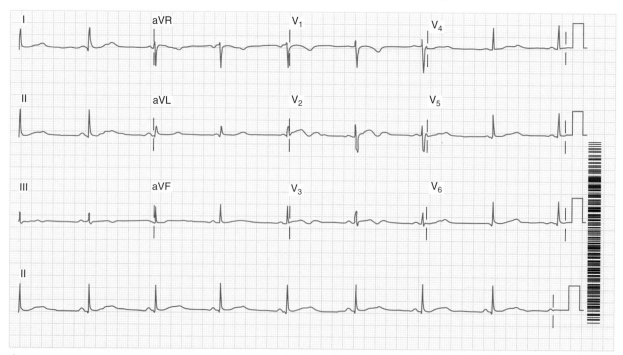

FIGURE 48-1 ECG showing sinus bradycardia at 48 beats per minute. There is a broad-based, notched T wave with a prolonged QT and T-wave inversions in anterior leads. Note that the T-wave notching can be seen in ≥3 leads.

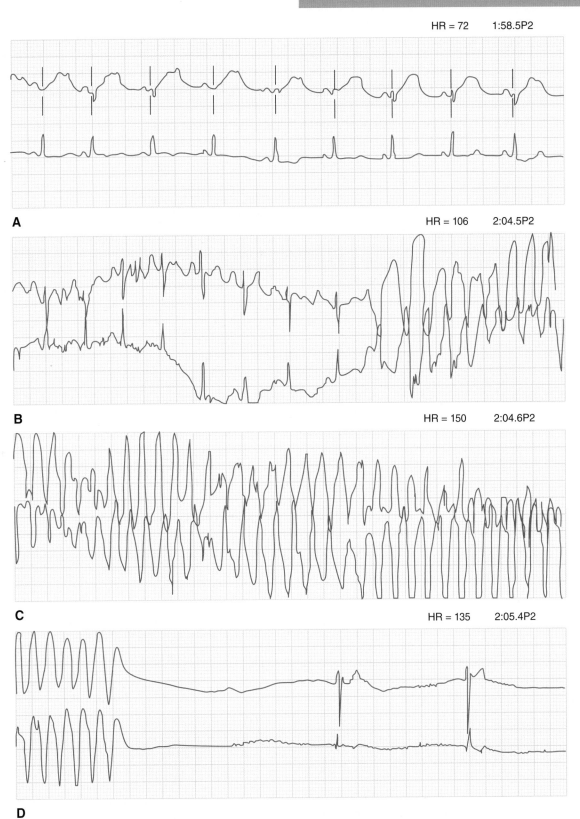

FIGURE 48-2 This tracing starts in sinus rhythm with a prolonged QT. The T wave is broad-based and notched. Polymorphic VT is initiated after a premature ventricular contraction (PVC). This then self-terminates with a junctional escape rhythm.

TABLE 48-1 Features of Cardiac and Noncardiac Syncope

	Neurocardiogenic	Seizure	Arrhythmic
Situational factors	Fear, fright, dehydration, upright posture	Occasional, triggered by flickering or flashing lights	Exertional, unrelated to posture
Prodrome	Light-headedness, warmth, nausea	Visual and auditory auras	None or brief light-headedness
Event Characteristics	Slump to the ground, injury unusual	Motor activity simultaneous with LOC, injury common, may last several minutes to even hours	Acute LOC, injury common, brief <15 secs
Post Syncope Symptoms	Fatigue, nausea	Postictal state, confusion, urinary or stool incontinence, tongue biting, Todd's paralysis	Usually none
Number of episodes	Multiple	Many	Few or one
Underlying disease	Unusual	Neurologic disease common	Heart disease common

Data from Bader Y, Link M. Syncope in the Athlete. Cardiac Electrophysiology Clinics 2013; 5(1):85-96.

TABLE 48-2 Differential Diagnosis

Benign causes of syncope

- Neurocardiogenic syncope

- Postexertion collapse

Life-threatening cardiac causes of syncope

- Long QT syndrome (LQTS)

- Catecholaminergic polymorphic ventricular tachycardia (CPVT)

- Right ventricular outflow tract ventricular tachycardia (RVOT VT)

- Brugada syndrome

- Arrhythmogenic right ventricular dysplasia (ARVD)

- Hypertrophic cardiomyopathy (HCM)

- Coronary anomalies

- Commotio cordis

structural heart disease or a primary arrhythmic condition and account for approximately 1% of all causes of syncope in the athlete. Details of incidence, prevalence, and geographic distribution are seen in Table 48-3.[2-4]

- SCD is two and a half times more common in the competitive athlete than the general population, demonstrating its direct relationship to competitive sports.

- The leading cause of SCD is hypertrophic cardiomyopathy (HCM) accounting for approximately 37% of cases followed by coronary anomalies and ion channelopathies, including long QT syndromes, which account for about 4% (Figure 48-3).

ETIOLOGY AND PATHOPHYSIOLOGY

The majority of cardiac causes of syncope are either congenital or inherited (either autosomal recessive or autosomal dominant).

Long QT Syndrome

- This group of disorders is genetically inherited, affecting cardiac ion channels, which result in prolonged ventricular repolarization, which may lead to polymorphic ventricular tachycardia.

- There are 13 different types of inherited prolonged QT, all of which involve a different genetic mutation. The most common forms of long QT are types 1, 2, and 3 accounting for the majority cases.

  ○ LQT1 results from a mutation in the α-subunit of the slow delayed rectifier potassium channel KCNQ1. These mutations result in reducing the amount of repolarizing current, thereby prolonging the action potential. This is the most common form of congenital long QT, making up one-third of cases. LQT1 is often triggered by exercise and has a specific association with swimming.

  ○ LQT2 results from a mutation in the α-subunit of the rapid delayed rectifier potassium channel KCNH1. Similar to LQT1, the mutations of LQT2 result in prolongation of the action potential. LQT2 can be triggered by exercise but is more commonly triggered by an emotional event or an auditory stimulus.

TABLE 48-3 Causes of Syncope in Athletes

	Incidence/Prevalence	Geographic Distribution
LQTS	• Affects 1:7000 of general population • 4% of SCD	
CPVT	• Affects 1:10,000 of general population	• Age of onset is 7-9 y
RVOT VT	• Most common cause of VT	• Diagnosed in the 3rd to 5th decade of life
Brugada Syndrome	• Affects 1:2000 • Mean age of SCD is 40 y	• Most prevalent in Southeast Asia
ARVD	• Affects 1:1000 of general population • 11% of SCD in general population	• 22% of SCD in athletes worldwide • 4% of SCD in athletes in United States
HCM	• 0.2%-0.5% of general population • Accounts for 35%-45% of SCD in athletes	• Yamaguchi syndrome (apical HCM) • 25% of HCM in Japanese • 1%-2% of HCM in Non-Japanese
Coronary Anomalies	• 17% of SCD in athletes	
Commotio Cordis	• 3% of SCD in athletes in United States	
Postexertion Collapse	• 70% of syncope in athletes	

○ LQT3 is result of a mutation in the α-subunit of the sodium channel SCN5A. This leads to failure of the sodium channel to remain inactivated, which results in a prolonged action potential duration.

○ LQT3 is less common than LQT1 and LQT2, but is more lethal.[5] As in LQT1 and 2, LQT3 can also be triggered by exercise but more commonly occurs during sleep. Characteristic features of LQT1, LQT2, and LQT3 are seen in Table 48-4.

Catecholaminergic Polymorphic Ventricular Tachycardia

• Another genetic disease that may result in polymorphic VT in athletes is catecholaminergic polymorphic ventricular tachycardia (CPVT). It is characterized by cardiac electrical instability due to activation of the sympathetic nervous system. Unlike LQT syndrome, it is not related to prolongation of the QT interval.

○ It is most commonly inherited in an autosomal dominant pattern resulting with mutations in the *RYR2* gene, which encodes for the ryanodine receptor channel. This accounts for about 55% of CPVT.

○ Autosomal recessive inheritance is by mutations in the *CASQ2* gene, which encodes calsequestrin, which is a calcium buffering protein of the sarcoplasmic reticulum and is responsible for about 2% of cases.[6]

• Mutations in the above receptors lead to calcium loading within myocardial cells and expose these patients to the risk of VT and ventricular fibrillation (VF) associated with acute emotion or exercise. Eighty percent of athletes with this disease have recurrent syncope, and thirty percent fall to sudden cardiac death.

Right Ventricular Outflow Tract Ventricular Tachycardia

• Right ventricular outflow tract ventricular tachycardia (RVOT VT) is the most common idiopathic VT in athletes. It most frequently occurs during emotional stress or exercise. Athletes usually present with palpitations and presyncope; however, it can infrequently present with syncope and exceptionally rarely present with sudden cardiac death.

Causes of SCD in the athlete

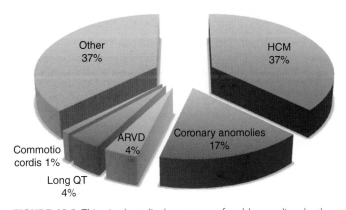

FIGURE 48-3 This pie chart displays causes of sudden cardiac death in athletes and their incidence.

TABLE 48-4 The Long QT Syndromes

	Gene Affected	Ion Current Change	Frequency	ECG Appearance
LQT1	KCNQ1	$\downarrow I_{Ks}$	45%	
LQT2	KCNH2	$\downarrow I_{Kr}$	45%	
LQT3	SCN5A	$\uparrow I_{Na}$	5%	

- Similar to CPVT, the principal mechanism of RVOT VT is due to intracellular calcium overload. One of cyclic adenosine monophosphate's (cAMP) roles is regulation of intracellular calcium. During exercise, cAMP levels rise, leading to an increase in intracellular calcium. This in turn, by a mechanism of triggered activity, leads to VT.

- There are two main phenotypic types of RVOT VT:
  - Nonsustained repetitive monomorphic VT.
  - Paroxysmal exercise-induced sustained RVOT VT, which more commonly affects athletes.[7]

Brugada Syndrome

- Although Brugada syndrome may be acquired, it is most commonly inherited in an autosomal dominant fashion and is due to a loss of function mutation in the SCN5A gene.

- Athletes with Brugada syndrome usually present with unexplained syncope and, less frequently, as sudden cardiac death.

- VF in Brugada patients is usually triggered by hyperthermia and during times of higher vagal tone, often occurring during sleep.[8] Because of their extensive training, athletes may have a higher baseline vagal tone, and during exercise rises in temperature may explain why athletes with Brugada are more likely to suffer from ventricular arrhythmias than nonathlete Brugada patients.

Arrhythmogenic Right Ventricular Dysplasia

- Arrhythmogenic right ventricular dysplasia (ARVD) is a genetic disorder with mutations in gene coding for desmosomal proteins, leading to fibrofatty replacement of myocardium. It is most often inherited in an autosomal dominant pattern.

- The right ventricle (RV) is affected in all but 5% of cases. There is left ventricular (LV) involvement in about 50% of cases and in a minority of cases only LV involvement.

- The "triangle of dysplasia" which is between the RV apex, the RV inflow tract, and the RV outflow tract is notoriously involved in ARVD.

- RVOT VT is the most common VT seen in these patients.[3]

Hypertrophic Cardiomyopathy

- Hypertrophic cardiomyopathy (HCM) is the most common cause of SCD in athletes and is caused by a number of mutations in genes coding proteins of the cardiac sarcomere most notably β-myosin heavy chain. Its familial form is inherited in an autosomal dominant pattern, but HCM can also be acquired as a de novo mutation.

- It is typically characterized by hypertrophy of the left ventricle in an asymmetric fashion with the anterior LV septum being the most commonly affected region.

- Thickening of the LV septum and systolic motion of the mitral valve can lead to left ventricular outflow tract (LVOT) obstruction, and in some cases a high gradient can lead to syncope.

- Ventricular arrhythmias occurring in patients with HCM are commonly the first clinical presentation of HCM and usually occur during strenuous physical activity.

Coronary Anomalies

- Athletes with anomalous coronaries may be completely asymptomatic, suffer from recurrent angina or syncope, and occasionally present with myocardial infarctions or sudden cardiac death.

- The most common coronary anomaly is a left anomalous coronary artery arising from the right coronary sinus, and this is associated with ischemia and sudden cardiac death (Figure 48-4).

- The course of an anomalous coronary is occasionally between the main pulmonary artery and the ascending aorta, and at times of exercise, an increase in the cardiac output may lead to compression of the coronary artery between them.

- A large territory of myocardium supplied by the anomalous coronary, the presence of an intramural segment within the aortic wall, and in particular a slit-like orifice of the coronary ostium are all high-risk features associated with increased mortality.

Commotio Cordis

- Commotio cordis is defined as VF resulting secondary from blunt chest injury and is seen in high-impact sports such as baseball, hockey, and boxing.
- For this to occur, the precordial impact must occur at a 10 to 30 ms interval just before the peak of the T wave as seen in Figure 48-5.
- The mechanism of commotio cordis is believed to be secondary to a series of events following impact of a blunt object. Blunt trauma → increase in left ventricular pressure → the myocardial cell membrane stretches → activation of stretch sensitive K^+_{ATP} ion channels → ventricular fibrillation.[9]

DIAGNOSIS

Patients with symptoms and signs suggestive of a cardiac cause for syncope should undergo a thorough, thoughtful, and systematic diagnostic approach, which begins with a detailed history and physical examination.

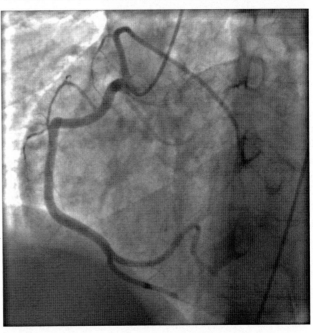

FIGURE 48-4 This is a left anterior oblique slightly cranial angiographic view of the right coronary artery with an anomalous left coronary artery arising from the ostium of the right coronary artery.

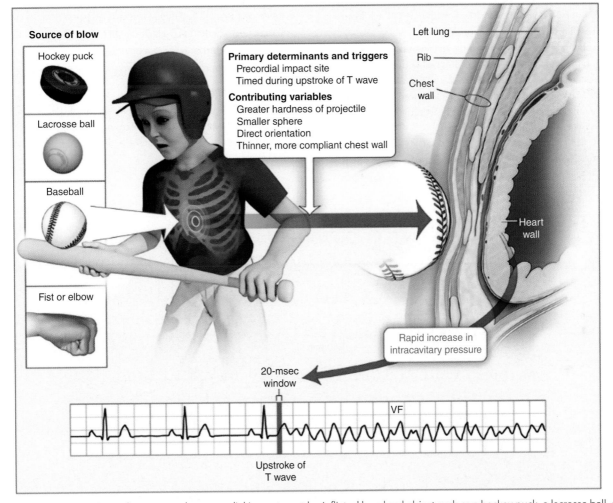

FIGURE 48-5 For commotio cordis to occur, the precordial impact must be inflicted by a hard object such as a hockey puck, a lacrosse ball, or a fist. This must occur within a 20 ms interval during the upstroke of the T wave resulting in ventricular fibrillation.

An electrocardiogram (ECG) should be performed on all patients and may be sufficient to provide a diagnosis. Echocardiography (Echo) should be performed in all patients with selective use of magnetic resonance imaging (MRI). Exercise treadmill testing (ETT) is a valuable tool in reproducing a patient's symptoms and detecting exertional ventricular arrhythmias. If noninvasive testing is diagnostic, electrophysiology studies are of no added value. If noninvasive testing is unfruitful, and there is a high index of suspicion for an arrhythmic cause, an EP study should be performed. The induction of nonsustained ventricular tachycardia, polymorphic ventricular tachycardia, and VF are not useful during an EP study as these findings are nonspecific and can be found in healthy individuals.[10] The role of genetic testing in confirming some of the above diagnoses is controversial because genetic mutations do not always have phenotypic consequences. Being aware of the implications of a positive or negative result is crucial.

Long QT Syndrome

- ECG: The ECG changes in long QT syndrome are often dynamic, and therefore their absence does not rule out the diagnosis. If absent, ECG changes can be provoked by drug challenges with β-agonists including epinephrine and isoproterenol. Instead of normal physiologic shortening of the QT interval with these provoking agents, patients with LQT1 and LQT2 experience prolongation of the corrected QT.

- ETT: When tachycardic young adults and children should shorten their QT interval; however, in patients with long QT syndrome, their QT will often fail to shorten or prolong.
  - LQT1: Diminished shortening of the QT interval, followed by exaggerated lengthening of the QT interval as the heart rate declines during recovery.
  - LQT2: Marked QT interval shortening followed by exaggerated lengthening of the QT interval as the heart rate declines during late recovery (4 minutes after exercise).
  - LQT3: Marked decrease in the QT interval.[11]
  - Long QT should be <450 ms in males and <470 ms in females.

- Genetic testing: In long QT syndrome, genetic testing will identify a specific mutation in 75% to 80% of cases. Traditionally, a clinical diagnostic criteria and a point system was used to assess probability of the diagnosis. This scoring system has a high specificity but low sensitivity; therefore, clinicians are leaning away from the scoring system and depending more on the length of the QT and genetic testing.[12]

Catecholaminergic Polymorphic VT

- ECG: The ECG is usually normal at rest. Isoproterenol infusion can be used to trigger VT in patients with CPVT.[13] The characteristic VT of CPVT is bidirectional with an alternating 180 degree QRS axis on a beat-to-beat basis as seen in Figure 48-6.

- ETT: Because CPVT is associated with increased sympathetic activity, it is often exposed during ETT, and the severity of the tachycardia is directly related to the level of exertion.

- Genetic testing: This is indicated in patients with a clinical presentation that is highly suspicious for CPVT but is not reproducible by ETT. Mutations in *RYR2* are inherited in an autosomal dominant pattern, whereas *CASQ2* gene mutations are inherited autosomal recessive.[7]

Right Ventricular Outflow Tract VT

- ECG: The ECG is usually normal at rest. Patients may have PVCs arising from the RVOT, which would have a left bundle branch block pattern and an inferior axis as seen in Figure 48-7.

- ETT: Similar to CPVT this may trigger the VT in patients.

- Echo: Normal.

- MRI: Focal thinning and fatty replacement of the right ventricular outflow tract is sometimes seen in patients with RVOT VT, although they are generally described as having structurally normal hearts.[14]

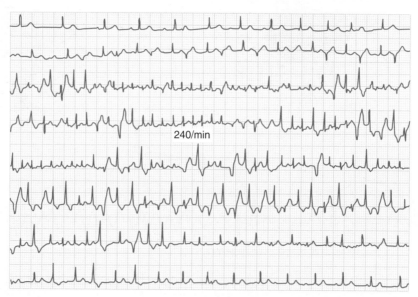

240/min

FIGURE 48-6 This ECG displays the typical pattern of bidirectional VT seen in CPVT.

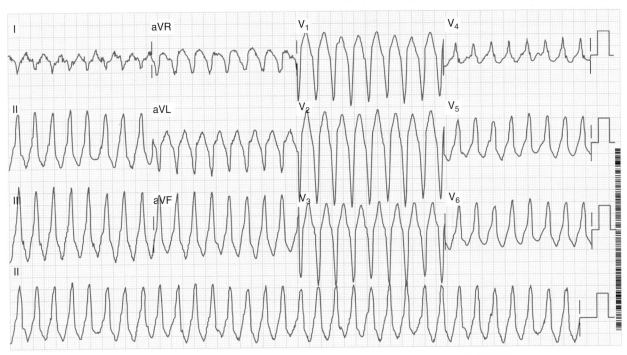

FIGURE 48-7 Wide complex tachycardia with an LBBB morphology and an inferior axis most consistent with RVOT VT.

Brugada Syndrome

- ECG: As in long QT, the ECG changes seen in Brugada syndrome are dynamic, so their absence does not rule out the diagnosis. There are three types of repolarization patterns seen in Brugada syndrome mainly affecting right-sided precordial leads (V_1-V_3). Type 1 Brugada pattern is the only diagnostic pattern of this disease.
    - Type 1 is characterized by a ≥2-mm coved ST-segment elevation followed by a negative T wave as seen in Figure 48-8.
    - Type 2 has a saddleback appearance with a downsloping ST segment with a takeoff that is ≥2 mm tapering to ≥1 mm and ending with an upright or biphasic T wave.
    - Type 3 has either a coved or saddleback ST segment with <1 mm ST elevation.[15]

- Raising right precordial leads to the second intercostal space can increase the sensitivity of the ECG for detecting a Brugada pattern in some patients. If that fails, flecainide and procainamide can be used to induce a Brugada pattern. Patients must develop a type 1 Brugada pattern for the ECG to be diagnostic.[16]

- Genetic testing: This involves sequencing *SCN5A* genes, which are the most common mutations in Brugada; however, only 15% to 30% of Brugada patients have *SCN5A* mutations, and not all patients with *SCN5A* mutations have Brugada.[17]

- Based on the Heart Rhythm Society consensus report, a diagnosis of Brugada syndrome is highly likely based on the presence of a spontaneous or provoked type 1 ECG pattern and one of the following: VF, polymorphic VT, family history of SCD at an age of <45 years, inducible VT with programmed stimulation, unexplained syncope, or nocturnal agonal respiration.

Arrhythmogenic Right Ventricular Dysplasia

- ECG: The most common ECG finding in patients with ARVD is T-wave inversion in leads V_1-V_3 as seen in Figure 48-9. This is a normal finding in only 4% of women and 1% of men greater than 14 years of age, so it is relatively specific and considered a diagnostic finding. Epsilon waves are seen in 50% of cases of ARVD.[18]

- Signal averaged ECGs: (SAECGs) have a diagnostic role in patients lacking typical ECG findings. SAECG is positive if two of the following three parameters are abnormal:
    - Fltered QRS duration (fQRS) ≥114 ms
    - Root-mean-square-voltage of the terminal 40 ms of the QRS of ≤20 μV
    - Duration of the terminal QRS signal <40 μV of ≥38 ms[19]

- Echo: Echo findings in ARVD include an enlarged hypokinetic RV and a thin RV free wall. Morphologic abnormalities of the RV are not uncommon, and these include heavy trabeculations 55% of the time, a prominent moderator band 35% of the time, and sacculations in about 20% of patients.

- MRI: This is useful when echo is nondiagnostic. It can demonstrate fatty infiltration, thinning of the RV free wall, and regional or global dilation of the RV and late gadolinium enhancement.

- Cardiac catheterization: May be useful in suspected cases without enough diagnostic evidence based on noninvasive approaches. RV angiography would demonstrate a dilated RV with transversely arranged and hypertrophic trabeculae.[20] RV biopsy can also be used to aid in the diagnosis; however, it is not commonly performed or recommended. This is because the presence of fat within the RV does not confirm ARVD due to the low specificity, and the absence of fat does not exclude it due to the patchy nature of the disease.

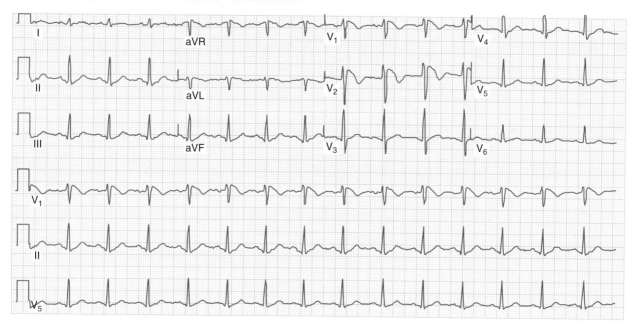

FIGURE 48-8 This is the typical type 1 Brugada pattern which is the only diagnostic Brugada pattern with >2 mm ST-segment elevation in V_2 followed by T-wave inversions.

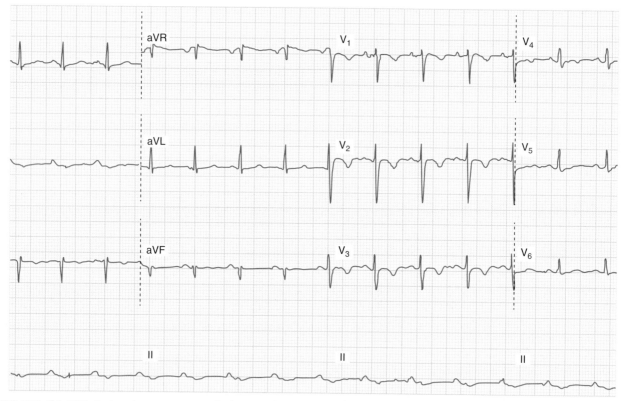

FIGURE 48-9 This ECG displays the most common findings in ARVD, which are precordial T-wave inversions extending to anterior leads.

- Genetic testing: This can be used to screen family members of those with ARVD. Although genetic testing will detect 50% of patients with ARVD, the diagnosis is clinical, and therefore the role for it is very limited in this disease.[21]

- The Arrhythmogenic Right Ventricular Dysplasia/Cardiomyopathy (ARVD/C) Task Force diagnostic criteria are seen in Table 48-5.[19]

HCM

- ECG: LVH with ST-segment depression and deep T-wave inversion is seen in 75% of cases. Left axis deviation is seen in about 25% of cases. Abnormal Q waves are seen in II, III, aVF, V_5, or V_6 in 20% to 25% of cases. Figure 48-10 demonstrates a typical HCM pattern.

TABLE 48-5 Arrhythmogenic Right Ventricular Dysplasia/Cardiomyopathy (ARVD/C) Task Force Criteria for ARVD

Major Criteria	Minor Criteria
Right ventricular dysfunction • Severe right ventricular (RV) dilation with reduced RV ejection fraction • Localized RV aneurysms • Severe segmental RV dilation	**Right ventricular dysfunction** • Mild global RV dilation • Regional RV hypokinesis • Mild segmental RV dilation
Tissue characterization • Fibrofatty replacement of myocardium by RV biopsy	**Tissue characterization** • Not meeting major criteria
Conduction abnormalities • Epsilon waves V_1-V_3 • QRS prolongation >110 ms V_1-V_3	**Conduction abnormalities** • T-wave inversions in V_2 and V_3 in an individual >12 years of age in the absence of a right bundle branch block • Late potentials on SAECGs • VT with left bundle branch block morphology • >1000 PVCs in 24 hours
Family history • Confirmed at autopsy or surgery	**Family history** • Family history of SCD before 35 years of age • Family history of ARVD

The diagnosis of ARVD requires either 2 major criteria, 1 major and 2 minor criteria, or 4 minor criteria.

- Echo: Increased LV wall thickness (>15 mm with no other cause for LVH), systolic anterior motion of the mitral valve, and mitral regurgitation are the cardinal findings seen in HCM. Hypertrophy may involve the septum, apex, LV free wall, and even the RV. Echo is sensitive in detecting HCM, but if there are no echocardiographic findings suggestive of HCM but a high index of suspicion for the disease, further testing may needed to rule it out. Figure 48-11 demonstrates massive LVH in a patient with HCM.

- MRI: Because of the superior views of MRI, it is more sensitive in detecting increases in LV wall thickness particularly in the anterolateral left ventricular free wall as well as estimating the degree of hypertrophy in the basal anterolateral free wall. The use of MRIs to evaluate for late myocardial enhancement is gaining an increasing role in HCM by quantifying scar burden and risk for ventricular arrhythmias.[2]

- Genetic testing: There may be a role for genetic testing in phenotypically negative family members of those with HCM. The proband or affected family member should have genetic testing done first to identify a possible gene mutation. Once that mutation is identified, it may be checked in phenotypically negative

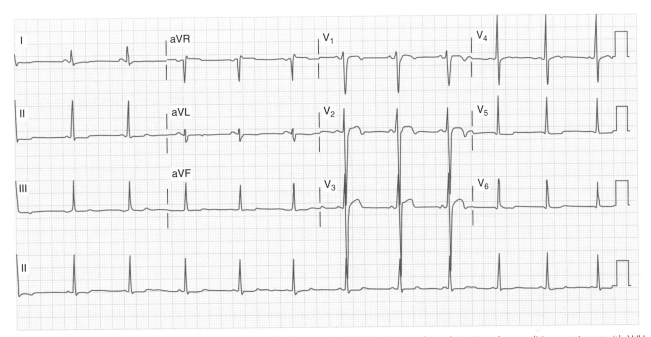

FIGURE 48-10 This ECG demonstrates NSR with left ventricular hypertrophy (LVH) criteria and repolarization abnormalities consistent with LVH.

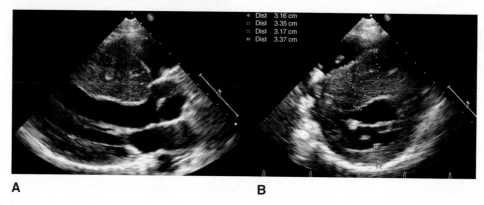

FIGURE 48-11 (A) Shown is a parasternal long axis echocardiographic view of a patient with HCM demonstrating massive LVH in the anterior septum. (B) Shown is a parasternal short axis view of the same patient quantifying the severity of LVH, which is seen in the anterior septum extending toward the anterior wall. The presence of massive LVH defined as ≥ 3 cm is considered massive and is a risk factor for sudden cardiac death.

TABLE 48-6 Management of Cardiac Causes of Syncope

Condition	Management	Sport Participation
Long QT syndrome	LQT1: β-Blockers LQT2: β-Blockers LQT3: mexilitine shortens the QT. ICD is indicated in patients with LQT who have had SCD. ICD is reasonable in patients with LQT and syncope refractory to medical therapy.	BC #36: Men with QT >470 and women with >480 should be excluded from competitive sport. Genotype (+), phenotype (−) can participate in sport. ESC: Men with QT>440 and women with >460 and genotype (+) should be excluded from competitive sport. Genotype (+), phenotype (−) are discouraged from participating in competitive sport.
CPVT	β-Blockers to suppress arrhythmia. All phenotype-positive patients should have an ICD implanted.	BC#36: Phenotype (+) patients (even only with symptoms) should be excluded from sport. Genotype (+) phenotype (−) patients (including a negative EP study) can participate in sport. ESC: All patients should be excluded from competitive sport.
RVOT VT	Adenosine (6-24 mg IV) is effective in termination by lowering cAMP levels. β-Blockers are also effective by inhibiting adenylatecyclase, which in turn decreases cAMP levels. Verapamil (10 mg IV) inhibits L-type calcium channels, thereby decreasing intracellular calcium levels. (Medical therapy for suppression has a 25%-50% success rate.) Radiofrequency ablation is the definitive management (90% cure rates).	

TABLE 48-6 Management of Cardiac Causes of Syncope (*Continued*)

Condition	Management	Sport Participation
Brugada syndrome	Symptomatic patients displaying the type 1 Brugada ECG (either spontaneously or after sodium channel blockade) who present with aborted sudden death, syncope, seizure, or nocturnal agonal respiration should undergo ICD implantation. Asymptomatic patients displaying a type 1 Brugada ECG (spontaneously or after sodium channel block) should undergo EPS if there is a family history of sudden cardiac death suspected to be due to Brugada syndrome. EPS may be justified when the family history is negative for sudden cardiac death if the type 1 ECG occurs spontaneously. If inducible for ventricular arrhythmia, the patient should receive an ICD. Asymptomatic patients who have no family history and who develop a type 1 ECG only after sodium channel blockade should be closely followed up.	BC#36: Phenotype (+) patients should be excluded from sport. Genotype (+) phenotype (−) patients (including a negative EP study) can participate in sport. ESC: All patients should be excluded from competitive sport.
ARVD	ICD indications: • Secondary prevention of SCD in patients who have had sustained VT or VF • Those with extensive disease • One or more affected family members with SCD, or unexplained syncope. (Syncope was an important predictor of life-saving ICD intervention in patients who received a prophylactic ICD.)	Exclusion from sport
HCM	LVOT obstruction: • β-Blockers • Nondihydropyridine calcium channel blocker • Disopyramide Septal myectomy or alcohol septal ablation in symptomatic patients refractory to medical therapy. Arrhythmia: ICD Indications • Secondary prevention of SCD • Family history of SCD • Syncope, not attributed to another cause • Abnormal blood pressure response to exercise • Massive LVH (≥30 mm) • Frequent, nonsustained VT	BC #36 Phenotypically (+): exclusion from sport. Genotypically (+), phenotypically (−): can participate in sport. ESC: Exclusion from all competitive sport.
Coronary anomalies	Reimplantation of the anomalous coronary in the correct sinus or unroofing the myocardium that covers the intramyocardial segment.	Exclusion from sports, but may resume if a normal stress study is obtained 3 months after successful corrective surgery.
Commotio Cordis	ACLS management of acute ventricular arrhythmia.	

Bethesda Conference (BC) # 36 and the European Society of Cardiology (ESC) agree that all patients with ICD should be excluded from competitive sport.
Modified with permission from Bader Y, Link M. Syncope in the Athlete. Cardiac Electrophysiology Clinics 2013;5(1):85-96.

family members. This can identify family members who may be at less risk of the disease and those who need closer follow-up.

Coronary Anomalies

- Computed tomography angiography (CTA): Using multislice CT scanners, patients can be evaluated noninvasively for coronary anomalies with high accuracy. CTA is also useful in mapping the course taken by these anomalous coronaries.[23]

Commotio Cordis

- Diagnosing commotio cordis is one of exclusion if the clinical scenario is consistent.

REFERENCES

1. Bader Y, Link M. Syncope in the athlete. *Card Electrophysiol Clin.* 2013;5(1):85-96.

2. Maron BJ. Hypertrophic cardiomyopathy. In: *Braunwald's Heart Disease.* 9th ed. Philadelphia, PA: Elsevier Saunders; 2012:1582-1594.

3. Dalal D, Nasir K, Bomma C, et al. Arrhythmogenic right ventricular dysplasia: a United States experience. *Circulation.* 2005;112:3823-3832.

4. Antzelevitch C, Brugada P, Brugada J, et al. Brugada syndrome: a decade of progress. *Circ Res.* 2002;91:1114-1118.

5. Moss AJ, Schwartz PJ, Crampton RS, et al. The long QT syndrome. Prospective longitudinal study of 328 families. *Circulation.* 1991;84:1136-1144.

6. Priori SG, Napolitano C, Memmi M, et al. Clinical and molecular characterization of patients with catecholaminergic polymorphic ventricular tachycardia. *Circulation.* 2002;106:69-74.

7. Leenhardt A, Lucet V, Denjoy I, Grau F, Ngoc DD, Coumel P. Catecholaminergic polymorphic ventricular tachycardia in children. A 7-year follow-up of 21 patients. *Circulation.* 1995;91:1512-1519.

8. Antzelevitch C, Brugada P, Brugada J, et al. Brugada syndrome from cell to bedside. *Curr Probl Cardiol.* 2005;30(1):9-54.

9. Maron B, Estes NA. Commotio cordis. *N Engl J Med.* 2010;362:917-927.

10. European Heart Rhythm Association, Heart Rhythm Society, Zipes DP, Camm AJ, Borggrefe M, et al. ACC/AHA/ESC 2006 guidelines for management of patients with ventricular arrhythmias and the prevention of sudden cardiac death: a report of the American College of Cardiology/American Heart Association Task Force and the European Society of Cardiology Committee for Practice Guidelines (Writing Committee to Develop Guidelines for Management of Patients With Ventricular Arrhythmias and the Prevention of Sudden Cardiac Death). *J Am Coll Cardiol.* 2006;48:247-346.

11. Napolitano C, Schwartz PJ, Brown AM, et al. Evidence for a cardiac ion channel mutation underlying drug-induced QT prolongation and life-threatening arrhythmias. *J Cardiovasc Electrophysiol.* 2000;11:691-696.

12. Sy RW, van der Werf C, Chattha IS, et al. Derivation and validation of a simple exercise-based algorithm for prediction of genetic testing in relatives of LQTS probands. *Circulation.* 2011;124:2187-2194.

13. Katagiri-Kawade M, Ohe T, Arakaki Y, et al. Abnormal response to exercise, face immersion, and isoproterenol in children with the long QT syndrome. *Pacing Clin Electrophysiol.* 1995;18:2128-2134.

14. Carlson MD, White RD, Trohman RG, et al. Right ventricular outflow tract ventricular tachycardia: detection of previously unrecognized anatomic abnormalities using cine magnetic resonance imaging. *J Am Coll Cardiol.* 1994;24:720-727.

15. Krishnan SC, Josephson ME. ST segment elevation induced by class IC antiarrhythmic agents: underlying electrophysiologic mechanisms and insights into drug-induced proarrhythmia. *J Cardiovasc Electrophysiol.* 1998;9:1167-1172.

16. Antzelevitch C, Brugada P, Borggrefe M, et al. Brugada syndrome: report of the second consensus conference: endorsed by the Heart Rhythm Society and the European Heart Rhythm Association. *Circulation.* 2005;111:659-670.

17. Miura D, Nakamura K, Ohe T. Update on genetic analysis in Brugada syndrome. *Heart Rhythm.* 2008;5:1495-1496.

18. Marcus FI, Zareba W. The electrocardiogram in right ventricular cardiomyopathy/dysplasia. How can the electrocardiogram assist in understanding the pathologic and functional changes of the heart in this disease? *J Electrocardiol.* 2009;42:136 e1-5.

19. Marcus FI, McKenna WJ, Sherrill D, et al. Diagnosis of arrhythmogenic right ventricular cardiomyopathy/dyplasia: proposed modification of the task force criteria. *Circulation.* 2010;121:1533-1541.

20. Daliento L, Rizzoli G, Thiene G, et al. Diagnostic accuracy of right ventriculography in arrhythmogenic right ventricular cardiomyopathy. *Am J Cardiol.* 1990;66:741-745.

21. Quarta G, Muir A, Pantazis A, et al. Familial evaluation in arrhythmogenic right ventricular cardiomyopathy: impact of genetics and revised task force criteria. *Circulation.* 2011;123:2701-2709.

22. Rickers C, Wilke NM, Jerosch-Herold M, et al. Utility of cardiac magnetic resonance imaging in the diagnosis of hypertrophic cardiomyopathy. *Circulation.* 2005;112:855-861.

23. Srinivasan KG, Gaikwad A, Kannan BR, et al. Congenital coronary artery anomalies: diagnosis with 64 slice multidetector row computed tomography coronary angiography: a single-centre study. *J Med Imaging Radiat Oncol.* 2008;52:148-154.

49 THE IMPLANTABLE LOOP RECORDER

Blair P. Grubb, MD, FACC

CASE PRESENTATION

A 71-year-old woman presents with complaints of multiple syncopal episodes. She describes these events as sudden in onset with little or no prodrone, accompanied by a rapid fall to the ground. She has suffered multiple traumas during falls. The loss of consciousness lasts anywhere from a few seconds to 5 minutes. Several episodes have been associated with urinary incontinence, and she is often confused afterwards. The patient has undergone electroencephalography, magnetic resonance imaging of the brain, echocardiography, a 12-lead electrocardiogram, coronary angiography, and electrophysiology study, all of which have been unremarkable. Multiple attempts at recording episodes by both Holter monitor and external event monitor have been unsuccessful. She therefore underwent placement of an implantable loop recorder. Five weeks later she suffered another syncopal episode, and a download of the event disclosed an episode of asystole that coincided with the syncope (Figure 49-1). She thereafter underwent dual chamber pacemaker implantation and has had no further syncopal episodes.

EPIDEMIOLOGY

Syncope, defined as the transient loss of postural tone and consciousness and spontaneous recovery, is a common clinical problem.[1] Approximately 3% of all emergency department visits and 1% to 6% of hospital admissions are for syncope. While a complete history and physical examination combined with direct laboratory testing can adequately establish a diagnosis in many patients, there are nonetheless patients who experience episodic cardiac arrhythmias that are not apparent on initial evaluation. They are often intermittent and transient and therefore difficult to detect. In these patients prolonged ambulatory monitoring using both external and now implantable electrodiagnostic recorders has been of great use in establishing a diagnosis. Indeed, by allowing for prolonged electrocardiographic monitoring, the implantable loop recorder (ILR) is able to provide a more certain correlation between observed rhythm experiences and the patient's symptoms. While external monitoring is only practical for relatively short periods of time, the ILR is capable of monitoring for up to 3 years. In addition, the ILR has the ability to auto-activate when a rhythm disturbance is present, thereby allowing episodes to be recorded independent of the patient having to activate the device. There are two ILRS that are presently available in the United States.[2] These are the Reveal (DX and XT) made by Medtronic (Minneapolis, MN) and the Confirm by St. Jude Medical (St. Paul, MN). Each of these is a small rectangular device that measures roughly $62 \times 19 \times 8$ mm and weighs approximately 17 grams. Two built-in sensing leads are located in the shell of the device, allowing for the recording of a single-lead, bipolar electrogram. These recordings can be stored and downloaded by means of a radiofrequency signal through a special programmer. The unit is usually implanted in the left pectoral area under local anesthesia. A study conducted at our institution evaluated the utility of an anatomic-based implant location based on a modified ECG lead II access.[3] Placement was determined by drawing an imaginary line between the substernal notch and the approximate area of the left nipple. An area in the inferior middle segment of the line was prepped and draped and anesthetized with 1% zylocaine solution. A 2-cm incision was made with a #15 scalpel along the lower one-third of the aforementioned line. Meticulous blunt dissection was used to create a subcutaneous pocket into which was inserted one of the aforementioned ILR devices. A telemetry wand (in a sterile cover) was then used to determine adequate signal size and strength. Very clearly visible P and QRS complexes were seen in all 63 patients at the time of initial placement. In none of the patients was it necessary to change the location or shape of the pocket. The average P-wave amplitude was 0.12 ± 0.2 mV and the mean peak-to-peak QRS amplitude was 0.48 ± 0.15 mV. Over a mean follow-up period of 10 ± 4 months, only 2 patients were noted to have a loss of P-wave amplitude (3.2%) while 1 patient had QRS under sensing (1.6%). We did not stitch the ILR in place as we found that this increased the amount of artifact present; rather, the subcutaneous pocket was made purposefully small to hold the device in place. (This also facilitates later removal.)

CLINICAL EXPERIENCE

A number of clinical trials have demonstrated the utility of the ILR in determining the etiology of syncope. Krahn et al found that in a group of 16 patients with syncope of unknown case (despite extensive

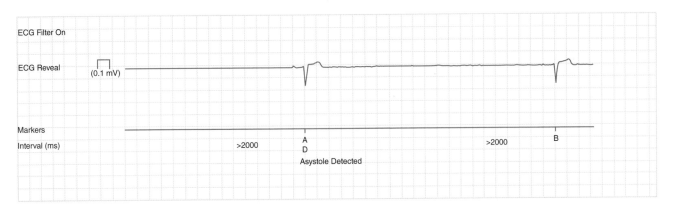

FIGURE 49-1 ILR recorded asystole.

evaluation) the ILR showed that in 60% of them syncope occurred due to an arrhythmic event.[4] Additional studies have shown that the device is equally effective in patients who had not undergone as extensive an amount of preimplant testing.[5] The recent ISSUE studies have clearly demonstrated the utility of the ILR in not only the diagnosis of syncope but also in guiding its treatment.[6] The recent ISSUE-3 trial showed that in patients with recurrent neurocardiogenic syncope associated with ILR documented asystole that permanent pacemaker implantation significantly reduced the recurrence rate of syncope.[7] The ILR has also been shown to be an effective means of detecting paroxysmal atrial fibrillation in patients with cryptogenic stroke.

REFERENCES

1. Grubb BP. Clinical Practice. Neurocardiogenic syncope. *N Engl J Med*. 2005;352(10);1004-1010.

2. Kanjwal K, Figueredo V, Karabin B, Grubb BP. The implantable loop recorder: current uses, future directions. *J Innov Card Rhythm Manage*. 2011;2:215-222.

3. Grubb BP, Welch M, Kanjwal K, Karabin B, Kanjwal Y. An anatomic-based approach for the placement of implantable loop recorders. *Pacing Clin Electrophysiol*. 2010;33(9):1149-1152.

4. Krahn AD, Klein GJ, Norris C, Yee R. The etiology of syncope in patients with a negative tilt table test and electrophysiologic testing. *Circulation*. 1995;92:1819-1824.

5. Krahn AD, Klein GJ, Yee R, Hoch JS, Skanes AC. Cost implications of testing strategy in patients with syncope: randomized assessment of syncope trial. *J Am Coll Cardiol*. 2003;42:495-501.

6. Brignole M, Sutton R, Menozzi C, et al. Early application of an implantable loop recorder allows effective specific therapy in patients with recurrent suspected neurally mediated syncope. *Eur Heart J*. 2006;27:1085-1092.

7. Brignole M, Menozzi C, Moya A, et al. Pacemaker therapy in patients with neurally-medicated syncope and documented asystole. Third International Study on Syncope of Uncertain Etiology (ISSUE-3): a randomized trial. *Circulation*. 2012;125: 2566-2571.

50 EVALUATION OF UNEXPLAINED SUDDEN CARDIAC DEATH

Clarence Khoo, MD, FRCPC, Shubhayan Sanatani, MD, FRCPC, Laura Arbour, MD, FRCPC, Andrew Krahn, MD, FRCPC

CASE PRESENTATION

A 40-year-old man of Asian descent is being assessed following an aborted sudden cardiac arrest. His wife had found him with agonal respirations while sleeping and was unable to wake him. Upon arrival of the paramedics, his initial rhythm was determined to be ventricular fibrillation (VF), and he was successfully defibrillated with a single DC shock by an external defibrillator. His initial 12-lead ECG showed down-sloping ST-elevation in the inferior and lateral leads (Figure 50-1), and he thus proceeded to coronary angiography. This did not demonstrate any flow-limiting coronary artery stenosis. Echocardiography showed normal biventricular systolic function.

EXPERT PRESENTATION

- Prior to the evaluation of any episode of sudden cardiac death (SCD), prompt resuscitation and the stabilization of any electrical or hemodynamic instability is imperative. If the patient is unable to

follow commands following return of spontaneous circulation, or a substantial period of cerebral hypoxia is suspected, then therapeutic hypothermic cooling should be considered.

- The initial evaluation of SCD should include:
  - A thorough history collected from the patient, first responders, witnesses, and family members regarding preexisting cardiovascular disease, cardiac symptoms, previous syncopal events, medications (both prescription and over-the-counter), and a family history of SCD. Included in the latter should be a screen for suspicious deaths in the family, that is, epilepsy, drownings, single motor vehicle accidents, and sudden infant death syndrome (SIDS).
  - A 12-lead ECG and rhythm strip to assess for any evidence of ischemia, ongoing arrhythmia, or suggestive findings of a cardiomyopathy or ion channelopathy.
  - In adults, coronary angiography to rule out an acute coronary syndrome as the cause of SCD. Computed tomography in younger patients may be considered.
  - Echocardiography to assess for any structural cardiac abnormalities.
- In the event that a diagnosis is not evident after this preliminary screen, the following potential etiologies for a ventricular tachyarrhythmia must be entertained:
  - Primary electrical causes/inherited ion channelopathies: Long QT syndrome (LQTS), short QT syndrome (SQTS), Brugada syndrome (BrS), catecholaminergic polymorphic ventricular tachycardia syndrome (CPVT).
  - Subclinical structural disease: Coronary vasospasm, anomalous coronary arteries and cardiomyopathies including arrhythmogenic

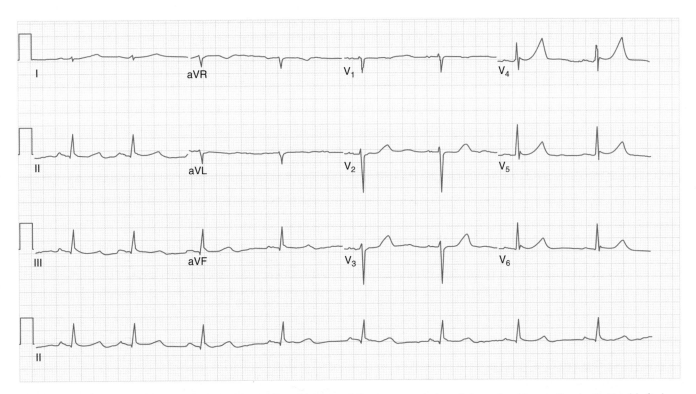

FIGURE 50-1 Twelve-lead electrocardiogram obtained from the patient following resuscitation of aborted sudden cardiac death. Notable findings include down-sloping J-point elevation of 0.1 mV in the inferior and lateral leads. There is also marked associated notching of the QRS in the affected leads. While the QT is prolonged, the QTc corrected for bradycardia is normal at 445 ms.

right ventricular cardiomyopathy (ARVC), hypertrophic cardiomyopathy (HCM), noncompaction, infiltrative cardiomyopathies.

- Further evaluation may include:
  - Consultation with a center with expertise in nonischemic sudden death conditions.
  - Exercise ECG testing to assess for failure of the QT interval to shorten with exercise (LQTS) or initiation of polymorphic or bidirectional ventricular tachycardia (CPVT).
  - Modified ECG with V_1 and V_2 leads placed 1 or 2 interspaces higher to improve the sensitivity of detecting a Brugada pattern.
  - Signal-averaged ECG (SAECG), which has utility in diagnosing ARVC.
  - Cardiac MRI (with contrast) to assess for cardiomyopathies with subtle structural abnormalities.
  - Pharmacologic challenge: Epinephrine infusion may make latent LQTS and CPVT apparent; procainamide infusion can unmask a Brugada pattern.
  - Genetic testing: If an inherited ion channelopathy or cardiomyopathy (eg, ARVC) is suspected, then genetic testing may reveal a mutation associated with the condition. A negative result does not exclude any of these conditions; the finding of a gene mutation of uncertain significance is much less helpful both diagnostically and with regards to screening of family members (see Chapter 51, Genetic Testing for Assessment of Inherited Arrhythmias).

DIAGNOSIS AND MANAGEMENT

- The patient demonstrated excellent neurologic recovery once extubated, and a comprehensive history was obtained from him with corroborative details from family members.
  - He had no previous history of cardiac diagnoses or symptoms.
  - There is no family history of unexplained syncope or cardiac arrest.

- A comprehensive diagnostic evaluation was performed in order to elucidate the etiology of the patient's aborted sudden cardiac arrest:
  - Exercise treadmill test: The patient exercised to 10.4 METS (9 minutes) with no inducible arrhythmias and no abnormal prolongation of the corrected QT interval (QTc) at peak exercise or recovery.
  - ECG with elevated precordial leads: no evidence of a Brugada pattern.
  - Cardiac MRI: No structural abnormalities or myocardial scar visualized.
  - Drug infusion challenge: Epinephrine and procainamide infusion did not reveal any ECG evidence of LQTS or BrS.

Due to the otherwise negative work-up, and the finding of J-point elevation in the inferolateral leads shortly after his cardiac arrest, a potential diagnosis of SCD associated with an early repolarization pattern (ERP) was entertained. An implantable cardioverter defibrillator (ICD) was implanted for secondary prevention purposes.

EVALUATION OF UNEXPLAINED SUDDEN CARDIAC DEATH

- In the absence of structural heart disease, SCD may be the result of a primary electrical disorder, subclinical structural cardiac disease,

TABLE 50-1 Causes of Unexplained Sudden Cardiac Death

1. Idiopathic ventricular fibrillation (44%)

2. Primary electrical disorder/inherited channelopathy (39%)
   a. Long QT syndrome (13%)
   b. Catecholaminergic polymorphic VT syndrome (13%)
   c. Early repolarization (8%)
   d. Brugada syndrome (5%)

3. Subclinical structural cardiac disease (17%)
   a. Arrhythmogenic right ventricular cardiomyopathy (10%)
   b. Coronary spasm (6%)
   c. Myocarditis (1%)

Data from Krahn AD, Healey JS, Chauhan V, et al. Systematic assessment of patients with unexplained cardiac arrest: Cardiac Arrest Survivors With Preserved Ejection Fraction Registry (CASPER). Circulation 2009;July28;120(4):278-285.

or idiopathic VF (Table 50-1). With rigorous screening, approximately 50% of cases will have an identifiable cause.[1]

- While implantation of an ICD for secondary prevention purposes is warranted for most survivors of SCD with adequate neurologic recovery, identifying a cause for SCD may allow for the addition of pharmacologic therapy and appropriate lifestyle modification for patients. Identification of a genetic cause for SCD may also be of significant value in the screening of family members.

- A step-wise evaluation strategy involving electrocardiography, imaging modalities, provocative testing, and genetic screening should be employed (Figure 50-2).[1]

- LQTS may be suspected if prolongation of the QTc is seen on the resting ECG, or during exercise testing at peak exercise or early in recovery (Figure 50-3).

- Automated computer-derived QTc measurements should be verified with manual measurements using the following standardized method (Figure 50-4)[2]:

  1. Measurements should be obtained in either lead II or V_5.

  2. The intersection of the tangent of the steepest slope of the last portion of the T wave to the baseline defines the end of the T wave.

  3. Corrected QT (QTc) is calculated by the Bazett formula ($QTc = QT/\sqrt{RR}$).

- ECG changes diagnostic for BrS are often transient and require either serial ECGs or provocative testing to unmask a type I Brugada pattern (2 mm ST elevation in V_1 and V_2 with an inverted T wave). Shifting the V_1 and V_2 ECG leads up 1 or 2 interspaces may suffice[3]; alternatively, a procainamide infusion can be used (Figure 50-5).

- CPVT should be suspected with the reproducible development of polymorphic ventricular extrasystoles or bidirectional VT with exercise (Figure 50-6).

- The diagnosis of ARVC requires multiple testing modalities that satisfy the ARVC task force criteria.[4] Dilatation of the right ventricle on imaging ± regional wall motion abnormalities

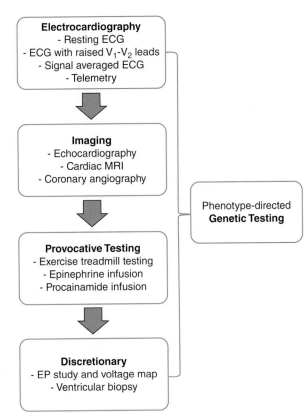

FIGURE 50-2 Suggested step-wise evaluation strategy for patients with unexplained sudden cardiac death. Abbreviations: ECG, electrocardiogram; EP, electrophysiology; MRI, magnetic resonance imaging. Adapted with permission from Krahn AD, Healey JS, Chauhan V, et al. Systematic assessment of patients with unexplained cardiac arrest: Cardiac Arrest Survivors With Preserved Ejection Fraction Registry (CASPER). Circulation 2009;July 28;120(4):278-285.

(Figure 50-7), an abnormal SAECG, or the finding of epsilon waves and extensive T-wave inversion in the anterior precordial leads (Figure 50-8) all contribute to the diagnosis.

- ERP can be identified by the finding of J-point elevation of ≥ 1.0 mV in association with QRS slurring or notching in two contiguous leads, excluding V_1 to $V_{3.}$[5]

EARLY REPOLARIZATION PATTERN AND SUDDEN CARDIAC DEATH

- Inferolateral J-point elevation of ≥ 0.1 mV has been identified in 14% to 41% of individuals without an etiology for SCD after rigorous diagnostic testing.[6]

- At present, the causality of ERP and SCD remains unclear, but there is a clear association between the two. This likely represents an imbalance of early currents I_{Na} and I_{to}. Some investigators believe that a channelopathy related to BrS may be responsible, while others believe that ERP may identify individuals more prone to developing fatal arrhythmias in the presence of various triggers.[7]

- ERP is common in the general population and in the majority of cases is a benign finding. Individuals at higher risk for SCD may include[6,8]:
  - J-point elevation ≥ 0.2 mV.
  - Distribution in multiple leads, especially if inferior leads involved.
  - Presence of QRS notching.
  - Dynamic fluctuation of J-point amplitude.
  - Horizontal or down-sloping ST segments.
  - Persistent J-point elevation with exercise.

- Secondary prevention patients should be offered an ICD unless contraindications exist. No validated risk stratification strategy

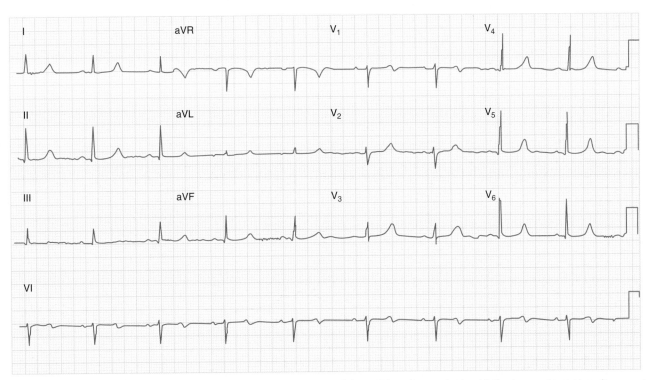

FIGURE 50-3 Representative 12-lead electrocardiogram from a patient with long QT syndrome obtained following an aborted cardiac arrest. The corrected QT (QTc) is prolonged at 530 ms with biphasic T waves in V_1.

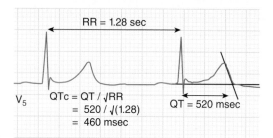

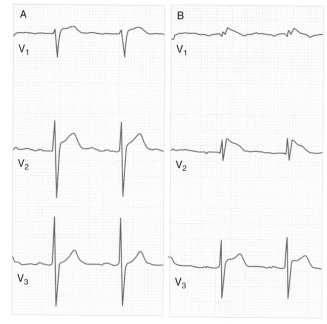

FIGURE 50-4 Standardized method of assessing the QT interval. In either lead II or V_5, the tangent from the steepest portion of the down-sloping portion of the T wave is taken to the baseline to mark the end of the T wave. The measured QT is then corrected by the preceding RR interval as per Bazett formula.

FIGURE 50-5 Anterior precordial leads (V_1-V_3) obtained from a patient with diagnosed Brugada syndrome and prior aborted sudden cardiac death. (A) Standard precordial lead placement with nonspecific J-point elevation in V_1-V_3. (B) Tracings from identical patient taken 1 minute later with V_1 and V_2 each moved up one interspace. Note the dramatic alteration in ST morphology that is now consistent with type I Brugada syndrome.

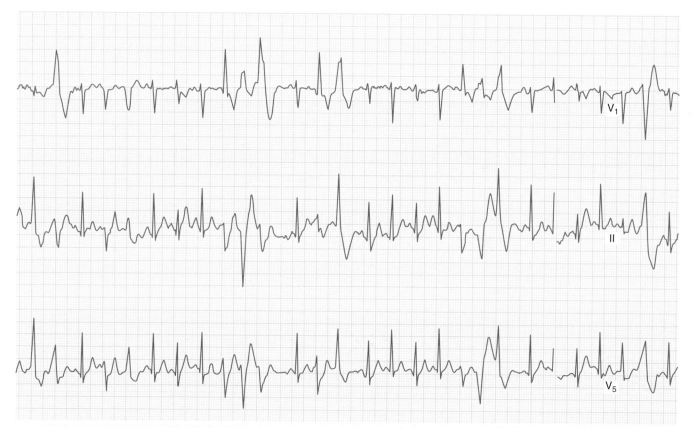

FIGURE 50-6 Representative rhythm strip during an exercise treadmill test in a patient later diagnosed with catecholaminergic polymorphic ventricular tachycardia syndrome. Runs of polymorphic ventricular ectopy are seen here at peak exercise and are diagnostic for this condition.

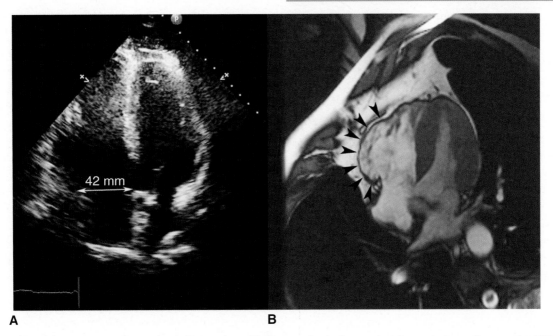

A   **B**

FIGURE 50-7 Multimodality imaging studies performed in a patient with diagnosed arrhythmogenic right ventricular cardiomyopathy. (A) Echocardiographic apical four-chamber view demonstrating dilatation of the right ventricle at end-diastole. (B) Magnetic resonance imaging in the same patient revealing an aneurysmal segment of the basal right ventricle during systole (arrowheads).

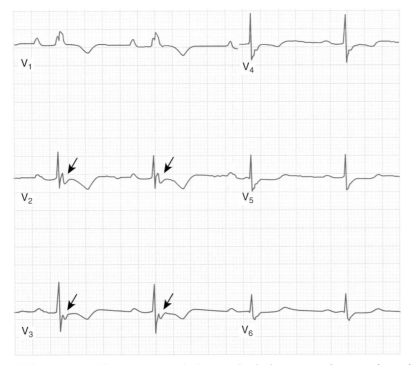

FIGURE 50-8 Selected precordial leads obtained from a patient with diagnosed arrhythmogenic right ventricular cardiomyopathy. Both epsilon waves (arrowheads) and diffuse T-wave inversions up to V_4 are present and qualify as major diagnostic criteria for this condition.

exists for primary prevention patients with ERP, and thus the appropriate management of these individuals remains largely uncertain.

- Recurrence of VF in patients with ERP may be reduced with infusion of isoproterenol or oral quinidine.[5]

REFERENCES

1. Krahn AD, Healey JS, Chauhan V, et al. Systematic assessment of patients with unexplained cardiac arrest: Cardiac Arrest Survivors With Preserved Ejection Fraction Registry (CASPER). *Circulation*. 2009;120(4):278-285.

2. Postema PG, De Jong JS, Van der Bilt IA, et al. Accurate electrocardiographic assessment of the QT interval: teach the tangent. *Heart Rhythm*. 2008;5(7):1015-1018.

3. Sangwatanaroj S, Prechawat S, Sunsaneewitayakul B, et al. New electrocardiographic leads and the procainamide test for the detection of the Brugada sign in sudden unexplained death syndrome survivors and their relatives. *Eur Heart J*. 2001;22(24):2290-2296.

4. Marcus FI, McKenna WJ, Sherrill D, et al. Diagnosis of arrhythmogenic right ventricular cardiomyopathy/dysplasia: proposed modification of the task force criteria. *Circulation*. 2010;121(13):1533-1541.

5. Stern S. Clinical aspects of the early repolarization syndrome: a 2011 update. *Ann Noninvasive Electrocardiol*. 2011;16(2):192-195.

6. Derval N, Simpson CS, Birnie DH, et al. Prevalence and characteristics of early repolarization in the CASPER registry: cardiac arrest survivors with preserved ejection fraction registry. *J Am Coll Cardiol*. 2011;58(7):722-728.

7. Benito B, Guasch E, Rivard L, et al. Clinical and mechanistic issues in early repolarization of normal variants and lethal arrhythmia syndromes. *J Am Coll Cardiol*. 2010;56(15):1177-1186.

8. Bastiaenen R, Raju H, Sharma S, et al. Characterization of early repolarization during ajmaline provocation and exercise tolerance testing. *Heart Rhythm*. 2013;10(2):247-254.

EVALUATION AND MANAGEMENT OF INHERITED ARRHYTHMIAS

51 GENETIC TESTING FOR ASSESSMENT OF INHERITED ARRHYTHMIAS

Clarence Khoo, MD, FRCPC, Shubhayan Sanatani, MD, FRCPC, Laura Arbour, MD, FRCPC, Andrew Krahn, MD, FRCPC

CASE PRESENTATION

The family members of a victim of sudden cardiac death (SCD) are being evaluated for their risk of an inherited arrhythmia. The proband was a 16-year-old girl who was found dead in her bed by her family one morning. She had returned home late from a party the night before. Following a negative autopsy, the immediate suspicion was that illicit substances were involved in her death, although the toxicology screen was subsequently negative. The family thus sought further medical evaluation after concerns were raised that an inherited cause may have contributed.

There was no history of syncope or other illness in the proband. She had been otherwise well up to the time of her demise. Her only medication was an over-the-counter antihistamine.

The family history was significant for multiple incidents of SCD. Her mother had experienced a previous syncopal episode and had four siblings who suffered SCD between the ages of 20 and 40 years. The proband's maternal grandmother had also died shortly after the birth of her youngest child. ECGs from the proband's mother and older sister demonstrated a prolonged corrected QT interval (Figure 51-1).

EXPERT OPINION

- Up to 30% of cases of sudden death in young individuals have no identifiable etiology for death at autopsy, thus raising the possibility of a primary arrhythmic disorder.[1]

- The acquisition and retention of tissue samples from the deceased in such cases may help in identifying mutations responsible for an inherited channelopathy.

- At present, genetic testing can identify known pathogenic mutations associated with channelopathies such as long QT syndrome (LQTS), short QT syndrome (SQTS), Brugada syndrome (BrS), catecholaminergic polymorphic ventricular tachycardia (CPVT), and certain cardiomyopathies including arrhythmogenic right ventricular cardiomyopathy (ARVC) and hypertrophic cardiomyopathy (HCM).

- If a causal mutation is identified, all first-degree relatives should be tested.
  - The finding of the same mutation in a relative along with clinical testing for the relevant clinical condition to establish the severity of the phenotype to conduct risk stratification should be followed by appropriate interventions when necessary.
  - Mutation carriers without an expressed phenotype may be observed on a q 1 to 3 year basis for development of phenotypic changes requiring intervention. Relatively benign interventions such as lifestyle modification, avoidance of arrhythmia-provoking drugs (in the case of LQTS and Brugada syndrome), or the use of certain pharmacologic therapies (ie, β-blockers) may be employed in specific situations.[2]
  - Relatives without the causal mutation require no further evaluation.

- If no causal mutation is identified in the proband, then the role of further genetic testing in first-degree relatives is limited.

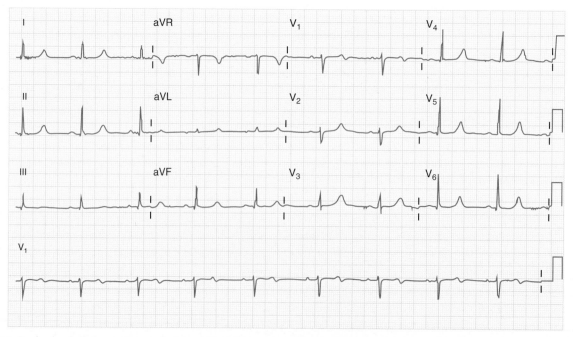

FIGURE 51-1 Twelve-lead electrocardiogram from a relative of the proband demonstrating prolongation of the QT interval at baseline.

GENETIC TESTING FOR ASSESSMENT
OF INHERITED ARRHYTHMIAS

SECTION VIII
EVALUATION AND MANAGEMENT
OF INHERITED ARRHYTHMIAS

359

- The lack of a causal mutation in the proband does not mean that an inherited etiology for SCD is absent, as genetic testing cannot identify all possible pathogenic mutations.
- If an inherited channelopathy or cardiomyopathy is still suspected, then follow-up of relatives on a regular basis should be performed to detect for the development of an overt phenotype. The interval between assessments is unknown, but likely every 3 to 5 years unless there is rapid development at the adolescent stage.

DIAGNOSIS AND MANAGEMENT

- Suspicion of LQTS was raised based on the strong family history of SCD and the ECG findings from the decedent's relatives. The family members were counselled with regards to genetic testing and were agreeable to proceed.
- Genetic testing performed from blood collected from the mother identified a pathogenic nonsense mutation in the *KCNH2* gene (c. 1184C>T; p.Gln391X).
- Splenic tissue had been frozen following the autopsy, and DNA was isolated. The same mutation found in the family was identified in the decedent, suggesting it contributed to her sudden death.
- A pedigree of affected members is depicted in Figure 51-2.

GENETIC TESTING IN THE SETTING OF SUDDEN UNEXPLAINED DEATH CASES

- Genetic testing for an inherited arrhythmic cause of death may be considered in autopsy-negative individuals who experience sudden death, especially if the circumstances are suggestive of primary arrhythmic conditions, for example, exercise induced, auditory stimuli, nocturnal death (particularly in Asian men) (Table 51-1), and if family members have evidence of a clinical phenotype.[3]
- In cases of unexplained SCD, tissue from the decedent should be obtained and stored using "DNA-friendly" preservation methods where possible.
- EDTA-preserved blood, fresh frozen tissue, and dried (Guthrie) blood spot cards, allow for the most ideal degree of DNA preservation for further analysis. However, the majority of specimens are currently archived as formalin-fixed tissue embedded in paraffin. Although extraction of DNA is still feasible from paraffin-embedded specimens, the yield of vital segments of DNA may be reduced by at least a third, thus hampering genetic analysis.[1] Extraction from formalin fixed tissue is typically unsuccessful.
- Up to 35% of cases of sudden death may have an underlying arrhythmic etiology.[4] This extends to suspect causes of death, including drownings and single-vehicle accidents.
- Genetic testing in family members should be reserved to cases where a pathogenic mutation is established in the decedent or a phenotype has been recognized in the relative, as in the described case scenario.

THE ROLE OF GENETIC TESTING OF HERITABLE ARRHYTHMIAS

- As the diagnostic yield of genetic testing for any condition is suboptimal, a negative test does not exclude the diagnosis of an inheritable arrhythmia.

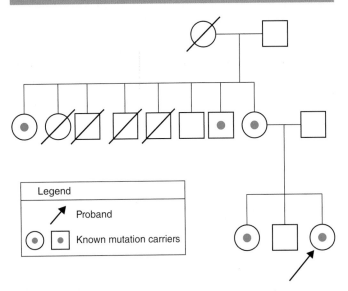

FIGURE 51-2 Pedigree constructed from detailed family history taken from relatives of the proband. Results of genetic screening for mutation in *KCNH2* causing phenotypic long QT syndrome are also depicted on the pedigree.

TABLE 51-1 Specific Circumstances Surrounding the Time of Death of the Decedent May Point to Certain Inheritable Arrhythmic Diagnoses

Specific Circumstances of Death	Potential Inheritable Arrhythmic Etiology
Exercise	LQT1, CPVT, HCM, ARVC
Swimming	LQT1
During sleep	LQT3, Brugada syndrome (especially if male, Asian)
Sudden auditory stimuli	LQT2

Abbreviations: ARVC, arrhythmogenic right ventricular cardiomyopathy; BrS, Brugada syndrome; CPVT, catecholaminergic polymorphic ventricular tachycardia; HCM, hypertrophic cardiomyopathies; LQT1-3, long QT syndromes.

TABLE 51-2 Summary of the Role of Genetic Testing of Inheritable Arrhythmias

	LQTS	SQTS	CPVT	BrS	HCM	ARVC
Commonly tested genetic mutations	*KCNQ1, KCNH2, SCN5A*	*KCNQ1, KCNH2, KCNJ2*	*RyR2, CASQ2*	*SCN5A*	*MYH7, MYBPC3, TNNI3, TNNT2, TPM1*	*DSC2, DSG2, DSP, JUP, PKP2, TMEM43*
Estimated yield of genetic testing	70%-80%	?	65%	25%	60%	50%
Testing recommended if clinically suspected in index case	+++	+	+++	++	+++	++
Screening of family members if index case is positive	+++	+++	+++	+++	+++	+++

Abbreviations: +, weak recommendation; ++, moderate recommendation; +++, strong recommendation; ARVC, arrhythmogenic right ventricular cardiomyopathy; BrS, Brugada syndrome; CPVT, catecholaminergic polymorphic ventricular tachycardia; HCM, hypertrophic cardiomyopathy; LQTS, long QT syndrome; SQTS, short QT syndrome.

Data from Ackerman MJ, Priori SG, Willems S, et al. HRS/EHRA expert consensus statement on the state of genetic testing for the channelopathies and cardiomyopathies this document was developed as a partnership between the Heart Rhythm Society (HRS) and the European Heart Rhythm Association (EHRA). Heart Rhythm 2011; Aug 8;8(8):1308-1339.

- In most cases, the primary role of genetic testing is in screening family members for subclinical disease. However, in specific situations, genetic testing may also aid in diagnosis of equivocal cases by providing extra evidence for a disease process (Table 51-2).

- Genetic testing for a specific condition should be reserved for individuals with a reasonable clinical suspicion for that condition to minimize the risk of false-positives.

- Family screening of all first-degree relatives should be offered if a causative mutation is identified in the index case.

- The finding of a potentially disease-causing mutation in an otherwise asymptomatic family member may prompt initiation of preventative measures including avoidance of triggers or the use of pharmacologic therapy (ie, β-blockers in LQTS or CPVT).

- Due to the numerous subtleties in ordering and interpreting the results of genetic tests, this should be reserved for physician experts and specialized inherited arrhythmia clinics. Genetic counselling is imperative prior to the consideration of any genetic testing because of personal, employment, and insurance implications.

Long QT Syndrome (LQTS)

- LQTS is usually inherited in an autosomal-dominant pattern (Romano-Ward syndrome) but in rare cases may be autosomal-recessive (Jervell and Lange-Nielsen syndrome). Spontaneous *de novo* mutations leading to LQTS may account for <10% of cases.[5]

- While mutations in ≥13 genetic loci have been attributed to LQTS, the majority result from mutations in the slow delayed rectifier potassium current (*KCNQ1*; LQT1), the rapid delayed rectifier potassium current (*KCNH2*; LQT2), or the inward sodium current (*SCN5A*; LQT3).

- Genetic testing should be performed in all patients with a confirmed diagnosis of LQTS to allow appropriate risk stratification and gene-specific therapies. There is evidence for mutation-specific therapeutic

and prognostic implications; mutation details predict response to β-blockade and may influence exercise recommendations.

- Genetic testing is also recommended for asymptomatic adult patients with prolongation of the QTc (in the absence of secondary causes) >500 ms and may be considered if >480 ms. In prepubescent patients, cut-offs of >460 to 480 ms are suggested.[5]

- As QT-prolonging medications may unmask latent LQTS, patients with drug-induced torsades de pointes (TdP) may be considered for genetic testing as well.

- Diagnostic yield of genetic testing for LQTS may be improved to 70% to 80% by reserving genetic testing for only those with a high clinical suspicion for LQTS.[6]

- Among patients with clinically definite LQTS, 75% to 80% will have mutations in genes responsible for LQT1 to LQT3. Less than 5% are due to mutations in other LQTS-associated genes.[5]

Short QT Syndrome (SQTS)

- SQTS is caused by autosomal-dominant mutations in genes encoding cardiac potassium channels (*KCNH2*/SQT1, *KCNQ1*/SQT2, *KCNJ2*/SQT3) caused by much less common gain of function mutations.

- Genetic testing may be offered for individuals with a high clinical index of suspicion for SQTS.

- No specific QT cut-offs currently exist to prompt investigation of asymptomatic individuals, although diagnostic criteria incorporating QTc measurements, clinical history, and family history have been proposed.[7]

Catecholaminergic Polymorphic VT (CPVT) Syndrome

- The genetic cause for CPVT has been attributed to either autosomal-dominant mutations in the cardiac ryanodine receptor gene (*RYR2*) or autosomal-recessive mutations in the cardiac

GENETIC TESTING FOR ASSESSMENT
OF INHERITED ARRHYTHMIAS

SECTION VIII
EVALUATION AND MANAGEMENT
OF INHERITED ARRHYTHMIAS

361

calsequestrin gene (*CASQ2*) as well as other proteins involved in calcium handling.

- Genetic testing identifies a mutation in up to 65% of CPVT patients, with the highest yield in those with documented bidirectional VT.[5]

- All patients with confirmed CPVT or a high clinical index of suspicion should be offered genetic testing.

Brugada Syndrome (BrS)

- Genetic testing is able to identify a causative mutation in as low as 5% of cases if the pattern is sporadic (as is the norm) or 20% to 25% of cases of BrS if familial. Of these, a mutation in the inward sodium channel gene (*SCN5A*) is responsible in >75% of cases.[5]

- Patients with a high clinical suspicion for BrS may benefit from genetic testing.

- Genetic testing is not indicated in patients with either an isolated type 2 or type 3 Brugada pattern.

Hypertrophic Cardiomyopathy (HCM)

- Autosomal-dominant mutations in sarcomeric proteins are responsible for HCM.

- Patients with a high clinical suspicion for HCM should be offered genetic testing.

- At present, the diagnostic yield of genetic testing for established HCM is ~60%.[5]

- There is as yet no evidence for mutation-specific prognostic implications.

Arrhythmogenic Right Ventricular Cardiomyopathy (ARVC)

- ARVC is transmitted as an autosomal-dominant condition with variable penetrance. Numerous genetic mutations largely involving desmosomal proteins (see Table 51-2) are implicated.[5]

- Genetic testing can be considered in patients with either a probable or possible diagnosis of ARVC based on task force diagnostic criteria.[8]

- There is also utility of genetic testing in confirming the diagnosis of ARVC in those who do not meet task force criteria but exhibit some features consistent with ARVC.

- The current diagnostic yield of genetic testing in probable cases of ARVC is ~50%.[5]

- ARVC is the most likely of the inherited arrhythmia conditions to return a variant of unknown significance genetic test result.

REFERENCES

1. Carturan E, Tester DJ, Brost BC, et al. Postmortem genetic testing for conventional autopsy-negative sudden unexplained death: an evaluation of different DNA extraction protocols and the feasibility of mutational analysis from archival paraffin-embedded heart tissue. *Am J Clin Pathol.* 2008;129(3):391-397.

2. Vincent GM, Schwartz PJ, Denjoy I, et al. High efficacy of beta-blockers in long-QT syndrome type 1: contribution of noncompliance and QT-prolonging drugs to the occurrence of beta-blocker treatment "failures." *Circulation.* 2009;119(2):215-221.

3. Gollob MH, Blier L, Brugada R, et al. Recommendations for the use of genetic testing in the clinical evaluation of inherited cardiac arrhythmias associated with sudden cardiac death: Canadian Cardiovascular Society/Canadian Heart Rhythm Society joint position paper. *Can J Cardiol.* 2011;27(2):232-245.

4. Tester DJ, Ackerman MJ. Postmortem long QT syndrome genetic testing for sudden unexplained death in the young. *J Am Coll Cardiol.* 2007;49(2):240-246.

5. Ackerman MJ, Priori SG, Willems S, et al. HRS/EHRA expert consensus statement on the state of genetic testing for the channelopathies and cardiomyopathies this document was developed as a partnership between the Heart Rhythm Society (HRS) and the European Heart Rhythm Association (EHRA). *Heart Rhythm.* 2011;8(8):1308-1339.

6. Modell SM, Bradley DJ, Lehmann MH. Genetic testing for long QT syndrome and the category of cardiac ion channelopathies. *PLoS Curr.* 2012;e4f9995f9969e9996c9997. doi:10.1371/4f9995f69e6c7.

7. Gollob MH, Redpath CJ, Roberts JD. The short QT syndrome: proposed diagnostic criteria. *J Am Coll Cardiol.* 2011;57(7):802-812.

8. Marcus FI, McKenna WJ, Sherrill D, et al. Diagnosis of arrhythmogenic right ventricular cardiomyopathy/dysplasia: proposed modification of the task force criteria. *Circulation.* 2010;121(13):1533-1541.

52 GENETIC COUNSELING

Amy C. Sturm, MS, CGC

A 17-year-old boy was referred to the Inherited Arrhythmia Clinic after suffering an aborted sudden cardiac death episode while running at school. The patient's past medical history was significant for epilepsy diagnosed at 6 years of age. A teacher reported the patient had no pulse and was not breathing during the event, and an automated external defibrillator detected a shockable rhythm, which was converted with a shock from the device. The baseline ECG was normal, an echocardiogram showed a structurally normal heart with normal left ventricular systolic function, and a stress test documented exercise-induced ventricular ectopy. Because of the patient's presentation, he underwent implantation of an implantable cardioverter defibrillator (ICD) for secondary prevention, and β-blocker therapy was initiated.

During the arrhythmia clinic appointment, a genetic counselor constructed a three-generation pedigree (Figure 52-1). The family history was significant for sudden death in a maternal uncle, but no other relatives had a concerning history. Given the family history and documentation of exercise-induced ventricular ectopy, catecholaminergic polymorphic ventricular tachycardia (CPVT) was considered a possible diagnosis, and genetic testing was discussed with the family. Informed consent was obtained, and a blood sample was collected for CPVT genetic testing. The patient tested positive for a novel, likely

pathogenic mutation in the *RYR2* gene (c.6916G>C; Val2306Leu). This result confirmed the diagnosis of autosomal-dominant CPVT in the patient and also allowed for subsequent cascade genetic testing in his at-risk relatives. His mother was identified to have the *RYR2* mutation while his father and sister both tested negative; this allowed the patient's paternal relatives to learn they were not at increased risk for CPVT. During follow-up visits, it was noted that the patient was suffering from insomnia and depression; his prior career goal before his diagnosis was to become a police officer, and he was having a difficult time adjusting to the idea that he would no longer be able to pursue such a path.

CASE EXPLANATION

Genetic testing was able to confirm a diagnosis of CPVT in a patient with a prior, likely misdiagnosis of epilepsy. Genetic counseling is recommended for all patients with CPVT (and other inherited heart diseases) and their at-risk relatives in the Heart Rhythm Society/ European Heart Rhythm Association expert consensus statement on genetic testing for channelopathies and cardiomyopathies.[1] Through a multidisciplinary clinical approach that included genetic counseling, the patient and his family were able to:

- Receive an accurate diagnosis and appropriate management.
- Determine their risk status through cascade, mutation-specific genetic testing.
- Receive information regarding the inheritance pattern of CPVT and recurrence risk.
- Learn about future reproductive options.
- Receive psychosocial support and resources.

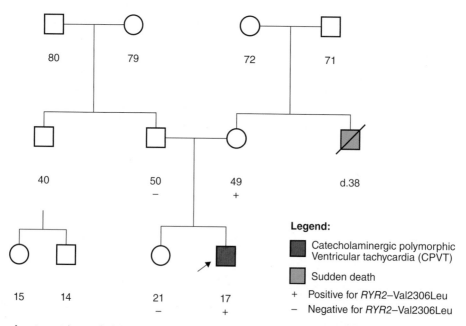

FIGURE 52-1 Pedigree of patient with catecholaminergic polymorphic ventricular tachycardia (CPVT). This three-generation pedigree utilizes standard pedigree symbols (men are represented by squares; women are represented by circles). The pedigree was constructed by the genetic counselor during the proband's first appointment in the Inherited Arrhythmia Clinic. A major "red flag" for risk assessment was present in the pedigree; the proband's maternal uncle died suddenly at 38 years of age. Genetic testing in the proband identified a causative mutation in the *RYR2* gene. Subsequently, the proband's first-degree at-risk relatives (parents and sister) underwent cascade genetic testing, and his mother was identified to also have the *RYR2* mutation.

GENETIC COUNSELING AND GENETIC COUNSELORS

Genetic Counseling

Genetic counseling is the process of helping individuals and their families understand and adapt to the medical, psychological, and familial implications of a genetic condition.[2] The genetic counseling process for patients with inherited heart disease includes multiple components, listed and explained in further detail below. Genetic counseling is indicated regardless of the availability of genetic testing for a specific cardiac disorder.

- Collection of ≥3 generation family medical history information, with special attention to "red flags" for inherited heart disease (Table 52-1).
  ○ Includes confirmation with medical records, autopsy reports, and death certificates.
- Performance of risk assessment utilizing medical and family history information.
- Analysis and discussion of inheritance patterns and recurrence risk.
- Facilitation of genetic testing process.
  ○ Pre- and posttest genetic counseling.
- Facilitation of family-based care.
  ○ Cascade genetic testing (Figure 52-2).
  ○ Coordination of family clinical screening.
- Discussion of reproductive options.
- Provision of written documentation of medical, genetic, and counseling information to referring health care providers and patients, including family letters.
- Provision of psychosocial counseling and anticipatory guidance.
- Provision of education, resources, and advocacy to patients and families.
- Discussion of available genetics research study options.
- Discussion of the availability of DNA banking, when applicable.

Genetic Counselors

Genetic counselors are health care professionals with specialized graduate degrees and expertise in medical genetics and counseling. Many genetic counselors work as members of a health care team and provide information and support to families with inherited conditions. Cardiovascular genetic counselors are an important resource and integral health care team members for patients and families with inherited heart disease, including those families who have suffered a sudden death in a young person.[3] It has been suggested that a master's-trained, board-certified genetic counselor, preferably with specialized training in cardiovascular genetics, be part of the multidisciplinary team involved in the care of families with heritable cardiovascular diseases.[4] The types of patients that should be referred to for cardiovascular genetic counseling and potentially genetic testing are listed in Table 52-2. Genetic counselors can be located by utilizing the "Find a Genetic Counselor" tool on the National Society of Genetic Counselors Web site, www.nsgc.org.

TABLE 52-1 "Red Flags" in Pedigree That May Signify Underlying Inherited Cardiovascular Disease

Red Flag	Possible Inherited Cardiovascular Disease
Sudden death, unexplained and/or accidental (eg, drowning, single motor vehicle accident)	Arrhythmia, cardiomyopathy, aortic dissection
Syncope or presyncope	Arrhythmia, cardiomyopathy
Exercise intolerance	Arrhythmia, cardiomyopathy
Relative(s) with pacemaker and/or implantable cardioverter defibrillator	Arrhythmia, cardiomyopathy
Sudden infant death syndrome (SIDS)	Emerging data suggests ~10%-15% of SIDS deaths are associated with mutations in several genes associated with cardiac ion channelopathies.
Seizures	May be misdiagnosed and represent syncopal episodes.
Premature "heart attack" (<55 years of age in a man; <65 years of age in a woman)	Arrhythmia, cardiomyopathy, aortic dissection
Heart transplantation	Cardiomyopathy
Heart failure <60 years of age	Cardiomyopathy

TAKING AN INFORMATIVE PEDIGREE: ESSENTIAL TOOL FOR CARDIOVASCULAR GENETIC MEDICINE

A careful family history for at least three generations should be collected and assessed for all patients with potential hereditary heart disease. The individual collecting the family history should actively inquire about the presence of "red flags" while constructing the pedigree since the patient themselves may not know to offer certain information important to risk assessment (eg, the presence of sudden infant death syndrome [SIDS] in a blood relative may represent the presence of a cardiac ion channel gene mutation). For a list of "red flags" and what inherited heart condition they may represent, see Table 52-1. The collection of family history is imperative in (1) aiding diagnosis, (2) identifying at-risk relatives, (3) selecting the most informative family member for genetic testing initiation, and (4) determining inheritance pattern.

While most inherited cardiac diseases follow an autosomal-dominant pattern of inheritance, there are important exceptions, and this information is necessary for the provision of accurate recurrence risks. Also complicating matters is the fact that many inherited cardiac

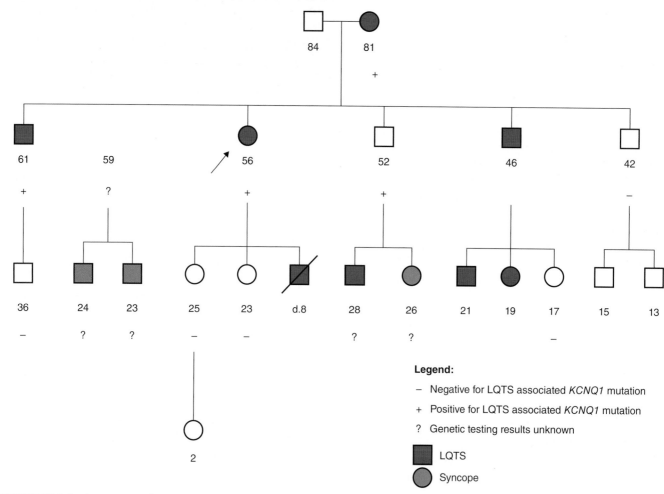

FIGURE 52-2 Implementation of cascade genetic testing in a large family with long QT syndrome (LQTS). This pedigree shows a large family with long QT syndrome (LQTS). The proband, designated by an arrow, is a 56-year-old woman who presented to the Inherited Arrhythmia Clinic due to her previous clinical diagnosis of LQTS after her 8-year-old son died suddenly while swimming. The genetic counselor met with the proband as part of her multidisciplinary consultation and this four-generation pedigree was constructed. Genetic testing had not been performed in the family to date, so the genetic counselor explained the potential benefits and limitation of LQTS genetic testing to the proband, who decided to proceed with full panel LQTS genetic testing. A pathogenic *KCNQ1* mutation was identified in the proband, which allowed predictive genetic testing to be offered to her at-risk relatives. Both of her daughters tested negative for the mutation, which meant her granddaughter was not at risk for LQTS. The proband utilized a family letter provided by the genetic counselor to inform the rest of her at-risk siblings and their children about the option of cascade genetic testing. Multiple additional individuals in the family were able to determine their accurate risk level based on the genetic testing information. Several additional individuals, marked with question marks, could still benefit from this predictive genetic testing information.

conditions, especially the heritable arrhythmia syndromes including long QT syndrome, Brugada syndrome, and arrhythmogenic right ventricular cardiomyopathy, display both incomplete and age-related penetrance and variable expressivity of clinical signs and symptoms. Small, or limited, family structures may also mask a genetic pattern of disease (eg, smaller sibships including only children may limit the number of affected individuals in the family; higher number of female relatives in a family can hide an X-linked disease). Because patients' self-reported family history information can have both reduced sensitivity and specificity, it is important to collect medical records, including autopsy reports, whenever possible so that diagnoses can be confirmed. In some cases, it is not until clinical screening commences through a family that a familial, or genetic, condition is able to be diagnosed, as has recently been shown with isolated atrioventricular block.[5] Also, family history is not static, but changes over time, and should therefore be updated periodically.

CARDIOVASCULAR GENETIC TESTING

Technological advances and cardiovascular genetics research discoveries have steadily and rapidly increased the number of clinically available genetic testing options for patients and their families with heritable heart diseases.[6] Because of the dramatic locus (multiple genes involved) and allelic (multiple mutations within a gene) heterogeneity observed in almost every heritable cardiac condition, most cardiovascular genetic tests involve multigene DNA sequencing panels that have been developed by commercial genetic testing laboratories. Most laboratories utilize next-generation DNA sequencing technologies, which provide fast and more cost-efficient analyses of multiple genes at one time. Up-to-date information on clinical and research genetic testing options can be located in two main online genetic testing databases: the National Institutes of Health Genetic Testing Registry (http://www.ncbi.nlm.nih.gov/gtr) and GeneTests (genetests.org).

TABLE 52-2 Indications for Referral for Cardiovascular Genetic Counseling and Testing

Patients with a suspected or definite diagnosis or family history of the following:

Inherited arrhythmias and channelopathies

- Long QT syndrome
- Short QT syndrome
- Brugada syndrome
- Catecholaminergic polymorphic ventricular tachycardia
- Familial atrial fibrillation
- Familial conduction system disease
- Idiopathic ventricular fibrillation

Cardiomyopathies

- Hypertrophic cardiomyopathy
- Idiopathic or familial dilated cardiomyopathy
- Arrhythmogenic right ventricular cardiomyopathy
- Left ventricular noncompaction cardiomyopathy
- Restrictive cardiomyopathy

Hereditary conditions affecting the aorta and other blood vessels

- Marfan syndrome
- Loeys-Dietz syndrome
- Ehlers-Danlos syndrome
- Familial thoracic aortic aneurysm and dissections
- Premature coronary artery disease (<55 years of age in a man; <65 years of age in a woman)
- Familial hypercholesterolemia
- Congenital heart disease
- Family history of sudden cardiac (or unexplained) death <50 years of age

While great strides have been made in the field of cardiovascular genetics, the fact that not all disease loci and genes associated with heritable cardiac conditions have been discovered means that currently available genetic tests have incomplete clinical sensitivities. Therefore, when currently available clinical disease-specific genetic testing panels (ie, Brugada syndrome gene panel) fail to identify the cause for a patient's likely genetic condition, health care providers can (1) consider large-scale genomic sequencing tests for their patients (ie, whole exome or whole genome sequencing) and (2) should inform the patient and potentially their family members about the option of participating in research studies focused on novel gene discovery.

The Clinical Utility and Value of Diagnostic and Predictive Genetic Testing

The clinical utility of genetic testing for multiple inherited cardiac diseases is now well recognized,[1] with applications including diagnostic confirmation, "phenocopy" identification which may target treatment (eg, Fabry disease, a phenocopy of hypertrophic cardiomyopathy, is treated with enzyme replacement therapy), therapeutics (eg, β-blocker initiation for the management of most long QT syndrome patients; implantable cardioverter defibrillator versus pacemaker consideration in patients with a *LMNA* mutation causing conduction system disease and dilated cardiomyopathy[7]), predictive genetic testing for at-risk relatives when the causative familial mutation(s) is identified, and the ability to provide patients with family planning information and reproductive options, including preimplantation and prenatal genetic diagnosis. Preimplantation genetic diagnosis allows couples the option to select mutation-negative embryos for implantation after in vitro fertilization. Prenatal genetic testing involves testing a sample of fetal DNA to determine whether the fetus carries the disease-associated mutation. Genetic counseling in these clinical settings is essential for the discussion of available testing options, risks (including miscarriage with certain prenatal sampling techniques), and to facilitate decision-making through supportive and nondirective counseling.

One of the main values of diagnostic genetic testing in an affected proband is that once their causative mutation(s) has been identified, all living first-degree relatives (parents, siblings, and children) can undergo predictive genetic testing. As additional mutation-positive individuals in the family are identified, genetic testing should continue to proceed in a stepwise, cascade fashion, moving through the pedigree in sequential steps until all at-risk relatives have been identified: this is termed cascade genetic testing (Figure 52-2). Predictive genetic testing also identifies those individuals in the family who did not inherit the genetic predisposition and therefore do not require serial clinical screening. This approach (using predictive genetic testing compared to serial lifetime clinical screening alone) has been shown to be highly cost-effective in families with hypertrophic cardiomyopathy.[8] Further, cascade genetic screening in families with inherited arrhythmia syndromes including long QT syndrome, Brugada syndrome, and CPVT through genetic testing and follow-up cardiac testing has been shown to result in treatment initiation with drugs and/or cardiac devices as well as counseling regarding lifestyle and drugs to avoid.[9]

The cardiac phenotype in some patients is due to the presence of multiple mutations; therefore, the best approach to genetic testing includes ordering the first, most comprehensive genetic testing panel on the most severely affected person in the family, since this will provide the highest likelihood of identifying all of the family's disease-associated mutations and will allow for the most accurate risk assessment and predictive genetic testing for at-risk relatives.[10]

Interpretation of Genetic Testing Results

Genetic testing results interpretation can be complex and challenging in many cases, with novel variants frequently identified whose clinical significance is not often clear. Variants identified through clinical genetic testing may be highly penetrant disease-causing mutations, lower penetrance modifiers of the clinical phenotype, or benign polymorphisms. Laboratories consider multiple factors in the interpretation of genetic testing results and whether a variant is actually pathogenic or not; this classification may change over time as new knowledge regarding the variant is gained. In order to fully realize the benefits and value of predictive genetic testing, accurate interpretation and application of genetic testing results is of the utmost importance, as clinicians must be sure they are testing at-risk relatives for the causative mutation and not a benign variant, especially when the stakes are high as with these inherited cardiovascular diseases that have risks for sudden cardiac death. In the absence of in vivo and/or in vitro models to examine these variants' functional significance, additional approaches, including analyzing cosegregation of the variant with the phenotype through large kindreds, amino acid conservation across species, variant frequency in large, ethnically matched control populations, and the use of in silico prediction tools, can be utilized. Variants with the highest likelihood of pathogenicity are those that cosegregate with the phenotype, are highly conserved, located in significant protein domains, and absent from matched controls.

Pretest Genetic Counseling

Pretest genetic counseling should include information on the indications for genetic testing as well as a discussion regarding the benefits, limitations, familial implications, and potential risks of genetic testing to insure informed decision-making. Pretest counseling should also include a discussion anticipating all possible results scenarios, including positive, negative, and/or uninformative genetic testing results and what each type of result would mean for the patient and his/her family. Pretest probabilities and clinical sensitivities should be shared with the patient (eg, a patient with a clinical diagnosis of Brugada syndrome should be informed that the current clinical sensitivity, or chance to find the disease-causing mutation, is approximately 25% to 40%). Possible psychological ramifications of genetic testing as well as baseline levels of risk perception, anxiety, and health beliefs should be assessed.[11] Questions regarding genetic discrimination are raised by many patients, and providers should therefore be prepared to discuss the protections afforded by, yet also the limitations of, the Genetic Information Nondiscrimination Act (GINA), which was signed into law on May 21, 2008. This federal law prohibits health insurers and employers from discriminating against individuals on the basis of their genetic information; however, life, disability, and long-term care insurance discrimination are not covered under GINA.

Posttest Genetic Counseling

Posttest genetic counseling should include a full discussion of genetic testing results and their implications for the index patient as well as at-risk relatives. Information regarding "duty to warn" should also be communicated; index patients should be counseled to inform their relatives of their risk as well as clinical screening recommendations. Family letters have been shown to be an effective tool to inform relatives of their risk and promote screening; these letters should include information about the family's diagnosis, inheritance pattern, risks, genetic testing, clinical screening, and preventative options.[12] If a pathogenic mutation is identified through clinical genetic testing, then family-specific single-site genetic testing is recommended for all living at-risk first-degree relatives. If genetic testing does not identify a causative mutation or if a variant of uncertain clinical significance is identified, the index patient should be informed that his/her condition may have an undetected underlying genetic/familial cause, that additional genetic testing may be warranted in the future as clinical sensitivities continue to improve, and that while at-risk relatives cannot pursue predictive genetic testing at this time, they should undergo clinical screening evaluations.

During posttest genetic counseling, an assessment of the psychological and emotional response to results should also be performed.[11] A positive result in a clinically affected individual may eliminate doubt and uncertainty, but for those who test positive through predictive testing (ie, they are genotype-positive, phenotype-negative)

it may have potential negative impacts including feelings such as increased worry, distress, anxiety, anger, fear of discrimination, alteration of self-esteem, and elimination of autonomy.[11] Genetic testing results can also impact family dynamics and relationships. Parents in particular may have feelings of guilt related to passing their mutation to their children. In this situation, it may be helpful to emphasize the benefits provided by this type of genetic information (ie, knowledge is power); specifically, clinicians can utilize this information to initiate clinical screening that may lead toward the earliest possible detection of disease and that may provide the opportunity for prophylactic treatment and lifestyle modifications.[13] Because many of the heritable cardiovascular conditions have inherent risks for arrhythmias and sudden cardiac death, the implications of positive predictive genetic testing can also include alteration of the ability to participate in competitive sports and other athletic activities, as well as additional lifestyle restrictions and modifications, which can be difficult for patients to cope with.

A negative genetic testing result can provide reassurance to patients regarding their personal risk level and that of their children and can also eliminate their need for follow-up cardiac screening. Patients in this category should be counseled that while they may have tested negative for their family's specific mutation, they can still develop heart disease, so they should not ignore or minimize cardiac symptoms they may have in the future. Patients who test negative may also experience feelings of so-called "survivor guilt," particularly in families where other siblings are clinically affected or have tested positive and are at risk.[11,13] It has been proposed that follow-up counseling within 3 to 6 months time to assess for persistent or amplified levels of distress over results should be offered to families with inherited cardiovascular diseases.[11]

CLINICAL SCREENING OF AT-RISK RELATIVES

Family member clinical screening is recommended for relatives who test positive via predictive genetic testing, those whose genetic status is unknown, and also for at-risk relatives in families where genetic testing has not identified the underlying molecular cause of a likely heritable disease. It is crucial for at-risk relatives to understand that a one-time normal echocardiogram, electrocardiogram, or other cardiac test does not clear them from the risk to develop the signs and symptoms, including sudden cardiac arrest or death, of a heritable cardiovascular disease in the future due to reduced and age-related penetrance and variable expressivity. For this reason, it must be communicated to the index patient that their at-risk relatives should undergo clinical screening, likely in a serial fashion, with personalized recommendations for follow-up from their health care providers. Similarly to cascade genetic testing, clinical screening should commence in a cascade fashion until all the first-degree relatives of affected individuals have undergone screening. Guidelines including recommended clinical screening approaches, modalities, and frequencies are available for certain inherited cardiac conditions.[7]

MULTIDISCIPLINARY APPROACH TO THE PATIENT AND FAMILY WITH INHERITED HEART DISEASE

An integrated, structured, multidisciplinary clinical approach to the care of families with inherited cardiac disease and sudden death has been recommended and should include the expertise of cardiologists, genetic counselors, clinical geneticists, nurses, pathologists, clinical and research molecular genetic testing centers, psychologists, and patient support groups.[3] Such multidisciplinary clinics need not require the actual physical presence of each and every subspecialty during every patient encounter, but instead involve strong, collaborative working relationships and communication between disciplines. Specialized cardiac genetics clinics have been shown to lead to better patient adjustment and less worry.[14] Many academic medical centers have established multidisciplinary inherited arrhythmia clinics as well as general cardiovascular genetic medicine clinics; community hospitals and other settings are also beginning to adopt this approach and are including genetic counseling and testing as part of their clinical service offerings. A timely American Heart Association policy statement on genetics and cardiovascular disease strongly advocates for the involvement of physicians and centers with expertise in cardiovascular genetics to guide the appropriate initiation, interpretation, and implementation of genetic testing.[15] Master's trained genetic counselors have been recommended as a solution to incorporate genetic medicine by providing genetic counseling and testing to applicable patients and by working in concert with subspecialty cardiovascular medicine physicians, such as electrophysiologists.[16]

CARDIOVASCULAR GENETIC COUNSELING AND TESTING: THE FUTURE

The past 10 years have been witness to an explosion of discovery in the field of cardiovascular genetics. This, along with the development of novel DNA sequencing technologies, has led to a steep increase in the number of clinical genetic testing options available to patients with, or at risk for, hereditary cardiovascular diseases. Patients have much better access to clinical genetic testing, with many health insurance companies and federally funded insurance plans covering genetic testing for their beneficiaries; practice guidelines and position statements also now exist that recommend genetic counseling and genetic testing and provide best practice approaches for the patient and family with a cardiovascular genetic condition.

With the costs of DNA sequencing continuing to drop, the $1000 whole genome sequence may very well be right around the bend for use in standard clinical care, and may even supersede the use of disease-specific gene panels. The health care provider, a cardiovascular *genomic* counselor, and the patient could potentially utilize information from each of the 3 billion nucleotides in the genetic code to personalize care (eg, tailored drug therapy) and more precisely predict future cardiovascular health status (ie, patient X will develop Y condition at 23 years of age without Z intervention). Future research will hopefully lead toward additional discoveries that could ameliorate or prevent these conditions altogether. This is the goal, and the promise, of individualized cardiovascular genetic medicine.

REFERENCES

1. Ackerman MJ, Priori SG, Willems S, et al. HRS/EHRA expert consensus statement on the state of genetic testing for the channelopathies and cardiomyopathies. This document was developed as a partnership between the Heart Rhythm Society (HRS) and the European Heart Rhythm Association (EHRA). *Heart Rhythm*. 2011;8(8):1308-1339.

2. Resta R, Biesecker BB, Bennett RL, et al. A new definition of genetic counseling: National Society of Genetic Counselors' Task Force report. *J Genet Couns*. 2006;15(2):77-83.

3. Ingles J, Yeates L, Semsarian C. The emerging role of the cardiac genetic counselor. *Heart Rhythm*. 2011;8(12):1958-1962.

4. Tester DJ, Ackerman MJ. Genetic testing for potentially lethal, highly treatable inherited cardiomyopathies/channelopathies in clinical practice. *Circulation*. 2011;123(9):1021-1037.

5. Baruteau AE, Behaghel A, Fouchard S, et al. Parental electrocardiographic screening identifies a high degree of inheritance for congenital and childhood nonimmune isolated atrioventricular block. *Circulation*. 2012;126(12):1469-1477.

6. Sturm AC, Hershberger RE. Genetic testing in cardiovascular medicine: current landscape and future horizons. *Curr Opin Cardiol*. 2013;28(3):317-325.

7. Hershberger RE, Lindenfeld J, Mestroni L, Seidman CE, Taylor MR, Towbin JA. Genetic evaluation of cardiomyopathy—a Heart Failure Society of America practice guideline. *J Card Fail*. 2009;15(2):83-97.

8. Ingles J, Mcgaughran J, Scuffham PA, Atherton J, Semsarian C. A cost-effectiveness model of genetic testing for the evaluation of families with hypertrophic cardiomyopathy. *Heart*. 2012;98(8):625-630.

9. Hofman N, Tan HL, Alders M, Van Langen IM, Wilde AA. Active cascade screening in primary inherited arrhythmia syndromes: does it lead to prophylactic treatment? *J Am Coll Cardiol*. 2010;55(23):2570-2576.

10. Sturm AC. Genetic testing in the contemporary diagnosis of cardiomyopathy. *Curr Heart Fail*. 2013;10(1):63-72.

11. Aatre RD, Day SM. Psychological issues in genetic testing for inherited cardiovascular diseases. *Circulation*. 2011;4(1):81-90.

12. Van Der Roest WP, Pennings JM, Bakker M, Van Den Berg MP, Van Tintelen JP. Family letters are an effective way to inform relatives about inherited cardiac disease. *Am J Med Genet A*. 2009;149A(3):357-363.

13. Ingles J, Zodgekar PR, Yeates L, Macciocca I, Semsarian C, Fatkin D. Guidelines for genetic testing of inherited cardiac disorders. *Heart Lung Circ*. 2011;20(11):681-687.

14. Ingles J, Lind JM, Phongsavan P, Semsarian C. Psychosocial impact of specialized cardiac genetic clinics for hypertrophic cardiomyopathy. *Genet Med*. 2008;10(2):117-120.

15. Ashley EA, Hershberger RE, Caleshu C, et al. Genetics and cardiovascular disease: a policy statement from the American Heart Association. *Circulation*. 2012;126(1):142-157.

16. Hershberger RE. Cardiovascular genetic medicine: evolving concepts, rationale, and implementation. *J Cardiovasc Trans Res*. 2008;1(2):137-143.

53 HYPERTROPHIC CARDIOMYOPATHY

James H. Hamilton, IV, MD, and S. Mark Borganelli, MD

CASE PRESENTATION

A 32-year-old man was referred to for evaluation of dyspnea on exertion and the finding of a systolic murmur on examination. He has begun to experience chest discomfort that is brought on with exertion and resolves with rest. He admits to frequent palpitations. Family history: father killed in a motor vehicle accident at age 35; paternal uncle died suddenly at age 40 of unknown cause.

Physical examination revealed a systolic murmur that worsens with rapidly standing, squatting, and standing again. A 12-lead ECG reveals prominent QRS voltage in the precordial leads with deep T-wave inversions (Figure 53-1). An echocardiogram was obtained demonstrating a nearly 5 cm ventricular septum and mitral regurgitation secondary to systolic anterior motion of the mitral valve (SAM) (Figures 53-2 to 53-5). A resting left ventricular outflow tract (LVOT) gradient of 45 mm Hg was recorded with a provocable gradient of >80 mm Hg (Figure 53-6).

The patient was started on metoprolol tartrate 50 mg twice daily and rapidly up titrated to 200 mg twice daily. Genetic counseling and genetic testing were performed, revealing a β-myosin heavy chain mutation and confirming the diagnosis of hypertrophic cardiomyopathy (HCM).

Based on a family history of unexplained sudden death and an LV wall thickness of greater than 3 cm, he underwent implantation of an ICD without complication for prevention of sudden cardiac death (SCD). Unfortunately, he had no improvement in symptoms despite high dose metoprolol and initiation of disopyramide. After 3 months of medical therapy and an attempt at pacing the right ventricle with the already implanted ICD, the LVOT gradient with provocation remained >50 mm Hg. Given his young age and refractory NYHA class III symptoms, he was referred to for myectomy. This operation was performed without complication and resulted in immediate improvement of symptoms. At follow-up 1 year later, the patient remains symptom-free with no resting or provocable LVOT gradient and no recorded arrhythmias.

EPIDEMIOLOGY

Inherited as an autosomal-dominant disorder, HCM is variably penetrant resulting in striking variations in phenotype even among first-degree relatives. Traditionally, the prevalence of HCM has been cited as 1:500, but due to the lack of symptoms in many individuals who may carry the genetic trait, the true prevalence may be much higher.[1,2]

ETIOLOGY AND PATHOPHYSIOLOGY

Clinically, hypertrophic cardiomyopathy (HCM) is generally described as left ventricular hypertrophy (LVH) with nondilated ventricular chambers in the absence of another cardiac or systemic disease that would be capable of producing the same degree of hypertrophy.[1,2] Patients may harbor nearly any diffuse or segmental pattern of hypertrophy and fibrosis with presentations ranging

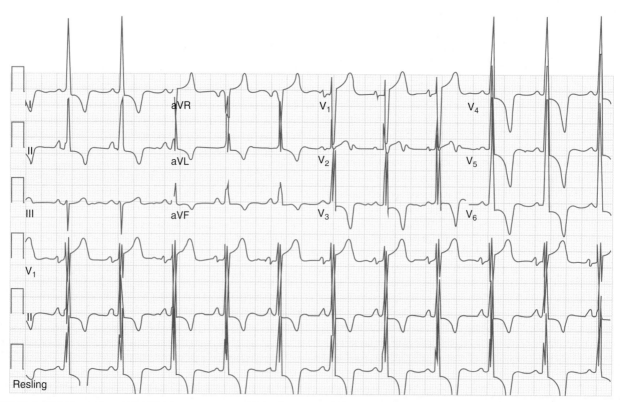

FIGURE 53-1 ECG in a patient with HCM. Note prominent QRS voltages and deep T-wave inversions.

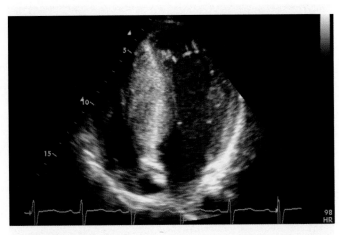

FIGURE 53-2 Echocardiogram demonstrating asymmetric hypertrophy with nearly a 5-cm septum.

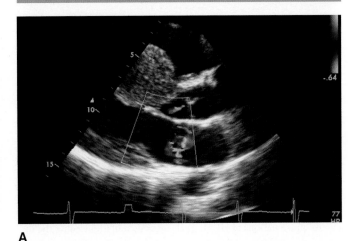

A

FIGURE 53-4A Parasternal long-axis view with color Doppler in diastole demonstrating normal opening of mitral valve.

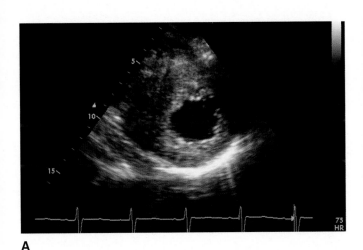

A

FIGURE 53-3A Parasternal short axis view of left ventricle in diastole.

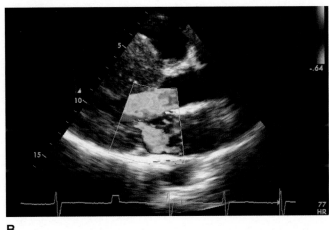

B

FIGURE 53-4B Parasternal long-axis view during systole with color Doppler demonstrating increased turbulent flow through the aortic valve with SAM and resulting mitral regurgitation.

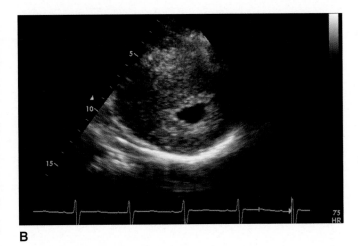

B

FIGURE 53-3B Parasternal short axis view of the left ventricle in systole.

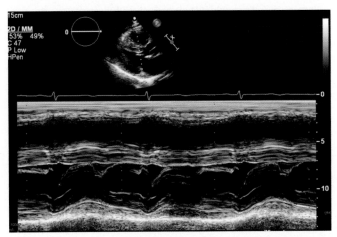

FIGURE 53-5 M-mode across the mitral valve demonstrating SAM with mitral-septal contact.

from completely asymptomatic to NYHA class II-IV heart failure to SCD.

The onset of symptoms and recognition of the disease may occur at any age from infancy to adulthood, but commonly develops during periods of accelerated body growth, such as adolescence. For that reason clinical screening is generally recommended in patients with genetically proven HCM beginning at age 12 and continuing yearly until age 18 to 21 followed by screening every 5 years thereafter.[1]

The availability of genetic testing has aided in the identification of an increasing number of genotype-positive, phenotype-negative patients. Indeed, there are now well over 1400 documented mutations that, when coupled with a sensitive genetic substrate and environmental triggering factors, are responsible for the variety of clinical presentations of HCM.[1,3] The genetic mutations allow the discrimination of HCM patients from patients with other genetic causes of LVH, such as Fabry disease, who would require much different management.

The original associations of genetic variants to HCM patients were isolated to myofilament (sarcomeric) proteins with the most common mutations occurring in the β-myosin heavy chain and cardiac myosin-binding protein C.[3] Recent investigations have focused not only on the sarcomeric proteins but on the associated contractile apparatus, as well, with new disease causing mutations classified as Z-disc HCM and calcium-handling HCM.[3] Ongoing investigations are trying to associate disease outcomes with various mutations and/or the affected protein subunits.[1,3] The cellular alterations caused by these mutations lead to varying degrees of hypertrophy and fibrosis in the heart. This in turn may eventually lead to systolic anterior motion of the mitral valve with LVOT obstruction; the resulting symptoms of dyspnea, congestive heart failure, and syncope; and the risk of cardiac arrhythmias including atrial fibrillation, ventricular tachycardia, and ventricular fibrillation.

DIAGNOSIS

Initial clinical evaluation of a patient includes a thorough personal and family history to elicit symptoms of syncope, exercise-induced chest discomfort, dyspnea, palpitations, and/or family history of SCD. The physical examination should include a careful auscultation of the patient with appropriate maneuvers such as stand-squat-stand to evaluate the characteristics of the murmur.

Initial screening should include each of the following:

- 12-lead ECG[1,2]

- Transthoracic echocardiogram

- 24-hour Holter monitoring

- Genetic assays if feasible

- Graded exercise test

The 12-lead ECG (see Figure 53-1) should demonstrate LVH and repolarization abnormalities. Incongruence between the ECG and echo findings should lead to definitive evaluation with either cardiac magnetic resonance imaging (CMRI)(Figure 53-7A and 53-7B) or invasive hemodynamic studies in the cath lab. In order to help assess the risk of SCD, HCM patients should also have 24-hour Holter monitoring and a graded exercise test performed at the time of diagnosis to evaluate for the presence of asymptomatic arrhythmias and determine the blood pressure response during exercise.[1,4]

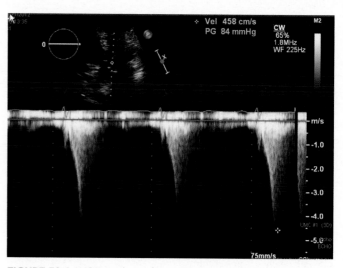

FIGURE 53-6 LVOT gradient after provocation with peak gradient recorded as 84 mm Hg.

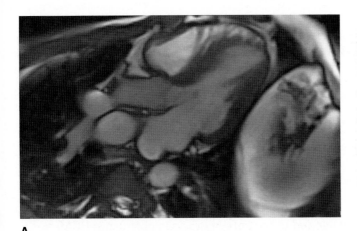

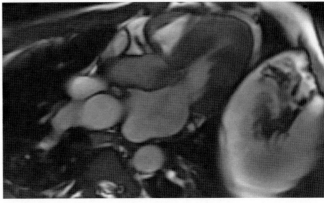

FIGURE 53-7A Cardiac MR with open mitral inflow during diastole. (Used with permission of Dr. Andrew Rivard at University of Mississippi Medical Center, Jackson, MS.)

FIGURE 53-7B Cardiac MR with obstruction of the LVOT during systole due to SAM of the mitral valve. (Used with permission of Dr. Andrew Rivard at University of Mississippi Medical Center, Jackson, MS.)

Screening with transthoracic echocardiogram should be performed at the time of the initial evaluation and yearly thereafter in known HCM patients and is recommended at the time of initial screening of first-degree relatives to assess left ventricular systolic and diastolic function, wall thickness, and outflow tract gradients.[1-3,5] The obstruction that occurs in HCM has been shown to be due to mitral valve systolic anterior motion (SAM) with mitral-septal contact (best illustrated in Figures 53-5 and 53-7B), muscular obstruction in the midcavitary region, or anomalous papillary muscle insertion into the anterior mitral leaflet.[1,2,6] The peak LVOT or midcavitary gradient should be measured at rest, and if <50 mm Hg, the test should be repeated with provocative measures such as exercise, Valsalva maneuver, or potentially amyl nitrate, with the latter rarely required in the current era. Provocation with dobutamine infusion during echo is no longer recommended. Upon testing, one-third of patients will have a resting LVOT gradient >30 mm Hg (obstructive HCM), one-third will have resting gradients <30 mm Hg (nonobstructive HCM), and a final one-third will have normal resting gradients but provoked gradients >30 mm Hg (labile obstruction).[1,2,6]

Genetic screening has become an important part of the work-up of HCM patients. Identifying a specific genetic mutation associated with HCM allows for easier screening stratification of first-degree relatives into a positive disease group or no disease group. Although all first degree relatives of HCM patients require initial clinical assessment with ECG and echocardiogram, if these relatives have normal clinical assessments and are free of the familial mutation, that individual patient does not need repeat assessment in the future.[1,3,5] Multiple studies are ongoing to determine whether specific mutation(s) lead to increased risk of SCD or severity of disease.[1,3]

MANAGEMENT

Management of HCM includes efforts to decrease heart failure and angina symptoms related to left ventricular diastolic dysfunction

and LVOT obstruction (Table 53-1), evaluating the risk of SCD and assessing for and treating cardiac arrhythmias.

Initial therapy for symptomatic and asymptomatic patients is generally with a β-blocker unless contraindications exist.[1,2,7] High doses of β-blockers may be required for symptom relief and can be pushed to maximum drug doses unless limited by bradycardia. Directly reducing contractility due to the negative inotropic effect of β-blockers improves the dynamic LVOT gradient, while the negative chronotropic effect improves diastolic filling times.

Alternatively, patients who cannot take β-blockers may be tried on verapamil.[1,2,7] Due to the pharmacologic properties of verapamil (and diltiazem), some patients may develop a more profound vasodilatory effect than the desired negative inotrope effect, in essence, worsening the dynamic LVOT obstruction/gradient and symptoms. Therefore, initiation of verapamil (or diltiazem) in patients with signs of severely elevated pulmonary capillary wedge pressure, low systemic blood pressure, and high LVOT gradients should be performed with extreme caution.[1,2,7] For patients with symptoms refractory to initial medical therapy, disopyramide may be considered as an adjunct agent.[1,2,7] The clinical benefits of disopyramide are related to its negative inotropic effect on the heart. Initiation of disopyramide should be done in a hospital setting with patients monitored for excessive QT prolongation and proarrhythmia.

For patients who remain medically refractory with continued NYHA class III-IV symptoms, additional therapeutic interventions must be considered. For patients who are younger and are felt to be suitable candidates, invasive septal reduction therapy is recommended at this point in management. This type of treatment is only effective for patients whose symptoms are attributable to increased peak LVOT gradients >50 mm Hg, whether at rest or with provocation, and is not intended for patients with symptoms related to severe diastolic dysfunction or angina related to subendocardial ischemia in the absence of a high LVOT gradient.[1,8-10] For patients who are not suitable candidates for invasive septal reduction and who already have dual chamber ICDs in place for prevention of SCD, attempts at RV pacing

TABLE 53-1 Summary of Guideline Pharmacologic Recommendations

Medication/Class	Recommendation
Class I	
β-blockers	To alleviate symptoms of heart failure and angina.
Verapamil	To alleviate symptoms of heart failure and angina in patients who cannot take β-blockers.
Phenylephrine	Treatment of acute hypotension in obstructive HCM unresponsive to fluids.
Vitamin K antagonists	Antithrombotic in HCM patients with atrial fibrillation.
Class IIa	
Disopyramide	Add to a β-blocker or verapamil if needed to control symptoms in obstructive HCM.
Amiodarone	Reasonable alternative to disopyramide for the treatment of HCM related atrial fibrillation.
Class IIb	
Diltiazem	Reasonable to consider in patients who cannot tolerate verapamil.
ACE Inhibitors/ARB	Usefulness in preserved LV ejection fraction is not well established.
Diuretics	Use with caution if required for congestive symptoms despite use of β-blockers and/or verapamil.
Phosphodiesterase inhibitors	Use with caution for patients with erectile dysfunction as may cause deleterious symptoms in patients with resting or provocable gradient.
Class III	
Dihydropyridine CCB	In patients with resting or provocable LVOT gradient.
Nitroglycerine	
Digoxin	For treatment of dyspnea in patients with HCM without atrial fibrillation.
Dopamine	For acute hypotension in patients with obstructive HCM.
Dobutamine	
Norepinephrine	

Data from Gersh BJ, Maron BJ, Bonow RO, et al. 2011 ACCF/AHA Guideline for the Diagnosis and Treatment of Hypertrophic Cardiomyopathy. Journal American College of Cardiology 2011;58:e212-260.

may be tried to reduce the LVOT gradient.[1,11] This concept was thought to be a potential therapeutic intervention for patients in the past with initial reports of symptomatic improvement and decreased LVOT gradients; however, three randomized controlled trials were published refuting the effectiveness of RV pacing as a means to decrease the LVOT gradient.[1,11,12] Based on the results of those trials, it appears that there is a symptomatic improvement in a majority of patients (30%-80%) but an objective reduction in LVOT gradient in a much smaller percentage of patients (25%-40%).[1,11,12] This indicates both a placebo effect and training effect of pacemaker therapy on the symptoms of these patients. With the current level of evidence, the guidelines give dual chamber pacing a class IIa indication to reduce LVOT gradients in patients who already have a dual chamber pacing device for non-HCM indications and a class IIb recommendation to improve symptoms in patients who have medically refractory symptoms but are poor candidates for invasive septal reduction.[1,11,12]

Invasive therapeutic options include surgical myectomy and alcohol septal ablation. Surgical myectomy procedures have been performed for nearly 5 decades with high volume centers reporting excellent success rates. Indeed, in patients who are deemed candidates for surgical myectomy, it has emerged as the treatment of choice for patients with obstructive HCM with operative success achieved in 90% to 95% of patients with operative mortality reported to be <1% and nonfatal complication rates of 2% to 3% in certain high volume centers.[1,8-10] In addition, myectomy has the advantage of being able to correct other causes of LVOT obstruction other than septal hypertrophy alone, such as aberrant papillary muscle implantation or abnormal elongation of the anterior mitral leaflet.[1,8-10] Following surgical myectomy, long-term survival did not differ from the age-matched, general U.S. population and was superior to that of HCM patients with LVOT obstruction who did not undergo myectomy. The reported incidence of SCD or appropriate ICD discharge following surgical myectomy is reported as <0.9%; however, surgical myectomy does not eradicate the need for SCD risk assessment and possible ICD implantation.[1,8-10]

In comparison, alcohol septal ablation is also of benefit in the right patient cohort and results in an immediate fall in gradient due to decreased septal contraction in >90% of patients.[1,9,10] Success rates are dependent on individual anatomy with an inherent need for a septal perforator artery that supplies the area of SAM-septal contact; in its absence, the procedure cannot be performed. Over half of patients undergoing alcohol septal ablation require temporary pacing during the procedure and between 10% and 20% require permanent pacing.[1,13] In addition, the reported rate of sustained ventricular arrhythmias and SCD following alcohol septal ablation is 3% to 10%.[1,13] Despite the complications, the data suggest that the 4-year survival is similar for both surgical myectomy and alcohol septal ablation procedures.[1,9,10,13]

Due to diastolic dysfunction and accompanying enlargement of the left atrium in HCM, atrial fibrillation is a common finding in patients older than 30 years old and ultimately occurring in up to 20% to 25% of HCM patients.[1,2] Even with short episodes of paroxysmal atrial fibrillation, the risk of thrombus formation and systemic embolization is high in HCM patients and results in a class I indication for anticoagulation with vitamin-K antagonists.[1,2] β-Blockers and verapamil are recommended for rate control, but symptoms may warrant attempts at rhythm control. Amiodarone or disopyramide (along with β-blockers or verapamil) have shown potential use as rhythm controlling agents with amiodarone being the preferred rhythm control agent.[1,2] Pulmonary vein isolation can be done in appropriate subsets of HCM patients with early success and complication rates similar to other forms of heart disease.[1]

Risk assessment for SCD must be performed in each patient at the time of initial evaluation and repeated at appropriate clinical intervals (usually yearly) for individuals who do not initially receive an ICD. The overall rate of SCD in HCM patients is approximately 1% per year; although, it appears that when patients have at least one of the following conventional risk markers, the rate of appropriate ICD therapy is approximately 3% to 4% per year.[1,4,14]

1. History of ventricular fibrillation, ventricular tachycardia, or aborted SCD

2. Family history of SCD related to HCM

3. Unexplained syncope (higher weight to events <6 months from evaluation)

4. Documented NSVT on ambulatory ECG monitoring

5. Maximal LV wall thickness greater than or equal to 30 mm

Of the above risk markers, prior aborted SCD carries the highest future risk, with a 10% per year event rate.[1,4,14]

The decision for ICD placement must be based upon the risk-benefit ratio in an individual patient. This is due to the high incidence of ICD complications in cohorts of HCM patients, reportedly up to 4% per year.[1,4,14] As such, the only class I indication for ICD implantation in HCM patients is survival of SCD.[1,14] There is a class II indication that ICD implantation is reasonable in patients with a family history of SCD, unexplained syncope, and LV wall thickness >30 mm.[1,14] In remaining patients, it is important to identify the presence of further risk factors, such as an abnormal blood pressure response to exercise or episodes of NSVT on continuous ECG monitoring that may sway the decision towards or away from ICD implantation.

FUTURE DIRECTIONS

Management of HCM continues to evolve. Of particular interest is the development of subcutaneous ICDs and their upcoming entrance into widespread clinical practice. Subcutaneous ICD effectiveness will need to be verified in HCM patients with the extremes of LV hypertrophy, but given the long-term complication rate of intravascular ICDs, these may prove to be quite beneficial, especially in young patients. Considering the long-term complications of intravascular hardware, implanters should choose the proper device to minimize the number of intravascular leads, with consideration given to single coil ICD leads and VDD leads when appropriate. Additionally, technology in the areas of cardiac MR and genetic testing may improve and, potentially, redefine SCD risk assessment and management of HCM.

REFERENCES

1. Gersh BJ, Maron BJ, Bonow RO, et al. 2011 ACCF/AHA Guideline for the Diagnosis and Treatment of Hypertrophic Cardiomyopathy: a report of the American College of Cardiology Foundation/American Heart Association Task Force on Practice Guidelines. *J Am Coll Cardiol.* 2011;58(25):e212-260.

2. Maron BJ, McKenna WJ, Danielson GK, et al. American College of Cardiology/European Society of Cardiology Clinical Expert Consensus Document on Hypertrophic Cardiomyopathy. A report of the American College of Cardiology Foundation Task Force on Clinical Expert Consensus Documents and the European Society of Cardiology Committee for Practice Guidelines. *J Am Coll Cardiol.* 2003;42(9):1687-1713.

3. Bos JM, Towbin JA, Ackerman MJ. Diagnostic, prognostic, and therapeutic implications of genetic testing for hypertrophic cardiomyopathy. *J Am Coll Cardiol.* 2009;54(3):201-211.

4. Maron BJ. Contemporary insights and strategies for risk stratification and prevention of sudden death in hypertrophic cardiomyopathy. *Circulation.* 2010;121(3):445-456.

5. Maron BJ, Seidman JG, Seidman CE. Proposal for contemporary screening strategies in families with hypertrophic cardiomyopathy. *J Am Coll Cardiol.* 2004;44(11):2125-2132.

6. Maron MS, Olivotto I, Zenovich AG, et al. Hypertrophic cardiomyopathy is predominantly a disease of left ventricular outflow tract obstruction. *Circulation.* 2006;114(21):2232-2239.

7. Fifer MA, Vlahakes GJ. Management of symptoms in hypertrophic cardiomyopathy. *Circulation.* 2008;117(3):429-439.

8. Ommen SR, Maron BJ, Olivotto I, et al. Long-term effects of surgical septal myectomy on survival in patients with obstructive hypertrophic cardiomyopathy. *J Am Coll Cardiol.* 2005;46(3):470-476.

9. Sorajja P, Valeti U, Nishimura RA, et al. Outcome of alcohol septal ablation for obstructive hypertrophic cardiomyopathy. *Circulation.* 2008;118(2):131-139.

10. Fernandes VK, Nielsen C, Nagueh SF, et al. Follow-up of alcohol septal ablation for symptomatic hypertrophic obstructive cardiomyopathy, the Baylor and Medical University of South Carolina experience 1996 to 2007. *JACC Cardiovasc Interv.* 2008;1(5):561-570.

11. Ommen SR, Nishimura RA, Squires RW, et al. Comparison of dual chamber pacing versus septal myectomy for the treatment of patients with hypertrophic obstructive cardiomyopathy: a comparison of objective hemodynamic and exercise end points. *J Am Coll Cardiol*. 1999;34(1):191-196.

12. Maron BJ, Nishimura RA, McKenna WJ, et al. Assessment of permanent dual-chamber pacing as a treatment for drug-refractory symptomatic patients with obstructive hypertrophic cardiomyopathy: a randomized, double-blind, crossover study (M-PATHY). *Circulation*. 1999;99(22):2927-2933.

13. Seggewiss H. Current status of alcohol septal ablation for patients with hypertrophic cardiomyopathy. *Curr Cardiol Rep*. 2001;3(2): 160-166.

14. Maron BJ, Spirito P, Shen WK, et al. Implantable cardioverter-defibrillators and prevention of sudden cardiac death in hypertrophic cardiomyopathy. *JAMA*. 2007;298(4):405-412.

ARRHYTHMOGENIC RIGHT VENTRICULAR
DYSPLASIA/CARDIOMYOPATHY (ARVD/C)

SECTION VIII
EVALUATION AND MANAGEMENT
OF INHERITED ARRHYTHMIAS

375

54 ARRHYTHMOGENIC RIGHT VENTRICULAR DYSPLASIA/CARDIOMYO-PATHY (ARVD/C)

Brittney Murray, MS, CGC, and Hugh Calkins, MD

CASE PRESENTATION

A 21-year-old competitive triathlete was brought into the emergency department after collapsing during a local race. She reported the onset of a rapid heart rate near the finish line of the cycling portion and suddenly collapsed. Upon arrival, the emergency medical services found her to be in sustained ventricular tachycardia (VT) at 260 ms (Figure 54-1), and she was converted to sinus rhythm with a 200 J external shock. Upon arrival to the emergency room, she was found again to be in VT at 263 bpm with left bundle branch block (LBBB), superior axis morphology. She lost consciousness and was again externally cardioverted (Figure 54-2). A 12-lead electrocardiogram (ECG) (Figure 54-3) demonstrated T-wave inversions across the precordium. An echocardiogram revealed no evidence of structural heart disease. Due to her ECG abnormalities, this was followed up with cardiac MRI, which revealed a dilated right ventricle (RV) with akinetic segments in the RV free wall and base (Figure 54-4). She was taken for electrophysiology study (EPS) which demonstrated easily inducible VT with two different morphologies (LBBB superior axis, and LBBB indeterminate axis) (Figure 54-5). Ablation was attempted but was unsuccessful in eliminating all inducible VTs. An epicardial focus was suspected. Based upon her evaluation, she was found to meet diagnostic criteria for arrhythmogenic right ventricular dysplasia/cardiomyopathy (ARVD/C). She was implanted with a single chamber ICD and discharged on β-blockers. During follow-up, frequent symptomatic runs of NSVT were recorded by her ICD. Antiarrhythmic drug therapy was discussed with the patient, but she preferred not to take more medications. For this reason, an epicardial VT ablation procedure was performed. Her VT was mapped to the anterior lateral RV free wall and ablated successfully (Figure 54-6). She did well following her ablation procedure and remained VT-free. She was advised to give up participation in athletic activities. She was also referred to a genetic counselor for genetic counseling and testing. Upon inquiry, it was noted that her maternal grandfather died suddenly

of a "heart attack" in his 40s. No other details were known, and there was no other history of cardiomyopathy or sudden death. Genetic testing returned a pathogenic mutation in the *plakophilin-2(PKP2)* gene: 2146-1G>C. Her older brother, also an athlete, was tested and found also to carry this mutation and was scheduled for appropriate cardiac screening.

ETIOLOGY AND PATHOPHYSIOLOGY OF ARVD/C

ARVD/C is an inherited cardiomyopathy characterized by fibro-fatty replacement of the myocardium, life-threatening ventricular arrhythmias and ventricular dysfunction (right > left ventricle). The disease has a prevalence estimated 1 per 5000, though some reports estimate the real prevalence could be as high as 1 in 1000 due to under-recognition. Sudden cardiac death (SCD) is the first manifestation in up to 50% of cases.[1]

Subsequent to the discovery of pathogenic mutations in the desmosomal genes (Table 54-1) in families with ARVD/C, the disruption of the desmosomal structure as the key factor in many cases leading to ARVD/C development has been widely accepted in the field.[2,3] The desmosomes not only provide structural attachment among cells, they also mediate intracellular signal transduction pathways as part of the intercalated disc[4] (Figure 54-7). The specific mechanism by which the mutations in these genes may translate into the variety of disease expression seen clinically, however, has been the subject of many hypotheses.

Proposed mechanisms include that desmosomal mutations disrupt a triad between gap junction, voltage-gated sodium channel complex, and desmosomes, or intercalated disc.[5] It is thought that the desmosomal proteins may have two roles: signal molecules that may promote cardiac myocyte apoptosis and also structural connections in the gap junction.[6] Disruption of the desmosomes leaves the cardiomyocytes unable to handle mechanical stress, which leads to the cells being ripped apart and cell death.[7] Evidence in mouse models and new clinical evidence from patient data have indicated that strenuous exercise in ARVD/C patients may play a pivotal role in advancing disease as mechanical stress of stretch in the heart disrupts these weakened connections.[8,9]

DIAGNOSIS

An ARVD/C diagnosis is made by meeting a set of major and minor diagnostic criteria (Table 54-2). There is no gold-standard test or criterion in the diagnostic criteria that is pathognomonic for ARVD/C, and a diagnosis of ARVD/C should not be made based on a single clinical test. The first diagnostic criteria for ARVD/C were published

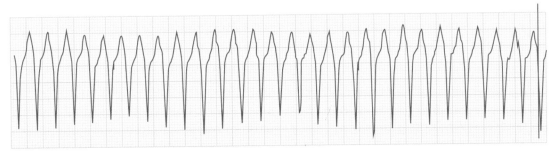

FIGURE 54-1 Patient's presenting VT upon arrival of EMS, recorded at 260 ms.

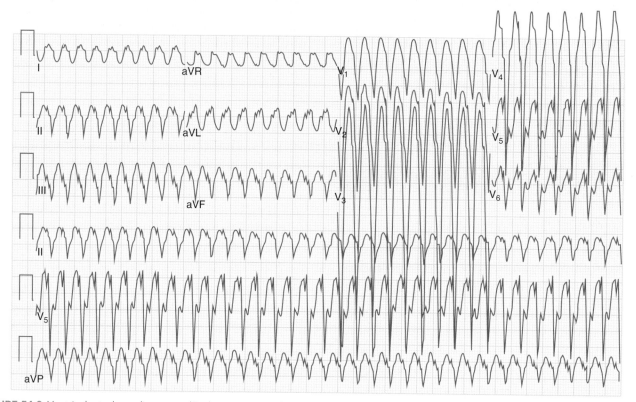

FIGURE 54-2 Ventricular tachycardia recurred in the emergency department, recorded on 12-lead ECG, revealed LBBB, superior axis morphology.

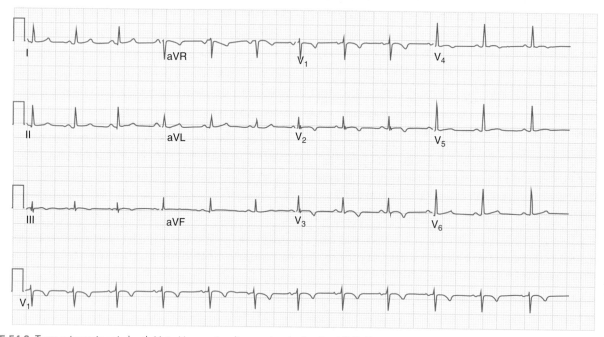

FIGURE 54-3 T-wave inversions in leads V_1 to V_4, a major diagnostic criterion for ARVD/C.

in 1994.[10] Over time, however, they were shown to lack sensitivity for the identification of early/mild disease, and they did not include the newly discovered utility of genetic testing for ARVD/C. Revised diagnostic criteria were proposed by a working task force in 2010.[11] In the revised criteria, a definite diagnosis of ARVD/C is fulfilled by two major or one major and two minor criteria, or four minor criteria.

An important specification is that criterion must be from separate categories. A borderline diagnosis is made by one major and one minor, or three minor criteria, and a possible diagnosis by one major or two minor criteria.

The diagnostic criteria are based on assessment of the extent of ventricular structural alterations and dysfunction, tissue characterization

ARRHYTHMOGENIC RIGHT VENTRICULAR
DYSPLASIA/CARDIOMYOPATHY (ARVD/C)

SECTION VIII
EVALUATION AND MANAGEMENT
OF INHERITED ARRHYTHMIAS

377

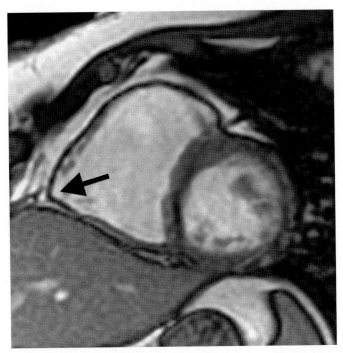

FIGURE 54-4 Cardiac MRI notes a dilated RV with akinesis of the base of the RV. Outpouching of the angle of the RV (denoted by arrow) is a classic MRI finding in ARVD/C.

on biopsy, repolarization and depolarization abnormalities on ECG and signal averaged ECG (SAECG), arrhythmias and ventricular ectopy, and family history and genetic criteria. Recommended noninvasive testing when evaluating for ARVD/C includes 12-lead ECG, SAECG, echocardiogram, cardiac MRI, exercise stress testing, and ambulatory ECG monitoring (24-hour Holter monitoring). Cardiac MRI has a much higher specificity and sensitivity for diagnosis than echocardiogram, especially in detecting early disease.[11] The revised diagnostic criteria remain limited in that it does not include those with left sided dominant disease. Left dominant disease in ARVD/C (LDAC) can be differentiated from DCM by a marked electrical instability that exceeds the degree of dysfunction. Up to one-third of genotyped individuals with an LDAC presentation had an identifiable pathogenic desmosomal mutation.[12]

Microscopic evaluation of samples at necropsy, surgery, or biopsy may reveal interstitial and replacement fibrosis and fatty infiltration. Pure fat infiltration of the RV is reported in >50% of normal hearts in elderly patients.[13] Furthermore, those with exclusively fatty infiltration of the RV on autopsy were older, lacked any family history of sudden cardiac death (SCD), and died during nonstrenuous activities. These studies have led to the conclusion that fibrofatty histology and not solely adipose replacement is associated with ARVD/C.[14] Autopsies and endomyocardial biopsy as part of a diagnosis of ARVD/C should be evaluated carefully.

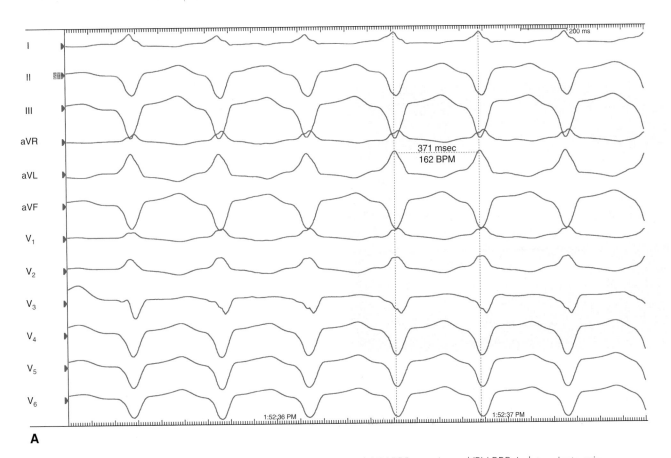

FIGURE 54-5 During electrophysiology study and ablation two VTs were noted: (A) LBBB superior and (B) LBBB, indeterminate axis.

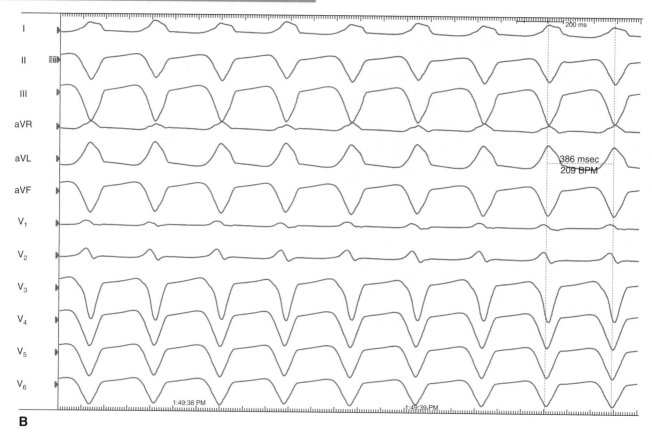

B

FIGURE 54-5 (Continued)

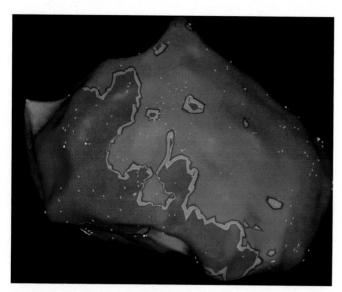

FIGURE 54-6 Epicardial three-dimensional voltage mapping created on a CARTO system demonstrating significant RV scar from the anterior to inferior RV extending from base to apex. Late potentials were also clearly present on the epicardial sites of scar.

TABLE 54-1 Genes Currently Associated with ARVD/C

Gene	Phenotype
JUP	Cardiocutaneous, Naxos syndrome
DSP (recessive)	Cardiocutaneous, Carvajal disease
DSP	
DSC2	
PKP2	
DSG2	
ARVD/C Phenotype	
Nondesmosomal	
RYR2	Catecholemingergic polymorphic VT, ARVD/C phenocopy
TGFβ3	Implication in disease pending
TMEM43	Fully penetrant, highly lethal
DES	Overlap syndrome with DCM
TTN	Overlap syndrome with DCM
PLN	Overlap syndrome with DCM

ARRHYTHMOGENIC RIGHT VENTRICULAR
DYSPLASIA/CARDIOMYOPATHY (ARVD/C)

SECTION VIII
EVALUATION AND MANAGEMENT
OF INHERITED ARRHYTHMIAS

379

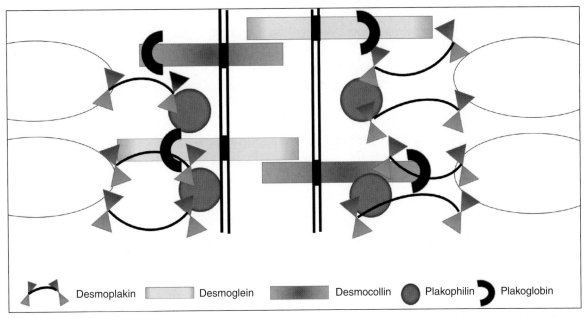

FIGURE 54-7 Schematic representation of the structure of the cardiac desmosome and intercalated disc. The desmosome links in the intermediate filament of the heart muscle (oval) and is embedded in the cell membrane (vertical line).

TABLE 54-2 Revised 2010 Task Force Criteria for Diagnosis of ARVD/C

Imaging

Major   By 2-D Echo

- Regional RV akinesis, dyskinesia, or aneurysm *and* 1 of the following (end diastole):
  - PLAX RVOT ≥32 mm (correct for body size [PLAX/BSA] ≥19 mm/m^2)
  - PSAX RVOT ≥36 mm (correct for body size [PSAX/BSA] ≥21 mm/m^2)
  - or fractional area change ≤33%

By MRI
- Regional RV akinesia or dyskinesia or dyssynchronous RV contraction *and* 1 of the following:
  - Ratio of RV end-diastolic volume to BSA ≥110 mL/m^2 (male) or ≥100 mL/m^2 (female)
  - or RV ejection fraction ≤40%

By RV Angiography
- Regional RV akinesia, dyskinesia, or aneurysm

Minor

By 2-D Echo
- Regional RV akinesia or dyskinesia *and* 1 of the following (end diastole):
  - PLAX RVOT ≥29 to <32 mm (correct body size PLAX/BSA ≥16 to <19 mm/m^2)
  - PSAX RVOT ≥32 to <36 mm (correct body size [PSAX/BSA] ≥18 to <21 mm/m^2)
  - or fractional area change >33% to ≤40%

By MRI
- Regional RV akinesia or dyskinesia or dyssynchronous RV contraction *and* 1 of the following:
  - Ratio of RVEDV to BSA ≥100 to <110 mL/m^2 (male) or ≥90 to <100 mL/m^2 (fem)
  - or RV EF >40% to ≤45%

TABLE 54-2 Revised 2010 Task Force Criteria for Diagnosis of ARVD/C

Imaging

Biopsy/necropsy/surgery

Major	• Residual myocytes < 60% by morphometric analysis (or <50% if estimated), with fibrosis replacement of RV free wall myocardium in ≥1 sample, with or without fatty replacement of tissue on endomyocardial biopsy
Minor	• Residual myocytes 60% to 75% by morphometric analysis (or 50% to 60% if estimated) with fibrous replacement of the RV free wall in ≥1 sample, with/without fatty replacement of tissue on endomyocardial biopsy

Depolarization abnormalities

Major	• Inverted T wave (V_1, V_2, V_3) or beyond; >14 y; in absence of complete RBBB QRS ≥120 ms
Minor	• Inverted T wave in V_1 and V_2; >14 y; in absence of complete RBBB or in V_4, V_5, or V_6 • Inverted T waves in leads V_1, V_2, V_3, and V_4 in individuals >14 y of age in the presence of complete RBBB

Repolarization abnormalities

Major	• Epsilon wave (reproducible low-amp signals between end of QRS complex to onset of T wave) in right precordial leads (V_1-V_3)

Minor	• Late potentials by SAECG in ≥1 of 3 parameters in absence of QRS duration of ≥110 ms on ECG
	  ○ Filtered QRS duration (fQRS) ≥114 ms
	  ○ Duration of terminal QRS <40µV (LAS duration) ≥38 ms
	  ○ Root-mean-square voltage (RMS) of terminal 40 ms ≤20µV
	• Terminal activation duration of QRS ≥55 ms measured from nadir of S wave to end of QRS, including R', in V_1, V_2, or V_3, in absence of complete RBBB

Arrhythmias

Major	• LBBB, superior axis NSVT or sustained VT (negative or indeterminate QRS in II, III, and aVF and positive in aVL)
Minor	• NSVT or sustained VT of RVOT configuration, LBBB inferior axis (positive QRS in II, III, and aVF and negative in aVL) or of unknown axis • >500 ventricular extrasystoles per 24 hours (Holter)

Family history/genetics

Major	• ARVD/C confirmed in first-degree relative who meets TFC • ARVD/C confirmed pathologically at autopsy or surgery in first-degree relative • Pathogenic mutation (associated or probably associated w/ ARVD/C) in individual under evaluation • History of ARVD/C in first-degree relative in whom not possible or practical to determine if relative meets TFC • Premature SCD (>35 yrs) due to suspected ARVD/C in first-degree relative • ARVD/C confirmed pathologically or by current TFC in second-degree relative

Data from Marcus, FI, McKenna, WJ, Sherrill, D, et al: Diagnosis of arrhythmogenic right ventricular cardiomyopathy/dysplasia: proposed modification of the Task Force Criteria. Eur Heart J 2010;31(7):806-814.

Family history is an important component of evaluation for ARVD/C. First-degree relatives of an individual diagnosed with ARVD/C are at 50% risk also to inherit the genetic predisposition to ARVD/C. A negative family history does not exclude the possibility of ARVD/C. Up to 50% of ARVD/C index cases have no family history of SCD or cardiomyopathy. Families should also be cautioned regarding the high variable expressivity of ARVD/C. Even within the same family and same known pathogenic mutation, severity of disease and type of presentation may vary greatly.[1]

Differential diagnosis in ARVD/C includes idiopathic premature ventricular contractions or ventricular tachycardia, myocarditis, and cardiac sarcoidosis. Patients presenting with ventricular arrhythmias should be first evaluated for more common idiopathic right ventricular outflow tract (RVOT) ectopy or VT.[1] Misdiagnosis is common in ARVD/C. Most commonly, over-read and over-reliance on cardiac MRI is part of the error.[15] There are also other diseases that may mimic ARVD/C. Many patients who present with right-sided cardiac sarcoidosis meet diagnostic criteria for ARVD/C. This can be

ARRHYTHMOGENIC RIGHT VENTRICULAR
DYSPLASIA/CARDIOMYOPATHY (ARVD/C)

SECTION VIII
EVALUATION AND MANAGEMENT
OF INHERITED ARRHYTHMIAS

381

differentiated in the involvement of the septum in the disease, presence of high-grade atrioventricular conduction block on ECG at presentation, which is unusual in ARVD/C, and rapid progression of disease.[16,17] Differentiation between myocarditis and ARVD/C is sometimes difficult, and the role of inflammation of the heart in the disease process of ARVD/C has yet to be fully clarified.[18,19]

MANAGEMENT

Definite ARVD/C Per Task Force Criteria

Hallmarks of ARVD/C clinical management include arrhythmia management, prevention of further structural progression, and adjustment to life with a chronic genetic condition. An important management decision to consider is the placement of an implantable cardioverter defibrillator (ICD) for protection from sustained ventricular arrhythmias and SCD. This decision should be made slowly and with consideration as these are young patients who are expected to live many years with a device that is not complication-free. It is currently recommended that ARVD/C patients presenting with sustained VT and/or ventricular fibrillation (VF) should undergo placement of an ICD because of a high risk of recurrent VT and/or SCD.[20,21] In contrast, there is much more uncertainty regarding placing an ICD for primary prevention.[22] We also recommend ICD implantation for most probands diagnosed with ARVD/C and also family members with high-risk features. Factors which have been identified as predictors of increased risk for development of a sustained ventricular arrhythmia include severity of structural heart disease and ECG abnormalities, frequent PVCs and runs of NSVT, cardiac syncope, proband status (probands are at higher risk than family members), inducible VT at EP testing, and the continuation of competitive or high level athletics. It is also important to consider patient preference when considering implantation of an ICD.[23-26]

ARVD/C traditionally disproportionately affects the right ventricle, save for left dominant forms described previously. The left ventricle may be involved in more advanced stages of the disease. Cardiac transplantation, however, is rare. Patients with early age presentation of the disease are those who are more likely to be considered for cardiac transplantation.[27]

Once a decision is reached regarding ICD placement and heart failure symptoms are managed, management should continue on a minimum annual basis. We currently advise that patients with ARVD/C be seen in follow-up at least on an annual basis at which time we recommend that an ECG, echocardiogram, device interrogation, and 24-hour Holter monitor are obtained. β-blockers and class III antiarrhythmic agents (sotalol and amiodarone) are commonly used to reduce arrhythmia burden and avoid ICD discharge.[22,28] We also routinely recommend that patients with ARVD/C, and especially those with significant RV or LV dysfunction, be treated with an angiotensin-converting enzyme inhibitor.

Catheter ablation has increasingly become a useful management tool for arrhythmias that are not controlled by medication.[29] Catheter ablation is generally used to decrease the frequency of episodes of sustained and nonsustained VT. For most patients, one or more antiarrhythmic medications are used initially. But if these medications are ineffective or poorly tolerated, catheter ablation is a reasonable next step. Although endocardial catheter ablation is effective in some, patients often require an epicardial approach. For this reason, our

current approach is to offer patients a combined endocardial/epicardial ablation procedure when catheter ablation is considered. Using this approach, VTs can be controlled in more than 80% of patients.[30]

Exercise and ARVD/C

Competitive athletes with ARVD/C have a five fold relative risk of SCD compared to nonathletes.[24] Individuals diagnosed with ARVD/C are recommended to avoid competitive and most recreational athletics.[31] Even if an ICD has been implanted, physical activity, especially strenuous activity, endurance, and highly competitive athletics, have been associated with an increased risk for acceleration of the disease phenotype.[8,32] Experimental evidence has shown that endurance training in heterozygous JUP-deficient mice accelerates the development of RV dysfunction and arrhythmias.[8] Recently, in the first study in patients, desmosomal mutations carriers that participated in more vigorous activity were more likely to present with ARVD/C, and once diagnosed, more likely to develop arrhythmias and stage C heart failure.[9] Patients should be counseled that significantly reducing physical exercise will not only reduce the risk of ventricular arrhythmias, but also moderate disease progression.[31] There is no evidence of a "safe" heart rate or level of exertion, and further studies are needed to clarify restrictions for patients and their families.

Family Member Screening

First-degree relatives of an ARVD/C proband should have screening with cardiac MRI, ECG, SAECG, exercise stress testing, and 24-hour Holter monitoring. Current recommendations state that this screening should be repeated every 2 to 3 years. Cascade genetic screening of a known genetic mutation in a family is useful to make screening recommendations for relatives. Genetic counseling by a trained professional is also recommended to discuss this option and benefits, limitations, and psychosocial concerns.[33] Mutation carriers should have complete screening described above every 1 to 2 years dictated by level of physical activity. Those who have tested negative for the family mutation have a significantly decreased risk of ARVD/C but are not completely risk-free considering the amount of families known with digenic inheritance of mutations and ambiguity regarding additional genetic and environmental factors contributing to disease.[34] Those testing negative for the family mutation may consider baseline screening with ECG and should have a low threshold to evaluate any symptoms.[1,35]

Age-related penetrance is well established in ARVD/C. Presentation in childhood is exceedingly rare.[1] Screening is recommended to begin around puberty. There is no guaranteed cutoff age at which clinical evaluation may be terminated; however, guidelines suggest that adolescents should be evaluated every 6 to 12 months through the second decade of life, and annually through the fourth decade, with less frequent evaluation afterwards.[1] Regardless, family members should have a low threshold for evaluation of symptoms.

OTHER MANAGEMENT CONSIDERATIONS

Pregnancy

Most individuals with mild to moderate ARVD/C and no symptoms of heart failure tolerate pregnancy well and have uneventful deliveries.[36] Increased evaluation is recommended, including echocardiogram and 24-hour Holter monitoring at baseline, 24-hour Holter monitoring at 7 months gestation, and echocardiogram and 24-hour Holter monitoring at 3 months postpartum. Potential teratogenic effects of medications should be considered. Genetic counseling should be offered regarding risk to offspring.

Psychosocial Counseling

Individuals with ARVD/C have been found to be at significant risk for anxiety and depression, especially in regards to adaptation to living with disease. This is complicated by their young age at presentation and high frequency of arrhythmias, often requiring device shocks.[37] Those without a prior family history have a particularly difficult time. Providers should consider referral for psychological counseling and referral to patient/family support organizations as part of clinical management.

CONCLUSION

In conclusion, ARVD/C is a rare but important cause of life-threatening cardiac arrhythmias resulting from an inherited defect in one or more desmosomal proteins. Patients with ARVD/C generally present with symptoms of the disease after puberty and before the age of 50 years with a mean age at presentation of 31 years. Diagnosis of ARVD/C is made after performing a number of diagnostic tests and is based on the 2010 Task Force Criteria. Important components of management include placement of an implantable defibrillator in high risk patients, antiarrhythmic drug therapy, catheter ablation, and exercise restriction. Cardiac transplantation is rarely required. With appropriate treatment, most patients with ARVD/C live long and high quality lives.

REFERENCES

1. Sen-Chowdhry S, Syrris P, Pantazis A, et al. Mutational heterogeneity, modifier genes, and environmental influences contribute to phenotypic diversity of arrhythmogenic cardiomyopathy. *Circ Cardiovasc Genet.* 2010;3(4):323-330.

2. McKoy G, Protonotarios N, Crosby A, et al. Identification of a deletion in plakoglobin in arrhythmogenic right ventricular cardiomyopathy with palmoplantar keratoderma and woolly hair (Naxos disease). *Lancet.* 2000;355(9221):2119-2124.

3. Sen-Chowdhry S, Syrris P, Ward D, et al. Clinical and genetic characterization of families with arrhythmogenic right ventricular dysplasia/cardiomyopathy provides novel insights into patterns of disease expression. *Circulation.* 2007;115(13):1710-1720.

4. Garcia-Gras E, Lombardi R, Giocondo MJ, et al. Suppression of canonical Wnt/beta-catenin signaling by nuclear plakoglobin recapitulates phenotype of arrhythmogenic right ventricular cardiomyopathy. *J Clin Invest.* 2006;116(7):2012-2021.

5. Delmar M. Desmosome-ion channel interactions and their possible role in arrhythmogenic cardiomyopathy. *Pediatr Cardiol.* 2012;33(6):975-979.

6. Oxford EM, Musa H, Maass K, et al. Connexin43 remodeling caused by inhibition of plakophilin-2 expression in cardiac cells. *Circ Res.* 2007;101(7):703-711.

7. Li D, Liu Y, Maruyama, M, et al. Restrictive loss of plakoglobin in cardiomyocytes leads to arrhythmogenic cardiomyopathy. *Hum Mol Genet.* 2011;20(23):4582-4596.

8. Kirchhof P, Fabritz L, Zwiener M, et al. Age- and training-dependent development of arrhythmogenic right ventricular cardiomyopathy in heterozygous plakoglobin-deficient mice. *Circulation.* 2006;114(17):1799-1806.

9. James CA, Bhonsale A, Tichnell C, et al. Exercise increases penetrance and arrhythmic risk in arrhythmogenic right ventricular dyplasia/cardiomyopathy (ARVD/C). *J Am Coll Cardiol.* 2013;62(14):1290-1297.

10. McKenna WJ, Thiene G, Nava A, et al. Diagnosis of arrhythmogenic right ventricular dysplasia/cardiomyopathy. Task Force of the Working Group Myocardial and Pericardial Disease of the European Society of Cardiology and of the Scientific Council on Cardiomyopathies of the International Society and Federation of Cardiology. *Br Heart J.* 1994;71(3):215-218.

11. Marcus FI, McKenna WJ, Sherrill D, et al. Diagnosis of arrhythmogenic right ventricular cardiomyopathy/dysplasia: proposed modification of the Task Force Criteria. *Eur Heart J* 2010;31(7):806-814.

12. Sen-Chowdhry S, Syrris P, Prasad SK, et al. Left-dominant arrhythmogenic cardiomyopathy: an under-recognized clinical entity. *J Am Coll Cardiol.* 2008;52(25):2175-2187.

13. Gallo P, d'Amati G, and Pelliccia F. Pathologic evidence of extensive left ventricular involvement in arrhythmogenic right ventricular cardiomyopathy. *Hum Pathol.* 1992;23(8):948-952.

14. Burke AP, Farb A, Tashko G, Virmani R. Arrhythmogenic right ventricular cardiomyopathy and fatty replacement of the right ventricular myocardium: are they different diseases? *Circulation.* 1998;97(16):1571-1580.

15. Bomma C, Rutberg J, Tandri H, et al. Misdiagnosis of arrhythmogenic right ventricular dysplasia/cardiomyopathy. *J Cardiovasc Electrophysiol.* 2004;15(3):300-306.

16. Dechering DG, Kochhauser S, Wasmer K, et al. Electrocardiographic characteristics of ventricular tachyarrhythmias in cardiac sarcoidosis versus arrhythmogenic right ventricular cardiomyopathy. *Heart Rhythm.* 2013;10(2):158-164.

17. Steckman DA, Schneider PM, Schuller J, et al. Utility of cardiac magnetic resonance imaging to differentiate cardiac sarcoidosis from arrhythmogenic right ventricular cardiomyopathy. *Am J Cardiol.* 2012;110(4):575-579.

18. Basso C, Thiene G, Corrado D, et al. Arrhythmogenic right ventricular cardiomyopathy. Dysplasia, dystrophy, or myocarditis? *Circulation.* 1996;94(5):983-991.

19. Corrado D, Basso C, Thiene G, et al. Spectrum of clinicopathologic manifestations of arrhythmogenic right ventricular cardiomyopathy/dysplasia: a multicenter study. *J Am Coll Cardiol.* 1997;30(6):1512-1520.

20. Corrado D, Leoni L, Link MS, et al. Implantable cardioverter-defibrillator therapy for prevention of sudden death in patients with arrhythmogenic right ventricular cardiomyopathy/dysplasia. *Circulation.* 2003;108(25):3084-3091.

ARRHYTHMOGENIC RIGHT VENTRICULAR
DYSPLASIA/CARDIOMYOPATHY (ARVD/C)

SECTION VIII
EVALUATION AND MANAGEMENT
OF INHERITED ARRHYTHMIAS

383

21. Corrado D, Calkins H, Link MS, et al. Prophylactic implant-able defibrillator in patients with arrhythmogenic right ventricular cardiomyopathy/dysplasia and no prior ventricular fibrillation or sustained ventricular tachycardia. *Circulation*. 2010;122(12):1144-1152.

22. Wichter T, Paul TM, Eckardt L, et al. Arrhythmogenic right ventricular cardiomyopathy. Antiarrhythmic drugs, catheter ablation, or ICD? *Herz*. 2005;30(2):91-101.

23. Bhonsale A, James CA, Tichnell C, et al. Incidence and predictors of implantable cardioverter-defibrillator therapy in patients with arrhythmogenic right ventricular dysplasia/cardiomyopathy undergoing implantable cardioverter-defibrillator implantation for primary prevention. *J Am Coll Cardiol*. 2011;58(14):1485-1496.

24. Corrado D, Leoni L, Link MS, et al. Implantable cardioverter-defibrillator therapy for prevention of sudden death in patients with arrhythmogenic right ventricular cardiomyopathy/dysplasia. *Circulation*. 2003;108(25):3084-3091.

25. Piccini JP, Dalal D, Roguin A, et al. Predictors of appropriate implantable defibrillator therapies in patients with arrhythmogenic right ventricular dysplasia. *Heart Rhythm*. 2005;2(11):1188-1194.

26. Dalal D, Molin LH, Piccini J, et al. Clinical features of arrhythmogenic right ventricular dysplasia/cardiomyopathy associated with mutations in plakophilin-2. *Circulation*. 2006;113(13):1641-1649.

27. Tedford RJ, James C, Judge DP, et al. Cardiac transplantation in arrhythmogenic right ventricular dysplasia/cardiomyopathy. *J Am Coll Cardiol*. 2012;59(3):289-290.

28. Wichter T, Borggrefe M, Haverkamp W, Chen X, Breithardt G. Efficacy of antiarrhythmic drugs in patients with arrhythmogenic right ventricular disease. Results in patients with inducible and non-inducible ventricular tachycardia. *Circulation*. 1992;86(1): 29-37.

29. Basso C, Bauce B, Corrado D, Thiene G. Pathophysiology of arrhythmogenic cardiomyopathy. *Nat Rev Cardiol*. 2011;9(4):223-233.

30. Philips B, Madhavan S, James C, et al. Outcomes of catheter ablation of ventricular tachycardia in arrhythmogenic right ventricular dysplasia/cardiomyopathy. *Circ Arrhythm Electrophysiol*. 2012;5(3):499-505.

31. Maron BJ, Chaitman BR, Ackerman MJ, et al: Recommendations for physical activity and recreational sports participation for young patients with genetic cardiovascular diseases. *Circulation*. 2004;109(22):2807-2816.

32. Fabritz L, Hoogendijk MG, Scicluna BP, et al. Load-reducing therapy prevents development of arrhythmogenic right ventricular cardiomyopathy in plakoglobin-deficient mice. *J Am Coll Cardiol*. 2011;57(6):740-750.

33. Ackerman MJ, Priori SG, Willems S, et al. HRS/EHRA Expert Consensus Statement on the State of Genetic Testing for the Channelopathies and Cardiomyopathies. *Heart Rhythm*. 2011;8(8):1308-1339.

34. Kapplinger JD, Landstrom AP, Salisbury BA, et al. Distinguishing arrhythmogenic right ventricular cardiomyopathy/dysplasia-associated mutations from background genetic noise. *J Am Coll Cardiol*. 2011;57(23):2317-2237.

35. Corrado D, Thiene G. Arrhythmogenic right ventricular cardiomyopathy/dysplasia: clinical impact of molecular genetic studies. *Circulation*. 2006;113(13):1634-1637.

36. Bauce B, Daliento L, Frigo G, Russo G, Nava A. Pregnancy in women with arrhythmogenic right ventricular cardiomyopathy/dysplasia. *Eur J Obstet Gynecol Reprod Biol*. 2006;127(2):186-189.

37. James CA, Tichnell C, Murray B, et al. General and disease specific psychosocial adjustment in patients with arrhythmogenic right ventricular dysplasia/cardiomyopathy with implantable cardioverter defibrillators: a large cohort study. *Circ Cardiovasc Genet*. 2012;5(1):18-24.

55 ECG CRITERIA AND DRUG CHALLENGE AS DIAGNOSIS FOR BRUGADA SYNDROME

Ruben Casado Arroyo, MD, PhD, Kristel Wauters, MD,
Pedro Brugada, MD, PhD.

CASE PRESENTATION

A 7-year-old child with a family history of sudden cardiac death (SCD) was admitted in our center because of several episodes of syncope. Due to the clinical history, an ajmaline test was performed. The test was stopped early (0.4 mg/kg) due to a positive result (Figures 55-1A and 55-1B). During the following minutes, the ECG shows severe abnormalities of the ventricular repolarization and some episodes of nonsustained ventricular tachycardia (Figure 55-1C). The patient was asymptomatic. An infusion of isoprenaline was started reversing the abnormalities in the ECG.

CONCEPT

Brugada syndrome is an autosomal-dominant, inherited channelo-pathy characterized by ST-segment elevation or J wave in the right precordial leads. First described in 1992,[1] the syndrome is associated with a high incidence of SCD secondary to a rapid polymorphic VT or VF in patients with structurally normal hearts.

EPIDEMIOLOGY

The prevalence of the Brugada ECG pattern is variable, ranging from 3% in endemic areas of Southeast Asia to 0.61% in Europe. In the United States, the prevalence ranges from 0.012% to 0.43%. However, because the diagnostic ECG pattern can be intermittently present or concealed, it is difficult to estimate the true prevalence of the disease in the general population.[2-4] In up to 60% of patients the

disease can be sporadic. Although the disease is inherited as an autosomal-dominant, there is a male predominance in its phenotype. It suggests that gender- and age-related factors (eg, sex hormones) may play a role in triggering the arrhythmia in Brugada syndrome. The age of onset of clinical manifestations (syncope or cardiac arrest) is the third to fourth decade of life.[5]

ETIOLOGY AND PATHOPHYSIOLOGY

The ST-T wave changes in Brugada syndrome likely reflect a profound change in the process of ventricular repolarization. Three different theories have attempted to explain the syndrome: the depolarization theory, the repolarization theory, and the neural crest theory.[6-8]

DIAGNOSIS

The diagnosis of Brugada syndrome (BS) requires the presence of a type 1 BS pattern in the right precordial leads (ie, V_1-V_3), either spontaneous or unmasked by class I antiarrhythmic drugs (Table 55-1), characterized by a prominent coved ST-segment elevation displaying J-point amplitude or ST-segment elevation ≥2 mm, followed by a negative T wave. The type 2 BS pattern (≥2 mm J-point elevation, ≥1 mm ST-segment elevation, and a saddleback appearance, followed by a positive or biphasic T wave), and type 3 BS pattern (either a saddleback or coved appearance, but with an ST segment elevation <1 mm) are considered to be suggestive but not confirmatory of the disease (Figure 55-2).

The diagnosis of BS is based on clinical diagnostic criteria (Table 55-2). Right bundle branch block may be associated with BS, but its presence is not required for the diagnosis (Figure 55-3). The drug challenge test involves administration of ajmaline, flecainide, procainamide, or pilsicainide under close cardiac monitoring and in a setting that is equipped for resuscitation. Procainamide remains the only choice for intravenous pharmacological induction protocols in the United States, despite consensus that both ajmaline and flecainide appear to be more efficacious. The drug challenge test is finished when (1) the diagnostic type 1 ST-segment elevation develops, (2) the ST segment elevation in type 2 ECG pattern increases by at least 2 mm, (3) PVCs or other arrhythmias develop, or (4) the QRS widens by 30% or more. Although the drug challenge test is generally

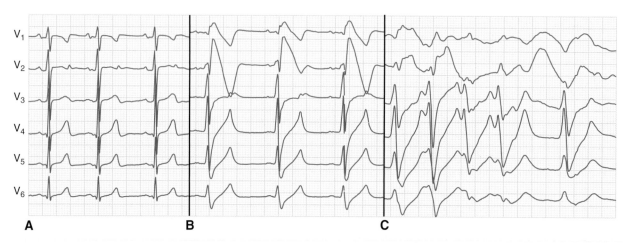

FIGURE 55-1 (A) Basal ECG of a 7-year-old child (type 2). (B) ECG positive for Brugada syndrome (type 1) during ajmaline infusion. The infusion was stopped after the positive result. (C) NSVT observed two minutes after stopping the infusion of ajmaline.

ECG CRITERIA AND DRUG CHALLENGE AS
DIAGNOSIS FOR BRUGADA SYNDROME

SECTION VIII
EVALUATION AND MANAGEMENT
OF INHERITED ARRHYTHMIAS

385

TABLE 55-1 Drugs Used to Unmask Brugada Syndrome

Drug	Dosage	Administration
Ajmaline	1 mg/kg over 5 min	IV
Flecainide	2 mg/kg over 10 min	IV
	400 mg	PO
Procainamide	10 mg/kg over 10 min	IV
Pilsicainide	1 mg/kg over 10 min	IV

safe, it can potentially precipitate malignant cardiac arrhythmias or advanced AV block, particularly in patients with preexisting intraventricular conduction disturbances (wide QRS complex) or infranodal AV conduction delay. Isoproterenol and sodium lactate can be effective antidotes in this setting.

Diagnostic genetic testing may be considered for patients who clinically manifest with symptoms of Brugada syndrome. Although the knowledge of a specific mutation may not provide guidance for determining prognosis or treatment, identification of a disease-causing mutation in the family can lead to genetic identification of at-risk family members who are clinically asymptomatic and who may have normal ECGs. However, it is important to remember that a negative result of genetic testing does not exclude the presence of the disease and, therefore, only a positive genetic diagnosis is informative.

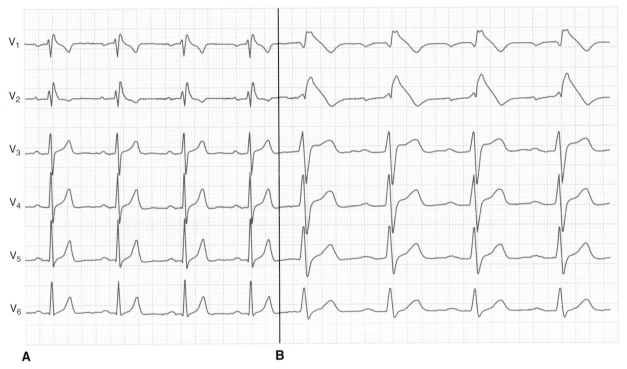

FIGURE 55-2 ECG patterns associated with Brugada syndrome. (A) Type 2 ECG (suspicious); (B) Type 1 ECG (diagnostic).

DIFFERENTIAL DIAGNOSIS

A group of diseases may cause development of ST-segment elevation in the right precordial leads, mimicking the BS ECG pattern (Table 55-3). Exposure to some drugs and ionic imbalance may produce a Brugada-like pattern, which may represent a genetic predisposition to BS (Table 55-4). Fever also modulates the phenotype and risk of arrhythmias in BS patients by causing accentuation of the inactivation of the Na+ channel, showing a type 1 ECG pattern and triggering ventricular arrhythmias.

MANAGEMENT

Currently, an ICD is the only proven effective treatment for Brugada syndrome. ICD implantation is recommended in patients with type 1 Brugada ECG (either spontaneously or after Na+ channel

blockade) and a history of aborted SCD or related symptoms such as syncope, seizure, or nocturnal agonal respiration, given that noncardiac causes of these symptoms have been carefully excluded. ICD devices need to be carefully programmed in Brugada syndrome patients in order to avoid inappropriate shocks, given the high incidence of supraventricular arrhythmias in this population. Programming a single VF zone of more than 210 beats/min with a monitor is preferable.

PATIENT EDUCATION

Fever may induce the appearance of a type 1 BS ECG pattern and may trigger episodes of ventricular arrhythmias in BS patients. In the case of fever, close ECG monitoring is appropriate in combination with lowering body temperature. BS patients should be advised to avoid all drugs that may induce a type 1 ECG or trigger

TABLE 55-2 Diagnostic Criteria of Brugada Syndrome.

Appearance of a type 1 ST-segment elevation (coved-type) ≥2 mm in more than one right precordial lead (V₁-V₃):

- Either spontaneously
- Or after sodium-blocker exposure

And one of the following:

• Documented ventricular fibrillation • (Self-terminating) polymorphic ventricular tachycardia • Inducibility of ventricular arrhythmias with programmed electrical stimulation.	Documented ventricular arrhythmias
Family history of sudden death before 45 y • Presence of a coved-type ECG in family members	Family history
• Syncope • Nocturnal agonal respiration	Arrhythmia-related symptoms

Other factor(s) accounting for the ECG abnormality should be ruled out.

CHAPTER 55

TABLE 55-3 Differential Diagnosis of ECG Abnormalities That Can Lead to ST-Segment Elevation in V₁-V₃

Atypical right bundle branch block	Dissecting aortic aneurysm
Acute myocardial infarction, especially of RV	Central and autonomic nervous system disorders
Hemopericardium	Duchenne muscular dystrophy
Acute pericarditis/ myopericarditis	Friedreich Ataxia
Pulmonary embolism	LV hypertrophy
Mechanical compression of RV outflow tract	Arrhythmogenic RV cardiomyopathy
Mediastinal tumor	Pectus excavatum
After electrical cardioversion	Early repolarization, especially in athletes
Hypothermia	Hyperkalemia
Hypercalcemia	

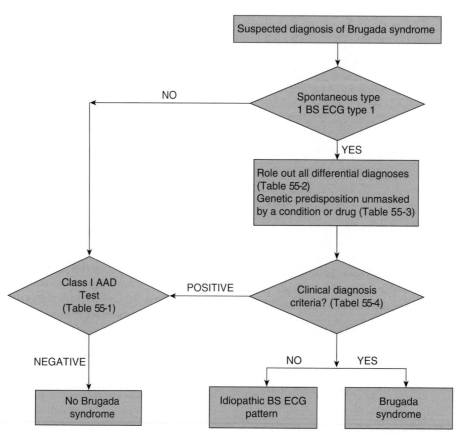

FIGURE 55-3 Diagnostic algorithm for Brugada syndrome.

ECG CRITERIA AND DRUG CHALLENGE AS
DIAGNOSIS FOR BRUGADA SYNDROME

SECTION VIII
EVALUATION AND MANAGEMENT
OF INHERITED ARRHYTHMIAS

387

TABLE 55-4 Drugs That Can Lead to ST-Segment Elevation in V_1-V_3.

Cocaine intoxication

Alcohol intoxication

Treatment with:

Antiarrhythmic drugs:

- Na channel blockers (class Ic, class Ia)

- Calcium channel blockers

- β-Blockers

Antianginal drugs:

- Calcium channel blockers

- Nitrates

Psychotropic drugs:

- Tricyclic antidepressants

- Tetracyclic antidepressants

- Phenothiazines

- Selective serotonin reuptake inhibitors

- Lithium

ventricular arrhythmias.[9] All BS patients must be followed-up on a regular basis, in order to identify the development of symptoms.

REFERENCES

1. Brugada P, Brugada J. Right bundle branch block, persistent ST segment elevation and sudden cardiac death: a distinct clinical and electrocardiographic syndrome. A multicenter report. *J Am Coll Cardiol*. 1992;20(6):1391-1396.

2. Rossenbacker T, Priori SG. The Brugada syndrome. *Curr Opin Cardiol*. 2007;22(3):163-170.

3. Campuzano O, Brugada R, Iglesias A. Genetics of Brugada syndrome. *Curr Opin Cardiol*. 2010;25(3):210-215.

4. Morita H, Zipes DP, Wu J. Brugada syndrome: insights of ST elevation, arrhythmogenicity, and risk stratification from experimental observations. *Heart Rhythm*. 2009;6(Suppl 11):S34-S43.

5. Antzelevitch C, Brugada P, Borggrefe M, et al. Brugada syndrome: report of the second consensus conference: endorsed by the Heart Rhythm Society and the European Heart Rhythm Association. *Circulation*. 2005;111(5):659-670.

6. Coronel R, Casini S, Koopmann TT, et al. Right ventricular fibrosis and conduction delay in a patient with clinical signs of Brugada syndrome: a combined electrophysiological, genetic, histopathologic, and computational study. *Circulation*. 2005;112(18):2769-2777.

7. Antzelevitch C. The Brugada syndrome: ionic basis and arrhythmia mechanisms. *J Cardiovasc Electrophysiol*. 2001;12(7):268-272.

8. Elizari MV, Levi R, Acunzo RS, et al. Abnormal expression of cardiac neural crest cells in heart development: a different hypothesis for the etiopathogenesis of Brugada syndrome. *Heart Rhythm*. 2007;4(3):359-365.

9. www.brugadadrugs.org

56 CATECHOLAMINERGIC POLYMORPHIC VENTRICULAR TACHYCARDIA

Matthew Needleman, MD, and Mark Haigney, MD

CASE PRESENTATION

A 16-year-old boy presents for evaluation after a syncopal episode associated with exercise in gym class. Further questioning reveals that the patient has had two syncopal episodes in the 3 years prior to his current presentation, one during a track meet, and the other during a soccer game. The patient is otherwise healthy, has no medical problems, and is not taking any medications. His family history is significant for a younger brother with a "seizure" disorder. The patient also has a maternal uncle who died after he "lost control" and fell off a bicycle during a cycling race.

Physical examination was normal. The baseline electrocardiogram revealed sinus bradycardia with a normal QT interval and no pathologic changes. Echocardiography revealed a structurally normal heart with no abnormalities. An exercise test was then performed. In early stages of exercise, there were frequent monomorphic PVCs, but in later stages of exercise the patient developed bidirectional VT. The patient became presyncopal during the treadmill test, and the test was stopped.

The patient was started on nadolol after the treadmill test. An implantable loop recorder was placed. Genetic testing was ordered, and the patient was found to have a ryanodine receptor (RyR2) mutation confirming the diagnosis of catecholaminergic polymorphic ventricular tachycardia (CPVT). Despite being on nadolol therapy, the patient experienced another syncopal episode during an episode of emotional stress, which correlated with ventricular tachycardia (Figures 56-1 and 56-2). Given his arrhythmogenic syncope despite β-blocker therapy, it was felt that an implantable cardioverter defibrillator would be appropriate, and this was placed. In addition, the patient was started on flecainide therapy with no recurrent syncopal events in follow-up.

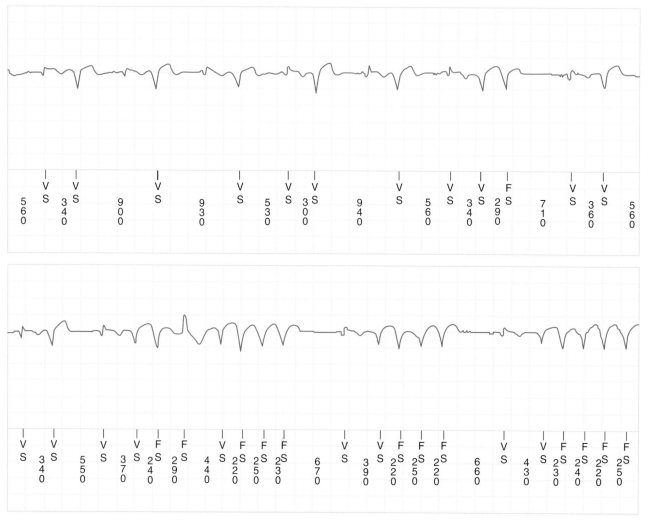

FIGURE 56-1 Implantable loop recorder in early exercise showing monomorphic premature ventricular contractions followed by salvos of polymorphic ventricular tachycardia.

CATECHOLAMINERGIC POLYMORPHIC
VENTRICULAR TACHYCARDIA

SECTION VIII
EVALUATION AND MANAGEMENT
OF INHERITED ARRHYTHMIAS

389

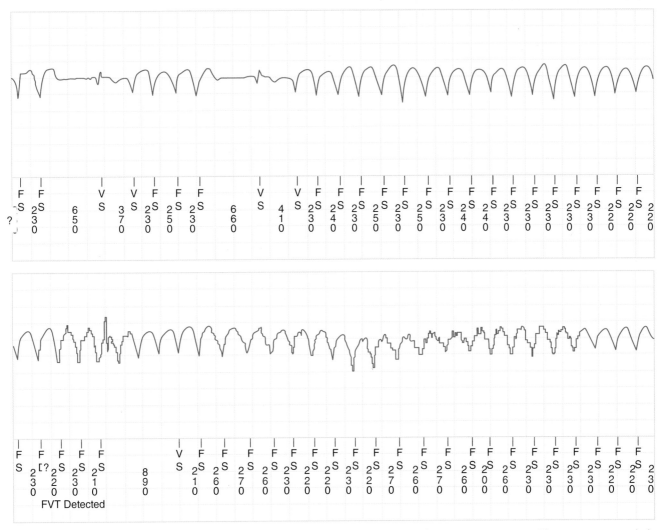

FIGURE 56-2 Implantable loop recorder showing sustained polymorphic ventricular tachycardia as exercise continues. This event was recorded as presyncope by the patient.

CASE EXPLANATION

Syncope during exercise is always concerning and requires a thorough evaluation. In patients with a structurally normal heart, the differential for a genetic electrical disorder includes the long QT syndromes, the short QT syndrome, Brugada syndrome, the Haissaguerre syndrome (idiopathic ventricular fibrillation associated with early repolarization), and CPVT. Of these syndromes, only CPVT has a normal baseline electrocardiogram with a normal QT interval. In addition to the baseline normal electrocardiogram, hallmarks of this syndrome include polymorphic or bidirectional VT that is reproducible with exercise and a family history of sudden death or syncope in an autosomal-dominant pattern. Based on recent investigations into the genetics of intracellular calcium regulation, the understanding of this disease has expanded, and this chapter will review the molecular genetics and discuss management of this newly described disease.

EPIDEMIOLOGY

- The first case report of CPVT was reported in 1975. A case series of four children with bidirectional ventricular tachycardia that was catecholamine-induced was reported in 1978.

- Multiple different cases series have now been reported, and currently it is estimated that the prevalence of the disease in 1:10,000 in Europe.[1]

- The syndrome is usually diagnosed in children and adolescents, although typically not before 2 years of age.

- The mortality of CPVT is 31% in untreated adults by the age of 30.[1]

PATHOPHYSIOLOGY

Calcium leakage from the sarcoplasmic reticulum (SR) is the mechanism of cellular cystolic calcium overload, resulting in CPVT. Normal calcium regulation during cardiac muscle contraction occurs in the SR and is controlled by the macromolecule called the calcium release complex (CRC)[2] which is composed of the following:

The Cardiac Ryanodine Receptor (RyR2)[3]

- This is the main calcium release channel present in the SR.
- RyR2 is a large protein with a large cytoplasmic footprint that allows regulatory proteins to modulate its function.

- The channel works though calcium-induced calcium release.
  - Calcium binds to RyR2 and triggers opening of L-type calcium channel, allowing rapid calcium to efflux from the SR.

Calsequestrin (CASQ2)

- Calsequestrin is a large acidic protein that serves as a calcium buffer within the SR.
- Mechanistically, CASQ2 though interactions with triadin and junction confer RyR2 calcium luminal sensitivity such that CASQ2 inhibits RYR2 calcium release at low luminal calcium levels.[4]

Triadin and Junctin[2]

- Trisk 32 is an isoform of triadin found in cardiac muscle.
- Two isoforms of junctin are found in both skeletal muscle and cardiac muscle.
- Knockout mice of both Trisk 32 and junctin have resulted in fatal arrhythmias.
- These proteins anchor CSQ2 to RyR2 and work though a complex mechanism with CASQ2 to regulate SR calcium through the RYR2 membrane channel.
- Mutations in RyR2, CASQ2, and triadin lead to cystolic calcium overload, which generates delayed after depolarizations (DADs), triggered activity, and ventricular arrhythmias.
- Adrenergic stimulation results in an increased open probability of the RYR2 though phosphorylation of regulatory component of the RYR2, leading to higher levels of cytosolic calcium.
- In mouse models of CPVT, it appears that there is Purkinje origin of the ventricular premature beats resulting from calcium overload.[5]

ETIOLOGY

As our understanding of molecular genetics increases, mutations in the RyR2 membrane channel, calsequestrin, and tritan have been identified.

Mutations in RyR2

- RyR2 mutations are the most frequent mutations identified in CPVT.
- The typical pattern identified was found to be autosomal dominant and was found on chromosome 1q42-43.[6]
- RyR2 is a 4967-amino acid protein, one of the largest genes in the human genome, with 105 exons.
- At least 50 mutations have been identified in RYR2 that are likely associated with CPVT, although some mutations have been found in arrhythmogenic right ventricular cardiomyopathy.
- Most mutations occur in the N-terminal region, the central zone, or in the c-terminal region and are missense mutations.
- Despite having a disease-associated mutation, relatives carrying an RYR2 mutation have marked phenotypic variability, and no genetic genotype-phenotype correlations have been established.[7]

Mutations in CASQ2

- Mutations in CASQ2 are less common and have been described to map to chromosome 1p13-21.[8]

- CASQ2 is a 399 amino acid protein, and over 20 unique disease-causing mutations in this protein have been described.
- Approximately half the mutations are missense mutations, and the other half lead to premature stop codons, leading to a truncated protein.
- Phenotypically, patients with a single CASQ2 mutation have less severe symptoms than CPVT patients with RYR2 mutations, but patients with multiple mutations have been described and are susceptible to ventricular arrhythmias.

Mutations in Triadin[2]

- Three unique mutations of triadin have been identified in patients with clinical CPVT who do not have mutations in RYR2 or CASQ2. Two of these mutations resulted in a premature stop codon, and another led to a missense mutation.
- As some of these mutations affect all triadin isoforms, skeletal muscle could be affected, and muscle weakness has been observed in at least one patient with a triadin stop codon mutation.

Other Described Mutations

- A mutation on chromosome 7p14-p22 has also been described in an autosomal recessive Arab family with an early onset lethal form of CPVT, but no specific gene or protein in calcium regulation has been identified.[9]
- Despite the known mutations previously described, a genetic cause is only found in 60% of cases of CPVT.

DIAGNOSIS

Clinical Presentation

- Syncope typically occurs during the first or second decade of life.
- Syncope is triggered by emotional stress or exercise.
- In children and young adults, syncope with seizure is often seen, and epilepsy is frequently misdiagnosed. Often, there may be a 2-year delay in the correct diagnosis.
- Depending on the causative mutation, there is usually a family history of syncope, seizure, or sudden death in approximately 30% of patients. An autosomal-dominant pattern suggests a RYR2 mutation whereas an autosomal-recessive pattern suggests a CASQ2 mutation.
- Exercise or emotional syncope with muscle weakness suggests a possible triadin mutation.[2]

Objective Findings

- The baseline resting electrocardiogram is normal with a normal QT interval.
- A low resting heart rate has been described in some patients with a RyR2 mutation. Mechanistically, it appears that increased RyR2 activity decreases sinus node activity by calcium dependent decrease in diastolic calcium, which decreases automaticity.[10]
- Atrial fibrillation is also seen in patients with CPVT. In a similar mechanism, RyR2 diastolic SR calcium leak appears to be associated with AF development in patients with CPVT.[11]

CATECHOLAMINERGIC POLYMORPHIC
VENTRICULAR TACHYCARDIA

SECTION VIII
EVALUATION AND MANAGEMENT
OF INHERITED ARRHYTHMIAS

391

Symptoms

-Exercise- or emotion-induced syncope
-Family history of sudden cardiac death
-Frequent misdiagnosis of child with a "seizure" disorder
-Diagnosis usually occurs within the first and second decade of life

Diagnostics

-Normal baseline electrocardiogram with normal baseline QT interval
-A lower than normal heart rate is typically recorded
-Exercise treadmill test with monomorphic ventricular ectopy followed by either polymorphic or bidirectional ventricular tachycardia
-Holter monitoring and/or implantable loop recorders frequently increase diagnostic yield
-Genetic testing-RyR2 mutations and CASQ2 mutations are found in 60% of patients with CPVT

FIGURE 56-3 Summary of historical and objective findings in CPVT.

- The heart is structurally normal on echocardiogram and cardiac MRI.

- Exercise testing or Holter monitoring during exercise typically reveals monomorphic ventricular premature beats at low heart rates. As the heart rate accelerates, the ventricular ectopy becomes more polymorphic and can become bidirectional (see Figures 56-2 and 56-3).

- The premature ventricular beats usually have right bundle branch block morphology with a left axis deviation, consistent with a left ventricular source.[12]

- If exercise continues, salvos of polymorphic ventricular tachycardia can occur and be sustained, leading to syncope.

- There is mixed evidence for the diagnostic benefit of an epinephrine infusion for inducing polymorphic ventricular tachycardia. In one study, the sensitivity of an epinephrine infusion was 28% and should not be considered routinely as a diagnostic alternative to exercise testing.[13]

- Polymorphic or biventricular tachycardia is usually not induced with programmed stimulation.

- In younger patients who may be noncompliant with exercise testing or Holter monitoring, there may be a diagnostic benefit to placement of an implantable loop recorder.

- The differential diagnosis for bidirectional ventricular tachycardia includes CPVT, Andersen-Tawil syndrome, and digoxin toxicity. Only CPVT should have normal baseline electrocardiogram, whereas Andersen-Tawil syndrome patients typically have a distinct T-U wave morphology that may aid in diagnosis.

Genetic Testing

- Commercially available genetic testing is currently available for mutations in RyR2 and calsequestrin only. Genetic mutations are found in approximately 60% of patients with CPVT, suggesting that there are other genes and mutations involved that have not been discovered yet.[1]

MANAGEMENT (FIGURE 56-4)

Exercise restriction is required in all patients with CPVT.

Medical Therapies

β-Blockers

- β-Blockers without sympathomimetic activity are the first-line medical therapy.

- Nadolol is the preferred prophylactic therapy, and the dose typically required to reduce symptoms such as syncope is 1.8 mg/kg.[1]

- Even in patients on adequate dosage of β-blockers, there is a 27% cardiac event rate. In this study, independent predictors of cardiac events were younger age at time of diagnosis and absence of β-blockers.[14]

- After an appropriate β-blocker titration, repeat exercise testing and/or Holter monitoring should be performed to document appropriate prevention of heart rates that may result in ventricular arrhythmias.

- Couplets and higher degree of ventricular arrhythmias on Holter monitoring suggest a higher cardiac event rate and indicate that medical therapy should be intensified.

- The importance of daily compliance with β-blockers should be stressed with patients and their families.

Flecainide

- Flecainide likely prevents spontaneous calcium release by inhibiting RyR2 and also prevents triggering of action potentials by inhibiting sodium channels. Both properties allow Flecainide to significantly reduce ventricular arrhythmias.

- In a study of 33 patients who had ventricular arrhythmias despite β-blocker therapy, 76% of patients had either partial or complete relief of ventricular arrhythmias when Flecainide was added to a β-blocker.[15]

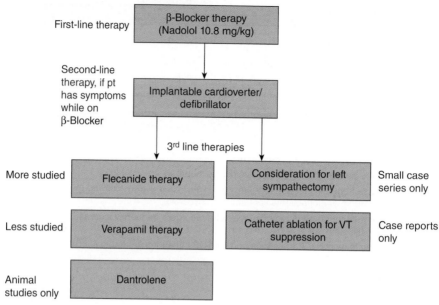

FIGURE 56-4 Summary of treatment options available in CPVT.

- Flecainide has also been shown to be useful in terminating defibrillator-induced storming of ICD discharges resulting from the hyperadrenergic state of the post-shock period.[16]

Verapamil

- In a small study of 5 patients with CPVT, adding verapamil to a β-blocker reduced ventricular arrhythmias better than β-blockers alone in short-term follow-up.[17]

Dantrolene

- Dantrolene reduces calcium leakage though skeletal muscle RyR1 and has been found to have effect on the RyR2 cardiac channel as well. In a mouse model, dantrolene was shown to have some benefit in reduction of arrhythmias, but human studies are in progress.[18]

Other Available Therapies

Implantable Cardioverter Defibrillator (ICD) Therapy

- ICD therapy is generally recommended for patients with CPVT and syncope despite β-blocker therapy, or documented sustained VT despite β-blocker therapy.

- ICD therapy is also indicated for secondary prevention of sudden cardiac death in patients with CPVT.

- Because ICD shocks provoke adrenaline release, ICDs can have proarrhythmic effects and induce a dangerous vicious cycle of shocks with additional sympathetic stimulation leading to defibrillator-induced storming.[19]

- Placement of ICDs in children and adolescents also carries a higher risk than typically described in adults such as multiple interventions for lead complications and revisions for growing.

Left Cardiac Sympathetic Denervation

- In small case series of 13 CPVT patients with refractory arrhythmias, despite β-blocker therapy left cardiac sympathetic denervation

has proven beneficial in reducing ventricular arrhythmias.[20] Longer term multicenter studies are still needed.

Catheter Ablation

- Successful catheter ablation for bidirectional ventricular tachycardia associated with CPVT in patients with recurrent ventricular ectopy has been described in case reports.[12]

Figure 56-4 summarizes the treatment options available for CPVT.

FOLLOW-UP AND LONG-TERM COMPLICATIONS

- A family history of syncope, a seizure disorder, or sudden cardiac death is reported in 30% of family members of patients with CPVT.

- Given that RyR2 mutations are inherited in an autosomal dominant pattern, screening of asymptomatic family members is necessary.

- In a large study, the event rates in "asymptomatic" family members with genetic mutations were similar to that of the index case in the family.[14]

- Despite the phenotypic variability, frequent reevaluation with exercise testing, Holter monitoring, and/or implantable loop recorder and consideration of β-blocker therapy should occur in all genetic mutation patients regardless of initial symptoms.

REFERENCES

1. Leenhardt A, Denjoy I, Guicheney P. Catecholaminergic polymorphic ventricular tachycardia. *Circ Arrhythm Electrophysiol.* 2012;5(5):1044-1052.

2. Roux-Buisson N, Cacheux M, Fourest-Lieuvin A, et al. Absence of triadin, a protein of the calcium release complex, is responsible for cardiac arrhythmia with sudden death in human. *Hum Mol Genet.* 2012;21(12):2759-2767.

3. Kushnir A, Marks AR. The ryanodine receptor in cardiac physiology and disease. *Adv Pharmacol.* 2010;59:1-30.

CATECHOLAMINERGIC POLYMORPHIC
VENTRICULAR TACHYCARDIA

SECTION VIII
EVALUATION AND MANAGEMENT
OF INHERITED ARRHYTHMIAS

393

4. Gyorke I, Nester N, Jones LR, Gyorke S. The role of calsequestrin, triadin, and junction in conferring cardiac ryanodine receptor responsiveness to luminal calcium. *Biophys J.* 2004;86(4): 2121-2128.

5. Herron TJ, Milstein ML, Anumonwo J, et al. Purkinje cell calcium dysregulation is the cellular mechanism that underlies catecholaminergic polymorphic ventricular tachycardia. *Heart Rhythm.* 2012;7(8):1122-1128.

6. Priori SG, Napolitano C, Tiso N, et al. Mutations in the cardiac ryanodine receptor gene (hRyR2) underlie catecholaminergic polymorphic ventricular tachycardia. *Circulation.* 2001;103(2): 196-200.

7. Van der Werf C, Nederend I, Hofman N, et al. Familial evaluation in catecholaminergic polymorphic ventricular tachycardia: disease penetrance and expression in cardiac ryanodine receptor mutation-carrying relatives. *Circ Arrhythm Electrophysiol.* 2012;5(4):748-756.

8. Lahat H, Eldar M, Levy-Nissenbaum E, et al. Autosomal recessive catecholamine- or exercise-induced polymorphic ventricular tachycardia: clinical features and assignment of the disease gene to chromosome 1p13-21. *Circulation.* 2001;103(12):2822-2827.

9. Bhuiyan ZA, Hamdan MA, Shamsi ETA, et al. A novel early onset lethal form of catecholaminericpolymprphic ventricular tachycardia maps to chromosome 7p14-p22. *J Cardiovasc Electrophysiol.* 2007;18(10):1060-1066.

10. Neco P, Torrente AG, Mesirca P, et al. Paradoxical effect of increased diastolic Ca2+ release and decreased sinoatrial node activity in a mouse model of catecholaminergic polymorphic ventricular tachycardia. *Circulation.* 2012;126(4):392-401.

11. Shan J, Xie W, Betzenhauser M, et al. Calcium leak though ryanodine receptors leads to atrial fibrillation in 3 mouse models of catecholaminergic polymorphic ventricular tachycardia. *Circ Res.* 2012;111(6):708-717.

12. Kaneshiro T, Naruse Y, Nogami A, et al. Successful catheter ablation of bidirectional ventricular premature contractions triggering ventricular fibrillation in catecholaminergic polymorphic ventricular tachycardia with RyR2 mutation. *Circ Arrhythm Electrophysiol.* 2012;5(1):e14-e17.

13. Marjamaa A, Hiippala A, Arrhenius B, et al. Intravenous epinephrine infusion test in diagnosis of catecholaminergic polymorphic ventricular tachycardia. *J Cardiovasc Electrophysiol.* 2012;23(2): 194-199.

14. Hayashi M, Denjoy I, Extramiana F, et al. Incidence and risk factors of arrhythmic events in catecholaminergic polymorphic ventricular tachycardia. *Circulation.* 2009;119(18):2426-2434.

15. Van der Werf C, Kannankeril PJ, Sacher F, et al. Flecanide therapy reduces exercise-induced ventricular arrhythmias in patients with catecholaminergic polymorphic ventricular tachycardia. *J Am Coll Cardiol.* 2011;57(22):2244-2254.

16. Hong RA, Rivera KK, Jittirat A, Choi JJ. Flecanide suppresses defibrillator-induced storming in catecholaminergic polymorphic ventricular tachycardia. *PACE.* 2012;35(7):794-979.

17. Rosso R, Kalman JM, Rogowski O, et al. Calcium channel blockers and beta-blockers versus beta-blockers alone for preventing exercise-induced arrhythmias in catecholaminergic polymoprphic ventricular tachycardia. *Heart Rhythm.* 2007;4(9):1149-1154.

18. Kobayashi S, Yano M, Uchinoumi H, et al. Dantroline, a therapeutic agent for malignant hyperthermia, inhibits catecholaminergic polymorphic ventricular tachycardia in RyR2(R2474s/+) knock-in mouse model. *Circ J.* 2010;74(12):2579-2584.

19. Mohamed U, Gollob MH, Gow RM, Krahn AD. Sudden cardiac death despite an implantable cardioverter-defibrillator in a young female with catecholaminergic ventricular tachycardia. *Heart Rhythm.* 2006;31(12):1480-1489.

20. Coleman MA, Bos JM, Johnson JN, et al. Videoscopic left cardiac sympathetic denervation of patients with recurrent ventricular fibrillation/malignant ventricular arrhythmia syndromes besides congenital long-QT syndrome. *Circ Arrhythm Electrophysiol.* 2012;5(4):782-788.

IMPLANTABLE CARDIAC DEVICES FOR MANAGEMENT OF MALIGNANT VENTRICULAR ARRHYTHMIAS AND TREATMENT OF HEART FAILURE

57 MAGNETIC RESONANCE IMAGING AND CARDIAC IMPLANTABLE ELECTRONIC DEVICES

Troy Rhodes, MD, PhD, FHRS, CCDS

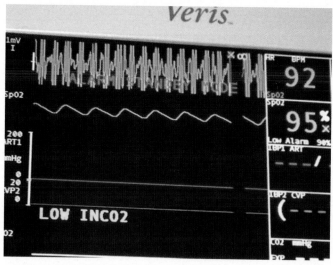

FIGURE 57-1 Patient monitor showing ECG lead artifact during MRI while pulse oximetry (SpO₂) is not affected. (Used with permission of Charles J. Love, MD.)

CASE PRESENTATION

A 67-year-old woman with a history of sick sinus syndrome underwent dual chamber pacemaker implantation in 1997. She developed persistent atrial fibrillation (AF) and underwent two left atrial ablations, but with recurrent AF had difficulty controlling ventricular rates leading to AV junction ablation. With chronic right ventricular pacing, she developed a nonischemic cardiomyopathy (LVEF 35%) and underwent upgrade to a biventricular pacemaker (Boston Scientific Contak Renewal) with the addition of St Jude Medical 1058T QuickSite XL in November 2008. Her existing right atrial and right ventricular leads (SJM 1188T Tendril, SJM 1246T Passive Plus TiN) had stable lead performance at upgrade. She is device-dependent with underlying sinus rhythm and complete AV block with ventricular asystole.

In 2010, she presented with retro-orbital headaches with head CT demonstrating a pituitary mass, followed by trans-sphenoidal resection with pathology showing an arachnoid cyst. Her headaches resolved following surgery, but she recently had recurrent headaches, and repeat CT imaging showed a residual mass in the left aspect of the sella turcica. Neurosurgery recommended brain magnetic resonance imaging (MRI) to further evaluate the residual mass and the association between arachnoid cysts and type 1 Chiari malformation.

Prior to MRI, device interrogation showed normal device and lead function. Unfortunately, an asynchronous mode (DOO) was not an available mode; therefore, her device was programmed DDI, magnet response was disabled, and the ventricular sensitivity was increased to 10 mV. Due to magnetic interference with ECG telemetry, the pulse oximetry waveform was monitored (Figure 57-1) with no ectopy, inhibition, or tracking noted. Following completion of her MRI, device interrogation showed stable sensing, capture thresholds, and impedances, and her initial device programming (DDDR) was restored.

MAGNETIC RESONANCE IMAGING FOLLOWING DEVICE IMPLANTATION

MRI is considered a relative contraindication for patients with conventional pacemakers and implantable cardioverter defibrillators (ICDs). As with this patient, it is anticipated that 50% to 75% of patients will have the need for a clinically indicated MRI during the lifetime of their device.[1]

There are multiple potential adverse interactions between a strong magnetic field and cardiac implantable electronic devices (CIEDs) including device movement, lead tip heating with thermal injury or changes in lead performance (sensing, capture thresholds, impedance),

MAGNETIC RESONANCE IMAGING AND CARDIAC
IMPLANTABLE ELECTRONIC DEVICES

SECTION IX
IMPLANTABLE CARDIAC DEVICES FOR
MANAGEMENT OF MALIGNANT

397

unpredictable magnetic sensor activation, reed-switch closure, rapid or asynchronous pacing, inhibition of pacing, inappropriate tachyarrhythmia therapies, programming alterations, battery consumption, damage to device circuitry, and arrhythmias.[2-10] Deaths associated with MRIs have been reported; all occurred during scans not supervised by a physician.[10-12] Hence the exact mechanism of death was not determined, although in one report, ventricular fibrillation was believed to the mechanism.[10]

The 2007 American Heart Association Guidelines outlined recommendations for device settings and safety monitoring during MRI but did not endorse MRI in patients with CIEDs.[13] MRI of patients with CIEDs should only be considered with compelling circumstances, and the risks and benefits for the patient should be established and documented. Several centers have offered MRI to patients with CIEDs but have excluded patients with abandoned or epicardial leads. Some centers have excluded device pacemaker-dependent patients due to the concern for power-on reset, in which the battery voltage decreases below a critical preset level, leading to unpredictable device operation. After the battery voltage recovers, the device typically resets to the manufacturer's nominal settings. The following recommendations are a compilation of the AHA Guidelines[13] and published protocols from academic centers.[14-18]

1. Patients with non-MR conditional pacemakers and ICDs ("legacy devices") with mature lead systems (>6 weeks) can be considered for MRI.

2. Prior to MRI, device interrogation should be performed to evaluate battery status, sensing, capture threshold, and lead impedances. Patients with devices that show abnormal or inadequate performance (ie, elevated capture threshold, pacing impedance, or depleted battery voltage) are not recommended to undergo scanning.

3. In patients who are not dependent upon pacing, some centers reprogram the device to an asynchronous mode (DOO, VOO) while others program a nonpacing mode (ODO, DDI, VVI). Reed switch activation by the magnetic field can result in magnet mode pacing; programming the device to an asynchronous mode should theoretically prevent this but it has still been seen in some patients.

4. Magnet, rate response, PVC, noise, ventricular sense, conducted atrial fibrillation (AF) response, and tachyarrhythmia therapies are disabled.

5. MR scanning should be performed at experienced centers with expertise in MRI and electrophysiology. A physician with MRI expertise should be involved optimally to plan the scan and minimize patient risk. MRI has been performed with a 1.5 Tesla magnet and the absorption rate is limited to 1.5 w/kg for a maximum of 30 minutes.

6. Informed consent should be obtained from the patient and should specifically list the risks including device dysfunction and/or damage, arrhythmia, and death.

7. The patient's vitals and heart rhythm should be monitored, and visual and voice contact should be maintained throughout the MRI. The patient should be instructed to report any concerns or unusual sensations. A physician with device expertise and a crash cart with external defibrillator and programmer should be present during scanning.

8. The device should be interrogated immediately after the MRI to evaluate lead and device performance and restore baseline programming.

MRI-CONDITIONAL PACEMAKER

In February 2011, the U.S. Food and Drug Administration (FDA) approved an MRI-conditional pacemaker for marketing in the United States (EnRhythm MRI SureScan Pacing System, Medtronic, Inc.) which utilizes a special lead system. The first- and second-generation devices are currently limited to 1.5 Tesla scanners. The MRI Surescan pacing system utilizes the Medtronic CapSureFix MRI Surescan (Model 5086) leads which were designed to minimize lead tip heating during MRI and impacts lead handling and patient complications. The materials, proximal and distal ends of the MRI-conditional 5086 leads are similar to the conventional bipolar Medtronic model 5076 leads; however, the 5086 leads use 2 filars (number of wires used in the conductor) instead of 4 (5076) to increase inductance and reduce lead tip heating during MRI.

The lead tip of the MRI-conditional 5086 leads are also stiffer (2.0 psi) than the 5076 lead (1.58 psi),[19,20] and this stiffness has been reported to be associated with increased risk of procedural complications.[21] A retrospective analysis of lead-related complications following implantation of 434 Surescan leads in 217 patients, reported an acute complication rate of 4.8% and an increased rate in women. Women accounted for 64 (64%) of cases requiring lead revision with all RV lead perforations occurring in women with apical lead placement. The higher complication rate was felt to be related in part to the stiffer design of the lead and the unique features of deploying the screw.

The 5086 lead requires special handling to minimize complications. The active fixation helix should be "exercised" (extended and retracted) on the surgical table prior to implant. The proximal lead segment should be straightened while extending the helix. During lead positioning, the stylet should be withdrawn 2 cm to reduce stiffness. After six to eight rotations, the lead tip should be monitored by fluoroscopy, since the helix may fully extend as built up torque is transferred to the lead tip. More rotations may be required for leads with tortuous path and atrial lead placement. RV septal lead placement should be considered, especially in women.[19]

Boston Scientific and St Jude Medical MRI-conditional pacemaker systems are currently in research trials.

The Centers for Medicare and Medicaid Services have approved reimbursement for MRI in patients with the MRI-conditional pacemaker system but does not reimburse MRIs performed in patients with other CIEDs.[22]

MRI AND IMPLANTABLE LOOP RECORDER

The Medtronic Reveal Plus Implantable Loop Recorder (ILR) is labeled "MR conditional," and patients may undergo MRI anytime following implantation.[13] Since the device contains ferromagnetic components, patients may feel slight movement of the device during scanning.[3] The electromagnetic field may adversely affect data stored on the device so interrogation should be performed prior to MRI; postscanning interrogation may reveal "arrhythmias" (Figure 57-2) recorded during the MRI due to artifact from the electromagnetic field.[12]

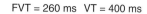

ID#	Type	Date	Time hh:mm	Duration hh:mm:ss	Max V. Rate	Median V. Rate
113	VT	22-Jun-2013	00:57	:57	353 bpm (170 ms)	222 bpm (270 ms)

FVT = 260 ms   VT = 400 ms

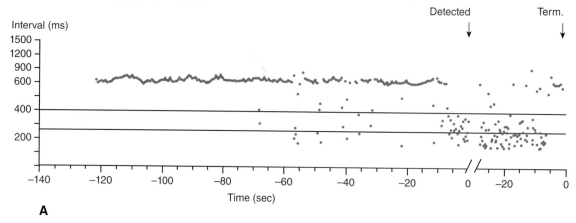

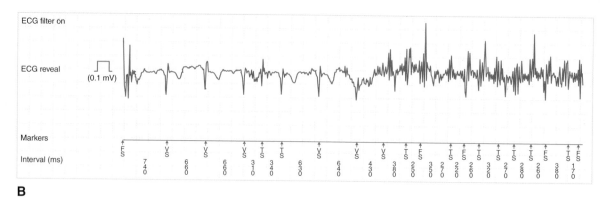

FIGURE 57-2 Interval plot (A) and stored EGM (B) recorded from a patient with a Medtronic Reveal ILR during a brain MRI. Noise recorded by the device was interpreted as VT.

CONCLUSIONS

- Magnetic resonance imaging is considered a relative contraindication for patients with conventional pacemakers and implantable cardioverter defibrillators (ICDs) due to the potential for multiple adverse interactions between a strong magnetic field and cardiac implantable electronic devices (CIEDs).

- MR scanning should be performed at experienced centers with expertise in MRI and electrophysiology.

- A physician with device expertise and a crash cart with external defibrillator and programmer should be present during scanning.

- The device should be interrogated prior to and after the MRI. Pacemaker-dependent patients should be programmed in an asynchronous mode (DOO, VOO) while a nonpacing mode (ODO, DDI, VVI) should be used for nondependent patients. Magnet, rate response, PVC, noise, ventricular sense, conducted atrial fibrillation (AF) response, and tachyarrhythmia therapies should be disabled.

- In February 2011, the FDA approved an MRI-conditional pacemaker for marketing in the U.S. (EnRhythm MRI SureScan Pacing System, Medtronic, Inc.) which utilizes a special lead system and requires special handling.

REFERENCES

1. Kalin R, Stanton MS. Current clinical issues for MRI scanning of pacemaker and defibrillator patients. *Pacing Clin Electrophysiol.* 2005;28(4):326-328.

2. Prasad SK, Pennell DJ. Safety of cardiovascular magnetic resonance in patients with cardiovascular implants and devices. *Heart.* 2004;90(11):1241-1244.

3. Shellock FG, Tkach JA, Ruggieri PM, Masaryk TJ. Cardiac pacemakers, ICDs, and loop recorder: evaluation of translational attraction using conventional ("long-bore") and "short-bore" 1.5- and 3.0-tesla MR systems. *J Cardiovasc Magn Reson.* 2003;5(2):387-397.

MAGNETIC RESONANCE IMAGING AND CARDIAC
IMPLANTABLE ELECTRONIC DEVICES

SECTION IX
IMPLANTABLE CARDIAC DEVICES FOR
MANAGEMENT OF MALIGNANT

399

4. Shellock FG, Crues JV. MR procedures: Biologic effects, safety, and patient care. *Radiology*. 2004;232(3):635-652.

5. Hayes DL, Holmes DR Jr, Gray JE. Effect of 1.5 tesla nuclear magnetic resonance imaging scanner on implanted permanent pacemakers. *J Am Coll Cardiol*. 1987;10(4):782-786.

6. Smith JM. Industry viewpoint: Guidant: Pacemakers, ICDs, and MRI. *Pacing Clin Electrophysiol*. 2005;28(4):264.

7. Stanton MS. Industry viewpoint: Medtronic: Pacemakers, ICDs, and MRI. *Pacing Clin Electrophysiol*. 2005;28(4):265.

8. Levine PA. Industry viewpoint: St. Jude Medical: Pacemakers, ICDs, and MRI. *Pacing Clin Electrophysiol*. 2005;28(4):266-267.

9. Faris OP, Shein MJ. Government viewpoint: U.S. food & drug administration: Pacemakers, ICDs, and MRI. *Pacing Clin Electrophysiol*. 2005;28(4):268-269.

10. Irnich W, Irnich B, Bartsch C, Stertmann WA, Gufler H, Weiler G. Do we need pacemakers resistant to magnetic resonance imaging? *Europace*. 2005;7(4):353-365.

11. Pohost GM, Blackwell GG, Shellock FG. Safety of patients with medical devices during application of magnetic resonance methods. *Ann N Y Acad Sci*. 1992;649:302-312.

12. Gimbel JR, Kanal E. Can patients with implantable pacemakers safely undergo magnetic resonance imaging? *J Am Coll Cardiol*. 2004;43(7):1325-1327.

13. Levine GN, Gomes AS, Arai AE, et al. Safety of magnetic resonance imaging in patients with cardiovascular devices: An American Heart Association scientific statement from the Committee on Diagnostic and Interventional Cardiac Catheterization, Council on Clinical Cardiology, and the Council on Cardiovascular Radiology and Intervention: endorsed by the American College of Cardiology Foundation, the North American Society for Cardiac Imaging, and the Society for Cardiovascular Magnetic Resonance. *Circulation*. 2007;116(24):2878-2891.

14. Gimbel JR, Kanal E, Schwartz KM, Wilkoff BL. Outcome of magnetic resonance imaging (MRI) in selected patients with implantable cardioverter defibrillators (ICDs). *Pacing Clin Electrophysiol*. 2005;28(4):270-273.

15. Gimbel JR, Bailey SM, Tchou PJ, Ruggieri PM, Wilkoff BL. Strategies for the safe magnetic resonance imaging of pacemaker-dependent patients. *Pacing Clin Electrophysiol*. 2005;28(10):1041-1046.

16. Burke PT, Ghanbari H, Alexander PB, Shaw MK, Daccarett M, Machado C. A protocol for patients with cardiovascular implantable devices undergoing magnetic resonance imaging (MRI): Should defibrillation threshold testing be performed post-(MRI). *J Interv Card Electrophysiol*. 2010;28(1):59-66.

17. Beinart R, Nazarian S. Magnetic resonance imaging in patients with implanted devices. *J Cardiovasc Electrophysiol*. 2012;23(9):1040-1042.

18. http://www.mayoclinic.org/medicalprofs/protocols-for-MRI-in-pacemaker-patients-cvuv9n3.html. Accessed June 30, 2013.

19. MRI SureScan Leads. http://www.medtronic.com/surescan/capsurefix.html. Accessed June 20, 2013.

20. Forleo GB, Santini L, Della Rocca DG, et al. Safety and efficacy of a new magnetic resonance imaging-compatible pacing system: early results of a prospective comparison with conventional dual-chamber implant outcomes. *Heart Rhythm*. 2010;7(6):750-754.

21. Rhodes T, McComb B, Augostini R, et al. Acute complications with MRI Surescan Leads. *Heart Rhythm*. 2013;10:S159.

22. MLN Matters. http://www.cms.gov/outreach-and-education/medicare-learning-network-MLN/MLNMattersArticles/downloads/MM7296.pdf. Updated August 14, 2012. Accessed June 30, 2013.

58 TECHNIQUE FOR DEVICE IMPLANTATION: CEPHALIC VEIN

Edmond M. Cronin, MB BCh BAO, Bruce L Wilkoff, MD, Niraj Varma, MA, DM, FRCP

CASE PRESENTATION

A 28-year-old man with a recent history of resuscitated cardiac arrest and long QT syndrome presents for implantation of an implantable cardioverter-defibrillator (ICD). Given recent media coverage of ICD lead recalls due to increased fracture rates, he asks whether his vulnerability to this problem can be reduced by any mechanism. The discussion includes using leads with a performance record proven over a chronic period and also routes of delivery during surgery.

PATHOPHYSIOLOGY

- Multiple access routes to the heart have been described for implantation of endovascular leads.

- The most commonly used are traditional subclavian vein puncture medial to the clavicle, extrathoracic subclavian or axillary vein puncture under fluoroscopic guidance,[1] and cephalic vein cut down.[2]

- The relative merits of traditional subclavian puncture and cephalic vein cut down have been long debated,[3] and all three have advantages and disadvantages (Table 58-1).

- A single-center randomized trial comparing cephalic and contrast-guided axillary vein techniques found no difference in early or late complications, but longer procedural time for cephalic vein implantation and implant success of only 64%.[4] Operators in this study were inexperienced, however.

- Intrathoracic subclavian vein puncture is discouraged due to the risk of complications including pneumothorax and an elevated likelihood of subclavian crush in between the clavicle and first rib.[5]

- Recent data from two ICD lead models with accelerated failure rates suggests that cephalic vein implantation may be associated with improved lead survival.[6,7] Whether this translates to other lead models is unknown. Slightly higher failure rates with subclavian implantation may be due to improper technique rather than the access route itself.

ANATOMY

- The cephalic vein is formed from the dorsal venous arch of the hand before ascending the lateral aspect of the upper limb.

- At the level of the shoulder it courses along the delto-pectoral groove, between the lateral border of the pectoralis major and medial aspect of the deltoid. This is the point of access for endovascular leads (Figure 58-1A).

- From the deltopectoral groove, the cephalic vein descends deeply, piercing the clavipectoral fascia, to join the axillary vein (itself a

TABLE 58-1 Comparison of Cephalic and Extrathoracic Subclavian Access

	Cephalic	Extrathoracic Subclavian Puncture
Procedure duration	Usually slightly longer (~5 mins).	Usually shorter.
Technical complexity	More difficult initially, but straightforward once experienced.	Simple.
Success rate	85%-90%.	Almost 100%.
Adjunctive techniques	May need to convert to puncture. This is more likely when multiple leads need to be delivered. Venogram rarely necessary.	May require contrast venogram.
Complications	Pneumothorax or inadvertent arterial puncture are virtually impossible. Arterial placement is not possible.	Pneumothorax possible. Inadvertent arterial puncture possible. Actual arterial placement possible though very rare.
Blood loss	Greater (eg, 10-30 cc) when venous pressure is high, but still clinically negligible. Advantage is that hemostasis can be secured under direct vision, which may be important in coagulopathies.	Approximately 5 mL (observable) per puncture. Actual venous puncture site usually is not visible and cannot be directly secured in coagulopathies, but since venous access is over the first rib, direct compression is very effective.
Late complications	May improve lead survival compared with subclavian access, although this may be related to subclavian puncture technique.	Subclavian crush if medial access (not extrathoracic). Arterio-venous fistula possible at extraction if puncture involves artery or vessels share common adventitia.

TECHNIQUE FOR DEVICE IMPLANTATION:
CEPHALIC VEIN

SECTION IX
IMPLANTABLE CARDIAC DEVICES FOR
MANAGEMENT OF MALIGNANT

401

continuation of the basilic vein from the same dorsal arch of the hand). This is illustrated in Figure 58-1B.

- The axillary vein ends at the lateral border of the first rib, where it becomes the subclavian vein (see Figure 58-1A).

- A medial site of entry into the subclavian vein risks passage through the costoclavicular ligament and/or the subclavius muscle, with subsequent "subclavian crush" leading to conductor fracture.[8]

- The relative courses of leads implanted via cephalic and axillary approaches are shown in Figure 58-2.

CEPHALIC VEIN CUT DOWN TECHNIQUE

In our practice, three routes for permanent endovascular lead implantation are used: extrathoracic subclavian vein puncture, cephalic vein cut down, and iliac vein puncture.

Cephalic vein cut down is performed as follows:

- The incision is made to expose the superior part of the deltopectoral groove (Figure 58-3A). This may be accomplished by a horizontal incision parallel and inferior to the clavicle, with its lateral margin overlying the deltopectoral groove. In some cases this may be displaced laterally relative to a conventional approach for subclavian access. The alternative approach, favored by our group, is to make a diagonal incision along the deltopectoral groove itself, extending superiorly to terminate approximately 1 cm below the inferior margin of the clavicle. The groove is easily visualized in thin or muscular patients. In obese patients, it is best palpated.

- Typically, we create a pocket first, since this provides more mobility in the space and permits assessment of hemostasis during the procedure. A conventional subcutaneous pocket may be formed, or submuscular if desired. The deltopectoral groove from this position is usually marked by a line of adipose tissue between pectoralis and deltoid, covered by a light condensation of fascia. These connective tissues are separated using blunt dissection to expose the cephalic vein in the groove.

- Further blunt dissection is performed to remove adherent connective tissues and thus mobilize several centimeters of the vein. It is important to expose the proximal aspect of the vein before it passes below the clavicle since this portion may deviate in direction or lead to branch vessels which may need to be tied off.

- The vein is controlled with two silk half-ties with long tails: one distally and one proximally (Figure 58-3C). These are passed below the vessel, which may be lifted with Gemini forceps (useful when the vein passes deep in the groove or in cases of marked obesity). The distal end is tied off at this stage, but this may be deferred until access is achieved in cases where patients are hypovolemic or the vein is collapsed or small.

- A small venotomy (about one-third of the circumference of the vein) is then performed on the anterior surface of the vein with an iris or Potts scissors. Alternatively, the vein can be cannulated with a needle.

- The venotomy is held open with a vein pick (Figure 58-3D).

- A lead (or a lead and guidewire in the case of dual chamber devices) is inserted directly into the vein (Figure 58-3E). The lead is advanced and positioned in the desired cardiac chamber in the usual fashion.

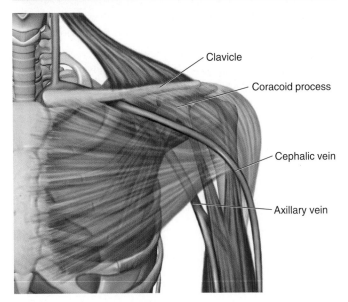

Clavicle

Coracoid process

Cephalic vein

Axillary vein

FIGURE 58-1A Anatomy of the venous drainage of the upper limb relevant to endovascular lead implant.

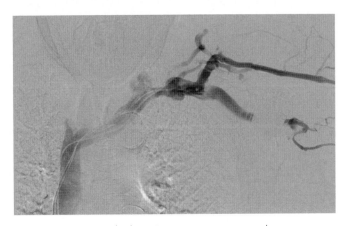

FIGURE 58-1B Digital subtraction contrast venogram demonstrating the radiographic anatomy of the cephalic, axillary, and subclavian veins. Note the pacemaker anterior to the axillary vein. The leads were implanted via the subclavian vein, which remains patent.

Peel-away sheaths can also be advanced over guidewires, usually with surprising ease since the cephalic vein is remarkably distensible.

- The proximal half-tie achieves hemostasis. Initially, slight tension may be applied as a temporary measure while leads are manipulated. For permanent hemostasis, it is tied over the anchoring sleeve once the lead(s) have been delivered. If possible, the tip of the anchoring sleeve is advanced partially into the venotomy. The suture is tied with enough tension to secure vein to lead and achieve hemostasis, avoiding excessive force, which may damage underlying lead insulation.

- The anchoring sleeve is secured medially to the pectoralis muscle with nonabsorbable ties (Figure 58-3F).

CLINICAL PEARLS

- Occasionally, a 5 Fr dilator and/or a hydrophilic wire is useful to direct and advance a guidewire through the cephalic vein in cases where it is narrow or tortuous. When encountered, this is typically at the point where the vessel pierces the clavipectoral fascia to join the axillary vein.

- Contrast venography can also be performed through this dilator to define the anatomy or diagnose a dissection if difficulty is encountered.

- Blunt dissection around and mobilization of the proximal part of the vein where it courses deeply toward the axillary vein facilitates passage of leads in many cases, and we perform this routinely. This also permits delivery of a purse-string (absorbable #0) suture below the vessel to draw pectoralis and deltoid together to secure hemostasis. This may be necessary when right sided filling pressures are elevated.

- Anchoring sleeves should be tied down to the pectoralis major. Wound closure remains unchanged to conventional. The deltopectoral area, following dissection and lead delivery, requires no additional closure after securing hemostasis.

- For CRT, a useful approach is to access the cephalic with a guidewire, and use this as a target to perform a single extrathoracic subclavian vein puncture for the left ventricular lead, which may be easier to implant from this route. The right ventricular and atrial leads are then implanted via the cephalic vein.

- When direct subclavian access is required, we prefer puncture over the lateral part of the first rib under fluoroscopic guidance. If the needle is not advanced past the first rib, pneumothorax is extremely unlikely. We also prefer to pass the needle directly to the vein at an angle dictated by the individual patient anatomy. While some have advocated a horizontal course until the needle tip is over the first rib, with subsequent tilting downward of the tip to advance to the vein, this results in an acutely angled track through the muscle, which may cause additional stress on the lead.

- Upgrading systems already implanted via the axillary or subclavian approach may be performed using the cephalic vein. The lead may be added with the approach described.

- Occasionally, the deltoid branch of the thoraco-acromial artery may course through the deltopectoral groove. Although inadvertent lead delivery is not possible in such a small vessel, laceration has to be carefully avoided. If this arterial branch shares connective

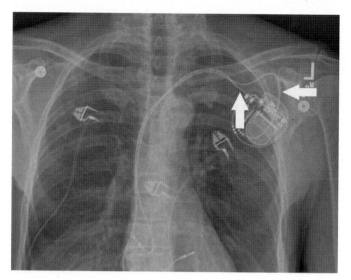

FIGURE 58-2 Postero-anterior chest x-ray demonstrating the radiographic correlates of cephalic and subclavian vein implant routes. The ventricular lead of this dual chamber pacemaker was implanted through the cephalic vein and advanced to the RV septum. This was not of sufficient caliber to accept two leads (which occurs uncommonly), so the atrial lead was implanted through the extrathoracic subclavian vein. Note the different initial angles of approach (marked by the arrowed anchoring sleeves); then both leads converge on the subclavian vein.

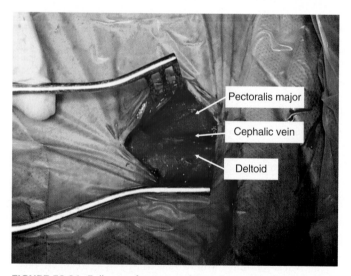

FIGURE 58-3A Following formation of the subcutaneous pocket and minor dissection of soft tissues, the cephalic vein is exposed in the delto-pectoral groove. In this series of intraoperative photographs, medial is at the top, and cephalad at right.

TECHNIQUE FOR DEVICE IMPLANTATION:
CEPHALIC VEIN

SECTION IX
IMPLANTABLE CARDIAC DEVICES FOR
MANAGEMENT OF MALIGNANT

403

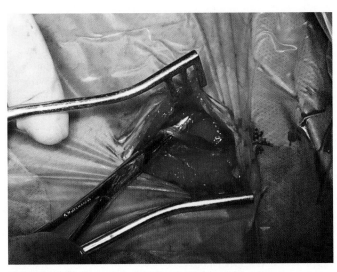

FIGURE 58-3B The vein is mobilized with blunt dissection.

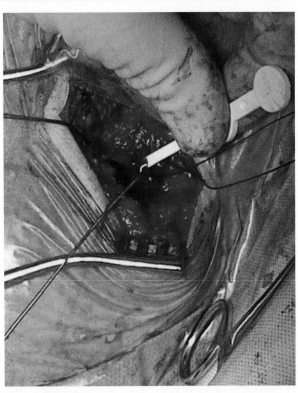

FIGURE 58-3D After a venotomy is made on the anterior surface of the vein, a vein pick can be used to hold the venotomy open while a guidewire is advanced. The pick can then be removed.

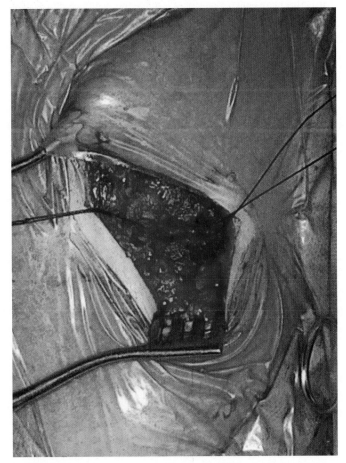

FIGURE 58-3C The vein is controlled proximally and distally with two silk half-ties. Tension applied to the proximal (cephalad) tie secures hemostasis yet permits passage of lead or sheath or guidewire. This is useful when venous pressures are high.

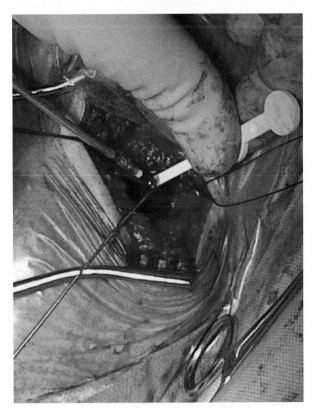

FIGURE 58-3E When implanting a dual-chamber system, a lead can usually be directly inserted beside the guidewire. If not, then a peel-away sheath can be passed over the guidewire and lead inserted conventionally.

time, we revert to the extrathoracic subclavian approach. However, when the relationship of bony landmarks is distorted with kyphosis (especially in elderly females), the accuracy of fluoroscopically guided sticks is reduced, and risks, such as pneumothorax, are increased. This may have severe consequences in some patients, for example, those with severe emphysema. Under these conditions, cephalic approach is preferred.

FOLLOW-UP

- Follow-up of leads implanted via the cephalic vein is identical to that for extrathoracic subclavian leads.

- Although ipsilateral pneumothorax is virtually impossible, postimplant postero-anterior and lateral chest X-ray is recommended to document lead position and assess for other complications.

LONG-TERM COMPLICATIONS

- The risk of ipsilateral venous thrombosis is not affected by cephalic or subclavian access.[12,13]

- Data on the impact of venous access on lead survival are conflicting, and it may be difficult to distinguish any effect of cephalic vein access from the known increased risk of lead fracture with suboptimal subclavian puncture technique.

- Nonetheless, cephalic access was associated with improved survival in two recently recalled ICD lead models.[6,7]

- The approach does not alter technique or success rate of subsequent transvenous lead extraction if this is necessary.

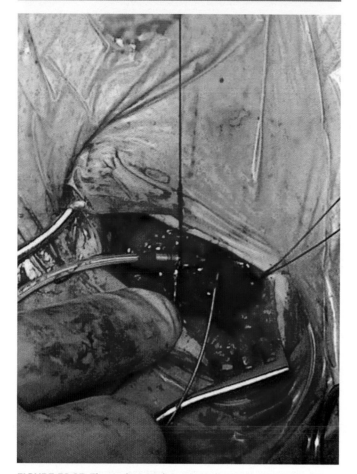

FIGURE 58-3F The anchoring sleeve is tied to pectoralis major.

tissues common with the cephalic vein, freeing the two structures from each other with blunt dissection is important.

- The cephalic vein is prone to displaying variations. If not visualized immediately, it may be found beneath the lateral border of pectoralis major. When branching, the medial branch vessel should be targeted for passage of lead/guidewire. Sometimes, the cephalic vein terminates within the deltopectoral groove in a mesh of small vessels, which may preclude passage of a wire. Rarely, the vein courses over the clavicle. Although this gains entry ultimately into the subclavian vein, this route should be avoided since a lead is heavily angled when taking this course and is vulnerable to trauma over the clavicle.

- Despite experience, cephalic vein access is not always possible. In our experience of 54 attempts over 1 year, access was successful in 45 (83.3%), consistent with another large experience.[9] Failure was due to:
  - Cephalic vein not visualized: 3 (5.5%)
  - Atretic: 3 (5.5%)
  - Aberrant course: 1 (1.9%)
  - Existing leads: 1 (1.9%)
  - Dissection: 1 (1.9%)

- With the use of additional guidewires and other techniques, success rates can be further extended; however, the operator has to balance this with prolonged procedure times.[10,11] Typically, in our practice, if the vein is not accessed within 5 minutes of incision

REFERENCES

1. Byrd CL. Clinical experience with the extrathoracic introducer insertion technique. *Pacing and Clin Electrophysiol.* 1993:16(9);1781-1784.

2. Parsonnet V, Zucker R, Gilbert L, Myers GH. Clinical use of an implantable standby pacemaker. *JAMA.* 1966:196(9);784-786.

3. Parsonnet V, Roelke M. The cephalic vein cutdown versus subclavian puncture for pacemaker/ICD lead implantation. *Pacing and Clin Electrophysiol.* 1999;22(5):695-697.

4. Calkins H, Ramza BM, Brinker J, et al. Prospective randomized comparison of the safety and effectiveness of placement of endocardial pacemaker and defibrillator leads using the extrathoracic subclavian vein guided by contrast venography versus the cephalic approach. *J Cardiovasc Electrophysiol.* 2001;24(4 Pt 1):456-464.

5. Jacobs DM, Fink AS, Miller RP, et al. Anatomical and morphological evaluation of pacemaker lead compression. *Pacing Clin Electrophysiol.* 1993;16(3 Pt 1):434-44.

6. Erkapic D, Duray GZ, Bauernfeind T, Rosa SD, Hohnloser SH. Insulation defects of thin high-voltage ICD leads: an underestimated problem? *J Cardiovasc Electrophysiol.* 2011;22(9):1018-1022.

7. Birnie DH, Parkash R, Exner DV, et al. Clinical predictors of Fidelis lead failure: report from the Canadian Heart Rhythm Society Device Committee. *Circulation.* 2012;125(10):1217-1225.

8. Magney JE, Flynn DM, Parsons JA, et al. Anatomical mechanisms explaining damage to pacemaker leads, defibrillator

TECHNIQUE FOR DEVICE IMPLANTATION:
CEPHALIC VEIN

SECTION IX
IMPLANTABLE CARDIAC DEVICES FOR
MANAGEMENT OF MALIGNANT

405

leads, and failure of central venous catheters adjacent to the sternoclavicular joint. *Pacing Clin Electrophysiol.* 1993;16(3 Pt 1): 445-57.

9. Tse HF, Lau CP, Leung SK. A cephalic vein cutdown and venography technique to facilitate pacemaker and defibrillator lead implantation. *Pacing Clin Electrophysiol.* 2001;24(4 Pt 1): 469-473.

10. Neri R, Cesario AS, Baragli D, et al. Permanent pacing lead insertion through the cephalic vein using a hydrophilic guidewire. *Pacing Clin Electrophysiol.* 2003:26(12);2313-2314.

11. Kolettis TM, Lysitsas DN, Apostolidis D, Baltogiannis GG, Sourla E, Michalis LK. Improved "cut-down" technique

for transvenous pacemaker lead implantation. *Europace.* 2010:12(9);1282-1285.

12. Rozmus G, Daubert JP, Huang DT, Rosero S, Hall B, Francis C. Venous thrombosis and stenosis after implantation of pacemakers and defibrillators. *J Interv Card Electrophysiol.* 2005;13(1):9-19.

13. Haghjoo M, Nikoo MH, Fazelifar AF, Alizadeh A, Emkanjoo Z, Sadr-Ameli MA. Predictors of venous obstruction following pacemaker or implantable cardioverter-defibrillator implantation: a contrast venographic study on 100 patients admitted for generator change, lead revision, or device upgrade. *Europace.* 2007;9(5);328-332.

59 TECHNIQUE FOR DEVICE IMPLANTATION: ILIAC VEIN

Edmond M. Cronin, MD MB BCh BAO,
Niraj Varma, MA, DM, FRCP, Bruce L. Wilkoff, MD

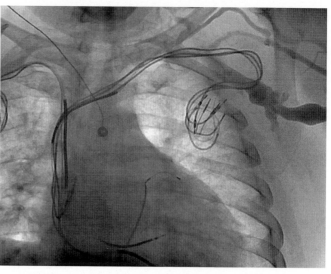

FIGURE 59-1 Multiple bilateral abandoned leads with contrast venogram demonstrating occlusion of the left subclavian vein. In this patient, a total of four leads have been implanted via the left subclavian vein, and two via the right subclavian vein. In this situation, if lead-related endocarditis occurs, all hardware must be extracted, and reimplant options are largely limited to the iliac or epicardial routes.

CASE PRESENTATION

A 45-year-old woman presents for reimplantation of a pacemaker. She has a history of congenital aortic stenosis and mitral valve prolapse and has had four open-heart surgeries, including mechanical aortic and mitral valve replacements. A dual-chamber pacemaker was implanted from the left due to postoperative complete heart block. The ventricular lead subsequently fractured, and as the left subclavian vein was found to be occluded, the system was abandoned, and a new pacemaker system was implanted via the right subclavian. She developed swelling of her pacemaker pocket, fever, and blood cultures positive for *Staphylococcus aureus* without vegetations identified by TEE. The active pacing system and the leads from both subclavian access sites were extracted percutaneously without complications. The patient retains a good atrial rhythm but has complete heart block without any ventricular escape rhythm and is supported by a temporary pacing electrode. As neither subclavian region is sterile, available transvenous routes are limited to the iliac vein.

PATHOPHYSIOLOGY

- The rise in cardiac implantable electronic device (CIED) implants over the past decade has been accompanied by an increasing number of patients with CIED-related infections and challenging lead management situations (Figure 59-1).

- Traditionally, leads have been implanted via the subclavian vein, which is accessed using either subclavian or axillary vein puncture or cephalic vein cut down.

- When there is obstruction to access through both subclavian veins or the superior vena cava, or when infected leads have recently been extracted from these veins, reimplantation is either precluded or inadvisable using these routes.

- Epicardial lead placement is often possible and may be the best choice if there are ongoing intracardiac vegetations or other concurrent indications for cardiac surgery. Nevertheless, it demands a more invasive procedure, is historically associated with inferior lead survival, and is often accompanied by higher capture thresholds.[1]

- A variety of alternative intracardiac approaches have been described, including a minithoracotomy with transatrial implant[2]; and transvenous access via the inferior vena cava, hepatic vein, femoral vein, and iliac vein.[3,4]

- The iliac vein approach (often mistakenly named "femoral vein" in the original description[3] and others) is the most widely accepted transvenous alternative to superior vein access and is particularly useful after extraction for infection.[5]

- Direct entry to the iliac vein is preferred since this approach avoids flexion of the lead as it crosses the inguinal ligament, which occurs with a true femoral vein approach (though this can also be performed).

ANATOMY

- The femoral vein ascends the thigh, accompanying the femoral artery, receiving several tributaries before reaching the level of the inguinal ligament.

- The inguinal ligament runs from the anterior superior iliac spine to the pubic tubercle.

- The femoral vein becomes the external iliac vein as it passes deep to the inguinal ligament into the abdomen; this is the site of venous access when using the iliac vein technique.

- The external iliac joins the internal iliac to become the common iliac vein; this joins with the contralateral common iliac to become the inferior vena cava.

ILIAC VEIN IMPLANT TECHNIQUE

- The right external iliac vein is most commonly used as this provides a more direct route to the heart, although both are suitable.

- The femoral vein is cannulated using the modified Seldinger technique, and a short 0.035 inch guidewire is introduced as a landmark and the external end secured to the drape using a mosquito or Kelly clamp.

- The inguinal ligament is identified by direct palpation using the bony landmarks described previously.

- A 2-cm incision is made just cephalad to the inguinal ligament, medial to the femoral arterial pulse.

- The incision is carried down to the fascia covering the external oblique.

- The external iliac vein is then cannulated using a direct stick from the fascia under fluoroscopic guidance using the guidewire as a target (Figure 59-2). It is important to keep the needle and attached syringe vertical to avoid puncturing too cephalad, which risks entering the peritoneal cavity, or too caudal, which would enter the femoral vein and produce a tight kink in the lead. This necessitates the operator's hand being briefly in the X-ray field of view.

- As with other transvenous routes of access, it is our practice to puncture the vein separately for each lead, to avoid lead-lead interaction, which can be experienced with the retained guidewire technique. However, this technique may also be used if it is the operator's preference.

- A long (24-cm) straight peel-away sheath is advanced over the guidewire (such as SafeSheath Long, Pressure Products, San Pedro, CA).

- Long, 75 to 100 cm, active fixation pace/sense or defibrillator leads are used.

- Active fixation leads are preferred as the risk of lead dislodgment is potentially higher with the iliac approach.[4]

- Atrial lead positioning is straightforward. The lead is advanced to the right atrial appendage or lateral wall, and the helix is deployed.

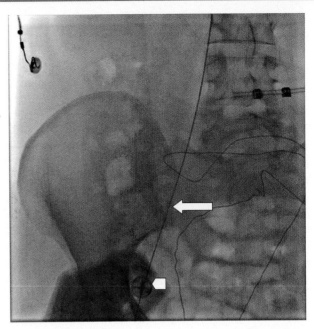

FIGURE 59-2 Puncture of the external iliac vein under fluoroscopic guidance, using a guidewire in the vein (introduced from the femoral vein caudal to the access site; arrow) as a target. Note the vertical orientation of the needle with a syringe attached (arrowhead), in the operator's hand. The site of puncture is just above the pelvic brim.

- Ventricular lead positioning is more complex. The stylet can be fashioned with a 90-degree angle approximately 5 cm from the tip to enable direct advancement to the right ventricular apex. Alternatively, an alpha loop can be created in the atrium, analogous to the technique used in cases of persistent left superior vena cava, and the lead advanced to the ventricle (Figure 59-3). With either technique, care should be taken to confirm that the lead is in the right ventricle and not in the coronary venous system. This necessitates fluoroscopy in both oblique projections.

- Coronary venous lead placement for cardiac resynchronization therapy has also been described from the iliac vein route.[6] Preshaped catheters can be used to engage the coronary sinus and perform venography, and a long peel-away sheath is used to deliver the lead using standard techniques. Both passive[6] and active fixation[7] coronary venous leads have been used, although the latter may present additional difficulty if subsequent lead extraction is required.[8]

- A generous degree of slack is necessary to account for abdominal and diaphragmatic excursions acting to draw the leads away from the heart.

- The leads and suture sleeves are reflected cephalad onto the abdominal fascia and are tied down to the muscle over the suture sleeves with nonabsorbable suture in the same fashion as with the superior approach. A purse-string or figure-of-eight suture may be used around the leads for hemostasis.

- The pocket is then fashioned. In our practice, it is created in the upper abdomen, on the ipsilateral side to venous access for pacemakers and on the left for implantable cardioverter defibrillators (ICDs). This facilitates defibrillation efficacy and allows for a placement of left posterior chest subcutaneous coil if defibrillation is not effective. A lower quadrant position for pacemaker implantation, utilizing a single incision, is also described.[9]

- The lead is then tunnelled from the access site to the pocket, using either a tunnelling tool or a Penrose drain (Figure 59-4).

- After irrigation (and defibrillation efficacy testing in the case of ICDs), the incisions are closed, and the final appearance is documented fluoroscopically (Figure 59-5).

SPECIAL CONSIDERATIONS FOR ICDs

- The iliac approach produces an altered vector from that seen with pectoral implants, as the can is in the upper abdomen, in the same position as was used for earlier, larger transvenous defibrillators.

- For single chamber ICDs, a single dual coil defibrillator lead with an alpha loop in the right atrium permits a good defibrillation vector with the SVC coil in the heart (Figure 59-3).

- For dual-chamber systems, two single coil defibrillator leads with one in the right ventricle and one in the right atrium permits the RA lead DF-1 pin to be used as the SVC port coil and the RV lead DF-1 pin as the RV port coil (Figure 59-6). This minimizes the amount of redundant lead length and the chances of lead-lead interactions.

- Defibrillation threshold is higher with abdominal compared with pectoral implant sites, and addition of a subcutaneous coil has been necessary to achieve an adequate safety margin in one-third of patients.[10] Defibrillation efficacy testing is required with this approach.

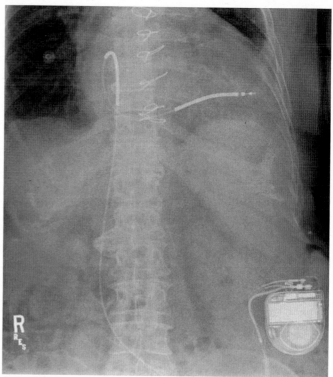

A

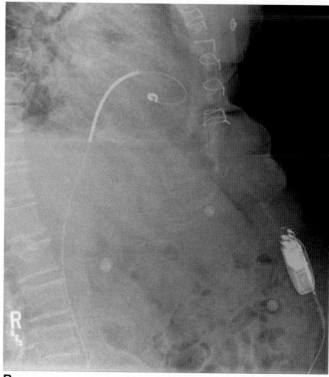

B

FIGURE 59-3 Postero-anterior (A) and left lateral (B) X-rays of a single-chamber ICD attached to a single-pass dual coil ICD lead implanted using the iliac vein technique, and utilizing an alpha loop in the right atrium to position the SVC coil in the heart. Note that slack must account for abdominal girth.

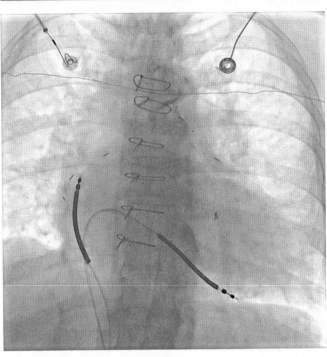

FIGURE 59-6 Dual-coil system using two ICD leads, each a single-coil lead. The ventricular electrode is deployed and connected conventionally. The defibrillation coil of the atrial lead is connected to the SVC port of the defibrillator, while the IS-1 component of the same lead is connected conventionally to the atrial port for pacing and sensing in the atrium.

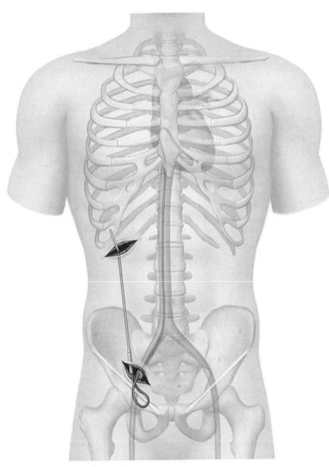

FIGURE 59-4 Tunneling of the lead. After the lead is secured to the fascia, it is tunneled to the pocket fashioned in the ipsilateral upper abdominal quadrant using a tunneling tool or a Penrose drain.

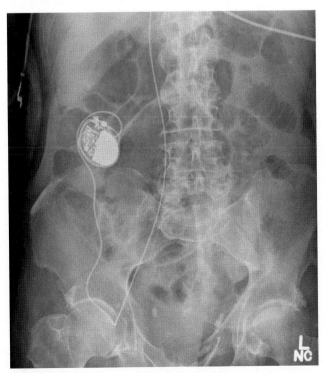

FIGURE 59-5 Fluoroscopic appearance of a single-lead pacemaker with the lead implanted using the iliac vein technique.

FOLLOW-UP

Follow-up is identical to that for devices placed via a superior venous approach. A high rate of lead dislodgement, especially atrial, has been described by some authors,[3,4,11] although not by others,[12] and is rare in our experience[5,10] of 115 iliac implants over 15 years. Routine use of active fixation leads, testing for current of injury by unfiltered electrograms recording,[13] and addition of adequate slack may all be contributors to a low rate of lead dislodgement. Nevertheless, maintaining a high degree of vigilance during follow-up is necessary. This may be aided by using generators with remote monitoring capability.[14] There is no evidence of an increased rate of venous thrombosis, phlebitis, or pocket infection following iliac vein implantation,[3-5,9-12] though the number of published cases is small. Deep venous thrombosis has not been a problem with iliac vein implantation, and patients return to full, active lifestyles.

REFERENCES

1. Belott PH, Reynolds DW. Permanent pacemaker and implantable cardioverter defibrillator implantation. In: Ellenbogen KA, Kay GN, Lau CP, Wilkoff BL, eds. *Clinical Cardiac Pacing, Defibrillation, and Resynchronization Therapy.* 4th ed. Philadelphia, PA: Elsevier; 2011;443-515.

2. Byrd CL, Schwartz SJ. Transatrial implantation of transvenous pacing leads as an alternative to implantation of epicardial leads. *Pacing Clin Electrophysiol.* 1990;13(12 Pt 2):1856-1859.

3. Ellestad MH, Caso R, Greenberg PS. Permanent pacemaker implantation using the femoral vein: a preliminary report. *Pacing Clin Electrophysiol.* 1980;3(4):418-423.

4. Ellestad MH, French J. Iliac vein approach to permanent pacemaker implantation. *Pacing Clin Electrophysiol.* 1989;12(7 Pt 1): 1030-1033.

5. Erdogan O, Augostini R, Saliba W, Juratli N, Wilkoff B. Transiliac permanent pacemaker implantation after extraction of infected pectoral pacemaker systems. *Am Heart J.* 1999:84(4);474-475.

6. Yousef Z, Paul V, Leyva F. Cardiac resynchronization via the femoral vein: a novel method in cases with contraindications to the pectoral approach. *Europace.* 2006;8(2):144-146.

7. Shandling A, Donohue D, Tobias S, Wu I, Brar R. Use of an active-fixation coronary sinus lead to implant a biventricular pacemaker via the femoral vein. *Tex Heart Inst J.* 2010;37(1):92-94.

8. Cronin EM, Ingelmo CP, Rickard J, et al. Active fixation mechanism complicates coronary sinus lead extraction and limits subsequent reimplantation targets. *J Interv Card Electrophysiol.* 2013;36(1):81-86.

9. Barakat K, Hill J, Kelly P. Permanent transfemoral pacemaker implantation is the technique of choice for patients in whom the superior vena cava is inaccessible. *Pacing Clin Electrophysiol.* 2000;23(4 Pt 1):446-449.

10. Ching CK, Elayi CS, Di Biase L, et al. Transiliac ICD implantation: defibrillation vector flexibility produces consistent success. *Heart Rhythm.* 2009;6(7):978-983.

11. Mathur G, Stables RH, Heaven D, Ingram A, Sutton R. Permanent pacemaker implantation via the femoral vein: an alternative in cases with contraindications to the pectoral approach. *Europace.* 2001;3(1):56-59.

12. García Guerrero JJ, De La Concha Castañeda JF, Fernández Mora G, et al. Permanent transfemoral pacemaker: a single-center series performed with an easier and safer surgical technique. *Pacing Clin Electrophysiol.* 2005;28(7):675-679.

13. Saxonhouse SJ, Conti JB, Curtis AB. Current of injury predicts adequate active lead fixation in permanent pacemaker/defibrillation leads. *J Am Coll Cardiol.* 2005;45(3):412-417.

14. Varma N, Michalski J, Epstein AE, Schweikert R. Automatic remote monitoring of implantable cardioverter-defibrillator lead and generator performance: the Lumos-T Safely RedUceS RouTine Office Device Follow-Up (TRUST) trial. *Circ Arrhythm Electrophysiol.* 2010;3(5):428-436.

MALIGNANT VENTRICULAR ARRHYTHMIAS
OCCURRING EARLY AFTER ACUTE MYOCARDIAL
INFARCTION AND REVASCULARIZATION

SECTION IX
IMPLANTABLE CARDIAC DEVICES FOR
MANAGEMENT OF MALIGNANT

411

60 MALIGNANT VENTRICULAR ARRHYTHMIAS OCCURRING EARLY AFTER ACUTE MYOCARDIAL INFARCTION AND REVASCULARIZATION

Byron K. Lee, MD, Nitish Badhwar, MBBS, Jeffrey E. Olgin, MD

CASE PRESENTATION

A 48-year-old man with no significant past medical history presented with coughing and shortness of breath and was diagnosed with a non-ST elevation myocardial infarction (MI). Cardiac catheterization found 3-vessel coronary artery disease. Echo showed an ejection fraction (EF) of 40% and a left ventricular apical thrombus. He underwent coronary artery bypass surgery and surgical removal of the apical thrombus. Postoperatively, atrial fibrillation (AF) was seen intermittently. He was discharged in sinus rhythm and in stable condition. An ambulatory ECG monitor was placed during an outpatient visit to assess AF frequency. Three months after his MI, while at the hospital cardiac rehabilitation unit, he had sudden loss of consciousness. He was found to be in ventricular fibrillation (VF). He was externally cardioverted, intubated, and brought to the cardiac care unit (CCU). The ambulatory ECG monitor caught the initiation of VF (Figure 60-1) and the external cardioversion (Figure 60-2).

EXPERT OPINION

- Patients who have had a recent MI are at high risk for sudden cardiac death, particularly if their EF is low.[1]
- The potential cardiac causes of sudden death following MI include:
  ○ Recurrent ischemia
  ○ Cardiac rupture
  ○ Tachyarrhymias (ie, ventricular tachycardia [VT] and VF)
  ○ Bradyarrhythmias (ie, complete heart block)
- Tachyarrhymias and bradyarrhythmias could be secondary to recurrent ischemia.
- Typically, VF or polymorphic VT is due to recurrent ischemia or cardiac rupture while monomorphic VT is due to a reentrant circuit from the MI scar.
- In the absence of evidence for cardiac rupture, the management of post-MI patients with syncope or life-threatening arrhythmias typically begins with ruling out recurrent ischemia, especially when the presenting rhythm is VF or polymorphic VT.

PATHOPHYSIOLOGY AND MANAGEMENT

- The patient had two more episodes of VF requiring external cardioversion in the CCU.
- Troponin was found to be positive.
- Emergent cardiac catheterization found a stenosis at the anastomosis of the LIMA to the LAD, which was opened by PTCA. The vessel was considered too small and tortuous for stent delivery.
- Echo following VF arrest showed an EF of 30% and no thrombus.
- An implantable cardioverter defibrillator (ICD) was later implanted.

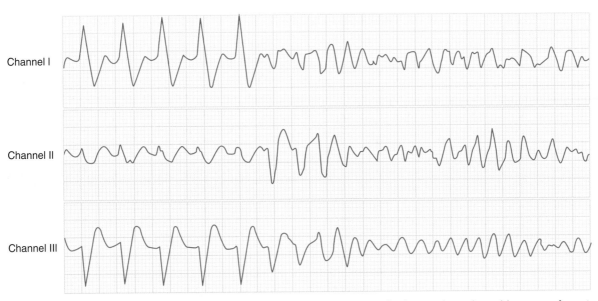

Channel I

Channel II

Channel III

FIGURE 60-1 Ambulatory ECG while patient was at the hospital cardiac rehabilitation unit for therapy shows the sudden onset of ventricular fibrillation.

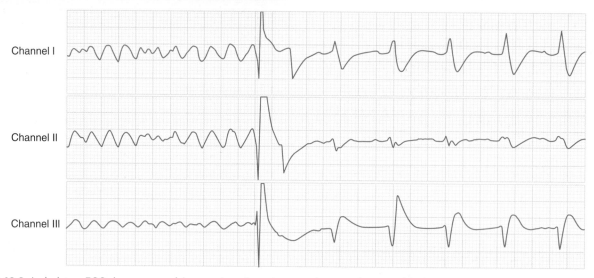

FIGURE 60-2 Ambulatory ECG shows successful external cardioversion to a slower and more stable rhythm.

FEATURES OF VENTRICULAR ARRHYTHMIAS OCCURRING EARLY AFTER ACUTE MYOCARDIAL INFARCTION

- The VALIANT study, which studied 14 609 patients for a median duration of 24.7 months after MI, demonstrated that 19% of all cardiac arrests occurred in the first 30 days after the infarct and that 83% of the patients who died suddenly in the first 30 days did so after hospital discharge. Patients with an EF ≤30% had a significantly higher incidence of early cardiac arrest, with a rate of 2.3% in the first month, followed by an additional 1.1% in the second month.[2]

- The EPHESUS study also investigated patients with low EF after MI and found that patients with an EF ≤40% had 5% mortality in the first 2 months, with more than half of the deaths sudden and likely due to arrhythmia.[3]

- Two randomized trials of ICDs implanted early in the post-MI period (<40 days) in patients with low EF showed no reduction in overall mortality.[4,5]

- Based on these two studies, the AHA/ACC/ESC Practice Guidelines for the Management of Patients with Ventricular Arrhythmias and the Prevention of Sudden Death recommends ICD implantation for the primary prevention of sudden death in patients with ischemic cardiomyopathy and EF of 30% to 40% only after waiting at least 40 days after MI and 90 days if revascularized.[6]

- Waiting 40 to 90 days before ICD implant means patients are unprotected from sudden death immediately post-MI.

- Some clinicians employ a wearable defibrillator vest in this waiting period to protect patients from ventricular tachyarrythmias. The most recent guidelines for management of post-MI patients state that the wearable defibrillator vest is investigational in this population. Currently there is no proof that this approach decreases sudden death and does no harm, although a randomized clinical trial (VEST trial) is currently underway.[7]

REFERENCES

1. Moss AJ, Hall WJ, Cannom DS, et al. Improved survival with an implanted defibrillator in patients with coronary disease at high risk for ventricular arrhythmia. Multicenter Automatic Defibrillator Implantation Trial Investigators. *N Engl J Med.* 1996;335(26):1933-1940.

2. Solomon SD, Zelenkofske S, McMurray JJ, et al. Sudden death in patients with myocardial infarction and left ventricular dysfunction, heart failure, or both. *N Engl J Med.* 2005;352(25):2581-2588.

3. Pitt B, et al. Eplerenone, a selective aldosterone blocker, in patients with left ventricular dysfunction after myocardial infarction. *N Engl J Med.* 2003;348(14):1309-1321.

4. Hohnloser SH, et al. Prophylactic use of an implantable cardioverter-defibrillator after acute myocardial infarction. *N Engl J Med.* 2004;351(24):2481-2488.

5. Steinbeck G, et al. Defibrillator implantation early after myocardial infarction. *N Engl J Med.* 2009;361(15):1427-1436.

6. Zipes DP, et al. ACC/AHA/ESC 2006 guidelines for management of patients with ventricular arrhythmias and the prevention of sudden cardiac death: a report of the American College of Cardiology/American Heart Association Task Force and the European Society of Cardiology Committee for Practice Guidelines (writing committee to develop Guidelines for Management of Patients With Ventricular Arrhythmias and the Prevention of Sudden Cardiac Death): developed in collaboration with the European Heart Rhythm Association and the Heart Rhythm Society. *Circulation.* 2006;114(10):e385-484.

7. O'Gara PT, et al. 2013 ACCF/AHA guidelines for the management of ST-elevation myocardial infarction: a report of the American College of Cardiology Foundation/American Heart Association Task Force on Practice Guidelines. *Circulation.* 2013;127(4):e362-425.

PREVENTION OF SUDDEN DEATH:
CHRONIC ISCHEMIC CARDIOMYOPATHY

SECTION IX
IMPLANTABLE CARDIAC DEVICES FOR
MANAGEMENT OF MALIGNANT

413

61 PREVENTION OF SUDDEN DEATH: CHRONIC ISCHEMIC CARDIOMYOPATHY

Khaled Awad, MD, and Andrew E. Epstein, MD, FAHA, FACC, FHRS

CASE PRESENTATION

A 56-year-old man collapsed in a park while attending an art show. Cardiopulmonary resuscitation (CPR) was performed by a bystander until the arrival of emergency medical services (EMS). The initial recordings showed ventricular fibrillation (Figure 61-1). Three direct current shocks were delivered, and amiodarone was given as an IV bolus (300 mg). On arrival at the emergency department, an electrocardiogram showed atrial fibrillation, probable inferior myocardial infarction (MI), and ventricular ectopy (Figure 61-2A). The presence of acute inferior MI became clear on a second electrocardiogram (Figure 61-2B). The patient was unresponsive, intubated, and CPR continued. He continued to have recurrent ventricular tachycardia and fibrillation treated with over 10 external shocks and repeat IV amiodarone. His past medical history was notable for cigarette use. On physical examination he remained unresponsive, had decorticate posturing, and his pupils were fixed and dilated. At emergent cardiac catheterization, an occluded right coronary artery was opened and stented (Figure 61-3). The following day he awoke with no memory defects. The left ventricular ejection fraction (LVEF) was 42%. On the day of discharge, the monitor tracing shown in Figure 61-4 was recorded. What should the next step be? Is an implantable cardioverter defibrillator (ICD) appropriate?

DISCUSSION

The patient under discussion suffered a cardiac arrest in the setting of acute MI. This does not represent a guideline-driven indication for implantation of an ICD.[1] The ventricular tachycardia recorded on the day of planned discharge, more than 48 hours after the infarction was nonsustained, accelerating, and likely automatic given the clinical circumstances. This suggests a changing substrate but not necessarily a fixed substrate with scar at risk for later ventricular tachycardia.

In the Multicenter Automatic Defibrillator Implantation Trial II (MADIT-II), patients with chronic ischemic heart disease, prior MI, LVEF ≤30%, and no requirement for ventricular arrhythmias or electrophysiologic study were randomized to receive either optimal medical therapy (OMT) or OMT with an ICD.[2] The study showed a clear benefit from ICD implantation (Figure 61-5). Exclusions to enrollment in MADIT-II included MI within 1 month or revascularization within 3 months of the index MI.

The device-based therapy guidelines state that primary prevention ICD therapy is indicated in patients with an LVEF of ≤35% due to prior MI who are at least 40 days post-MI and in NYHA functional class II or III.[1] Furthermore, since revascularization was performed, implicit in the guidelines is that a 3-month waiting period is indicated for this indication since recommendations were based on MADIT-II, which excluded patients from randomization within that time frame. In addition, the national coverage determination precludes reimbursement by Medicare for devices implanted within these waiting periods.[3] Notably, since the arrest occurred in the setting of acute MI, it does not represent an indication for secondary prevention ICD implantation either.

Additional evidence supporting the inadvisability of implanting an ICD within the first month following MI derives from the Defibrillator in Acute Myocardial Infarction Trial (DINAMIT)[4] and the Immediate Risk Stratification Improves Survival (IRIS) study.[5] In DINAMIT, patients with a LVEF ≤35% and abnormal autonomic function (decreased heart rate variability or heart rate >80 bpm on monitoring) were randomized between 6 and 40 days post-MI to OMT with or without an ICD. Survival in both groups was identical (Figure 61-6A). Notably, arrhythmic death was less in the ICD group compared to control, but exactly counterbalanced by nonarrhythmic death in the ICD group.[4] In IRIS, patients with an LVEF ≤40% and a heart rate >90 bpm or nonsustained ventricular tachycardia were randomized 5 to 31 days post-MI on OMT to receive an ICD or not. Identical to DINAMIT, the IRIS study showed no survival benefit with ICD therapy, and similarly the reduction in SCD by the ICD was completely offset by a parallel increase in nonsudden death, thereby replicating the DINAMIT results (Figure 61-6B).[5]

The Valsartan in Acute Myocardial Infarction Trial (VALIANT) has been cited as evidence that the risk of sudden arrhythmic death in the first month post-MI, especially in patients with left ventricular

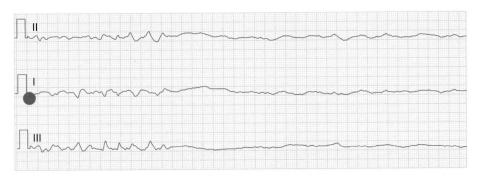

FIGURE 61-1 Presenting rhythm strip.

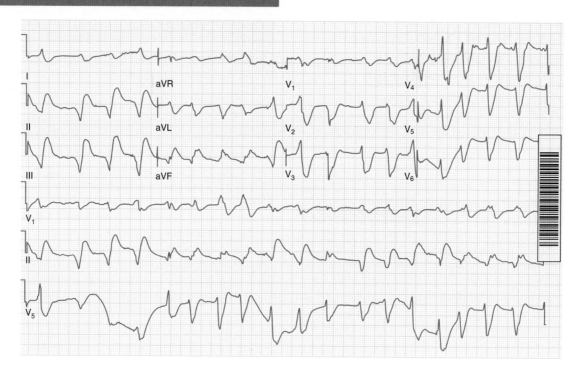

A Initial ECG

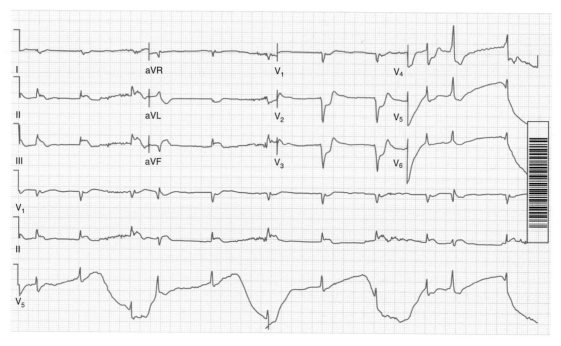

B Second ECG

FIGURE 61-2 ECGs on presentation after CPR. (A) The initial ECG. (B) The subsequent ECG.

dysfunction and an LVEF ≤30%, is such that ICD implantation early post-MI is advisable. In the study, 19% of all sudden deaths or cardiac arrest occurred in the first month, at a rate of 1.4% per month, and 83% of sudden deaths in the first month occurred after hospital discharge.[6] Despite these risks, in a subanalysis of patients who had died suddenly in VALIANT and who had autopsies, only 54 of 105 deaths could be attributed to an arrhythmic origin.[7] For the other

51 patients, causes for these nonarrhythmic but apparently sudden deaths included MI (31 patients), cardiac rupture (13), heart failure (4), stroke (1), pulmonary embolus (1), and overdose (1). Overall, autopsy results lead to reassignment of cause of death in 17% of the patients most commonly because of fatal MIs or ruptures that were not recognized in patients who died suddenly.[7] Although sudden death due to recurrent MI or rupture was highest in the first month in

PREVENTION OF SUDDEN DEATH:
CHRONIC ISCHEMIC CARDIOMYOPATHY

SECTION IX
IMPLANTABLE CARDIAC DEVICES FOR
MANAGEMENT OF MALIGNANT

415

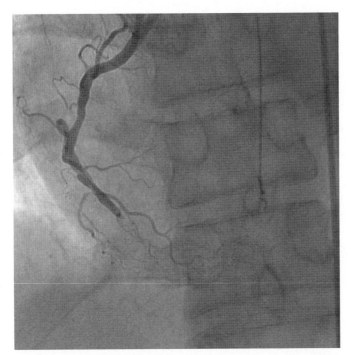

A

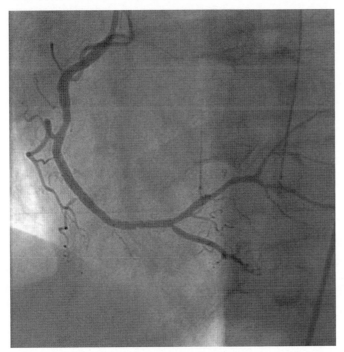

B

FIGURE 61-3 Angiograms of occluded and revascularized right coronary artery. (A) The initial angiogram of the right coronary artery, which is occluded. (B) The vessel after successful percutaneous intervention.

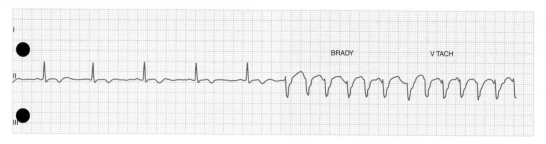

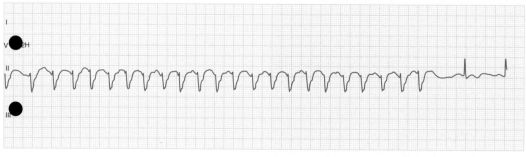

FIGURE 61-4 Monitor tracing while awaiting hospital discharge. Thirty-five beats of monomorphic ventricular tachycardia are shown. The irregularity and acceleration suggests an automatic mechanism from injured myocardium.

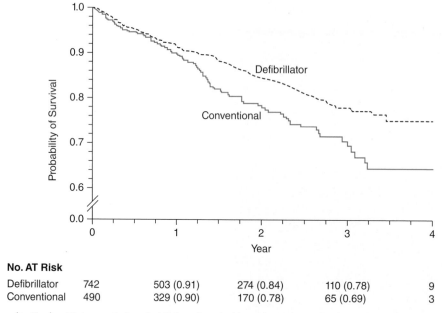

No. AT Risk					
Defibrillator	742	503 (0.91)	274 (0.84)	110 (0.78)	9
Conventional	490	329 (0.90)	170 (0.78)	65 (0.69)	3

FIGURE 61-5 MADIT-II results. Kaplan-Meier survival probabilities of survival in patients treated with an ICD and conventional medical therapy. There was a benefit from ICD therapy (P = 0.007). Reproduced with permission from Moss AJ, Zareba W, Hall WJ, et al. Prophylactic implantation of a defibrillator in patients with myocardial infarction and reduced ejection fraction. *N Engl J Med.* 2002;Mar21;346(12):877-883.

PREVENTION OF SUDDEN DEATH:
CHRONIC ISCHEMIC CARDIOMYOPATHY

SECTION IX
IMPLANTABLE CARDIAC DEVICES FOR
MANAGEMENT OF MALIGNANT

417

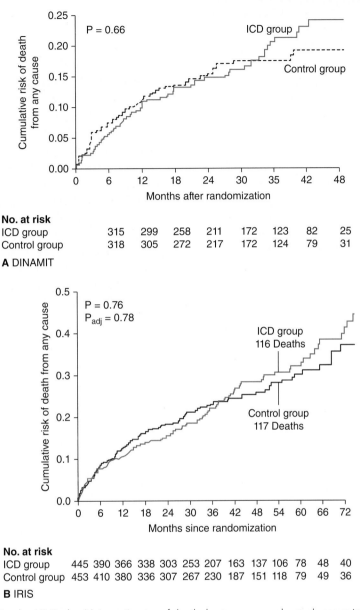

FIGURE 61-6 DINAMIT and IRIS Results. (A) Kaplan-Meier estimates of death due to any cause by study group in DINAMIT. (Reproduced with permission from Hohnloser SH, Kuck KH, Dorian P, et al. Prophylactic use of an implantable cardioverter-defibrillator after acute myocardial infarction. *N Engl J Med.* 2004;Dec 9;351(24):2481-2488.) (B) IRIS (Reproduced with permission from Steinbeck G, Andresen D, Seidl K, et al. Defibrillator implantation early after myocardial infarction. *N Engl J Med.* 2009;Oct 8;361(15):1427-1436.) In neither study was there a benefit from the addition of an ICD to optimal medical therapy. Furthermore, in both studies the decrease in sudden arrhythmic death provided by an ICD was exactly balanced by an increase in nonarrhythmic causes, virtually all cardiac.

VALIANT, it later declined.[7] However, arrhythmic death increased over time from 20% in the first month to 75% later in the study. Thus, the actual rate of early sudden death was overestimated in VALIANT.

The patient under discussion underwent emergent cardiac catheterization. Recent data show that resuscitated victims of SCA with or without known cardiac causes should undergo emergency angiography and percutaneous intervention if indicated.[8] If comatose they should also undergo therapeutic hypothermia. Kern reviewed the literature regarding outcomes of coronary angiography after resuscitation from cardiac arrest and showed that 60% may survive to hospital discharge with 86% having a favorable neurologic outcome.[8]

Finally, based on the above information, while the infarct is healing a life vest may be useful in situations as described in this case scenario in addition to OMT with β-blockade, an ACE inhibitor, and statin therapy.[8-10] In follow-up, the presented patient's LVEF increased to over 55% in one month, and no arrhythmia events were recorded by the life vest. An ICD was not implanted.

REFERENCES

1. Epstein AE, DiMarco JP, Ellenbogen KA, et al. ACC/AHA/HRS 2008 Guidelines for Device-Based Therapy of Cardiac Rhythm Abnormalities: a report of the American College of Cardiology/ American Heart Association Task Force on Practice Guidelines (Writing Committee to Revise the ACC/AHA/NASPE 2002

Guideline Update for Implantation of Cardiac Pacemakers and Antiarrhythmia Devices) developed in collaboration with the American Association for Thoracic Surgery and Society of Thoracic Surgeons. *J Am Coll Cardiol*. 2008;51(21):e1-62.

2. Moss AJ, Zareba W, Hall WJ, et al. Prophylactic implantation of a defibrillator in patients with myocardial infarction and reduced ejection fraction. *N Engl J Med*. 2002;346(12):877-883.

3. National Coverage Determination (NCD) for Implantable Automatic Defibrillators. 2005; http://www.cms.gov/medicare-coverage-database/details/ncd-details.aspx?NCDId=110&ncdver=3&bc=AAAAgAAAAAAAAA%3d%3d&. Accessed 10/21/2014.

4. Hohnloser SH, Kuck KH, Dorian P, et al. Prophylactic use of an implantable cardioverter-defibrillator after acute myocardial infarction. *N Engl J Med*. 2004;351(24):2481-2488.

5. Steinbeck G, Andresen D, Seidl K, et al. Defibrillator implantation early after myocardial infarction. *N Engl J Med*. 2009;361(15):1427-1436.

6. Solomon SD, Zelenkofske S, McMurray JJ, et al. Sudden death in patients with myocardial infarction and left ventricular dysfunction, heart failure, or both. *N Engl J Med*. 2005;352(25):2581-2588.

7. Pouleur AC, Barkoudah E, Uno H, et al. Pathogenesis of sudden unexpected death in a clinical trial of patients with myocardial infarction and left ventricular dysfunction, heart failure, or both. *Circulation*. 2010;122(6):597-602.

8. Kern KB. Optimal treatment of patients surviving out-of-hospital cardiac arrest. *JACC Cardiovasc Interv*. 2012;5(6):597-605.

9. Chung MK, Szymkiewicz SJ, Shao M, et al. Aggregate national experience with the wearable cardioverter-defibrillator: event rates, compliance, and survival. *J Am Coll Cardiol*. 2010;56(3):194-203.

10. Epstein AE, Abraham WT, Bianco N, et al. Wearable cardioverter-defibrillator use in patients perceived to be at high risk early post-myocardial infarction. *J Am Coll Cardiol*. 2013;62(21):2000-2007.

PREVENTION OF SUDDEN DEATH:
NONISCHEMIC CARDIOMYOPATHY

SECTION IX
IMPLANTABLE CARDIAC DEVICES FOR
MANAGEMENT OF MALIGNANT

419

62 PREVENTION OF SUDDEN DEATH: NONISCHEMIC CARDIOMYOPATHY

Khaled Awad, MD, and Andrew E. Epstein, MD, FAHA, FACC, FHRS

CASE PRESENTATION

A 37-year-old woman presented with 3 weeks of worsening exertional dyspnea and orthopnea. On evaluation, a nonischemic dilated cardiomyopathy (NIDCM) was diagnosed. The left ventricular ejection fraction (LVEF) was 33%. An ECG showed sinus rhythm with left bundle branch block (LBBB), QRS duration 130 ms, and a normal PR interval. Nonsustained ventricular tachycardia (NSVT) was recorded on monitoring. The patient was treated with a β-receptor blocker, an angiotensin converting enzyme inhibitor (ACEI), and spironolactone and referred to for implantable cardioverter defibrillator (ICD) implantation. Is this appropriate?

DISCUSSION

NICDM may result from viral infection, autoimmune or inflammatory disease, genetic or metabolic disorders, tachycardia (so-called tachycardia-mediated cardiomyopathy), or causes that are not readily apparent, and most are therefore labeled idiopathic. Regardless of cause, after any reversible cause is treated, most patients with NIDCM are treated with similar therapies including diuretics, β-receptor blockers, ACEIs, angiotensin receptor blockers (ARBs), aldosterone antagonists, and often an ICD sometimes combined with the capability for biventricular pacing. The prevalence of NIDCM as compared to ischemic cardiomyopathy has not been completely characterized but ranges from 2% to 13% in the ambulatory setting and up to 50% in large clinical trials.[1-3]

The patient presented has a newly diagnosed NIDCM. The Device-Based Therapy Guidelines from the American College of Cardiology, American Heart Association, and Heart Rhythm Society detail indications for ICD implantation in patients with NIDCM.[4] The primary class I indication is for patients who have an LVEF ≤35% and NYHA class II or III heart failure. Class II implantation indications are for those with unexplained syncope and "significant LV dysfunction" (class IIa indication), those who are outpatients awaiting transplantation (class IIa indication), and those with an LVEF ≤35% but who have NYHA functional class I heart failure (class IIb indication). These recommendations are based heavily on the Defibrillators in Nonischemic Cardiomyopathy Treatment Evaluation (DEFINITE) trial[5] and the Sudden Cardiac Death and Heart Failure Trial (SCD-HeFT),[3] and implicit in the recommendations is that patients have been treated with optimal medical therapy (OMT).

DEFINITE enrolled patients with NICDM, NYHA class I-III heart failure, LVEF<36%, and premature ventricular complexes or NSVT on monitoring.[5] All patients received OMT and randomized to OMT alone versus OMT with an ICD. The primary end point was death from any cause. The patients were well treated, 86% received ACEIs, and 85% received β-receptor blockers. The mean LVEF was 21%. Although the primary end point was not reached, albeit with a trend to benefit from an ICD (P = 0.08), there was an 80% reduction in sudden death from arrhythmia (P = 0.006) (Figure 62-1).

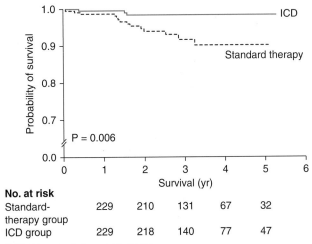

A Death from any cause

B Sudden death from arrhythmia

No. at risk					
Standard-therapy group	229	210	131	67	32
ICD group	229	218	140	77	47

FIGURE 62-1 Kaplan–Meier estimates of death from any cause (A) and sudden death from arrhythmia (B) among patients who received standard OMT and those who received an ICD. For the ICD group, as compared with the standard therapy group, the hazard ratio for death from any cause was 0.65 (95% confidence interval, 0.40 to 1.06) and the hazard ratio for sudden death from arrhythmia was 0.20 (95% confidence interval, 0.06 to 0.71). Reproduced with permission from Kadish A, Dyer A, Daubert JP, et al. Prophylactic defibrillator implantation in patients with nonischemic dilated cardiomyopathy. *N Engl J Med.* 2004;May 20; 350(21):2151-2158.

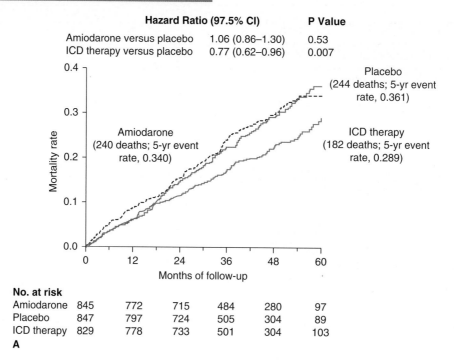

	Hazard Ratio (97.5% CI)	P Value
Amiodarone versus placebo	1.06 (0.86–1.30)	0.53
ICD therapy versus placebo	0.77 (0.62–0.96)	0.007

No. at risk

Amiodarone	845	772	715	484	280	97
Placebo	847	797	724	505	304	89
ICD therapy	829	778	733	501	304	103

A

FIGURE 62-2A Kaplan–Meier estimates of death from any cause in SCD-HeFT. Compared to OMT alone, ICD therapy resulted in a reduction in the primary end point of all-cause mortality (hazard ratio = 0.77). Note the curves continue to separate throughout the follow-up period of up to 5 years consistent with continued benefit drawn from ICD therapy. Reproduced with permission from Bardy GH, Lee KL, Mark DB, et al. Amiodarone or an implantable cardioverter-defibrillator for congestive heart failure. *N Engl J Med.* 2005;Jan 20;352(3):225-237.

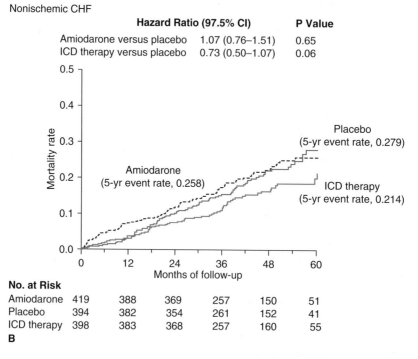

Nonischemic CHF

	Hazard Ratio (97.5% CI)	P Value
Amiodarone versus placebo	1.07 (0.76–1.51)	0.65
ICD therapy versus placebo	0.73 (0.50–1.07)	0.06

No. at Risk

Amiodarone	419	388	369	257	150	51
Placebo	394	382	354	261	152	41
ICD therapy	398	383	368	257	160	55

B

FIGURE 62-2B Kaplan–Meier estimates of death from any cause for patients with NIDCM in SCD-HeFT.[3] The benefit derived from ICD therapy in patients with NIDCM was no different from those with ischemic cardiomyopathy. Reproduced with permission from Bardy GH, Lee KL, Mark DB, et al. Amiodarone or an implantable cardioverter-defibrillator for congestive heart failure. *N Engl J Med.* 2005;Jan 20;352(3):225-237.

SCD-HeFT included patients with NIDCM, NYHA class II-III heart failure, and an LVEF ≤35%.[3] Randomization was between OMT, OMT with amiodarone, or OMT with an ICD. The primary end point was death from any cause. The median LVEF was 25%, and as in DEFINITE, the patients were well-treated medically. Compared to OMT, the addition of an ICD decreased the risk of death by 23%. Notably, patients on amiodarone experienced increased early mortality within the first year (Figure 62-2).

PREVENTION OF SUDDEN DEATH:
NONISCHEMIC CARDIOMYOPATHY

SECTION IX
IMPLANTABLE CARDIAC DEVICES FOR
MANAGEMENT OF MALIGNANT

421

With respect to when to consider ICD implantation in patients with NIDCM, a waiting period of at least 3 months is required. This waiting period was driven in large part by SCD-HeFT, which required a 3-month waiting period for medical therapy to be optimized,[3] and since many cardiomyopathies improve with OMT. Notably, McNamara et al showed that LVEF markedly improves after recent onset heart failure in nonischemic cardiomyopathy.[6] Stratified by LVEDD, those with LVEDDs <60 mm experienced a 19% improvement in the LVEF (from 27% to 45% at 6 months), for LVEDDs 60 to 70 mm, a 17% improvement in LVEF (from 23% to 40% at 6 months), and for LVEDDs >70 mm, a 13% improvement in LVEF (from 20% to 32% at 6 months). In DEFINITE, no heart failure duration was specified.[5] Since the primary end point was not reached ($P = 0.08$), including death or resuscitated cardiac arrest, no inference can be made about timing of ICD implantation. In addition, a third study, the Cardiomyopathy Trial (CAT) also addressed primary prevention ICD implantation in patients with NIDCM.[7] Patients with NIDCM, NYHA class II-III heart failure, a LVEF ≤30% and duration of heart failure ≤9 months were enrolled and randomized to OMT alone or OMT with an ICD. The trial was terminated early for futility when interim analysis indicated that with continued enrollment no survival benefit would be shown from ICD therapy added to OMT.

Although a DEFINITE substudy suggested that ICD implantation within 3 or 9 months following diagnosis provided benefit, as indicated above, the analysis violates the statistical principal that subanalyses cannot be used to draw conclusions when the overall study is negative.[8]

Furthermore, enrollment in SCD-HEFT required that heart failure must have been present for at least 3 months so there can be no inference made regarding early implantation from that study either.[3] Also, although SCD-HeFT showed benefit from ICD therapy, the benefit became apparent only after over a year. Thus, no study supports early implantation of an ICD in patients with newly diagnosed heart failure. And for Medicare patients, the Centers for Medicare and Medicaid Services (CMS) determined that clinical trial data was adequate to conclude that an ICD is reasonable and necessary for patients with NIDCM >3 months, NYHA class II or III heart failure, and measured an LVEF ≤35% after 3 months of diagnosis if the beneficiary is receiving the ICD for primary prevention, and is enrolled in either a clinical trial or registry such as the National Cardiac Data Registry (NCDR).[9] Otherwise, the waiting period is 9 months. For the reasons previously stated, ICD implantation within the first 3 months following the diagnosis of heart failure is not appropriate. This patient was followed, treated optimally, and the LVEF improved to 45%. She was not treated with an ICD.

Another point to consider is that our patient had LBBB. Multiple studies have shown that LBBB, as a marker for electrical dyssynchrony (QRS >120 ms), is associated with increased mortality and morbidity in subjects with LV systolic dysfunction.[10-12] LBBB

contributes to progressive pump failure and increases the risk of developing ventricular arrhythmias.[13] Cardiac resynchronization therapy (CRT) via biventricular pacing has changed the paradigm in management of systolic heart failure with LV dyssynchrony (usually identified by a prolonged QRS duration, especially LBBB) allowing for direct electrical intervention to restore interventricular synchrony, which is discussed in a separate chapter of this monograph. Though more often used in Europe compared with the United States, for patients with LV dysfunction, symptomatic heart failure, and a prolonged QRS duration, using CRT alone without defibrillation (a CRT pacemaker, CRT-P) may be considered, especially in situations where an there may be reasons why ICD implantation might not be desirable after open discussion with the patient and his or her family.

Two major studies addressed CRT-P in patients with severe LV dysfunction and evidence of dyssynchrony. The Comparison of Medical Therapy, Pacing, and Defibrillation in Heart Failure (COMPANION) study enrolled patients with either ischemic or nonischemic cardiomyopathy, a LVEF ≤35%, and a QRS duration ≥120 msec.[1] Patients in COMPANION were randomized to OMT alone, OMT with a CRT-P, or OMT with a biventricular ICD (CRT-D). In this study, patients with CRT (CRT-P and CRT-D groups combined) experienced a 20% reduction in mortality and hospitalization from any cause. The study was terminated early because of marked reduction in the primary and secondary endpoints with CRT. Although there was a clear trend towards lower mortality in the CRT-P group, 24% in relative terms when compared to the OMT group, that was not statistically significant ($P = 0.06$) (Figure 62-3). Had the study not been terminated early, CRT-P could have been associated with statistically significant reduction in mortality.

The Cardiac Resynchronization-Heart Failure (CARE-HF) study compared CRT-P to OMT in patients with LVEF of ≤35%, NYHA class III or IV heart failure, a left ventricular end-diastolic dimension of at least 30 mm (indexed to height), and a QRS duration ≥120 ms. For those with QRS durations 120 to 149 ms, evidence of dyssynchrony was also required.[14] This study showed marked reduction in the primary composite end point of death or cardiovascular hospitalization (39% in CRT-P group, 55% in OMT group, hazard ratio, 0.63; 95% confidence interval, 0.51 to 0.77; P < 0.001) (Figure 62-4). The relative risk reduction in mortality observed in the CARE-HF trial was not only similar to the CRT-D arm in COMPANION, but the mortality benefit was achieved without the defibrillation capabilities of the device. Indeed, in COMPANION the secondary endpoint of death or hospitalization from a cardiovascular cause (the primary endpoint in CARE-HF) was decreased only 1% by the addition of a defibrillator to CRT-P (Figure 62-3C). Thus, for patients who desire quality of life and improved longevity but do not desire an ICD, a CRT-P is completely appropriate and emphasizes the importance of discussing options and having patients share in the decision making process.[15]

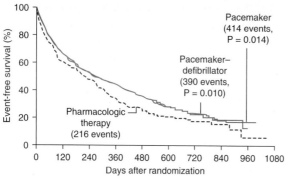

No. at risk

Pharmacologic therapy	308	176	115	72	46	24	16	6	1
Pacemaker	617	384	294	228	146	73	36	14	3
Pacemaker–defibrillator	595	385	283	217	128	61	25	8	0

A Primary end point

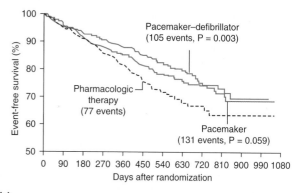

No. at risk

Pharmacologic therapy	308	284	255	217	186	141	94	57	45	25	4	2
Pacemaker	617	579	520	488	439	355	251	164	104	60	25	5
Pacemaker–defibrillator	595	555	517	470	420	331	219	148	95	47	21	1

B Secondary end point

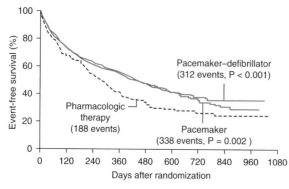

No. at risk

Pharmacologic therapy	308	199	134	91	56	29	20	8	2
Pacemaker	617	431	349	282	194	102	51	22	5
Pacemaker–defibrillator	595	425	341	274	167	89	45	20	3

C Death from or hospitalization for cardiovascular causes

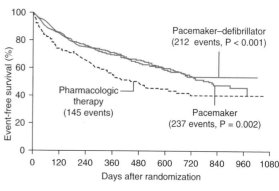

No. at risk

Pharmacologic therapy	308	216	161	118	76	39	28	11	2
Pacemaker	617	498	422	355	258	142	75	35	9
Pacemaker–defibrillator	595	497	411	343	228	131	71	27	5

D Death from or hospitalization for heart failure

FIGURE 62-3 Kaplan–Meier Estimates of the time to the primary endpoint of death from or hospitalization for any cause (A), the time to the secondary endpoints of death from any cause (B), the time to death from or hospitalization for cardiovascular causes (C), and the time to death from or hospitalization for heart failure (D). (A) The 12-month rates of death from or hospitalization for any cause (the primary end point) were 68% in the OMT group, 56% in the group that received CRT-P, and 56% in the group that received CRT-D. (B) The 12-month rates of death from any cause were 19% in the OMT group, 15% in the CRT-P group, and 12% in the CRT-D group. (C) The 12-month rates of death from or hospitalization for cardiovascular causes were 60% in the OMT group, 45% in the CRT-P group, and 44% in the CRT-D group. (D) The 12-month rates of death from or hospitalization for heart failure were 45% in the OMT group, 31% in the CRT-P group, and 29% in the CRT-Dgroup. P values are for the comparison with OMT. Reproduced with permission from Bristow MR, Saxon LA, Boehmer J, et al. Cardiac-resynchronization therapy with or without an implantable defibrillator in advanced chronic heart failure. *N Engl J Med.* 2004;May 20;350(21):2140-2150.

PREVENTION OF SUDDEN DEATH:
NONISCHEMIC CARDIOMYOPATHY

SECTION IX
IMPLANTABLE CARDIAC DEVICES FOR
MANAGEMENT OF MALIGNANT

423

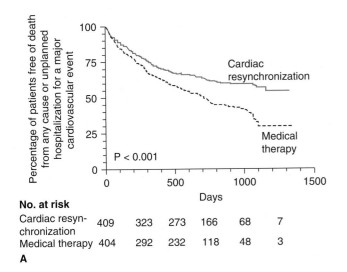

A

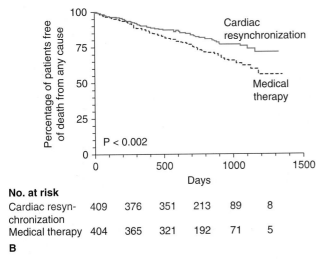

B

FIGURE 62-4 Kaplan–Meier estimates of the time to the primary end-point (A), and the principal secondary end point (B) in the CARE-HF trial. The primary end point was death from any cause or an unplanned hospitalization for a major cardiovascular event, significantly decreased by CRT-P (hazard ratio, 0.63, 95% confidence interval, 0.51 to 0.77; P<0.001). The principal secondary end point was death from any cause was also decreased by CRT-P (hazard ratio, 0.64; 95% confidence interval, 0.48 to 0.85; P<0.002). Reproduced with permission from Cleland JG, Daubert JC, Erdmann E, et al. The effect of cardiac resynchronization on morbidity and mortality in heart failure. *N Engl J Med*. 2005;April 14;352(15):1539-1549.

REFERENCES

1. Bristow MR, Saxon LA, Boehmer J, et al. Cardiac-resynchronization therapy with or without an implantable defibrillator in advanced chronic heart failure. *N Engl J Med*. 2004;350(21):2140-2150.

2. Follath F. Nonischemic heart failure: epidemiology, pathophysiology, and progression of disease. *J Cardiovasc Pharmacol*. 1999;33(Suppl 3):S31-35.

3. Bardy GH, Lee KL, Mark DB, et al. Amiodarone or an implantable cardioverter-defibrillator for congestive heart failure. *N Engl J Med*. 2005;352(3):225-237.

4. Epstein AE, DiMarco JP, Ellenbogen KA, et al. ACC/AHA/HRS 2008 Guidelines for Device-Based Therapy of Cardiac Rhythm Abnormalities: a report of the American College of Cardiology/American Heart Association Task Force on Practice Guidelines (Writing Committee to Revise the ACC/AHA/NASPE 2002 Guideline Update for Implantation of Cardiac Pacemakers and Antiarrhythmia Devices) developed in collaboration with the American Association for Thoracic Surgery and Society of Thoracic Surgeons. *J Am Coll Cardiol*. 2008;51(21):e1-62.

5. Kadish A, Dyer A, Daubert JP, et al. Prophylactic defibrillator implantation in patients with nonischemic dilated cardiomyopathy. *N Engl J Med*. 2004;350(21):2151-2158.

6. McNamara DM, Starling RC, Cooper LT, et al. Clinical and demographic predictors of outcomes in recent onset dilated cardiomyopathy: results of the IMAC (Intervention in Myocarditis and Acute Cardiomyopathy)-2 study. *J Am Coll Cardiol*. 2011;58(11):1112-1118.

7. Bansch D, Antz M, Boczor S, et al. Primary prevention of sudden cardiac death in idiopathic dilated cardiomyopathy—The "Cardiomyopathy Trial (CAT). *Circulation*. 2002;105(12):1453-1458.

8. Kadish A, Schaechter A, Subacius H, et al. Patients with recently diagnosed nonischemic cardiomyopathy benefit from implantable cardioverter-defibrillators. *J Am Coll Cardiol*. 2006;47(12):2477-2482.

9. National Coverage Determination (NCD) for Implantable Automatic Defibrillators. 2005; http://www.cms.gov/medicare-coverage-database/details/ncd-details.aspx?NCDId=110&ncdver=3&bc=A AAAgAAAAAAAAA%3d%3d&. Accessed Oct 21, 2014.

10. Baldasseroni S, Opasich C, Gorini M, et al. Left bundle-branch block is associated with increased 1-year sudden and total mortality rate in 5517 outpatients with congestive heart failure: a report from the Italian network on congestive heart failure. *Am Heart J*. 2002;143(3):398-405.

11. Silvet H, Amin J, Padmanabhan S, et al. Prognostic implications of increased QRS duration in patients with moderate and severe left ventricular systolic dysfunction. *Am J Cardiol*. 2001;88(2):182-185, A186.

12. Tabrizi F, Englund A, Rosenqvist M, et al. Influence of left bundle branch block on long-term mortality in a population with heart failure. *Eur Heart J*. 2007;28(20):2449-2455.

13. Horwich T, Lee SJ, Saxon L. Usefulness of QRS prolongation in predicting risk of inducible monomorphic ventricular tachycardia in patients referred for electrophysiologic studies. *Am J Cardiol*. 2003;92(7):804-809.

14. Cleland JG, Daubert JC, Erdmann E, et al. The effect of cardiac resynchronization on morbidity and mortality in heart failure. *N Engl J Med*. 2005;352(15):1539-1549.

15. Lin GA, Matlock DD. Less patient-centered care: an unintended consequence of guidelines? *JAMA Intern Med*. 2013;173(7):578-579.

63 AVID REGISTRY: REVERSIBLE CAUSES OF SUDDEN CARDIAC DEATH

Richard Bayer II, MD, and Michael Gold, MD

CASE PRESENTATION

A 20-year-old woman with a medical history of only a recent urinary tract infection presented to the emergency department for evaluation of palpitations. While in the waiting room the patient suffered a witnessed cardiac arrest. A code was called and cardiopulmonary resuscitation (CPR) was begun. Upon arrival of the code team, she was noted to be in ventricular tachycardia (Figure 63-1) and was externally defibrillated to normal sinus rhythm. Subsequent 12-lead ECG (Figure 63-2) demonstrated a prolonged QT interval with a QTc of 640 ms. She continued to have frequent episodes of ventricular tachycardia that were refractory to magnesium and amiodarone infusion but responsive to lidocaine. Further interviewing of the family revealed that the patient had been started on levofloxacin 3 days prior for a urinary tract infection. At this time the levofloxacin was discontinued, and trimethoprim/sulfamethoxazole was substituted. She was monitored in the cardiac critical care unit where she continued to have nonsustained runs of ventricular tachycardia of decreasing frequency over the next 48 hours. The lidocaine was discontinued, and her QTc shortened and eventually returned to normal (Figure 63-3). After 3 days of observation, she demonstrated no further episodes of ventricular tachycardia. She was discharged home and at follow-up had a normal 12-lead ECG including a normal QT interval.

A 60-year-old man with a known medical history of coronary artery disease, previous stent to the left anterior descending coronary artery with a chronically occluded right coronary artery, hypertension, hyperlipidemia, diabetes, and an ischemic cardiomyopathy with an ejection fraction (EF) of 40% presents after an out-of-hospital cardiac arrest. He was playing golf with a friend when he was noted to suddenly collapse. CPR was initiated and EMS was contacted. An automatic external defibrillator (AED) was available and was used to defibrillate the patient. Interrogation of the AED revealed the patient to be in ventricular tachycardia (Figure 63-4). Upon arrival to the emergency department, routine laboratory work revealed a low potassium level of 3.2 mmol/L. The patient was started on potassium replacement, and a single chamber implantable cardiac defibrillator (ICD) was placed. At follow-up, his potassium level had remained in the normal range; however, interrogation of his ICD revealed several episodes of ventricular tachycardia that were pace-terminated.

ETIOLOGY

There are several mechanisms by which sudden cardiac death (ventricular tachycardia/ventricular fibrillation [VT/VF]) can be can be caused by potentially reversible causes. The most common of these include electrolyte imbalances, drugs, and ischemia.[1]

Electrolyte Abnormalities

Hypokalemia

Hypokalemia is a common electrolyte abnormality that is encountered during clinical practice. It can be observed in as many as 20% of hospitalized patients.[2] This prevalence is notable among cardiac patients, as the most common cause of hypokalemia is the use of diuretics, mainstay therapy for hypertension and heart failure.[2] See Table 63-1 for major causes of hypokalemia.

Potassium is necessary in the maintenance of the cardiac myocyte resting transmembrane potential as well as repolarization of the cardiac action potential[3,4] (Figure 63-5). As such, alterations in the serum potassium concentration can have important cellular electrophysiolgic effects. Specifically, low serum potassium concentrations decrease the outward delayed rectifier current (I_{Kr}), prolonging repolarization.[3] This may occur through internalization and degradation of the HERG channels that are responsible for I_{Kr}, which has been demonstrated to occur at low serum potassium concentrations.[5] The electrocardiographic results of hypokalemia can be prolongation of the QT interval predisposing to malignant ventricular arrhythmias and torsades de pointes.[3,5]

Hyperkalemia

While not as common as hypokalemia, hyperkalemia can occur in up to 8% of hospitalized patients. Hyperkalemia is most commonly

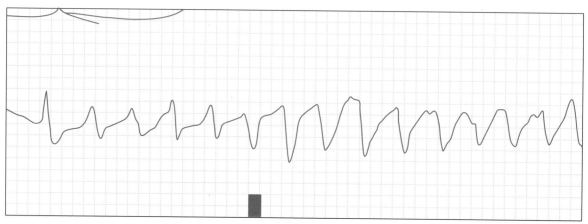

FIGURE 63-1 Initial rhythm seen on rhythm strip following witnessed arrest.

AVID REGISTRY: REVERSIBLE CAUSES
OF SUDDEN CARDIAC DEATH

SECTION IX
IMPLANTABLE CARDIAC DEVICES FOR
MANAGEMENT OF MALIGNANT

425

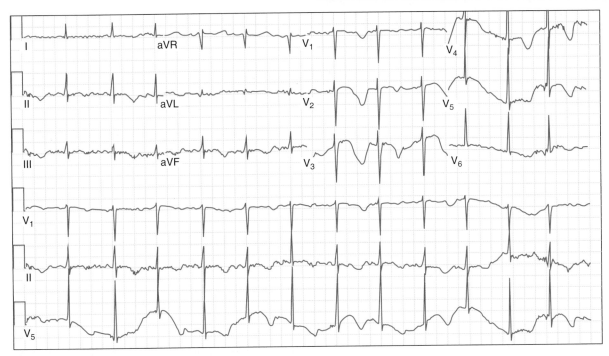

FIGURE 63-2 Initial 12-lead ECG following defibrillation.

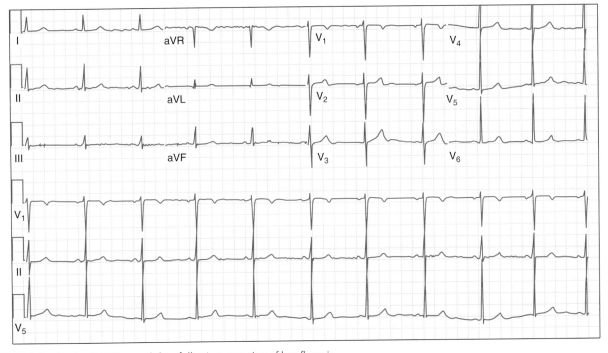

FIGURE 63-3 Twelve-lead ECG several days following cessation of levofloxacin.

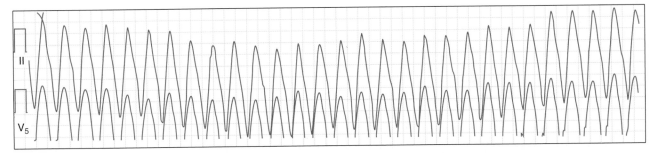

FIGURE 63-4 Rhythm strip of initial rhythm prompting defibrillation from AED.

TABLE 63-1 Major Causes of Hypokalemia

Causes of Hypokalemia

Renal losses

- Diuretic use
- Renal tubular acidosis
- Hypomagnesemia
- Mineralocorticoid excess

Gastrointestinal loses

- Diarrhea
- Emesis
- Laxatives
- Drainage (naso-gastric tube, G-tube, etc.)

Intracellular shift

- Alkalosis
- Excess insulin
- Hypothermia
- Use of beta-agonists

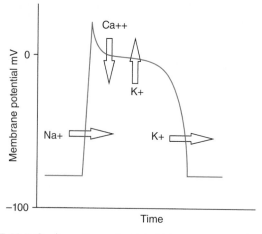

FIGURE 63-5 Cardiac action potential with ion movements during the various phases. Sodium and calcium ions entering the cell; potassium ions moving out of the cell during repolarization.

TABLE 63-2 Major Causes of Hyperkalemia

Causes of Hypokalemia

Reduced excretion

- Acute and chronic kidney disease
- Aldoseterone deficiency
- Volume depletion

Extracellular shift

- Acidosis
- Hyperglycemia
- Beta blockers
- Exercise

Drugs

- Digoxin
- Succinylcholine
- Calcineurin inhibitors
- Minoxidil

observed in patients with renal insufficiency and as a consequence of medications.[6] Please see Table 63-2 for causes of hyperkalemia.

The cardiac myocyte resting membrane potential is maintained at approximately −90 mV.[3] As extracellular potassium levels increase, as in the setting of hyperkalemia, the resting membrane potential decreases. This change in resting membrane potential affects the number of voltage gated sodium channels available for activation during phase 0 of the action potential. As the number of sodium channels available decreases, the magnitude of the inward sodium current decreases, resulting in slowing of impulse propagation and prolongation of membrane depolarization. As potassium levels continue to rise, membrane depolarization continues to lengthen with widening of the QRS and eventual merging with the T wave, producing a sine wave pattern. Once this is observed, without normalization of the potassium level, ventricular fibrillation and asystole are almost certain.[7]

Hypomagnesemia

Hypomagnesemia is another frequently occurring electrolyte abnormality, occurring in up to 12% of hospitalized patients.[8] Similar to potassium, the use of diuretics, both loop and thiazide-type, can result in renal magnesium wasting.[9] Other medications, such as the frequently prescribed proton pump inhibitors, can also cause hypomagnesaemia through decreased absorption.[10]

The effects of magnesium on the cardiac action potential most likely occurs through its interactions with the ion channels of other cations. Magnesium within the cardiac cell functions to block cellular potassium channels thus limiting efflux of intracellular potassium. This action is crucial in promoting the potassium flow that comprises the inward rectification current.[11] Magnesium also influences calcium movement through L-type Ca^{++} channels, which work with the rectification current to maintain the phase 2 plateau of the cardiac action potential.[3,11] Increase in either of these currents, resulting from magnesium depletion, decreases the cardiac action potential and thus increases susceptibility to arrhythmias.[12]

AVID REGISTRY: REVERSIBLE CAUSES
OF SUDDEN CARDIAC DEATH

SECTION IX
IMPLANTABLE CARDIAC DEVICES FOR
MANAGEMENT OF MALIGNANT

427

Hypocalcemia

Hypocalcemia is most frequently encountered in patients with chronic renal insufficiency.[6] During phase 2 of the cardiac action potential, influx of calcium though L-type Ca^{++} channels balances outward movement of potassium, which produces the plateau phase.[3] A low extracellular calcium level decreases this inward flow. This decreased inward flow of calcium works also to decrease the outward flux of potassium and functions to prolong the action potential. The end result is prolongation of the QT interval and risk for the development of torsades de pointes.[6]

Medications and Drugs

Both prescription medications as well as illicit drugs can cause VT and VF through a variety of mechanisms.

Acquired Long QT

The exact incidence of drug-induced long QT and subsequent development of torsades de pointes is largely unknown. According to data from the World Health Organization Drug Monitoring Centre, there were 761 cases of drug-induced torsades de pointes reported between 1983 and 1999. Of these 761 cases, 34 were fatal. However, there is some speculation that due to variable reporting this voluntary reporting system may underestimate the true incidence by as much as 10-fold.[13] A large population-based case-control study conducted in the Netherlands demonstrated a significant increase in the risk of sudden cardiac death with current use of any noncardiac QT-prolonging drug with an odds ratio of 2.7. However, the overall incidence was still quite low with only 24/775 cases currently using a noncardiac QT-prolonging drug.[14]

The most common mechanism by which medications prolong the QT interval is through blockade of the potassium channel encoded by the HERG gene.[3,13] Blockade of this channel results in decreased potassium efflux, I_{Kr}, prolonging repolarization and phase 3 of the action potential. Prolongation of repolarization in turn leaves myocardial cells susceptible to early afterdepolarizations, resulting in triggered activity. In the right environment, this triggered activity can then result in reentry and perpetuation of torsades de pointes.[13] This effect may be further modulated by serum potassium concentrations. As serum potassium levels decrease the blocking effect of the drug on I_{Kr} is enhanced. This results in a further increase in the duration of repolarization and a subsequent increase in the risk of development of torsades de pointes. However, at higher potassium concentrations the blocking effects on I_{Kr} are attenuated, less QT prolongation is seen, and the risk of torsades de pointes is lessened.[15]

Sodium Channel Blockers

Drugs that block sodium channels can perpetuate VT or VF via a different mechanism. By blocking sodium channels, conduction is slowed via prolongation of rapid depolarization, phase 0 of the action potential.[3,16] In this setting, reentry may be perpetuated because with slower conduction a propagating wavefront of depolarization is less likely to encounter refractory myocardium and in turn be quenched. In patients with circuits for reentry, such as scar formation from ischemic heart disease, this has the potential to sustain reentry and thus VT. While this VT is frequently slower, it has the potential to degenerate into slow VF that can be highly resistant to cardioversion.[16]

Cocaine

Cocaine is the most frequently abused illicit drug that results in emergency department visits in the United States. In 2011, it was responsible for just over 40% of the 1.25 million emergency department visits involving illicit drugs.[17]

Cocaine can cause sudden cardiac death through multiple mechanisms. Perhaps the most well known mechanism is myocardial ischemia precipitated by catecholamine-induced vasoconstriction.[18] However, cocaine also has a more direct proarrhythmic effect by interaction with both cardiac sodium and potassium channels.[18,19] Cocaine blocks the sodium channel and thus prolongs rapid depolarization, phase 0 of the action potential. Similar to class I antiarrhythmic medications, by prolonging the action potential there is a risk for perpetuating reentry, as it is less likely to encounter refractory myocardium.[18] Cocaine is also frequently used in conjunction with alcohol. In this setting a compound, cocaethylene, is formed which also functions to block sodium channels. Thus the arrhythmogenesis of cocaine may be enhanced when combined with alcohol.[18,19] The effects on the sodium channels also exhibit use dependence, and thus faster heart rates result in more potent blockade and further slowing of depolarization.[19] Given that cocaine increases circulating catecholamines and thus increases heart rate, it potentiates its own effects, thus increasing the risk for life-threatening arrhythmias.[18] Not only does cocaine block sodium channels, it also blocks potassium channels responsible for the rapid phase of the delayed rectified current, I_{Kr}.[18,19] Interestingly, its effects of repolarization are biphasic. At low concentration, it appears to selectively inhibit I_{Kr}, resulting in QT prolongation. However, at high concentrations it not only inhibits I_{Kr}, but also the inward sodium flow and possibly inward calcium movement resulting in a decrease in repolarization time. As a result, at low doses, one may expect to see more torsades de pointes, owing to I_{Kr} inhibition. While at higher doses, slow monomorphic VT may occur due to sodium channel blockade.[18]

Ischemia

Perhaps the most well-known cause of sudden cardiac death is that of myocardial ischemia and infarction. However, the overall incidence of sustained ventricular arrhythmias, VT or VF, still remains low. In a population of just over 40 000 ST-segment elevation myocardial infarction patients, sustained VT/VF occurred in just 10.2%, with approximately 80% of these occurring within the first 48 hours.[20] The frequency of these arrhythmias is even lower in patients with non–ST-segment elevation myocardial infarction (NSTEMI) or unstable angina (UA). In a population of just over 25 000 NSTEMI/UA patients, sustained VT/VF occurred in just 2.1%.[21]

The pathogenesis behind ischemia causing malignant ventricular arrhythmias is likely related to changes in the resting cardiac membrane potential as well as disruption of the normal ion currents. In the setting of ischemia, the resting membrane potential of the cardiac myocyte is reduced.[3] This reduction in trans-membrane potential is due to efflux of potassium ions. Some of this is attributed to ischemia-induced inhibition of the Na^+/K^+ cotransporter.[22] However, this alone does not explain the extent of potassium loss. With ischemia, the myocyte must switch to anaerobic metabolism, generating anion by-products such as lactate and phosphate, which diffuse out of the cell. Potassium may follow these anions in order to maintain electroneutrality.[23] The results of these changes are reduction in action potential velocity and slowing of conduction time. These areas of slowed conduction, in ischemic tissue, are adjacent to areas of normal conduction, in nonischemic myocardium. This creates an environment where unidirectional block can occur and reentry can be established, and the ultimate result is VT/VF.[3]

TREATMENT

The treatment of reversible sudden cardiac death should be directed to the underlying cause when possible. In the case of electrolyte abnormalities hypo/hyperkalemia, hypomagnesemia, and hypocalcemia should be corrected. In the case of QT-prolonging drugs, these should be discontinued. In these situations when torsades de pointes is likely the malignant arrhythmia, it is imperative that potassium be replaced and intravenous magnesium be administrated. Increasing extracellular potassium helps to increase the rapid component of the delayed rectifier current, I_{Kr} and decrease the drug-induced block. This accelerates repolarization, helping to shorten the QT interval. Magnesium does not shorten the QT interval, and its exact mechanism of decreasing arrhythmogenesis is unknown; however, it has been postulated to be related to blocking of calcium channels.[16] In cases that are refractory to potassium and magnesium, overdrive pacing at a rate of around 100 bpm may be beneficial by both shortening the QT interval and decreasing the development of early afterdepolarizations.[24] When ischemia is the inciting event, focus should be directed on reperfusion therapies.

ICD versus No ICD

Following successful resuscitation from sudden cardiac death, a decision will need to be made regarding the possible implantation of an ICD for secondary prevention. It has been convention that patients, with what was thought to be a transient or reversible cause of cardiac arrest, were at low risk of subsequent death and did not require ICD implantation.[1] This appears to be most apparent in the population of patients with an acute ST elevation myocardial infarction as the cause of their sudden cardiac death. In a series that evaluated 143 patients who were successfully resuscitated and then discharged following an out-of-hospital cardiac arrest, patients presenting with ECG evidence of a transmural infarction were at the lowest risk of mortality at follow-up. At 16 months of follow-up no patients in the acute transmural infarction group died, and after 2 years, the group had a mortality rate of 14%. This is compared to the group who had sudden cardiac death not related to an acute transmural MI who had mortality rates of 32% and 43% at 16 months and 2 years, respectively.[25] More recent studies have also demonstrated the relative lack of impact on mortality in the setting of recent MI. Two large randomized controlled trials looking at just over 1200 patients who were randomized to ICD versus medical therapy within 40 days of an acute MI with a reduced left ventricular ejection fraction showed no mortality benefit with early prophylactic ICD implantation. While both trials were able to show a reduction in the number of sudden cardiac deaths, this benefit was offset by an increased number of nonsudden cardiac death.[26,27]

Whereas the data are convincing that patients presenting with sudden cardiac death as a result of acute MI do not benefit from prophylactic ICD implantation, the other potential reversible causes have not been evaluated thoroughly. The Antiarrhythmics Versus Implantable Defibrillators Trial (AVID) clearly showed a benefit of ICD versus antiarrhythmic drug therapy (primarily amiodarone) among patients presenting with VT or VF. However, patients with what were felt to be reversible causes were excluded from the randomized portion of this trial. Yet, a secondary analysis of the nonrandomized registry revealed that at 3 years of follow-up the mortality of this group approached 30%. This was not statistically different from the mortality rate of those patients presenting with primary VT/VF, and when mortality was adjusted for age, ejection fraction, coronary artery disease, coronary artery bypass grafting, and aspirin usage, the mortality in the reversible causes subset was actually greater.[28] This illustrates that the determination of patients at low risk is difficult and that patients presenting with what is felt to represent a reversible cause of sudden cardiac death need to be evaluated rigorously and followed closely, given their high mortality rate.

CASE DISCUSSION

Both of the cases presented at the beginning of the chapter illustrate patients who presented with aborted sudden cardiac death and who had potential causes of their arrest that were reversible. In the case of the young woman, she was being treated with a known QT-prolonging drug, and discontinuation of this drug resulted in normalization of her QT interval. She was also found to have a structurally normal heart, and the presenting arrhythmia was torsades de pointes. She was cautioned to notify her physicians about future use of potential QT-prolonging medications. In this setting she was appropriately deemed to be at low risk for recurrent sudden cardiac death and did not undergo ICD implantation. The second case illustrates a patient with multiple cardiac risk factors who had a cardiac arrest in the setting of mild hypokalemia. He was deemed to be of higher risk for recurrent sudden cardiac death. This determination was made after careful review of his care. While indeed his potassium was low, his presenting sudden cardiac death was not secondary to torsades de pointes, as one would expect with hypokalemia. Also, given his reduced ejection fraction and that he requires chronic diuretic usage for heart failure symptoms, he was felt to be at high risk for recurrent VT/VF, and thus an ICD was implanted. In retrospect, this was the appropriate decision given that at follow-up he was noted to have several pace-terminated episodes of VT.

REFERENCES

1. Wyse DG, Friedman PL, Brodsky MA, et al. Life-threatening ventricular arrhythmias due to transient or correctable causes: high risk for death in follow-up. *J Am Coll Cardiol.* 2001;38(6):1718-1724.

2. Gennari FJ. Hypokalemia. *N Engl J Med.* 1998;339(7):451-458.

3. Zipes DP, Braunwald E. *Braunwald's Heart Disease: A Textbook of Cardiovascular Medicine.* 7th ed. Philadelphia, PA: W.B. Saunders; 2005:75.

4. Lilly LS and Harvard Medical School. *Pathophysiology of Heart Disease: A Collaborative Project of Medical Students and Faculty.*

AVID REGISTRY: REVERSIBLE CAUSES
OF SUDDEN CARDIAC DEATH

SECTION IX
IMPLANTABLE CARDIAC DEVICES FOR
MANAGEMENT OF MALIGNANT

429

5th ed. Baltimore, MD: Wolters Kluwer/Lippincott Williams & Wilkins; 2011:461.

5. Guo J, Massaeli H, Extracellular K+ concentration controls cell surface density of IKr in rabbit hearts and of the HERG channel in human cell lines. *J Clin Invest.* 2009;119(9): 2745-2757.

6. El-Sherif N, Turitto G. Electrolyte disorders and arrhythmogenesis. *Cardiol J.* 2011;18(3):233-245.

7. Parham WA, Mehdirad AA, Biermann KM, Fredman CS. Hyperkalemia revisited. *Tex Heart Inst J.* 2006;33(1):40-47.

8. Wong ET, Rude RK, Singer FR, Shaw ST Jr. A. A high prevalence of hypomagnesemia and hypermagnesemia in hospitalized patients. *Am J Clin Pathol.* 1983;79(3):348-352.

9. Siegel D, Hulley SB, Black DM, et al. Diuretics, serum and intracellular electrolyte levels, and ventricular arrhythmias in hypertensive men. *JAMA.* 1992;267(8):1083-1089.

10. Broeren MA, Geerdink EA, Vader HL, van den Wall Blake AW. Hypomagnesemia induced by several proton-pump inhibitors. *Ann Intern Med.* 2009;151(10):755-756.

11. Fazekas T, Scherlag BJ, Vos M, Wellens HJ, Lazzara R. Magnesium and the heart: antiarrhythmic therapy with magnesium. *Clin Cardiol.* 1993;16(11):768-774.

12. Agus ZS. Hypomagnesemia. *J Am Soc Nephrol.* 1999;10(7):1616-1622.

13. Yap YG, Camm AJ. Drug induced QT prolongation and torsades de pointes. *Heart.* 2003;89(11):1363-1372.

14. Straus SM, Sturkenboom MC, Bleumink GS, et al. Non-cardiac QTc-prolonging drugs and the risk of sudden cardiac death. *Eur Heart J.* 2005;26(19):2007-2012.

15. Yang T, Roden DM. Extracellular potassium modulation of drug block of IKr. Implications for torsade de pointes and reverse use-dependence. *Circulation.* 1996;93(3):407-411.

16. Roden DM. Mechanisms and management of proarrhythmia. *Am J Cardiol.* 1998;82(4A):49I-57I.

17. United States. Substance Abuse and Mental Health Services Administration. Office of Applied Studies. Drug Abuse Warning Network: national estimates of drug-related emergency department visits, in DHHS publication no (SMA) 2006, U.S. Dept. of Health and Human Services, Substance Abuse and Mental Health Services Administration: Rockville, MD.

18. O'Leary ME, Hancox JC. Role of voltage-gated sodium, potassium and calcium channels in the development of cocaine-associated cardiac arrhythmias. *Br J Clin Pharmacol.* 2010;69(5):427-442.

19. Bauman JL, DiDomenico RJ. Cocaine-induced channelopathies: emerging evidence on the multiple mechanisms of sudden death. *J Cardiovasc Pharmacol Ther.* 2002;7(3):195-202.

20. Newby KH, Thompson T, Stebbins A, et al. Sustained ventricular arrhythmias in patients receiving thrombolytic therapy: incidence and outcomes. The GUSTO Investigators. *Circulation.* 1998;98(23):2567-2573.

21. Al-Khatib SM, Granger CB, Huang Y, et al. Sustained ventricular arrhythmias among patients with acute coronary syndromes with no ST-segment elevation: incidence, predictors, and outcomes. *Circulation.* 2002;106(3):309-312.

22. Vermeulen JT, Tan HL, Rademaker H, et al. Electrophysiologic and extracellular ionic changes during acute ischemia in failing and normal rabbit myocardium. *J Mol Cell Cardiol.* 1996;28(1):123-131.

23. Kleber AG. Resting membrane potential, extracellular potassium activity, and intracellular sodium activity during acute global ischemia in isolated perfused guinea pig hearts. *Circ Res.* 1983;52(4):442-450.

24. Khan IA. Long QT syndrome: diagnosis and management. *Am Heart J.* 2002;143(1):7-14.

25. Baum RS, Alvarez H 3rd, Cobb LA. Survival after resuscitation from out-of-hospital ventricular fibrillation. *Circulation.* 1974;50(6):1231-1235.

26. Steinbeck G, Andresen D, Seidl K, et al. Defibrillator implantation early after myocardial infarction. *N Engl J Med.* 2009;361(15):1427-1436.

27. Hohnloser SH, Kuck KH, Dorian P, et al. Prophylactic use of an implantable cardioverter-defibrillator after acute myocardial infarction. *N Engl J Med.* 2004;351(24):2481-2488.

28. Anderson JL, Hallstrom AP, Epstein AE, et al. Design and results of the antiarrhythmics vs implantable defibrillators (AVID) registry. The AVID Investigators. *Circulation.* 1999;99(13):1692-1699.

64 PATIENT WITH ISCHEMIC CARDIOMYOPATHY PRESENTS WITH SUSTAINED STABLE VENTRICULAR TACHYCARDIA

Byron K. Lee, MD, and Jeffrey E. Olgin, MD

CASE PRESENTATION

A 90-year-old man with a history of previous myocardial infarction (MI), coronary artery bypass surgery, and recurrent right side pleural effusions was admitted for effusion drainage. During his hospitalization, he developed sudden onset of a wide complex tachycardia (Figure 64-1) requiring cardioversion. IV amiodarone was started. Troponins were found to be borderline positive. Catheterization showed total occlusion of both the right coronary artery and a saphenous vein graft to the LAD. Although neither occlusion appeared to be acute, both vessels were stented. Following percutaneous coronary intervention, despite continued IV amiodarone and multiple external cardioversions, the wide complex tachycardia was recurrent and then became incessant. At heart rates in the 140 to 180 bpm range, he maintained his systolic blood pressure at 90 to 110 mm Hg. He was transferred to our hospital for EP study and ablation.

EXPERT OPINION

- The differential diagnosis for a wide complex tachycardia include:
  - Ventricular tachycardia (VT)
  - Supraventricular tachycardia (SVT) with aberrancy (ie, LBBB or RBBB)
  - Paced tachycardia
  - Antidromicatrial ventricular reciprocating tachycardia (AVRT)
  - SVT with a bystander accessory pathway

- Patients with previous MI or impaired ejection fraction are at higher risk for VT.

- Paced tachycardias should have pacing spikes before each QRS.

- Antidromic AVRT and SVT with a bystander accessory pathway are seen in Wolff-Parkinson-White patients who should have a delta wave on baseline ECG.

- In this patient, VT was suspected based on the history of MI. Furthermore, there were more QRS complexes than P waves seen on the presenting ECG (see arrows in Figure 64-1), essentially clinching the diagnosis of VT. Rarely, SVTs such as AVNRT with upper common final pathway block or junctional tachycardia with retrograde block in the AVN can have more ventricular depolarizations than atrial depolarizations; however, one would not expect a wide QRS complex different than the native QRS in that case.

- For patients with incessant VT, antiarrhythmics are typically tried first to suppress the VT.

- When antiarrhythmics are not successful, emergent ablation is necessary.

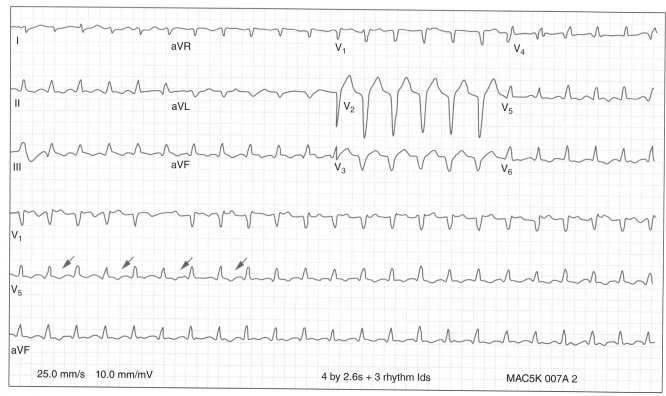

FIGURE 64-1 ECG of the wide complex tachycardia. There are more QRS complexes than P-wave complexes (arrow), essentially clinching that the mechanism of the wide complex tachycardia is ventricular tachycardia.

PATIENT WITH ISCHEMIC CARDIOMYOPATHY
PRESENTS WITH SUSTAINED STABLE
VENTRICULAR TACHYCARDIA

SECTION IX
IMPLANTABLE CARDIAC DEVICES FOR
MANAGEMENT OF MALIGNANT

431

- Although ICD implantation may be eventually necessary, it is not the next step in management of patients with incessant VT since it would lead to multiple shocks.

PATHOPHYSIOLOGY AND MANAGEMENT

- The patient was brought to the EP Laboratory in stable VT.

- A diagnosis of VT was confirmed with intracardiac recordings.

- Mapping of the tachycardia started in the LV since the patient had a scar in the LV from a previous anterior wall MI.

- Voltage mapping of the LV showed low voltages in the apical septum corresponding to scar from the previous MI (Figure 64-2).

- Activation mapping showed the VT was likely from a small circuit exiting from the mid septum basal to the scar (Figure 64-3).

- Mapping in this region discovered a site with a mid-diastolic potential (Figure 64-4), indicating that the catheter tip is at a protected area of slow conduction.

- Pace-mapping at this site led to conduction delay and a pace map matching perfectly the clinical VT (Figure 64-5), indicating that catheter tip is in a region of slow conduction that exits from the same region as the VT.

- The postpacing interval after pace-mapping matched the VT cycle length, indicating that this site was in the circuit.

- Ablation at this site promptly terminated the tachycardia. No VT was inducible after ablation.

- The patient had no recurrent VT subsequently.

- An ICD was placed prior to discharge.

FEATURES OF VENTRICULAR TACHYCARDIA IN ISCHEMIC CARDIOMYOPATHY

- VT in ischemic cardiomyopathy is typically due to a reentrant circuit involving the scar from a previous MI.

- When the VT is stable (not leading hemodynamic collapse), ablation of the targeted VT is successful in 71% to 79% of patients.[1-5]

- Three-dimensional mapping and more powerful ablation catheters have improved the ablation of VT.

- After acutely successful VT ablation, 31% of patients during follow-up of 9 to 25 months have recurrence of either the original VT or a new VT.[1-5]

- It is controversial whether patients with ischemic cardiomyopathy and ejection fraction >35% who have had successful VT ablation should get an ICD.[1-3]

- Even though the recurrence rate of VT is relatively high after ablation, most VT recurrences are not fatal.[1-3]

- ICDs are very effective in terminating VT. Frequently, the ICD can terminate the VT with antitachycardic pacing rather than a shock that might cause pain.

- Patients with frequent or incessant VT, even if they meet guidelines for ICD implantation will need therapy for the VT (either drugs or ablation) to prevent frequent ICD shocks.

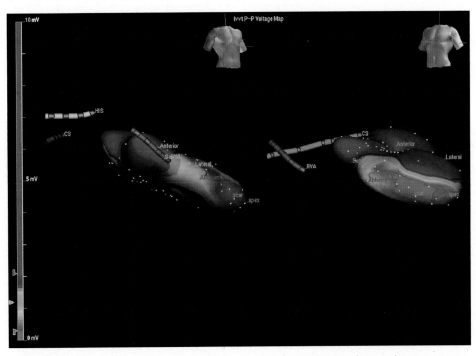

FIGURE 64-2 Voltage map of the LV during VT. The gray color indicates an area of low voltage in the apical septum corresponding to scar from the previous MI.

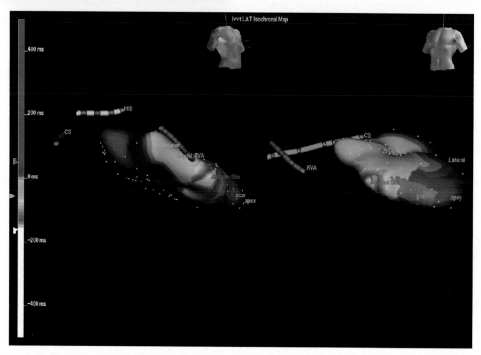

FIGURE 64-3 Activation map of the LV during VT. The white color indicates that the earliest site of ventricular activation is the mid-septum just basal to the scar. The reentry circuit is exiting from this region.

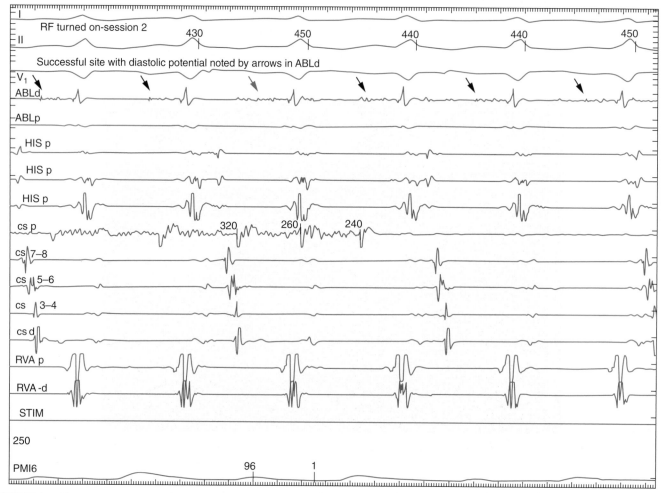

FIGURE 64-4 Activation mapping at the successful ablation site. The mid-diastolic potentials (arrows) indicate that the catheter tip is at a protected area of slow conduction, suggesting a good site for ablation.

PATIENT WITH ISCHEMIC CARDIOMYOPATHY
PRESENTS WITH SUSTAINED STABLE
VENTRICULAR TACHYCARDIA

SECTION IX
IMPLANTABLE CARDIAC DEVICES FOR
MANAGEMENT OF MALIGNANT

433

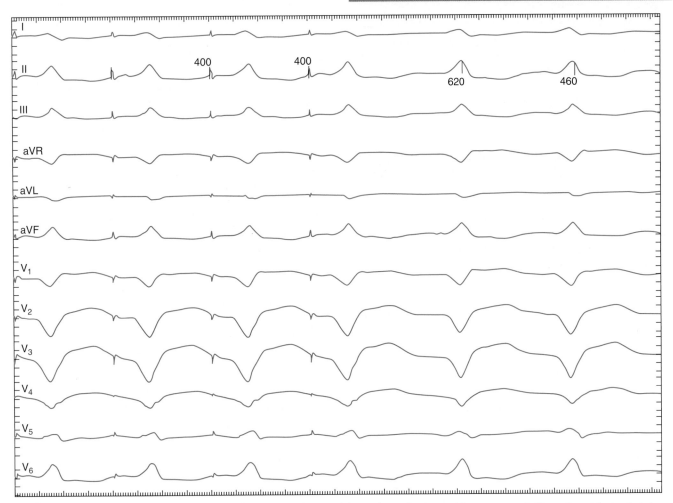

FIGURE 64-5 Pace-mapping at the successful ablation site. Conduction delay and a perfectly matching pace map indicate that catheter tip is in a region of slow conduction that exits from the same region as the VT, suggesting a good site for ablation.

REFERENCES

1. Borger van der Burg AE, de Groot NM, van Erven L, Bootsma M, van der Wall EE, Schalij MJ. Long-term follow-up after radiofrequency catheter ablation of ventricular tachycardia: a successful approach? *J Cardiovasc Electrophysiol*. 2002;13(5):417-423.

2. Delacretaz E, Stevenson WG. Catheter ablation of ventricular tachycardia in patients with coronary heart disease. Part II: Clinical aspects, limitations, and recent developments. Pacing Clin Electrophysiol. 2001;24(9 Pt 1):1403-1411.

3. Della Bella P, De Ponti R, Uriarte JA, et al. Catheter ablation and antiarrhythmic drugs for haemodynamically tolerated post-infarction ventricular tachycardia; long-term outcome in relation to acute electrophysiological findings. *Eur Heart J*. 2002;23(5): 414-424.

4. Nabar A, et al. Echocardiographic predictors of survival in patients undergoing radiofrequency ablation of postinfarct clinical ventricular tachycardia. *J Cardiovasc Electrophysiol*. 2002;13(1 Suppl):S118-121.

5. Strickberger SA, et al. A prospective evaluation of catheter ablation of ventricular tachycardia as adjuvant therapy in patients with coronary artery disease and an implantable cardioverter-defibrillator. *Circulation*. 1997;96(5):1525-1531.

65 MANAGING RECURRENT ICD THERAPIES: MEDICAL THERAPY

Paul L. Hess, MD, and Sana M. Al-Khatib, MD, MHS

CASE PRESENTATION

A 61-year-old man with ischemic cardiomyopathy, a left ventricular ejection fraction of 25%, and an implantable cardioverter defibrillator (ICD) presented for an ICD shock that occurred at home without any warning. The device fired 2 weeks prior to the current presentation without associated symptoms. After a second shock in the emergency department that was clearly delivered for ventricular tachycardia (VT) (Figure 65-1), a bolus of amiodarone was administered followed by a continuous infusion. On arrival to the floor, the patient initially denied symptoms but was concerned about whether he would receive another shock. Device interrogation confirmed two appropriate shocks. A cardiac catheterization demonstrated two patent bare metal stents in the left anterior descending artery and diffuse narrowing in all arteries largely unchanged from a cardiac catheterization done 3 years ago. Baseline thyroid and liver function profiles were obtained, and a 6-g load of amiodarone was completed. Defibrillation threshold testing was performed, and a >10-J safety margin was documented. Upon discharge, oral amiodarone was prescribed, and close follow-up was arranged with his cardiologist and electrophysiologist. He was instructed to call the clinic if he received a single shock and to proceed directly to the emergency department in the event of a second shock or if he had significant symptoms with one shock. During follow-up, thyroid and liver function profiles have remained stable, and no further ICD shocks have been delivered.

EPIDEMIOLOGY

- Claiming the lives of more than 400 000 patients in the United States annually, sudden cardiac death is a significant public health hazard.[1] The ICD improves the overall survival of many patients with left ventricular systolic function[2,3] by terminating malignant arrhythmias. The survival advantage observed in clinical trials translates to a benefit in real-world populations.[4]

- Broadening indications and technology dissemination have led to a rise in the number of patients with ICDs, and in turn, therapies delivered by devices. The incidence of shocks varies according to patient characteristics, including the original indication for ICD placement, as well as concomitant medical therapies and device programming. In the modern therapeutic era, approximately 10% to 20% of patients experience a shock within 1 year, and 40% to 50% experience a shock within 5 years after ICD placement.[5] Two in every three of these are appropriate.[5]

- The incidence of recurrent shocks is less understood.

ETIOLOGY AND PATHOPHYSIOLOGY

- Shocks delivered for VT or ventricular fibrillation are termed "appropriate," while those delivered for any other reason such as supraventricular arrhythmias, noise from electromagnetic interference, or a fractured lead are called "inappropriate."

- Appropriate shocks can occur in the setting of acute ischemia or myocardial scarring. Abrupt ischemia can trigger a number of ventricular arrhythmias, including monomorphic VT (Figure 65-2), polymorphic VT, or ventricular fibrillation. Chronic scarring and temporal dispersion of the surrounding myocardium can lead to VT whose mechanism is typically reentry.

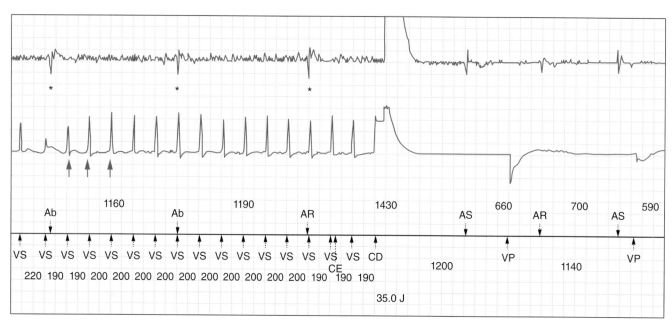

FIGURE 65-1 ICD shock delivery. After the ICD detected an arrhythmia with a higher number of ventricular (arrows) than atrial (*) depolarizations, it appropriately delivered a 35-J defibrillation.

MANAGING RECURRENT ICD
THERAPIES: MEDICAL THERAPY

SECTION IX
IMPLANTABLE CARDIAC DEVICES FOR
MANAGEMENT OF MALIGNANT

435

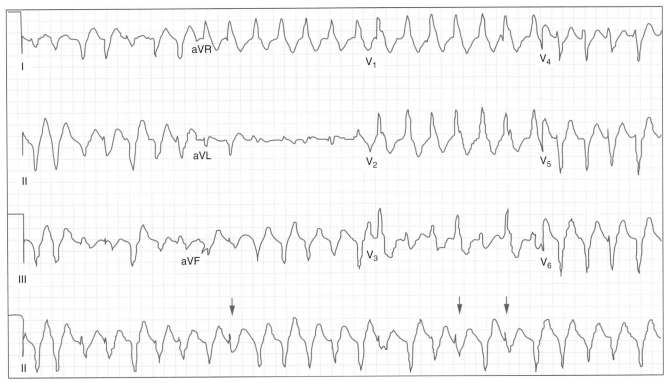

FIGURE 65-2 Monomorphic VT. Electrocardiographic features suggestive of ventricular tachycardia include atrioventricular dissociation, precordial QRS concordance, fusion beats, and capture beats. In this example, fusion beats (arrows) are readily observed in lead II.

- Appropriate shock-inducing arrhythmias are also observed in the setting of decompensated heart failure, electrolyte abnormalities, drug exposures, and genetic disorders.

- Inappropriate shocks are most commonly caused by atrial fibrillation, supraventricular tachycardia, or sinus tachycardia (Figure 65-3A), and abnormal sensing,[6] including T-wave oversensing (Figure 65-3B), double counting of the QRS complex, oversensing of diaphragmatic or skeletal myopotentials, electromagnetic interference, or a fractured lead. ICD programming is a key determinant of therapy delivery. Patients' heart rates must exceed a detection threshold chosen by the treating physician. The duration and number of intervals at heart rates above the threshold also play a role. Programming optimization is imperfect, however, and inappropriate shocks can occur despite it. Mechanical complications related to the ICD and leads per se may also lead to shocks. Problems relating to implantation include a loose set screw, periclavicular lead placement causing a fracture, or lead dislodgment. Manufacturing defects can cause lead fractures or insulation breaks, as has been observed with the Sprint Fidelis and Riata leads respectively. Twiddler's syndrome often occurs in the setting of psychiatric comorbidity and can cause lead dislodgement or failure.

DIAGNOSIS

- When a shock is reported, an assessment is indicated. When this is performed depends on the number of shocks and the associated symptoms. If the patient does not need immediate medical attention, transtelephonic transmission is useful. Patients experiencing ≥2 shocks or significant symptoms should be assessed promptly.

A careful history and physical examination is the cornerstone of any medical evaluation. A history consistent with anginal discomfort may prompt a work-up for ischemia. A history of vomiting or diarrhea may suggest an electrolyte abnormality. Review of prescribed medications may identify a culprit. Device interrogation is critical to differentiate appropriate from inappropriate therapies. VT may be differentiated from a supraventricular cause by comparing the atrial rate with the ventricular rate (see Figure 65-1). If only ventricular markers are available for analysis (such as the case in a single chamber device), a change in R-wave morphology from baseline may provide a clue.

- Noise on the electrogram may indicate electromagnetic interference, a loose set screw, or a lead fracture (Figure 65-4). Software upgrades are available for various lead models that allow early detection and management of lead fractures.

MEDICAL MANAGEMENT

- Potentially offending medications should be stopped. Conversely, evidence-based medications should be initiated or up-titrated barring contraindications, as they reduce mortality and heart failure hospitalizations in patients with left ventricular systolic function. β-Blockers, angiotensin converting enzyme inhibitors, and mineralocorticoid receptor antagonists also favorably impact the risk of sudden death.[7-9]

- In addition to optimizing heart failure therapies, consideration can be given to initiating antiarrhythmic medications. Antiarrhythmic options are dictated by the underlying cause, the two most common of which are atrial fibrillation and VT. Atrial fibrillation can be

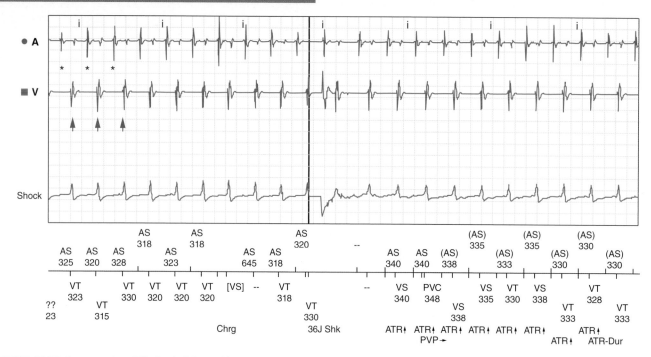

FIGURE 65-3A Inappropriate ICD shock delivered for sinus tachycardia. Atrial depolarizations (*) preceding ventricular depolarizations (arrows) with a 1:1 ratio, QRS morphology identical to that in normal sinus rhythm, and persistence of this rhythm after a shock indicate this tachyarrhythmia was sinus tachycardia. The patient was exercising heavily at the time of the shock.

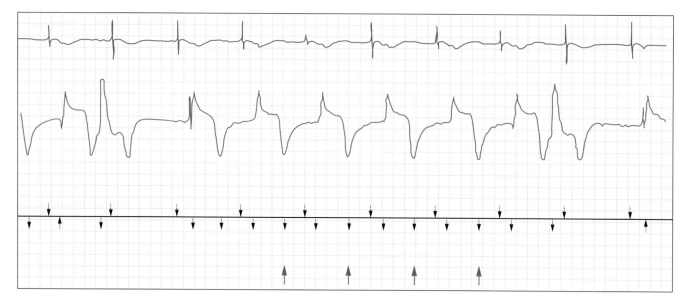

FIGURE 65-3B Inappropriate ICD shock delivered for T-wave over-sensing. Markers at the foot of the strip indicate that both QRS complexes and T waves (arrows) were sensed; this double counting led to shock delivery.

treated with amiodarone, sotalol (if LVEF >20%), or dofetilide.[10] VT can be treated with sotalol (if LVEF >20%) or amiodarone.

- In a multicenter trial of 302 ICD recipients, 160 to 320 mg of sotalol daily resulted in a 44% relative risk reduction in the composite endpoint of death or ICD shock.[11]

- In a different trial of 146 patients with inducible sustained VT or ventricular fibrillation, sotalol reduced the incidence of sustained ventricular tachyarrhythmias compared with no antiarrhythmic drug treatment.[12]

- The isolated enantiomer *d*-sotalol is associated with worse outcomes among patients with severe systolic dysfunction or advanced heart failure and is thus contraindicated in these instances.[13,14] However, the racemic mixture of sotalol (*d,l*-sotalol) is used in current clinical practice.

- Another clinical trial randomized 412 patients to amiodarone and β-blocker, sotalol alone, or β-blocker alone. Sotalol alone was superior to β-blockade in reducing the number of ICD shocks; amiodarone superimposed on background β-blockade was better still.[15]

MANAGING RECURRENT ICD
THERAPIES: MEDICAL THERAPY

SECTION IX
IMPLANTABLE CARDIAC DEVICES FOR
MANAGEMENT OF MALIGNANT

437

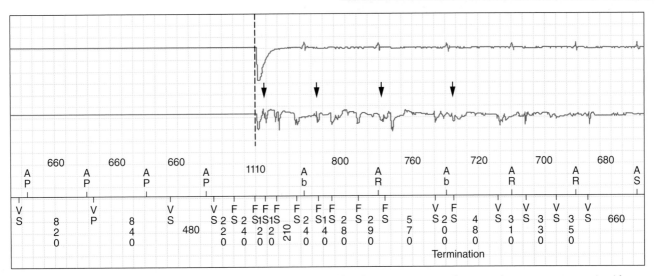

FIGURE 65-4 Electrogram noise. Electrogram noise (arrows) can be caused by electromagnetic interference, a loose set screw, or a lead fracture. The patient in this example had a ventricular lead fracture.

- Amiodarone has been shown to reduce arrhythmic death but not all-cause mortality in several trials.[16-18]

- If either sotalol or amiodarone prove ineffective, mexiletine is a viable alternative. However, a trend toward increased mortality was observed in one trial.[19]

- Mounting evidence suggests off-label use of dofetilide[20] and ranolazine[21] can be considered. The latter is often reserved for patients with ischemic heart disease. The Ranolazine in ICD trial was designed to assess whether ranolazine decreases the likelihood of a composite consisting of VT or ventricular fibrillation requiring antitachycardia pacing, ICD shocks, or death, and is ongoing. Further research on ranolazine and dofetilide is needed.

- In the event of serial shocks, amiodarone in its intravenous form is first-line treatment.

- When using antiarrhythmic drugs, the side effect profiles and potential toxicities must be weighed against the potential therapeutic benefit. Amiodarone toxicities can impact a number of organs, including the eye, thyroid gland, lungs, liver, and skin. Regular monitoring is required, but there are no rigorous data on the best means or optimal frequency. Mexiletine can adversely affect the gastrointestinal and central nervous systems in a dose-dependent fashion. Dofetilide and ranolazine are metabolized by the cytochrome P450 3A enzyme and thus interact with ketoconazole, diltiazem, verapamil, macrolide antibiotics, and grapefruit juice. Sotalol, amiodarone, dofetilide, and ranolazine can prolong the QT interval and potentially cause torsades de pointes. As a general rule, all antiarrhythmics can be viewed as proarrhythmic as well and must be used judiciously. In patients with renal dysfunction, particularly the elderly, sotalol, dofetilide, and ranolazine must be used with caution.

- ICD-antiarrhythmic drug interactions must also be taken into account. Most antiarrhythmic medications have a negative chronotropic effect. Prescribing physicians should therefore optimize bradycardic pacing mode parameters when such medications are started. DDD mode is generally preferred to maintain AV synchrony and minimize the likelihood of pacemaker syndrome. In addition to negative chronotropy, many antiarrhythmic drugs can also affect defibrillation thresholds. Whereas sotalol and dofetilide can decrease defibrillation thresholds, lidocaine and amiodarone increase it. Ranolazine, mexiletine, and propafenone do not appear to significantly affect it. Patients with borderline safety margins may benefit from defibrillation threshold testing after initiating drugs that increase defibrillation thresholds. The same drugs should prompt testing of pacing thresholds and sensing, though this space is less well-characterized.

- Finally, ICD programming should be optimized to prevent further shocks. Increasing the treatment threshold to ≥200 beats per minute reduces shocks and mortality in a primary prevention population.[22] This may also hold true among patients who have received an ICD shock. Increasing the number of intervals to detect VT in primary and secondary prevention ICD recipients also reduces the incidence of shocks but not mortality.[23] Further, the sensitivity of device leads to myocardial depolarization can be adjusted. If done properly, abnormal sensing can be minimized. Finally, detection algorithms differentiating lethal from nonlethal arrhythmias by taking into account the rapidity of rhythm onset, rhythm stability, and electrogram morphology (Figure 65-5) can also be employed.

LONG-TERM COMPLICATIONS AND FOLLOW-UP

- Appropriate shock recipients are at a higher risk of heart failure and death compared with those who do not experience a shock[24]; the latter risk doubles with one or more recurrent defibrillations.[25] Inappropriate shock recipients are also at greater risk of death.[25] Whether appropriate or inappropriate, defibrillations are associated with a reduced quality of life.[26]

- Accordingly, shock recipients should be closely monitored for imminent heart failure exacerbations. During clinical encounters, close attention should be paid to patients' volume status and evidence-based medication regimen. Further, patients' psychosocial distress should be carefully managed. This may take the form of education,

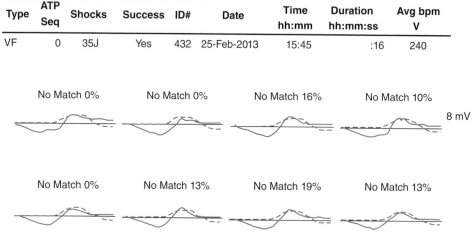

Type	ATP Seq	Shocks	Success	ID#	Date	Time hh:mm	Duration hh:mm:ss	Avg bpm V
VF	0	35J	Yes	432	25-Feb-2013	15:45	:16	240

No Match 0%   No Match 0%   No Match 16%   No Match 10%   8 mV

No Match 0%   No Match 13%   No Match 19%   No Match 13%

FIGURE 65-5 Electrogram morphology detection. ICDs can be configured to detect the degree of mismatch between the observed QRS complex during an arrhythmia and the morphology of the stored QRS template. The device administers a shock when the difference between the two exceeds a programmed value.

close follow-up, and concrete plans for management of a future shock. A full complement of health care providers, including a primary care physician, a heart failure specialist, an electrophysiologist, and a mental health specialist, may jointly aid in these undertakings.

REFERENCES

1. Zheng ZJ, Croft JB, Giles WH, Mensah GA. Sudden cardiac death in the United States, 1989 to 1998. *Circulation*. 2001;104(18): 2158-2163.

2. Moss AJ, Zareba W, Hall J, et al. Prophylactic implantation of a defibrillator in patients with myocardial infarction and reduced ejection fraction. *N Engl J Med*. 2002;346(12):877-883.

3. Bardy GH, Lee KL, Mark DB, et al. Amiodarone or implantable cardioverter-defibrillator for congestive heart failure. *N Engl J Med*. 2005;352(3):225-237.

4. Al-Khatib SM, Hellkamp A, Bardy GH, et al. Survival of patients receiving a primary prevention implantable cardioverter-defibrillator in clinical practice vs clinical trials. *JAMA*. 2013;309(1):55-62.

5. Saxon LA, Hayes DL, Gilliam FR, et al. Long-term outcome after ICD and CRT implantation and influence of remote device follow-up: the ALTITUDE survival study. *Circulation*. 2010;122(23):2359-2367.

6. Daubert JP, Zareba W, Cannom DS, et al. Inappropriate implantable cardioverter-defibrillator shocks in MADIT II: frequency, mechanisms, predictors, and survival impact. *J Am Coll Cardiol*. 2008;51(14):1357-1365.

7. McMurray J, Kober L, Roberton M, et al. Antiarrhythmic effect of carvedilol after acute myocardial infarction: results of the Carvedilol Post-Infarct Survival Control in Left Ventricular Dysfunction (CAPRICORN) trial. *J Am Coll Cardiol*. 2005;45(4): 525-530.

8. Domanski MJ, Exner DV, Borkowf CB, Geller NL, Rosenberg Y, Pfeffer MA. Effect of angiotensin converting enzyme inhibition on sudden cardiac death in patients following acute myocardial infarction: a meta-analysis of randomized clinical trials. *J Am Coll Cardiol*. 1999;33(3):598-604.

9. Bapoje SR, Bahia A, Hokanson JE, et al. Effects of mineralocorticoid receptor antagonists on the risk of sudden cardiac death in patients with left ventricular systolic dysfunction: a meta-analysis of randomized controlled trials. *Circ Heart Fail*. 2013;6(2):166-173.

10. Fuster V, Ryden LE, Cannom DS, et al. 2011 ACCF/AHA/HRS focused updates incorporated into the ACC/AHA/ESC 2006 guidelines for the management of patients with atrial fibrillation: a report of the American College of Cardiology Foundation/ American Heart Association task force on practice guidelines. *Circulation*. 2011;123(10):e269-367.

11. Pacifico A, Hohnloser SH, Williams JH, et al. Prevention of implantable-defibrillator shocks by treatment with sotalol. *N Engl J Med*. 1999;340(24):1855-1862.

12. Kuhlkamp V, Mewis C, Mermi J, Bosch RF, Seipel L. Suppression of sustained ventricular tachyarrhythmias: a comparison of d,l-sotalol with no antiarrhythmic drug treatment. *J Am Coll Cardiol*. 1999;33(1):46-52.

13. Waldo AL, Camm AJ, deRuyter H, et al. Effect of d-sotalol on mortality in patients with left ventricular dysfunction after recent and remote myocardial infarction. *Lancet*. 1996;348(9019):7-12.

14. Zipes DP, Camm AJ, Borggrefe M, et al. ACC/AHA/ESC 2006 guidelines for management of patients with ventricular arrhythmias and the prevention of sudden cardiac death: a report of the American College Of Cardiology/American Heart Association task force and the European Society Of Cardiology committee for practice guidelines (writing committee to develop guidelines for management of patients with ventricular arrhythmias and the prevention of sudden cardiac death). *J Am Coll Cardiol*. 2006;48(5):e247-346.

15. Connolly SJ, Dorian P, Roberts RS, et al. Comparison of betablockers, amiodarone plus beta-blockers, or sotalol for prevention of shocks from implantable cardioverter defibrillators: the optic study: a randomized trial. *JAMA*. 2006;295(2):165-171.

MANAGING RECURRENT ICD
THERAPIES: MEDICAL THERAPY

SECTION IX
IMPLANTABLE CARDIAC DEVICES FOR
MANAGEMENT OF MALIGNANT

439

16. Julian DG, Camm AJ, Frangin G, et al. Randomised trial of effect of amiodarone on mortality in patients with left-ventricular dysfunction after recent myocardial infarction: EMIAT. *Lancet*. 1997;349(9053):667-674.

17. Cairns JA, Connolly SJ, Roberts R, Gent M. Randomised trial of outcome after myocardial infarction in patients with frequent or repetitive ventricular premature depolarisations: CAMIAT. *Lancet*. 1997;349(9053):675-682.

18. Singh SN, Fletcher RD, Fisher SG, et al. Amiodarone in patients with congestive heart failure and asymptomatic ventricular arrhythmia. Survival trial of antiarrhythmic therapy in congestive heart failure. *N Engl J Med*. 1995;333(2):77-82.

19. Impact Research Group. IR: International mexiletine and placebo antiarrhythmic coronary trial: I. Report on arrhythmia and other findings. Impact Research Group. *J Am Coll Cardiol*. 1984;4(6):1148-1163.

20. Baquero GA, Banchs JE, Depalma S, et al. Dofetilide reduces the frequency of ventricular arrhythmias and implantable cardioverter defibrillator therapies. *J Cardiovasc Electrophysiol*. 2012;23(3):296-301.

21. Scirica BM, Morrow DA, Hod H, et al. Effect of ranolazine, an antianginal agent with novel electrophysiological properties, on the incidence of arrhythmias in patients with non ST-segment elevation acute coronary syndrome: results from the Metabolic Efficiency With Ranolazine for Less Ischemia in Non St-Elevation Acute Coronary Syndrome Thrombolysis in Myocardial Infarction 36 (MERLIN-TIMI 36) randomized controlled trial. *Circulation*. 2007;116(15):1647-1652.

22. Moss AJ, Schuger C, Beck CA, et al. Reduction in inappropriate therapy and mortality through ICD programming. *N Engl J Med*. 2012;367(24):2275-2283.

23. Gasparini M, Proclemer A, Klersy C, et al. Effect of long-detection interval vs standard-detection interval for implantable cardioverter-defibrillators on antitachycardia pacing and shock delivery: The ADVANCE III randomized clinical trial. *JAMA*. 2013;309(18):1903-1911.

24. Moss AJ, Greenberg H, Case RB, et al. Long-term clinical course of patients after termination of ventricular tachyarrhythmia by an implanted defibrillator. *Circulation*. 2004;110(25):3760-3765.

25. Poole JE, Johnson GW, Hellkamp AS, et al. Prognostic importance of defibrillator shocks in patients with heart failure. *N Engl J Med*. 2008;359(10):1009-1017.

26. Mark DB, Anstrom KJ, Sun JL, et al. Quality of life with defibrillator therapy or amiodarone in heart failure. *N Engl J Med*. 2008;359(10):999-1008.

66 MANAGING RECURRENT ICD THERAPIES: ABLATION THERAPY

Sean D. Pokorney, MD, MBA and Sana M. Al-Khatib, MD, MHS

CASE PRESENTATION

The patient is a 61-year-old man with a history of ischemic cardiomyopathy, a left ventricular ejection fraction (LVEF) of <15%, and a history of percutaneous coronary interventions on the mid-left anterior descending artery and the right coronary artery. He had a primary prevention implantable cardioverter-defibrillator (ICD) placed 3 years ago. He received an ICD shock for monomorphic ventricular tachycardia (VT) approximately 6 months after his ICD was implanted. He was started on sotalol at that time. The patient did not tolerate sotalol due to gastrointestinal symptoms, and he stopped taking the medication after a few doses. Approximately 2 years after his first ICD shock, the patient presented with electrical storm, having received 3 ICD shocks for monomorphic VT in the 24 hours prior to presentation. He had a cardiac catheterization that showed nonobstructive coronary artery disease with the most severe lesion being a 40% stenosis in the second diagonal artery. The patient was taken to the electrophysiology lab for an electrophysiology study and possible VT ablation.

The patient had two morphologies of easily inducible VT. The first VT had a tachycardia cycle length of 410 ms and right bundle branch block (RBBB) morphology with a superior axis and a transition at V_3. This VT was found to arise from the inferior apex (Figure 66-1). The second VT had a tachycardia cycle length of 410 ms and left bundle branch block (LBBB) morphology with an inferior axis and a transition at V_3. This VT was mapped to the anterior septum (Figure 66-2). Identical morphologies to the VTs were achieved by pacing in the respective scar border zones (Figure 66-3). Extensive ablation was performed at the scar border zones for each region, targeting areas of electrical excitability and diastolic potentials (Figure 66-4). The clinical VTs were noninducible at the completion of the procedure.

EPIDEMIOLOGY

- ICDs have been clearly demonstrated to improve the survival of patients at an increased risk of sudden cardiac death either due to prior cardiac arrest, VT, or significant left ventricular dysfunction.[1-5]

- A survey of ICD use in 61 countries in 2009 showed 222 407 new implants and 105 620 replacements worldwide, and the survey demonstrated a nearly 12% increase in ICD implantation in the United States between 2005 and 2009.[6]

- Primary prevention ICD trials demonstrated appropriate ICD shocks for VT/ventricular fibrillation (VF) in 18% of patients in Multicenter Automatic Defibrillator Implantation Trial II (MADIT-II) at 21 months[7] and 22% of patients in Sudden Cardiac Death in Heart Failure Trial (SCD-HeFT) at 45 months.[8]

- Secondary prevention trials found appropriate ICD shocks for VT/VF in 47% of patients in the Ventricular Tachycardia Ablation in Coronary Heart Disease (VTACH) study at 23 months[9] and 31% of

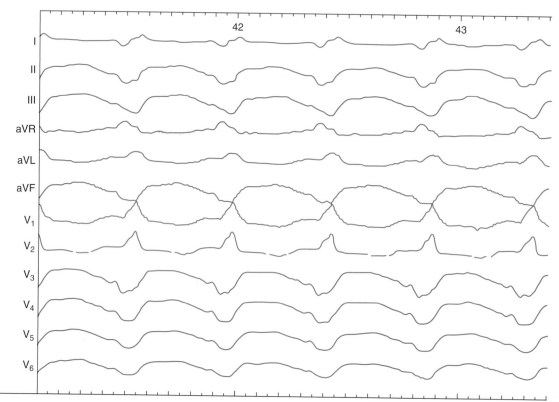

FIGURE 66-1 A 12-lead ECG of the patient's first VT (VT₁).

MANAGING RECURRENT ICD THERAPIES:
ABLATION THERAPY

SECTION IX
IMPLANTABLE CARDIAC DEVICES FOR
MANAGEMENT OF MALIGNANT

441

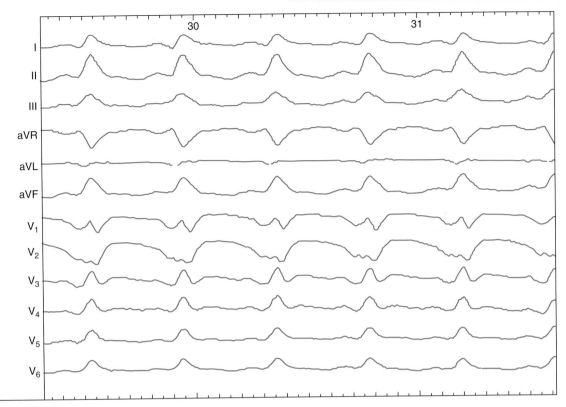

FIGURE 66-2 A 12-lead ECG of the patient's second VT (VT₂).

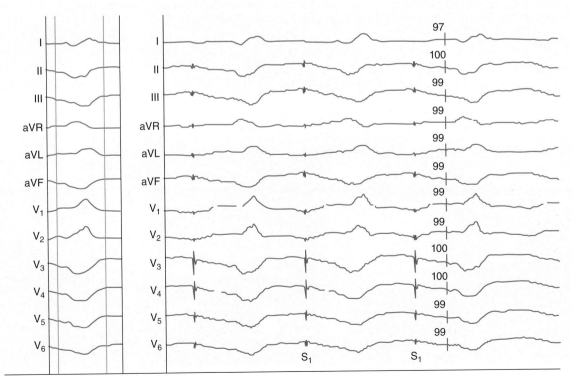

FIGURE 66-3A Pace map match for VT₁ from the inferior apex.

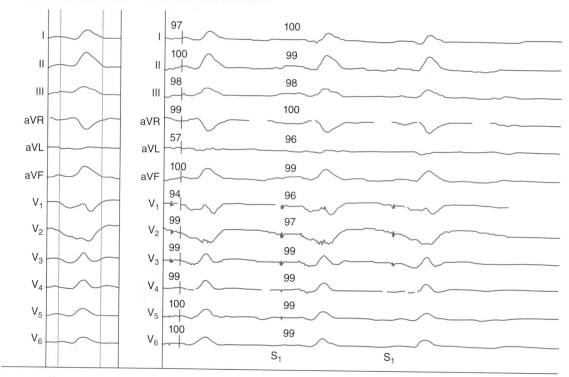

FIGURE 66-3B Pace map match for VT$_2$ from the anterior septum.

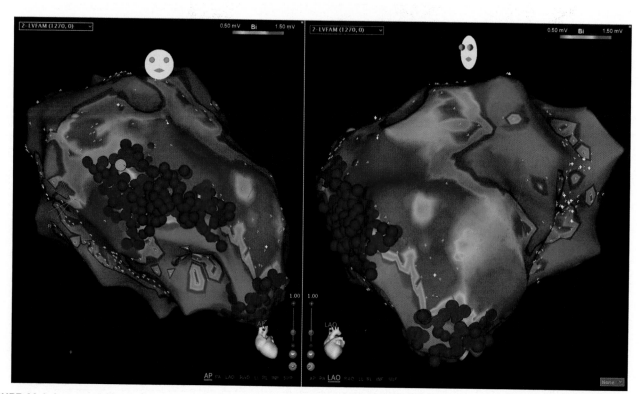

FIGURE 66-4 Activation/ablation map with straight anteroposterior view on the left and left anterior oblique view on the right. The grey dot is the dense scar. The aqua dot is the site of the pace map. The red dots are the ablation sites for the VT from the inferior apex (VT$_1$) and from the anterior septum (VT$_2$).

patients in the Substrate Mapping and Ablation in Sinus Rhythm to Halt Ventricular Tachycardia (SMASH-VT) trial at 23 months.[10]

- Appropriate ICD shocks have serious consequences, despite their proven, life-saving efficacy.
  - Long-term follow-up data from MADIT-II[11] and SCD-HeFT[8] found that patients have a significantly higher risk of death after appropriate ICD termination of VT or VF. Specifically, compared with patients who did not receive an appropriate ICD shock, those who did had a 3.5 times and 5.7 times higher risk of mortality in MADIT-II and SCD-HeFT, respectively.
  - Patients have a decline in physical functioning and mental well-being after one or more ICD shock.[12]

DIAGNOSIS

- If the VT rate is at or above the programmed detection rate of the ICD, the VT episode is captured by the device, which makes management easier as it is often difficult to capture the VT by any other modality. Multiple VT morphologies are commonly inducible during an electrophysiology (EP) study, and the stored electrograms (EGMs) may help one identify a patient's clinical VT.[13]
  - Stored EGM data provide the cycle length of the clinical VT.
  - In 13 postinfarct patients with an ICD and with 12-lead ECGs of the clinical VT, visual inspection and computer analysis of the ICD EGMs correctly differentiated the clinical VT in 96% and 98% of the cases, respectively. This was achieved despite the fact that 67% of patients had an inducible, previously undocumented VT with a cycle length within 10% of the cycle length of the clinical VT.
- The stored EGMs of VT episodes may also be useful in patients who are noninducible in the EP lab, which could be due to recent administration of an antiarrhythmic medication, and with normal voltage maps that preclude substrate modification.[14]
  - A target ablation area can be identified by pacing at the tachycardia cycle length and matching the morphology of the recorded paced tachycardia to the EGM morphology.

MANAGEMENT

Pharmacologic Treatment of VT in ICD Patients

- Medications can reduce ICD shocks, as seen in the Optimal Pharmacological Therapy in Cardioverter Defibrillator Patients (OPTIC) trial. OPTIC was a randomized controlled trial, in which 412 patients received β-blockers alone, sotalol, or a combination of amiodarone and β-blockers.[15]
  - Cumulative rates of shock over 1 year were 39% with β-blocker alone, 24% with sotalol, and 10% with amiodarone and a β-blocker.
  - Amiodarone reduced shocks by a statistically significant amount compared with a β-blocker alone or sotalol, while sotalol had a nonstatistically significant trend toward reduction in ICD shocks compared with a β-blocker.
- Antiarrhythmic medications have adverse events, despite their utility in preventing tachyarrhythmias.

  - In OPTIC, the discontinuation rates of amiodarone and sotalol were high even during the first year: 18% and 24%, respectively.[15]
  - Amiodarone increases defibrillation threshold by a statistically significant amount.[16]

Catheter Ablation in Electrical Storm

- Four analyses of VT ablation that included ≥10 patients with electrical storm have been published, and the details of these can be found in Table 66-1.[17-20]
- The largest evaluation of the efficacy of VT ablation in electrical storm was a prospective study with 95 patients.[18]
  - The patients were mostly men with ischemic cardiomyopathy.
  - The clinical VT was ablated in 89% of patients, and 72% of patients had no inducible VT postablation.
  - Patients were followed for a mean of 22 ± 13 months, and 66% of patients had no VT recurrence during follow-up, while only 8% of patients had recurrence of electrical storm.
  - There were no periprocedural deaths, but there were two transient ischemic attacks and two vascular complications.
- Similar rates of recurrence of VT at 62% to 69% and electrical storm at 6% to 13% were seen in the other smaller, retrospective studies.[17,19,20]
- The longest mean follow-up in the published studies was 28 months, and there were no long-term outcomes available on this patient population, so the durability of the effect of VT ablation remains unknown.

Catheter Ablation in Incessant Ventricular Tachycardia

- Endocardial and epicardial approaches to VT ablation have been effective in treating incessant VT with success rates of ablating the clinical VT of 90% to 94%, as shown in Table 66-2.[21,22]
- The two studies that examined catheter ablation in incessant VT had a minority (35%-40%) of patients with an ICD.
- In these two studies, there was only one procedure-related death, resulting in a 6% periprocedural death rate in that study with 17 patients.[22]
- There was a significant difference in VT recurrence rates between the two studies with 90% of patients having no recurrent VT after epicardial ablation and 65% having no recurrent VT after endocardial ablation. This may be due to the better durability of the epicardial approach compared with the endocardial one; however, unmatched patient populations, the relatively small number of patients in these studies, and the disparity in mean follow-up of 18 versus 30 months may also account for this difference.

Catheter Ablation After Appropriate ICD Therapy

- The available data on catheter ablation in ICD recipients have been summarized for retrospective studies in Table 66-3[23-28] and prospective studies in Table 66-4.[29-33]
- The majority of the studies have been conducted in patients with ischemic cardiomyopathy.

TABLE 66-1 VT Ablation in Patients with Electrical Storm[*]

	Kozluk et al[17]	Carbucicchio et al[18]	Arya et al[19]	Deneke et al[20]
Study type	Retrospective	Prospective	Retrospective	Retrospective
Number of patients	24	95	13	32
Age	63 ± 8	64 ± 13	57 ± 18	68 ± 10
Male patients	21 (88%)	85 (89%)	9 (69%)	NR
Patients with ICM/MI	18 (75%)	72 (76%)	0	17 (53%)
Number of ablations	28	113	17	40
Epicardial ablations (% of total ablations)	2 (7%)	10 (11%)	4 (24%)	3 (8%)
Complete success	NR	68 (72%)	8 (62%)	19 (59%)
Partial success	NR	17 (18%)	5 (38%)	11 (34%)
Failure	NR	10 (11%)	0	2 (6%)
Procedure-related death	0	0	0	1 (3%)
Follow-up period (months)	27.8 ± 15.9	22 ± 13	24.6 ± 20.9	15 (IQR 0-30)
Events during follow-up				
No VT	16 (66%)	63 (66%)	8 (62%)	22 (69%)
Any VT recurrence	5 (21%)	32 (34%)	5 (38%)	10 (31%)
Electrical storm recurrence	3 (13%)	8 (8%)	NR	2 (6%)
Death	3 (13%)	11 (12%)	4 (24%)	3 (9%)

NR = Not reported. All numbers have percent of patient population. Mean ± standard deviation. Median (Interquartile range or IQR)

[*]Included studies had to satisfy the following criteria: a published manuscript, in English, and with more than 10 patients.

- Postablation, the percentage of patients who were noninducible for any VT ranged from 22% to 78%.

- The rates of noninducible patients postablation and successfully ablated clinical VT in the two largest, prospective studies were 40% to 49% and 72% to 92%, respectively.[30-31] Despite the variation in success of ablation, both studies had similar rates of recurrence of VT at 46% to 47% with 6 to 8 months of follow-up.

- The Cooled RF Ablation trial found that 81% of patients had ≥75% reduction in VT events, when comparing the 2-month periods before and after VT catheter ablation, and the 1-year recurrence rate after ablation was 56%.[30]

- The Thremocool VT Ablation Study also showed a significant impact on VT events postablation with 67% of patients having ≥75% reduction in VT events, when comparing the 6-month periods before and after ablation. This 231 patient experience found that patients had a median of 11.5 episodes of VT in the 6 months prior to ablation, which was reduced to a median of 0 (interquartile range of 0-7) episodes of VT in the 6 months after ablation.[31]

- There are no randomized controlled trials of VT catheter ablation powered to assess mortality.

- There are no data available on the impact of reduction of VT events and ICD shocks with VT catheter ablation on quality of life.

- Periprocedure mortality rates range from 0% to 5%, and the most frequently experienced complications included heart failure, stroke, cardiac tamponade, and vascular injury.

Catheter Ablation as Prophylaxis for Appropriate ICD Therapy

- The only two randomized controlled trials of VT catheter ablation in ICD recipients are the VTACH and SMASH-VT trials. Both of these trials randomized patients with a secondary prevention indication for an ICD and ischemic cardiomyopathy to ICD with VT catheter ablation or ICD without VT catheter ablation (Table 5).[9-10]

- The primary end point of the VTACH trial was time to first recurrence of VT, which was longer (18.6 months) in the ablation arm compared with the control arm with (5.9 months) (p = 0.051).

TABLE 66-2 VT Ablation in Patients with Incessant VT*

	Brugada et al[21]	Cao et al[22]
Study type	Retrospective	Retrospective
Number of patients	10	17
Age	68 ± 9	65 ± 8
Male patients	9 (90%)	16 (94%)
Patients with ICM/MI	8 (80%)	15 (88%)
Number of ablations	11	20
Epicardial ablations (% of total ablations)	11 (100%)	0
Patients with ICD	4 (40%)	6 (35%)
Successful ablation of clinical VT	9 (90%)	16 (94%)
Failure	1 (10%)[a]	1 (6%)
Procedure-related death	0	1 (6%)
Follow-up period (months)	18 ± 18	30 ± 12
Events during follow-up		
No VT	9 (90%)	11 (65%)
Any VT recurrence	1 (10%)	6 (35%)
Recurrence of same VT	0	1 (6%)
Death	0	4 (24%)

All numbers have percent of patient population. Mean ± standard deviation.
[a] = 2 failures by epicardial approach but 1 was successfully abled endocardially.
*Included studies had to satisfy the following criteria: a published manuscript, in English, and with more than 10 patients.

Ablation resulted in a statistically significant improvement in the number of patients free from VT or VF at 2 years (47% in the ablation arm versus 29% of controls) (hazard ratio of 0.61 with 95% confidence interval [CI] of 0.37 to 0.99). The rate of appropriate ICD shocks per year during follow-up in the ablation group was 0.6% compared with 3.4% in the control group.[9]

- The primary endpoint in SMASH-VT was survival free from appropriate ICD therapy. The number of appropriate ICD therapies was significantly lower in the ablation arm (12%) compared with the control arm (33%) (hazard ratio 0.35 with 95% CI of 0.15 to 0.78 and p-value of 0.007). There was a 73% reduction in ICD shocks in the ablation group, as compared with controls. Overall survival was not different between treatment strategies.[10]

Timing of VT Ablation

- The optimal timing for VT ablation in patients with structural heart disease is unknown.
- Current guidelines give a class I recommendation for VT ablation in[34]:
  - Patients with sustained, monomorphic VT, who have failed an antiarrhythmic, do not tolerate an antiarrhythmic, or do not want to take long-term antiarrhythmic medications.

  - Patients with an ICD, who receive multiple shocks for sustained VT and are not willing to take long-term antiarrhythmic medications or are not controllable with reprogramming their ICD or adjusting antiarrhythmic medical therapy.

- Catheter ablation is also recommended for patients with incessant sustained monomorphic VT or electrical storm and patients with polymorphic VT or VF that is triggered by a targetable focus.[35]

- It has been suggested that earlier referral for VT ablation may result in more favorable outcomes, including lower rates of VT recurrence and reduced mortality, but this remains to be elucidated.

- One single center, retrospective analysis evaluated patients referred early after their first episode of VT (36 patients in early referral) compared with patients that had VT ablation after two or more VT episodes (62 patients in late referral).[36]

- Early referral patients had improved VT-free survival compared with the late referral group (p-value 0.01), and a multivariable analysis found that early referral was the only statistically significant, independent variable affecting VT-free survival.

TABLE 66-3 Retrospective Studies of VT Ablation in Patients after Appropriate ICD Therapy[*]

	Sauer et al[23]	Inada et al[24]	Segal et al[25]	O'Callaghan et al[26]	Kim et al[27]	Alzand et al[28]
Study type	Retrospective	Retrospective	Retrospective	Retrospective	Retrospective	Retrospective
Number of patients	208	285	40	55	21	27
Age	64 ± 13	68	65 ± 8	67 ± 8	67 ± 8	68 ± 8
Male patients	187 (90%)	247 (87%)	31 (78%)	50 (91%)	20 (95%)	25 (93%)
Patients with ICM/MI	144 (69%)	285 (100%)	40 (100%)	55 (100%)	21 (100%)	27 (100%)
Incessant VT	NR	NR	NR	NR	3 (14%)	4 (15%)
Number of ablations	327	NR	NR	NR	25	31
Epicardial ablations	NR	27	0	NR	0	0
Patients with ICD	208 (100%)	254 (89%)	26 (65%)	38 (69%)	9 (43%)	27 (100%)
Complete success	94 (45%)	159 (56%)	24 (60%)	11 (22%)	6 (29%)	21 (78%)
Partial success	298 (91%)	85 (30%)	9 (23%)	31 (60%)	11 (52%)	6 (22%)
Failure	29 (9%)	27 (9%)	7 (18%)	9 (18%)	4 (19%)	0
Peri-procedure death	0	11 (4%)	2 (5%)	1 (2%)	1 (5%)	0
Follow-up period (months)	51 ± 29	45 ± 33 (mortality) 19 ± 24 (VT recurrence)	36 ± 21	39 ± 23	13 ± 5	38 (IQR 12-72)
Events during follow-up						
Any VT recurrence	61 (29%)	39%	20 (50%)	NR	9 (45%)	18 (67%)
Death	89 (43%)	111 (39%)	13 (33%)	20 (36%)	1 (5%)	9 (33%)
Survival-free VT recurrence	NR	NR	75%, 53%, 37%, and 28% at 1, 2, 3, and 5 years	50%, 28%, and 28% at 1, 3, and 5 years	25% recurrence of ablated VT during follow-up	NR

NR = Not reported. All numbers have percent of patient population. Mean ± standard deviation. Median (Interquartile range or IQR).
[*]Included studies had to satisfy the following criteria: a published manuscript, in English, and with more than 10 patients.

- There are several ongoing randomized controlled studies investigating timing of ablation and/or comparing ablation with antiarrhythmic medications[37]:
  - Trial Comparing Ablation with Medical Therapy in Patients with Ventricular Tachycardia (VeTAMed).
  - Antiarrhythmic Medication versus MRI-Merge Ablation in the Treatment of Ventricular Tachycardia.
  - Early Ablation Therapy for the Treatment of Ischemic Ventricular Tachycardia in Patients with Implantable Cardioverter Defibrillators (ASPIRE).
  - Ventricular Tachycardia Ablation versus Enhanced Drug Therapy (VANISH).
  - A Study of Early Robotic Ablation by Substrate Elimination of Ventricular Tachycardia (ERASE-VT).
  - Pilot Study of Catheter Ablation for Ventricular Tachycardia in Patients with an Implantable Cardioverter Defibrillator (CALPYSO).
  - Does Timing of VT Ablation Affect Prognosis in Patients with an Implantable Cardioverter-Defibrillator? (PARTITA).

CONCLUSIONS

- ICD shocks for VT or VF are associated with poor prognosis and negative impact on quality of life.
- It is important to reassess the treatment plan for a patient after an appropriate ICD therapy.
- VT ablation can result in a low recurrence rate of VT or VF, and the procedure can decrease ICD therapies delivered in patients having frequent VT/VF episodes.
- Future studies should focus on understanding the long-term impact of this procedure on important outcomes like survival, health care utilization, and quality of life.
- Earlier referral for VT ablation has been suggested as a better approach to patients with VT and structural heart disease; however, more robust data on the optimal timing of VT ablation are needed.
- More data are also needed on selecting patients for VT ablation who are most likely to benefit from ablation.

TABLE 66-4 Prospective Studies of VT Ablation in Patients after Appropriate ICD Therapy*

	Jais et al[29]	Calkins et al[30]	Stevenson et al[31]	Tanner et al[32]	Henz et al[33]
Study type	Prospective	Prospective	Prospective	Prospective	Prospective
Number of patients	70	146	231	63	17
Age	67 ± 11	65 ± 13	68 (IQR 59-72)	64 ± 9	53 ± 11
Male patients	63 (90%)	134 (92%)	89%	89%	10 (59%)
Patients with ICM/MI	56 (80%)	119 (82%)	231 (100%)	63 (100%)	0
Incessant VT	NR	NR	16%	NR	NR
Number of ablations	84	171	251	70	17
Epicardial ablations (% of total ablations)	22 (31%)[a]	NR	NR	0	16 (94%)
Patients with ICD	53 (76%)	115 (79%)	94%	49 (78%)	17 (100%)
Complete success	49 (70%)[b]	59 (40%)	113 (49%)	NR	NR
Partial success	21 (30%)	47 (32%)	99 (43%)	51 (81%)	14 (83%)
Failure	0	40 (27%)	5 (2%)[c]	12 (19%)	3 (17%)
Peri-procedure death	2 (3%)	4 (3%)	7 (3%)	0	0
Follow-up period (months)	22 (IQR 14-27)	8.1 ± 5.1	6	12 ± 3	11 ± 3
Events during follow-up					
Any VT recurrence	32 (46%)	66 (46%)	108 (47%)	31 (49%)	6 (35%)
Death	13 (19%)	26 (18%)	24 (10%)	5 (8%)	1 (6%)
Survival-free VT recurrence	NR	Median 24 days	NR	NR	79% of success group at mean 11 months

NR = Not reported. All numbers have percent of patient population. Mean ± standard deviation. Median (Interquartile range or IQR).
[a] = one patient had non-percutaneous epicardial ablation during open chest surgery, [b] = VT noninducible at the end of the case,
[c] = 5 patients had no ablation lesions applied.
*Included studies had to satisfy the following criteria: a published manuscript, in English, and with more than 10 patients.

- The data from current ongoing studies, future trials, and analyses of durability of VT ablation and long-term outcomes of ablation patients will likely influence future recommendations.

REFERENCES

1. A comparison of antiarrhythmic-drug therapy with implantable defibrillators in patients resuscitated from near-fatal ventricular arrhythmias. The Antiarrhythmics versus Implantable Defibrillators (AVID) Investigators. *N Engl J Med.* 1997;337(22):1576-1583.

2. Connolly SJ, Gent M, Roberts RS, et al. Canadian implantable defibrillator study (CIDS): a randomized trial of the implantable cardioverter defibrillator against amiodarone. *Circulation.* 2000;101(11):1297-1302.

3. Moss AJ, Zareba W, Hall WJ, et al. Prophylactic implantation of a defibrillator in patients with myocardial infarction and reduced ejection fraction. *N Engl J Med.* 2002;346(12):877-883.

4. Bardy GH, Lee KL, Mark DB, et al. Amiodarone or an implantable cardioverter-defibrillator for congestive heart failure. *N Engl J Med.* 2005;352(3):225-237.

5. Kuck KH, Cappato R, Siebels J, Ruppel R. Randomized comparison of antiarrhythmic drug therapy with implantable defibrillators in patients resuscitated from cardiac arrest: the Cardiac Arrest Study Hamburg (CASH). *Circulation.* 2000;102(7):748-754.

6. Mond HG, Proclemer A. The 11th world survey of cardiac pacing and implantable cardioverter-defibrillators: calendar year 2009—a World Society of Arrhythmia's project. *Pacing Clin Electrophysiol.* 2011;34(8):1013-1027.

7. Daubert JP, Zareba W, Cannom DS, et al. Inappropriate implantable cardioverter-defibrillator shocks in MADIT II: frequency, mechanisms, predictors, and survival impact. *J Am Coll Cardiol.* 2008;51(14):1357-1365.

TABLE 66-5 Prophylactic VT Ablation to Minimize Appropriate ICD Therapy[*]

	Kuck et al[9]	Reddy et al[10]
Study type	Randomized controlled trial	Randomized controlled trial
Number of patients	107 total 52 ablation	128 total 64 ablation
Age	66 ± 8 total 67 ± 8 ablation	67 ± 9 ablation
Male patients	100 (93%) total 50 (96%) ablation	59 (92%) ablation
Patients with ICM/MI	100%	100%
Number of ablations	60 (12 crossover, 3 repeat)	61
Epicardial ablations	NR	0
Patients with ICD	100%	100%
Acute success	27 (60%)	NR
Undefined	12 (27%)	NR
Failure	6 (13%)	NR
Procedure-related death	0	0
Follow-up period (months)	23 ± 9	23 ± 6
Death	9 (8%) total 5 (10%) ablation	11 (17%) control 6 (9%) ablation
Survival free	18.6 months (ablation)	NR
ICD therapy	5.9 months (control)	
Reduction In VT frequency	At 2 years, 47% ablation group and 29% control free of VT	73% reduction in ICD shock in ablation group

NR = Not reported. All numbers have (Percent of patient population). Mean ± Standard Deviation.
[*]Included studies had to satisfy the following criteria: a published manuscript, in English, and with greater than 10 patients.

8. Poole JE, Johnson GW, Hellkamp AS, et al. Prognostic importance of defibrillator shocks in patients with heart failure. *N Engl J Med.* 2008;359(10):1009-1017.

9. Kuck KH, Schaumann A, Eckardt L, et al. Catheter ablation of stable ventricular tachycardia before defibrillator implantation in patients with coronary heart disease (VTACH): a multicentre randomised controlled trial. *Lancet.* 2010;375(9708):31-40.

10. Reddy VY, Reynolds MR, Neuzil P, et al. Prophylactic catheter ablation for the prevention of defibrillator therapy. *N Engl J Med.* 2007;357(26):2657-2665.

11. Moss AJ, Greenberg H, Case RB, et al. Long-term clinical course of patients after termination of ventricular tachyarrhythmia by an implanted defibrillator. *Circulation.* 2004;110(25):3760-3765.

12. Schron EB, Exner DV, Yao Q, et al. Quality of life in the antiarrhythmics versus implantable defibrillators trial: impact of therapy and influence of adverse symptoms and defibrillator shocks. *Circulation.* 2002;105(5):589-594.

13. Yoshida K, Liu TY, Scott C, et al. The value of defibrillator electrograms for recognition of clinical ventricular tachycardias and

for pace mapping of post-infarction ventricular tachycardia. *J Am Coll Cardiol.* 2010;56(12):969-979.

14. Tschabrunn CM, Anter E, Marchlinski FE. Identifying non-inducible ventricular tachycardia origin utilizing defibrillator electrograms. *J Interv Card Electrophysiol.* 2013;36(3):243-246.

15. Connolly SJ, Dorian P, Roberts RS, et al. Comparison of beta-blockers, amiodarone plus beta-blockers, or sotalol for prevention of shocks from implantable cardioverter defibrillators: the OPTIC Study: a randomized trial. *JAMA.* 2006;295(2):165-171.

16. Hohnloser SH, Dorian P, Roberts R, et al. Effect of amiodarone and sotalol on ventricular defibrillation threshold: the optimal pharmacological therapy in cardioverter defibrillator patients (OPTIC) trial. *Circulation.* 2006;114(2):104-109.

17. Kozluk E, Gaj S, Kiliszek M, Lodzinski P, Piatkowska A, Opolski G. Efficacy of catheter ablation in patients with an electrical storm. *Kardiol Pol.* 2011;69(7):665-670.

18. Carbucicchio C, Santamaria M, Trevisi N, et al. Catheter ablation for the treatment of electrical storm in patients with implantable

cardioverter-defibrillators: short- and long-term outcomes in a prospective single-center study. *Circulation.* 2008;117(4):462-469.

19. Arya A, Bode K, Piorkowski C, et al. Catheter ablation of electrical storm due to monomorphic ventricular tachycardia in patients with nonischemic cardiomyopathy: acute results and its effect on long-term survival. *Pacing Clin Electrophysiol.* 2010;33(12):1504-1509.

20. Deneke T, Shin DI, Lawo T, et al. Catheter ablation of electrical storm in a collaborative hospital network. *Am J Cardiol.* 2011;108(2):233-239.

21. Brugada J, Berruezo A, Cuesta A, et al. Nonsurgical transthoracic epicardial radiofrequency ablation. *J Am Coll Cardiol.* 2003;41(11):2036-2043.

22. Cao K, Gonska BD. Catheter ablation of incessant ventricular tachycardia: acute and long-term results. *Eur Heart J.* 1996;17(5):756-763.

23. Sauer WH, Zado E, Gerstenfeld EP, Marchlinski FE, Callans DJ. Incidence and predictors of mortality following ablation of ventricular tachycardia in patients with an implantable cardioverter-defibrillator. *Heart Rhythm.* 2010;7(1):9-14.

24. Inada K, Roberts-Thomson KC, Seiler J, et al. Mortality and safety of catheter ablation for antiarrhythmic drug-refractory ventricular tachycardia in elderly patients with coronary artery disease. *Heart Rhythm.* 2010;7(6):740-744.

25. Segal OR, Chow AW, Markides V, Schilling RJ, Peters NS, Davies DW. Long-term results after ablation of infarct-related ventricular tachycardia. *Heart Rhythm.* 2005;2(5):474-482.

26. O'Callaghan PA, Poloniecki J, Sosa-Suarez G, Ruskin JN, McGovern BA, Garan H. Long-term clinical outcome of patients with prior myocardial infarction after palliative radiofrequency catheter ablation for frequent ventricular tachycardia. *Am J Cardiol.* 2001;87(8):975-979;A4.

27. Kim YH, Sosa-Suarez G, Trouton TG, et al. Treatment of ventricular tachycardia by transcatheter radiofrequency ablation in patients with ischemic heart disease. *Circulation.* 1994;89(3):1094-1102.

28. Alzand BS, Timmermans CC, Wellens HJ, et al. Unmappable ventricular tachycardia after an old myocardial infarction. Long-term results of substrate modification in patients with an implantable cardioverter defibrillator. *J Interv Card Electrophysiol.* 2011;31(2):149-156.

29. Jais P, Maury P, Khairy P, et al. Elimination of local abnormal ventricular activities: a new end point for substrate modification in patients with scar-related ventricular tachycardia. *Circulation.* 2012;125(18):2184-2196.

30. Calkins H, Epstein A, Packer D, et al. Catheter ablation of ventricular tachycardia in patients with structural heart disease using cooled radiofrequency energy: results of a prospective multicenter study. Cooled RF Multi Center Investigators Group. *J Am Coll Cardiol.* 2000;35(7):1905-1914.

31. Stevenson WG, Wilber DJ, Natale A, et al. Irrigated radiofrequency catheter ablation guided by electroanatomic mapping for recurrent ventricular tachycardia after myocardial infarction: the multicenter thermocool ventricular tachycardia ablation trial. *Circulation.* 2008;118(25):2773-2782.

32. Tanner H, Hindricks G, Volkmer M, et al. Catheter ablation of recurrent scar-related ventricular tachycardia using electroanatomical mapping and irrigated ablation technology: results of the prospective multicenter Euro-VT-study. *J Cardiovasc Electrophysiol.* 2010;21(1):47-53.

33. Henz BD, do Nascimento TA, Dietrich Cde O, et al. Simultaneous epicardial and endocardial substrate mapping and radiofrequency catheter ablation as first-line treatment for ventricular tachycardia and frequent ICD shocks in chronic chagasic cardiomyopathy. *J Interv Card Electrophysiol.* 2009;26(3):195-205.

34. Zipes DP, Camm AJ, Borggrefe M, et al. ACC/AHA/ESC 2006 guidelines for management of patients with ventricular arrhythmias and the prevention of sudden cardiac death—executive summary: a report of the American College of Cardiology/American Heart Association Task Force and the European Society of Cardiology Committee for Practice Guidelines (Writing Committee to Develop Guidelines for Management of Patients with Ventricular Arrhythmias and the Prevention of Sudden Cardiac Death) Developed in collaboration with the European Heart Rhythm Association and the Heart Rhythm Society. *Eur Heart J.* 2006;27(17):2099-2140.

35. Aliot EM, Stevenson WG, Almendral-Garrote JM, et al. EHRA/HRS Expert Consensus on Catheter Ablation of Ventricular Arrhythmias: developed in a partnership with the European Heart Rhythm Association (EHRA), a Registered Branch of the European Society of Cardiology (ESC), and the Heart Rhythm Society (HRS); in collaboration with the American College of Cardiology (ACC) and the American Heart Association (AHA). *Europace.* 2009;11(6):771-817.

36. Frankel DS, Mountantonakis SE, Robinson MR, Zado ES, Callans DJ, Marchlinski FE. Ventricular tachycardia ablation remains treatment of last resort in structural heart disease: argument for earlier intervention. *J Cardiovasc Electrophysiol.* 2011;22(10):1123-1128.

37. National Institutes of Health Clinical Trials Website. http://www.clinicaltrials.gov. Accessed March 10, 2014.

67 PAUSE-DEPENDENT POLYMORPHIC VENTRICULAR TACHYCARDIA

Alaric Franzos, MD, Erich F Wedam, MD,
Mark Haigney, MD

CASE PRESENTATION

A 95-year-old man with coronary artery disease, an ischemic cardiomyopathy (left ventricular ejection fraction 45%), and atrial fibrillation (without anticoagulation) presented to the emergency department after multiple episodes of syncope. He was initially responsive but suddenly developed altered mental status. His Glasgow coma score fell from 15 (ie, fully awake and responsive) to 4 (indicating coma). The subject simultaneously developed fixed pinpoint pupils, extensor posturing, roving gaze, and Cheyne-Stokes breathing. Except for an elevated pro-BNP of 1386 ng/ml (reference range 5.0-450), laboratory analysis was normal including a serum potassium 4.5 mEq/L (3.6-5.0) and a serum digoxin level of 0.6 ng/ml (0.8-1.2). A noncontrast CT suggested an initial diagnosis of mid pons ischemic stroke due to basilar artery occlusion. Tissue plasminogen activator was administered with restoration of the patient basilar artatus to normal, and the patient transferred to the medical intensive care unit. A brain magnetic resonance imagery (MRI) showed no evidence of acute stroke. An electrocardiogram revealed atrial fibrillation, complete heart block, a QTc of 540 ms, and a right bundle branch morphology escape rhythm (Figure 67-1)—a significant change from prior electrocardiograms showing atrial fibrillation, a QTc of 450 ms, and left bundle branch block (Figure 67-2). Episodes of polymorphic ventricular tachycardia or "torsades de pointes" (TdP) were evident on telemetry (Figure 67-3). Magnesium sulfate (two grams) was administered, and the patient was emergently transported to the electrophysiology lab where a temporary pacemaker was placed, suppressing further episodes of TdP. Placement of a permanent pacemaker prevented further TdP.

CASE EXPLANATION

The patient presented with recurrent syncope complicated by a basilar artery thrombosis. While it is impossible to be certain, it seems likely that the syncope was caused by either the onset of complete heart block or the development of TdP, and the onset of coma appears to be attributable to the basilar artery occlusion. While the etiology of the complete heart block is likewise uncertain, the presence of preexisting left bundle branch block suggests significant infra-His conduction disease. The manifestation of a new right bundle branch block and regularization of the ventricular response is most consistent with complete atrioventricular block. The etiology of the polymorphic ventricular tachycardia is not mysterious, however, and is due to the new onset of severe bradycardia and resultant QT interval prolongation associated with the escape rhythm. The immediate and permanent resolution of the arrhythmia with the institution of ventricular pacing, the absence of a history of QT prolongation, and the lack of a QT-prolonging drug indicate that this is pause-dependent TdP, although some contribution from the cerebral insult cannot be ruled out.

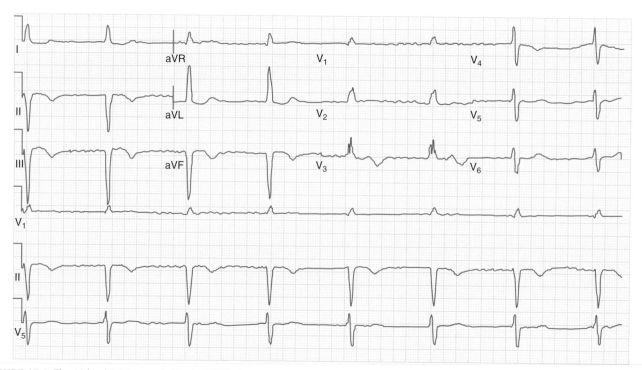

FIGURE 67-1 The 12-lead ECG recorded in the MICU showing complete heart block and QTc prolongation.

PAUSE-DEPENDENT POLYMORPHIC
VENTRICULAR TACHYCARDIA

SECTION IX
IMPLANTABLE CARDIAC DEVICES FOR
MANAGEMENT OF MALIGNANT

451

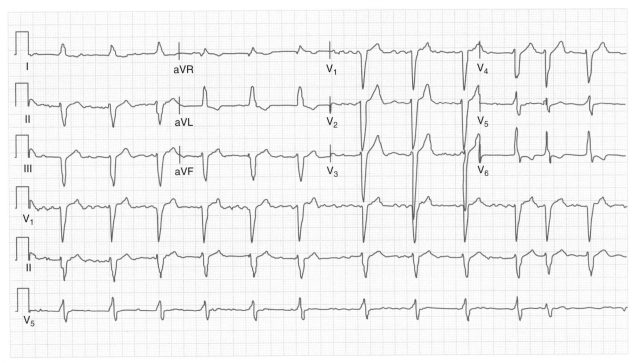

FIGURE 67-2 The 12-lead ECG recorded at prior visit showing LBBB and a QTc of 450 ms. In the presence of LBBB, this is a normal QTc.

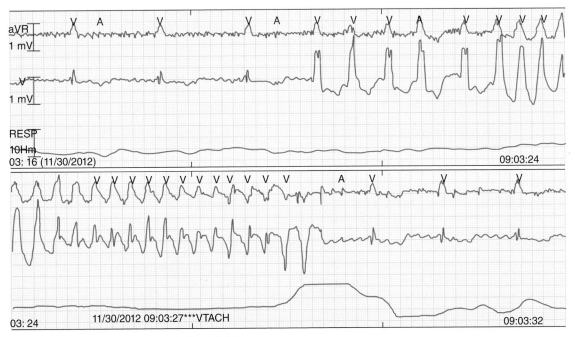

FIGURE 67-3 Telemetry strip showing onset and offset of TdP.

EPIDEMIOLOGY

- The prevalence of true pause-dependent TdP is unknown but is likely rare. Sporadic case reports document QT prolongation and TdP in children and adults after congenital or acquired complete heart block.[1-3]
  - In its "pure" form, it is associated with a normal QT interval prior to the pause.

- TdP commonly presents as two syndromes: syncope and sudden cardiac death (SCD).
  - Syncope is a common syndrome, with an incidence of 6.2 cases per 1000 person-years, with a cardiac cause identified in 9.5%, but the percentage of cases attributable to pause-dependent TdP is likely very small.[4]

○ At autopsy, a long QT (LQT) associated gene mutation (a congenital predisposition to TdP) was identified in approximately one-third of cases of SCD without structural heart disease.[5]

○ TdP is also associated with structural heart disease, with an odd's ratio of 3.9 in NYHA Class III or IV dilated cardiomyopathy exposed to dofetilide, a potent inhibitor of the rapid component of the delayed rectifier potassium current, IKr.[6]

○ In 60 cases collected over 11 years, the most common causes of TdP include QT-prolonging drugs (38%), hypokalemia (27%), and severe bradycardia (35%).[7]

ETIOLOGY AND PATHOPHYSIOLOGY

• Torsades de pointes (TdP) is a polymorphic ventricular tachycardia typified by continuous change in the QRS axis in the setting of a prolonged QT interval, often occurring in short bursts.

• The long QT interval can be congenital or acquired and reflects increased heterogeneity of repolarization, a necessary requirement for induction of reentrant arrhythmias.

• TdP is typically—perhaps always—multifactorial in origin, requiring interaction of depressed "repolarization reserve"[8] due to drugs, structural heart disease, ischemia, electrolyte imbalances, female gender, altered calcium handling, or bradycardia combined with a trigger in the form of a premature beat (Table 67-1).

• Pause-dependent TdP is an acquired cause of QT prolongation.

○ Some degree of heart rate slowing may contribute to the induction of arrhythmia in the presence of a preexisting long QT interval (acquired or congenital).

  ■ Even in normal individuals, substantial prolongation of the QT interval can be seen at slower heart rates (Figure 67-4).

  ■ In subjects with depressed repolarization reserve, slowing of the heart rate may be the final insult that allows TdP to occur.

  ■ Viskin and coworkers found that an increase of the RR interval of >100 ms preceded the onset of TdP in 82% of congenital long QT patients with documented pause-dependent TdP, and some degree of pause-dependence was manifested by 46 of 52 subjects above the age of 3.[9]

  ■ Subjects with congenital LQTS due to loss of function mutations in KCNH2 (IKr) appear to have a particular predisposition to pause-dependent TdP, seen in 68% of LQT2 subjects experiencing TdP but 0% of LQT1.[10]

  ■ In subjects receiving the IKr blocker quinidine, a "long-short" sequence whereby a premature beat followed by a compensatory pause resulted in a premature beat initiating TdP in 90% of cases[11]

○ Sudden iatrogenic reductions of heart rate may result in TdP after ablation of the atrioventricular node in atrial fibrillation for rapid ventricular rates, and maintaining ventricular pacing at 80 to 90 bpm suppresses the arrhythmia by shortening the QT and preventing premature beats.[12]

  ■ In a meta-analysis of 26 subjects experiencing cardiac arrest following atrioventricular node ablation, 23 were paced at a rate less than 80 bpm, and 19 had significant structural heart disease contributing to their reduced repolarization reserve.

○ Case reports suggest that bradycardia may be sufficient to cause enough loss of repolarization reserve to induce TdP. Proof of this concept in the animal model is lacking.

TABLE 67-1 Loss of Repolarization Reserve: Risk Factors for Torsades de Pointes

hERG mutation (0.1%-1% of population)
QT-prolonging drug use, particularly at high dose
Preexisting QTc >450 ms
Electrolyte disturbances ↓ K$^+$, ↓ Mg^{2+}
Female gender
Bradycardia
Atrial fibrillation
Combination of QT-prolonging drugs
Inhibition of drug metabolism
Cardiac ischemia/congestive heart failure
Liver disease, eg, cirrhosis
Anorexia nervosa/HIV

  ■ In dogs subjected to complete atrioventricular block and the IKr blocker dofetilide, TdP could not be induced acutely but only after development of chronic changes in ventricular chamber size and action potential prolongation due to down-regulation of IKr.[13]

  ■ Experimental data from rabbits shows that slow heart rates result in:

    • Increased calcium loading of the sarcoplasmic reticulum.[14]

    • Leakage of calcium from the sarcoplasmic reticulum.

    • Early and delayed afterdepolarizations through activation of sodium-calcium exchange.[15]

    • If large enough, this instability in the membrane potential can trigger premature beats that that can serve to initiate TdP.

○ Whether bradycardia-induced premature beats can be sufficient to trigger TdP alone is unclear, and in any suspected case of pause-dependent TdP, a search for other causes of reduced repolarization reserve should be undertaken.

DIAGNOSIS

• Torsades de pointes has characteristic morphologic features (Figure 67-5):

  ○ Wide, polymorphic QRS.

  ○ Three or more beats.

  ○ Alternating polarity (axis) in a sinusoidal pattern.

  ○ Prolonged QT interval (ie, at least >450 msecs but >500 msec more definitive).

  ○ Presence of a "long-short R-R interval" preceding the onset of tachycardia

  ○ If the arrhythmia is not preceded by a long QT interval, it is known simply as polymorphic ventricular tachycardia.

• Pause-dependent TdP is a diagnosis of exclusion, and the presence of other contributing factors such as an unrecognized ion channelopathy, QT-prolonging drug, or structural heart disease must be excluded, as ventricular pacing may not be adequate to prevent TdP in these conditions.

PAUSE-DEPENDENT POLYMORPHIC
VENTRICULAR TACHYCARDIA

SECTION IX
IMPLANTABLE CARDIAC DEVICES FOR
MANAGEMENT OF MALIGNANT

453

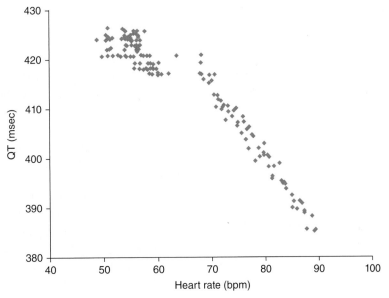

FIGURE 67-4 Decremental atrial pacing from a heart rate of 50 to 90 shortens the QT interval by 45 msec in a healthy subject.

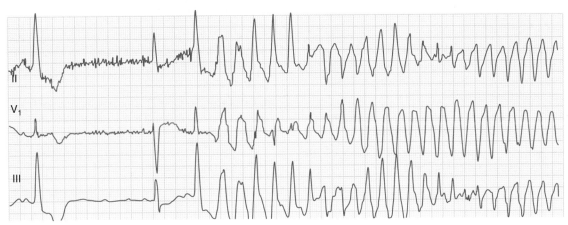

FIGURE 67-5. Intermittent high degree atrioventricular block resulting in a pause-dependent prolongation in the QT interval and initiation of triggering premature ventricular complex, followed by TdP. Note the "long-short" RR interval preceding the TdP.

DIFFERENTIAL DIAGNOSIS

- Acute myocardial ischemia
- Drug-induced or congenital long QT syndrome
- Catecholaminergic polymorphic ventricular tachycardia
- "Coarse" Ventricular fibrillation
- Takotsubo cardiomyopathy
- Atrial fibrillation and Wolff-Parkinson-White syndrome

MANAGEMENT

- Acute management of pause-dependent TdP focuses on elimination of pauses, which are usually a consequence of bradycardia or intermittent heart block.
- Continuous intravenous isoproterenol can be administered to achieve a goal heart rate >90 bpm.

- Increased heart rate decreases the QT interval, and therefore decreases the heterogeneity of repolarization and the likelihood of triggering premature complexes (Figure 67-5).
- Temporary transvenous pacing may be required.
- Intravenous magnesium has been shown to suppress after depolarizations with a small increase (0.5-1.0 mmol/liter) in extracellular magnesium, but magnesium is unlikely to completely suppress TdP in subjects with severe bradycardia.[16]
- Potentially treatable underlying causes include:
  ○ Excessive nodal blockade (via β-blockers or nondihydropyridine calcium channel blockers).
  ○ Lyme disease.
- Placement of a permanent pacemaker may be required if an underlying cause for the slow stimulation rate (bradycardia or pauses) cannot be identified and treated.

○ Placement of a permanent pacemaker effectively eliminates true pause-dependent TdP, but the clinician must be confident that other causes of reduced repolarization reserve have been addressed.

○ Implantation of cardioverter-defibrillator may be more appropriate if other causes of reduced repolarization reserve cannot be addressed.

REFERENCES

1. Nikolic G, Arnold J, Coles DM. Torsade de pointes and asystole in a child with complete heart block and prolonged QT interval. *Aust Paediatr J*. 1983;19(3):187-191.

2. Tan AT, Ee BK, Chia BL. Torsade de pontes and complete heart block in familial cardiomyopathy. *Singapore Med J*. 1984;25(2):84-86.

3. Gladman G, Davis AM, Fogelman R, Hamilton RM, Gow RM. Torsade de pointes, acquired complete heart block and inappropriately long QT in childhood. *Can J Cardiol*. 1996;12(7):683-685.

4. Soteriades ES, Evans JC, Larson MG, et al. Incidence and prognosis of syncope. *N Engl J Med*. 2002;347(12):878-885.

5. Tester DJ, Ackerman MJ. Postmortem molecular screening in unexplained sudden death. *J Am Coll Cardiol*. 2007;49(2):240-246.

6. Pedersen HS, Elming H, Seibaek M, et al. Risk factors and predictors of torsades de pointes ventricular tachycardia in patients with left ventricular systolic dysfunction receiving dofetilide. *Am J Cardiol*. 2007;100(5):876-880.

7. Salle P, Rey JL, Bernasconi P, et al. Torsades de pointe. Apropos of 60 cases. *Ann Cardiol Angeiol*. 1985;34(6):381-388.

8. Roden DM. Taking the idio out of idiosyncratic—predicting torsades de pointes. *PACE*. 1998;21(15):1029-1034.

9. Viskin S, Fish R, Zeltser D, et al. Arrhythmias in the congenital long QT syndrome: how often is torsade de pointes pause dependent? *Heart*. 2000;83(6):661-666.

10. Tan HL, Bardai A, Shimizu W, et al. Genotype-specific onset of arrhythmias in congenital long-QT syndrome: possible therapy implications. *Circulation*. 2006;114(20):2096-2103.

11. Bauman JL, Bauernfeind RA, Hoff JV, Strasberg B, Swiryn S, Rosen KM. Torsade de pointes due to quinidine: observations in 31 patients. *Am Heart J*. 1984;107(3):425-430.

12. Nowinski K, Gadler F, Jensen-Urstad M, Bergfeldt L. Transient proarrhythmic state following atrioventricular junction radiofrequency ablation: pathophysiologic mechanisms and recommendations for management. *Am J Med*. 2002;113(7):596-602.

13. Dunnink A, van Opstal JM, Oosterhoff P, et al. Ventricular remodelling is a prerequisite for the induction of dofetilide-induced torsade de pointes arrhythmias in the anaesthetized, complete atrio-ventricular-block dog. *Europace*. 2012;14(3): 431-436. doi: 10.1093/europace/eur311. Epub 2011 Sep 22.

14. Qi X, Yeh YH, Chartier D, et al. The calcium/calmodulin/kinase system and arrhythmogenic afterdepolarizations in bradycardia-related acquired long-QT syndrome. *Circ Arrhythm Electrophysiol*. 2009;2(3):295-304.

15. Kim JJ, Nemec J, Papp R, Strongin R, Abramson JJ, Salama G. Bradycardia alters Ca(2+) dynamics enhancing dispersion of repolarization and arrhythmia risk. *Am J Physiol Heart Circ Physiol*. 2013;304(6):H848-860.

16. Davidenko JM, Cohen L, Goodrow R, Antzelevitch C. Quinidine-induced action potential prolongation, early afterdepolarizations, and triggered activity in canine Purkinge fibers. Effects of stimulation rate, potassium and magnesium. *Circulation*. 1989;79(3):674-686.

OPTIMAL PROGRAMMING OF ICD
TO REDUCE UNNECESSARY THERAPY

SECTION IX
IMPLANTABLE CARDIAC DEVICES FOR
MANAGEMENT OF MALIGNANT

455

68 OPTIMAL PROGRAMMING OF ICD TO REDUCE UNNECESSARY THERAPY

Malini Madhavan, MBBS, Paul A. Friedman, MD, FACC, FHRS

CASE PRESENTATION

A 69-year-old woman received a single chamber Medtronic ICD for primary prevention of sudden death. The device was programmed to detect VF at 320 ms if 30/40 intervals met criteria. "Wavelet" morphology discrimination was turned on so that therapy would be withheld if tachycardia electrogram (EGM) matched with that of the normal rhythm template by 70% or more. The supraventricular tachycardia (SVT) limit was set at 280 ms, and high rate time out was off. The patient received shocks, and device interrogation is shown in Figure 68-1.

EXPERT OPINION

The arrhythmia seen is an SVT. The device compares the morphology of the far field EGM during tachycardia with that of a template stored during normal rhythm and finds that eight of the last eight complexes do not "match." The far field electrogram records the EGM between the pulse generator and the right ventricular coil, although other vectors are programmable. In contrast, the near field electrogram records the signal between the right ventricular tip and ring (or tip and coil) and generally contains less morphology information.

Since the morphology during tachycardia does not match the template, the device classifies the rhythm as ventricular fibrillation (VF) and delivers therapy. On closer examination, the top of the EGM appears to be "cut-off," or in other words, truncated. Figure 68-2 shows clipped and unclipped EGMs from the same patient. Saturation of the amplifiers results in clipping of the EGM that distorts the EGM resulting in misclassification of the SVT by the morphology algorithm as a VT with subsequent inappropriate shock delivery.

SVT-VT discrimination algorithms are designed to prevent inappropriate therapy for SVT. Morphology algorithms compare EGMs during tachycardia to a template acquired during normally conducted rhythm. If the tachycardia EGM differs from the template by more

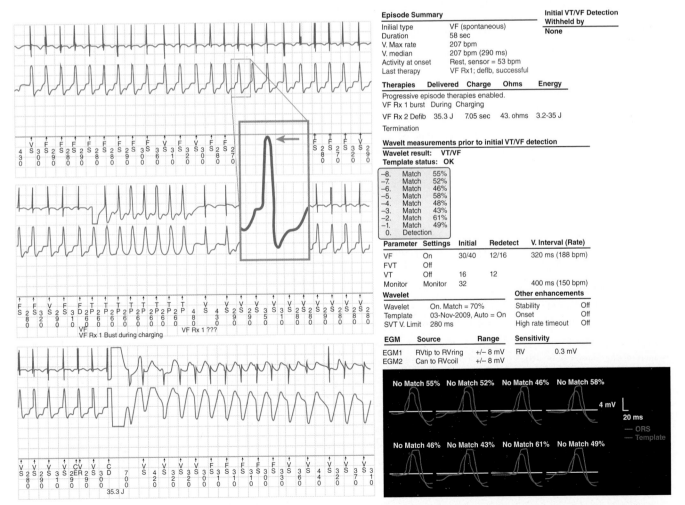

FIGURE 68-1 Inappropriate shock for supraventricular tachycardia. Misclassification by the morphology discrimination algorithm is seen due to clipping (inset) of the electrogram. (Reproduced with permission from Hayes DL, Asirvatham SJ, Friedman PA. Cardiac pacing, defibrillation and resynchronization: a clinical approach. 3rd ed.: Wiley-Blackwell; 2012.)

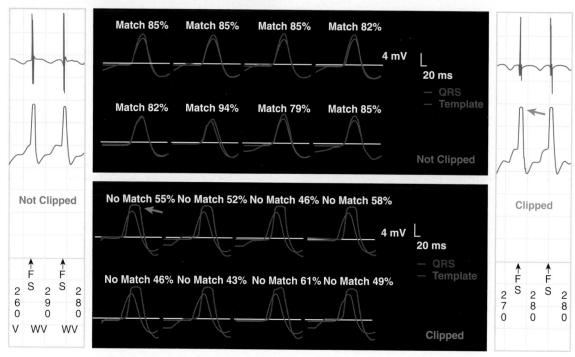

FIGURE 68-2 Morphology error due to clipping. Unclipped electrograms are shown on the left and top. (Left) The top electrogram is the near field channel, the bottom electrogram is far field, and the markers are at bottom. The letters "WV" indicate that SVT is diagnosed by the wavelet algorithm and therapy withheld. The electrogram matches with that of the template, and the rhythm is classified appropriately as SVT. (Right) Shown is the clipped electrogram. Clipping results in distortion of the electrograms, which do not match with that of the template (bottom) despite no physiologic change in the signal itself. It can be prevented by reprogramming the dynamic gain. (Reproduced with permission from Hayes DL, Asirvatham SJ, Friedman PA. Cardiac pacing, defibrillation and resynchronization: a clinical approach. 3rd ed.: Wiley-Blackwell; 2012.)

than a programmed threshold, the rhythm is classified as VT. Morphology is the only noninterval based single chamber algorithm for SVT-VT discrimination, and it is generally the most accurate. However, misclassification can occur due to truncation of EGM as seen in this case. This can be avoided by adjusting the amplitude gain so that the sensed EGM falls within 25% to 75% of the dynamic range. Other causes of morphology misclassification include:

- SVT with rate related aberrancy. To prevent this, a template can be acquired during atrial pacing at a rapid rate (eg, 120 bpm) and template updates disabled.

- Errors in alignment of EGM.

- Myopotential distortion of the EGM. This is a unique situation in which noise on the far field signal can result in inappropriate shock.

- Changes in morphology over time due to lead maturation or bundle branch block. These can be avoided by periodic automatic updating of the template.

- Recurrent arrhythmia shortly after shock delivery. The EGM is often distorted in the minutes immediately following shock delivery. While morphology is not applied during redetection, if an episode terminates and a new arrhythmia develops, the algorithm may be applied before physiologic recovery of the EGM.

UNNECESSARY VERSUS INAPPROPRIATE SHOCK

Delivery of ICD shock for rhythms other than ventricular tachycardia (VT) or VF is termed "inappropriate shock." Recent studies

have shown that programming the device to delay shocks for non-sustained VT or VF and programming antitachycardia pacing (ATP) can improve outcomes. The term "unnecessary shock" encompasses inappropriate shocks and therapy delivered for VT that would have responded to ATP or self-terminated given time. Optimal programming of ICDs prevents unnecessary shocks.

PROGRAMMING TO PREVENT UNNECESSARY SHOCKS

The detection and treatment of arrhythmia by an ICD involves a series of steps, each of which provides an opportunity to minimize shocks (Figure 68-3).

(1) Rate and Duration of Initial Detection

The ICD sense amplifier processes local EGMs to create discrete cardiac events. The time interval between these events defines the heart rate. Tachycardia is detected if the heart rate crosses the detection threshold for a programmable duration or number of intervals. Programming the ICD to delay detection will allow termination of nonsustained VT/VF; programming a higher cutoff rate avoids therapy for slower, better-tolerated rhythms. In contrast to secondary prevention patients, patients with a primary prevention ICD have VT rates that tend to be faster than SVT, so that programming a higher detection rate serves to discriminate VT from SVT, and thus prevent inappropriate detection of SVTs.[1]

The MADIT-RIT study (Multicenter Automatic Defibrillator Implantation Trial to Reduce Inappropriate Therapy) prospectively

OPTIMAL PROGRAMMING OF ICD
TO REDUCE UNNECESSARY THERAPY

SECTION IX
IMPLANTABLE CARDIAC DEVICES FOR
MANAGEMENT OF MALIGNANT

457

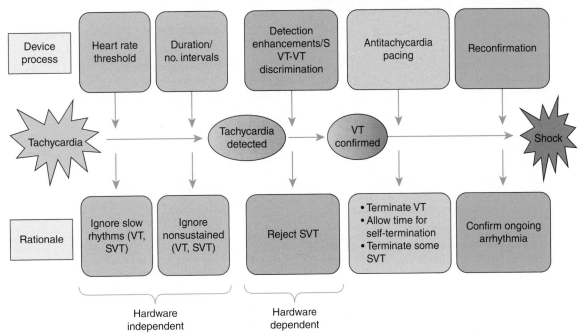

FIGURE 68-3 Overview of detection and treatment of ventricular arrhythmia by implantable cardioverter-defibrillator (ICD). The detection and treatment of ventricular arrhythmia by an ICD involves a sequence of events that provide opportunities to prevent unnecessary shocks using appropriate programming. (Reproduced with permission from Madhavan et al. Optimal programming of implantable cardiac-defibrillators, *Circulation.* 2013;Aug 6;128(6):659-672.)

randomized 1500 primary prevention ICD recipients to 1 of 3 groups: 1) High-rate therapy (detection at ≥200 bpm with a 2.5-second delay totherapy), 2) delayed therapy (60-second delay at 170-199 bpm, 12-second delay at 200-249 bpm, and 2.5-second delay at ≥250 bpm), and 3) conventional therapy (2.5-second delay at 170-199 bpm and 1-second delay at ≥200 bpm).[2] The high-rate and delayed-therapy groups had a lower risk of inappropriate therapy for SVT and death (Figure 68-4) with a similar incidence of syncope compared with conventional programming. These data indicate that programming primary prevention ICDs with a detection zone ≥200 bpm or with delayed therapy at >170 bpm is a preferred strategy. Although nuanced differences in determination of heart rate and duration exists among manufacturers, the fundamental concept of rate and duration triggering detection is similar across devices and therefore is hardware independent and broadly applicable.

(2) Detection Enhancements: SVT/VT Discrimination

Following initial tachycardia detection, the device utilizes algorithms to distinguish true VT from an SVT. These discriminators are hardware specific and differ between single and dual chamber devices and manufacturers. The algorithms used in single chamber devices are presented in Figure 68-5. Dual chamber algorithms incorporate atrial timing information with ventricular intervals and morphology to improve accuracy. These algorithms differ significantly between manufacturers. While dual chamber algorithms generally have improved accuracy, atrial under- or oversensing can lead to misclassification.

(3) Optimizing Ventricular Sensing

ICDs have to sense reliably both normal R waves and small fibrillatory waves while avoiding sensing of T waves and extracardiac signals. ICDs utilize dynamic sensitivity or gain wherein the sensitivity is

at the minimum after each R wave and progressively increased until a subsequent ventricular event. These prevent sensing of physiological events such as T waves and yet maintain sufficient sensitivity to detect small fibrillatory waves.

T-wave oversensing (TWOS) can occur in the setting of low R wave amplitude, large T waves and long QT interval. TWOS can lead to double counting and inappropriate therapy. Figure 68-6A shows TWOS during sinus rhythm leading to inappropriate shock. In this case the R- to T- wave ratio was sufficiently large to allow correction of the problem by reduction of ventricular sensitivity. This may however increase the risk of undersensing VF. However, decreasing ventricular sensitivity is not advisable if the T-wave amplitude is large in comparison to the R wave as in Figure 68-6B. Changing the sensing vector (dedicated versus integrated bipolar sensing) may sometimes provide a more favorable R to T ratio. Lead revision may sometimes be required.

(4) Antitachycardia Pacing

Antitachycardia pacing (ATP) is pacing at a cycle length shorter than VT that terminates VT by depolarizing the excitable gap to block reentry. ATP can reduce shocks, improve quality of life, and lengthen pulse generator life without significantly increasing the risk of VT acceleration or syncope. Although ATP has traditionally been used to terminate slow VT, it has also been subsequently shown to be effective for fast monomorphic VT (>180-200 bpm).[3,4] ATP during charge for fast VT reduces the time to shock if ATP is not successful.

(5) Reconfirmation and Noncommitted Shocks

If ATP fails to terminate VT, the device charges to deliver shock. VT may sometimes terminate during the charge. First generation ICDs delivered the shock regardless of arrhythmia termination. Hence the

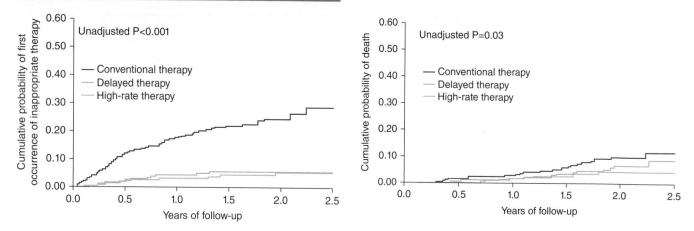

FIGURE 68-4 Extension of the intervals to detection and delaying time to detection of VT/VF in the MADIT-RIT trial resulted in reduction in number of inappropriate therapies (A) and mortality (B). (Reproduced with permission from Moss et al. Reduction in inappropriate therapy and mortality through ICD programming, *NEJM*. 2012; Dec 13;367(24):2275-2283.)

Algorithm	Function	Strengths	Limitations	Performance	Suggested parameter settings
Onset Inhibit therapy if gradual onset Rationale: Sinus tachycardia has gradual onset compared to abrupt onset of VT	Abrupt onset of VT Slow warm up of sinus tachycardia	High sensitivity for distinguishing sinus tachycardia from VT	Misclassify • AF, SVTs with abrupt onset as VT • Exercise-induced VT that follows sinus tachycardia under detected • PVCs before VT may misclassify VT as gradual onset • Applied only once at initial detection – misclassification cannot be corrected	• Accuracy in rejecting sinus tachycardia 98%, VT under detection in 0.5% • Specificity 64%	• Medtronic 84%-88% • Boston Scientific 9% • St. Jude 100 ms
Stability Inhibit therapy if ventricular rate is variable Rationale: RR intervals are irregular in AF compared to regular in VT	Stable RR intervals in VT Irregular RR intervals in AFib	High sensitivity for discriminating VT from AFib at rates <170 bpm	Misclassify • Stable SVT (eg, atrial flutter) as VT • Rapid AF where RR is less variable as VT • Irregular VT (such as in the setting of antiarrhythmic drugs) as AFib	• Sensitivity 95% specificity 77%-88% at rate <170 bpm • Sensitivity and specificity ↓ at rates >170 bpm; best applied to tachycardia <170 bpm	• Medtronic 40-50 ms • Boston Scientific 24-40 ms, 2.5 s • St. Jude 80 ms
Morphology Inhibit therapy if morphology of intracardiac electrogram matches template stored in normal rhythm Rationale: Discriminates SVT from VT based on comparison of morphology, independent of RR intervals	VT – morphology does not match template SVT – morphology matches template	• Discriminate abrupt onset stable SVT (eg, atrial flutter) from VT • Applied continuously, permits correction if initial misclassification occurs • Can be applied at rapid rates >200 bpm	• Misclassify SVT with aberrancy • Misclassification due to electrogram malalignment, truncation • Cannot be applied to redetection post shock	• Most accurate of the single chamber algorithms • Medtronic wavelet™ Sensitivity 100%, Specificity 78% • Boston Scientific Rhythm ID™ Sensitivity 99%-100% Specificity 92%-97% • St. Jude Morphology Discrimination™ in conjunction with dual chamber discriminators Sensitivity 100% Specificity 84%	• Medtronic - 3/8 electrograms > 70% match • Boston Scientific – Rhythm ID 'ON'* • St. Jude – 5/8 electrograms >60% match

FIGURE 68-5 Single chamber SVT-VT discrimination algorithms. (Reproduced with permission from Madhavan et al. Optimal programming of implantable cardiac-defibrillators, *Circulation*, 2013;Aug 6;128(6):659-672.)

OPTIMAL PROGRAMMING OF ICD
TO REDUCE UNNECESSARY THERAPY

SECTION IX
IMPLANTABLE CARDIAC DEVICES FOR
MANAGEMENT OF MALIGNANT

459

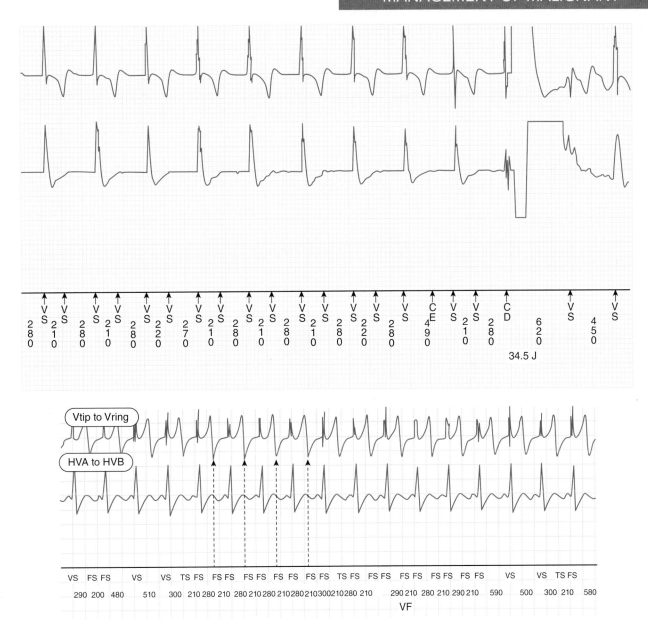

FIGURE 68-6 (A) Inappropriate shock due to T-wave oversensing. The R- to T-wave amplitude ratio is sufficiently large to allow programming of lower ventricular sensitivity. This was sufficient to prevent shocks in this patient. (B) Inappropriate detection of SVT as ventricular arrhythmia due to T-wave oversensing. In contrast to the tracing shown in Figure 68-6A, the R- to T-wave amplitude ratio is less than 1. Reprogramming of ventricular sensitivity will not be successful in avoiding T-wave oversensing and increases risk of VF undersensing. Hence this patient underwent revision of the ICD lead.

shock was "committed." Contemporary devices "reconfirm" the persistence of arrhythmia during and after charge. If arrhythmia terminates spontaneously the charge is painlessly dissipated and the shock is "noncommitted." Shocks should be programmed as noncommitted when possible to avoid unnecessary shocks. The process of reconfirmation is less specific than initial detection and has been reported to result in shocks despite VT termination.[5]

CONCLUSIONS

ICD programming to nonnominal settings prevents unnecessary shocks. Several strategies are available to minimize shocks.

The extension of detection intervals and duration, application of SVT-VT discriminators, and use of ATP have been shown to reduce shocks and should be routinely employed.

REFERENCES

1. Wilkoff BL, Hess M, Young J, et al. Differences in tachyarrhythmia detection and implantable cardioverter defibrillator therapy by primary or secondary prevention indication in cardiac resynchronization therapy patients. *J Cardiovasc Electrophysiol.* 2004;15(9):1002-1009.

2. Moss AJ, Schuger C, Beck CA, et al. Reduction in inappropriate therapy and mortality through ICD programming. *N Engl J Med.* 2012;367(24):2275-2283.

3. Wathen MS, DeGroot PJ, Sweeney MO, et al. Prospective randomized multicenter trial of empirical antitachycardia pacing versus shocks for spontaneous rapid ventricular tachycardia in patients with implantable cardioverter-defibrillators: pacing fast ventricular tachycardia reduces shock therapies (PainFREE Rx II) trial results. *Circulation.* 2004;110(17):2591-2596.

4. Wilkoff BL, Williamson BD, Stern RS, et al. Strategic programming of detection and therapy parameters in implantable cardioverter-defibrillators reduces shocks in primary prevention patients: results from the prepare (primary prevention parameters evaluation) study. *J Am Coll Cardiol.* 2008;52(7):541-550.

5. Bernier M, Essebag V. Inappropriate shock despite successful termination of supraventricular tachycardia by antitachycardia pacing during charging. *Pacing Clin Electrophysiol.* 2010;33(9):e81-83.

69 PACEMAKER PROGRAMMING TO MINIMIZE RIGHT VENTRICULAR PACING

Malini Madhavan, MBBS, Paul A. Friedman, MD, FACC, FHRS

CASE PRESENTATION

A 68-year-old man with ischemic cardiomyopathy, ejection fraction of 35%, and intermittent AV block underwent implantation of a Medtronic dual chamber ICD. The device was programmed DDDR 60-120 bpm, sensed AV delay of 150 ms, and paced AV delay of 120 ms. The patient presented after 1 year with worsening heart failure symptoms. Device interrogation revealed that 80% of ventricular events were paced. The patient's intrinsic rhythm was sinus rhythm with first degree AV block. Figure 69-1 was obtained during device interrogation.

EXPERT OPINION

Several manufacturer-specific algorithms exist to monitor for impending heart failure. Figure 69-1 shows the OptiVol fluid status monitoring algorithm available in Medtronic devices. The daily thoracic impedance trend is monitored and plotted at the bottom. The presence of pulmonary edema will decrease the daily thoracic impedance. The OptiVol fluid index is the difference between the daily impedance and the patient's reference impedance, which is an internal reference that is updated on a continuous basis. This index will increase as risk of incipient overt heart failure increases. Figure 69-1 shows an upward trend in the OptiVol index for a few weeks prior to presentation consistent with the clinical impression of worsening heart failure. Thoracic impedance drop can also be due to fluid in the pocket or lead revision and pleural effusion. Hence, clinical correlation is essential in interpreting heart failure monitoring tools. In the absence of other precipitants of heart failure, clinical worsening in our patient was suspected to be due to high percentage of RV apical pacing. RV pacing avoidance algorithm, managed ventricular pacing, was enabled. Subsequently, the rate of RV pacing declined to 10%, and his ejection fraction improved to preimplantation levels.

WHY SHOULD WE MINIMIZE RIGHT VENTRICULAR PACING?

The premise behind programming to minimize ventricular pacing is the finding that frequent right ventricular pacing may induce ventricular dyssynchrony and left ventricular dysfunction. The Dual Chamber and VVI Implantable Defibrillator (DAVID) trial randomized patients with LV dysfunction undergoing implantation of an implantable cardioverter defibrillator (ICD) to either DDD pacing at 70 bpm or backup VVI pacing at 40 bpm.[1] The trial noted a significant increase in death or hospitalization for heart failure in patients with DDD-70 compared to VVI-40. This was attributed

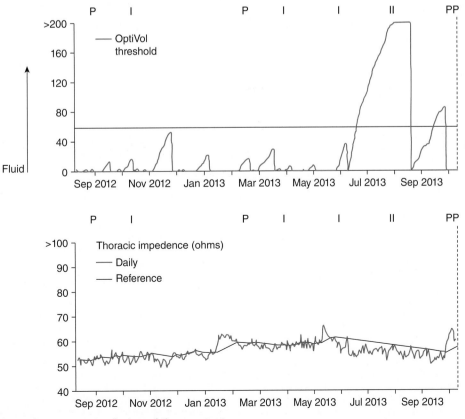

FIGURE 69-1 Thoracic impedance monitoring for heart failure monitoring.

to a significant reduction in the percentage of ventricular pacing in patients programmed to VVI-40 (4% versus 78%). The risk for heart failure increases with the percentage of RV pacing, with significant risk associated with >40% pacing. Post-hoc analysis of the Multicenter Automatic Defibrillator II (MADIT II) trial showed increased incidence of ventricular tachycardia with greater percentage of RV pacing.[2] Hence several algorithms and programming strategies have been developed to promote intrinsic ventricular rhythm and minimize RV pacing.

STRATEGIES TO MINIMIZE VENTRICULAR PACING

Several programming strategies can be employed to avoid unnecessary RV pacing. Atrial only pacemaker (AAI) can be considered in patients with sinus node dysfunction and normal AV node. This is generally not preferred in patients with a history or risk of dysfunction of AV conduction.

Programming a low ventricular "back-up" pacing rate (such as 40 bpm) is recommended in patients with single chamber ICD who do not require antibradycardia therapy. This is supported by the DAVID trial described previously. Moreover, trials such as INTRINSIC RV and MVP trial did not establish superiority of advanced ventricular avoidance algorithms such as AV search hysteresis and MVP respectively over VVI back-up pacing in this population.[3, 4]

Patients with ICDs and a traditional indication for pacing often receive a dual chamber device. Programming a long "fixed" AV delay can encourage intrinsic conduction in these patients. However, this can result in unfavorable hemodynamic effects and "upper rate behavior" and is generally not preferred. This has led to the introduction of several algorithms to minimize RV pacing, many of which are manufacturer specific. We provide a brief general description of these algorithms.

AV Search Hysteresis

AV hysteresis avoids the disadvantages of a long fixed AV delay by allowing the AV delay to vary. If a ventricular-sensed event occurs, the device extends the AV delay to a programmable long interval to promote intrinsic conduction. If there is failure to conduct with a ventricular-paced event for a programmed number of cycles, the device switches back to the shorter AV interval. The device then performs periodic search for intrinsic conduction by prolonging the AV delay for a programmed number of intervals. Figure 69-2 shows operation of the AV search+ algorithm (Boston Scientific).

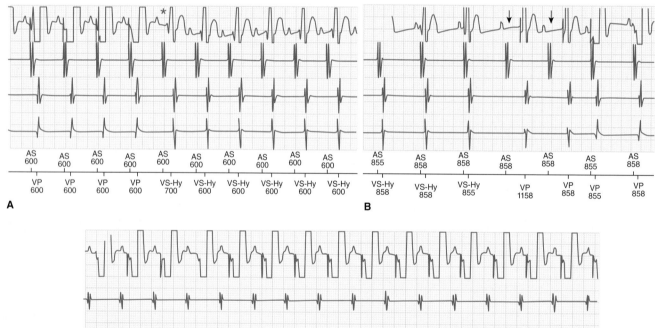

FIGURE 69-2 AV search hysteresis (AV Search+, Boston Scientific) in a 65-year-old with a dual chamber ICD and intermittent AV block. (A) Dual chamber pacing with a short AV interval of 120 ms is noted. The algorithm then extends the AV interval to "search" for intrinsic AV conduction (*). Since a sensed ventricular event occurs, the longer AV interval persists allowing intrinsic conduction until in (B) two consecutive P waves fail to conduct within a programmed interval of 400 ms (arrows). Following this, the short programmed AV interval takes effect. (C) The algorithm extends the AV interval again for a programmed number of eight beats. Since no intrinsic conduction is seen during this search the device reverts to a short AV delay. (Used with permission of Boston Scientific.)

PACEMAKER PROGRAMMING TO MINIMIZE RIGHT
VENTRICULAR PACING

SECTION IX
IMPLANTABLE CARDIAC DEVICES FOR
MANAGEMENT OF MALIGNANT

463

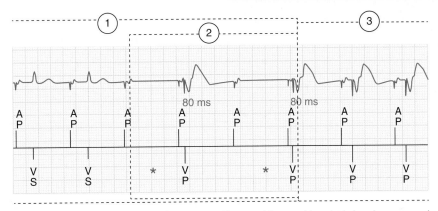

FIGURE 69-3 Operation of managed ventricular pacing (Medtronic) in a 68-year-old man with a dual chamber pacemaker implanted for intermittent AV block. The rhythm was observed on telemetry 1 day following the implantation. The device is programmed with lower rate limit of 70 bpm, upper rate limit of 110 bpm, and AV interval of 180 ms. There are two atrial paced beats (AP) that are not followed by a ventricular complex. This demonstrates functioning of managed ventricular pacing (MVP), an algorithm used by Medtronic devices to minimize ventricular pacing and does not represent device malfunction. The device is functioning in the AAI mode at the beginning of the tracing with "ventricular surveillance" (section 1). This allows intrinsic conduction of the first two atrial events with a long AV interval of 260 ms. The third atrial paced beat fails to conduct to the ventricle which triggers ventricular pacing with the next cycle at a short nonphysiologic AV delay of 80 ms. If a programmed number of atrial events fail to conduct to the ventricle as in section 2, the mode switches to DDD (section 3) resulting in ventricular pacing with the programmed AV delay. The device then checks periodically for intrinsic conduction. (Reproduced with permission from Hayes DL, Asirvatham SJ, Friedman PA. *Cardiac Pacing, Defibrillation and Resynchronization: A Clinical Approach.* 3rd ed. Wiley- Blackwell; 2012.)

AAI ←→ DDD Mode Switch

The dual chamber device operates in the functional AAI mode with active ventricular surveillance when there is intrinsic conduction. If AV block develops for a programmed number of atrial events, the device switches to DDD mode with the programmed AV delay. The device then periodically searches for intrinsic conduction using either the AV search hysteresis (RHYTHMIQ, Boston Scientific) or by mode switching to AAI (MVP, Medtronic). Figure 69-3 shows operation of the managed ventricular pacing (MVP) algorithm (Medtronic).

Proarrhythmia Due to Ventricular Pacing Avoidance Algorithms

While ventricular pacing avoidance algorithms are generally effective and safe in the majority of patients, proarrhythmia has been occasionally reported. We present a few examples.

Pacemaker-Mediated Tachycardia Due to AV Hysteresis

Figure 69-4 shows the AV hysteresis algorithm, ventricular intrinsic preference (VIP) operational in a St. Jude dual chamber pacemaker. The patient is initially paced in the atrium and ventricle sequentially with a short AV interval of 170 ms. The AV hysteresis algorithm then extends the AV interval to 290 ms to search for intrinsic conduction.

Since a sensed ventricular event does not occur, the ventricle is paced when the long AV interval expires. The lack of antegrade AV node conduction and the long AV delay promote retrograde VA conduction. If the retrograde atrial event is sensed outside the postventricular atrial refractory period, an episode of pacemaker mediated tachycardia is initiated.

Polymorphic Ventricular Tachycardia Due to AAI ←→ DDD Mode Switch

The AAI ←→ DDD mode switch algorithms permit single nonconducted P waves in contrast to standard dual chamber operation. A second nonconducted P wave is not allowed. Hence, following a nonconducted P wave, the device will pace the ventricle for one cycle in the DDD mode. As demonstrated in Figure 69-5, this results in a short-long-short coupling sequence, which in the vulnerable patient can lead to polymorphic VT.[5] This is a rare phenomenon.

CONCLUSIONS

High percentage of RV apical pacing can lead to ventricular dyssynchrony and increased incidence of heart failure. Several strategies are available to minimize RV pacing. The selection of device and AP programming should be tailored to the individual patient.

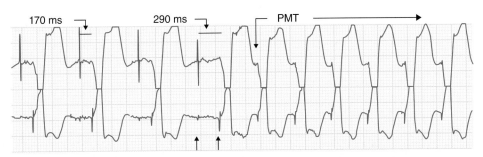

FIGURE 69-4 Initiation of pacemaker-mediated tachycardia due to AV hysteresis in dual chamber pacemaker.

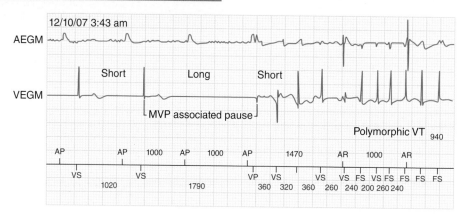

FIGURE 69-5 Polymorphic ventricular tachycardia initiated by short-long-short sequence due to operation of the managed ventricular pacing (MVP) algorithm in a dual chamber ICD. (Reproduced with permission from Hayes DL, Asirvatham SJ, Friedman PA. *Cardiac Pacing, Defibrillation And Resynchronization: A Clinical Approach.* 3rd ed. Wiley- Blackwell; 2012.)

REFERENCES

1. Wilkoff BL, Cook JR, Epstein AE, et al. Dual-chamber pacing or ventricular backup pacing in patients with an implantable defibrillator: the Dual Chamber and VVI Implantable Defibrillator (david) trial. *JAMA.* 2002;288(24):3115-3123.

2. Steinberg JS, Fischer A, Wang P, et al. The clinical implications of cumulative right ventricular pacing in the multicenter automatic defibrillator trial II. *J Cardiovasc Electrophysiol.* 2005;16(4):359-365.

3. Olshansky B, Day JD, Moore S, et al. Is dual-chamber programming inferior to single-chamber programming in an implantable cardioverter-defibrillator? Results of the INTRINSIC RV (Inhibition of Unnecessary RV Pacing With AVSH in ICDs) study. *Circulation.* 2007;115(1):9-16.

4. Sweeney MO, Ellenbogen KA, Tang AS, et al. Atrial pacing or ventricular backup-only pacing in implantable cardioverter-defibrillator patients. *Heart Rhythm.* 2010;7(11):1552-1560.

5. Vavasis C, Slotwiner DJ, Goldner BG, et al. Frequent recurrent polymorphic ventricular tachycardia during sleep due to managed ventricular pacing. *Pacing Clin Electrophysiol.* 2010;33(5):641-644.

70 CARDIAC RESYNCHRONIZATION THERAPY

Daniel J. Friedman, MD, and Jagmeet P. Singh, MD, DPhil

CASE PRESENTATION

A 63-year-old man with diabetes, hypertension, and ischemic cardiomyopathy presented to the emergency department with orthopnea, paroxysmal nocturnal dyspnea, and increased lower extremity edema over the past 2 weeks. He underwent placement of a cardiac resynchronization therapy device with defibrillator 8 months prior when he was noted to have an ejection fraction of 24% and NYHA class III symptoms despite maximal medical therapy. Exam demonstrated 86% room air saturation, mild respiratory distress, an irregularly irregular heart rhythm, bilateral rales, and 2+ pitting edema. An ECG demonstrated atrial fibrillation with multiple QRS morphologies: paced and native IVCD with left axis deviation (Figure 70-1). A PA and lateral radiograph demonstrated bilateral interstitial edema and an implanted device with three leads in the heart. The coronary sinus (left ventricular) lead was located in the apical region (Figure 70-2). The patient was admitted and diuresed. He was started on anticoagulation and underwent cardioversion with restoration of sinus rhythm after transesophageal echocardiogram excluded left atrial

appendage thrombus. Transthoracic echocardiogram demonstrated a diffusely hypokinetic left ventricle with a 21% ejection fraction, and he subsequently underwent echocardiogram guided AV and VV optimization. At the time of discharge, the patient continued to experience NYHA class III symptoms.

CRT: THE BASICS

CRT is an advanced pacing strategy able to restore electrical synchrony of both the atria and ventricles leading to improved chamber filling and pump function. Typical CRT systems include a right atrial lead, right ventricular lead, and left ventricular lead (Figure 70-2). The LV lead is typically implanted transvenously via the coronary sinus but can also be implanted epicardially via lateral thoracotomy. The 3-lead system allows for restoration of the AV and VV synchrony that is commonly lost in severe systolic heart failure with advanced conduction disease. Thus, CRT is more than simply biventricular pacing. CRT may be implanted with or without a defibrillator.

CRT has represented a significant advance in the treatment of severe symptomatic systolic heart failure with electrical dyssynchrony as evidenced by a prolonged QRS on the surface electrocardiogram. CRT has been associated with a significant reduction in heart failure symptoms, heart failure hospitalizations, and mortality[1-4] and has become a widely accepted device therapy for a variety of indications. It has additionally been associated with improvements in exercise capacity, oxygen consumption, NYHA symptom class, and quality of life. While CRT is currently approved by the United States Food and Drug Administration for patients with EF <35% and either 1) QRS >120 ms and NYHA class III/IV symptoms or 2) QRS >130 ms, LBBB, and NYHA II symptoms, major society guidelines define additional

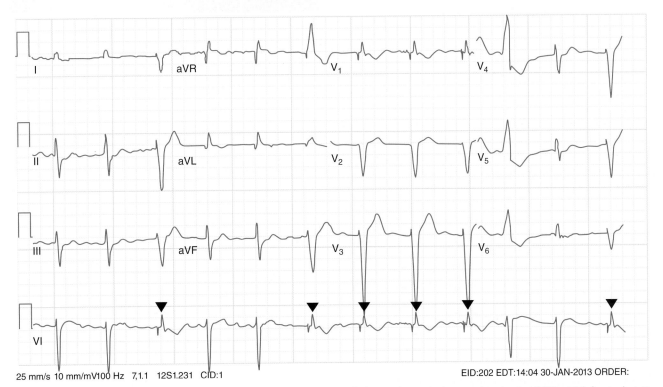

25 mm/s 10 mm/mV 100 Hz 7,1.1 12S1.231 CID:1   EID:202 EDT:14:04 30-JAN-2013 ORDER:

FIGURE 70-1 An ECG demonstrating atrial fibrillation with multiple QRS morphologies: biventricular paced and native IVCD with left axis deviation. Note the paced beats, marked with "▼" on the V$_1$ rhythm strip, are characterized by prominent R wave in V$_1$ and a narrower QRS compared to the native QRS.

appropriate patient subsets in whom the use of CRT is thought to be of benefit.[5] These subsets are largely dictated by the width of the QRS interval and morphology of the conduction defect. In most situations, CRT is considered appropriate for patients with a LBBB and a QRS width ≥120 ms, while in patients with a non-LBBB morphology, the QRS width should ideally be ≥150 ms.

IMPACT ON MYOCARDIAL STRUCTURE AND FUNCTION

CRT has been clearly linked to favorable changes in myocardial structural and functional parameters, termed reverse remodeling. Ongoing therapy has been associated with increased ejection fraction, reduced mitral regurgitation, and decreased chamber size, including LV dimension and volume. Patients manifesting these changes are often referred to as echocardiographic responders. Notably, some degree of echocardiographic response often occurs immediately after initiation of CRT, though the maximal extent of response typically requires approximately 6 months of therapy. Echocardiographic response is tightly linked to improvements in clinical outcomes and is felt to be an important mechanism underlying the clinical improvements afforded by CRT.[6]

IMPACT ON ELECTRICAL FUNCTION AND DYSFUNCTION

The initiation of CRT is associated with a number of changes in electrical activation, function, and stability. Simultaneous or near simultaneous depolarization of the ventricles via biventricular pacing decreases the electrical dyssnchrony associated with ventricular conduction delay, leading to an increasingly synchronous mechanical contraction. Favorable change in the ventricular activation sequence may be manifested by a narrowing of the QRS interval with biventricular pacing. CRT additionally involves optimization of the AV interval, allowing for improvements in diastolic filling with a reduction in diastolic mitral regurgitation. AV optimization often involves programming to reduce the AV interval, which is frequently prolonged in the context of cardiomyopathy.

Initial reports suggested that CRT might be associated with an increase in ventricular arrhythmias. Multiple mechanisms were postulated, including epicardial pacing leading to a reversal of the transmural gradient with increased heterogeneity of repolarization, functional reentry, and torsades de pointes, and biventricular pacing causing a collision of multiple wavefronts in close proximity to a susceptible anatomic substrate. While these mechanisms may lead to arrhythmogenesis in a minority of CRT patients, antiarrhythmic mechanisms typically predominate, outweighing the theoretical deleterious effects. The antiarrhythmic effects of CRT are likely related to favorable changes in wall tension, LV size, neurohormonal activation, LV mass, and oxygen consumption, which are likely important for arrhythmogenesis. CRT additionally decreases pauses and conduction delays, which are important mechanisms for pause dependent and macroreentrant arrhythmias, respectively. Thus, while CRT may exert a number of pro- and antiarrhythmic effects on the myocardium, it is now well accepted that the net effect of CRT is a reduction of ventricular arrhythmias and sudden death. Improvements in electrical stability have been linked with echocardiographic response. Some have suggested that the antiarrhyhmic effect of CRT is sufficient to preclude benefit from concomitant ICD implantation, though this remains controversial, and most CRT patients typically receive an ICD.

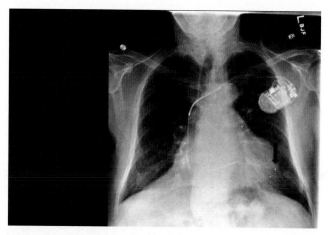

A

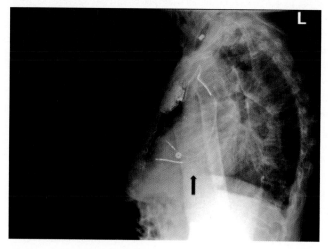

B

FIGURE 70-2 A posteroanterior and lateral radiograph demonstrating bilateral interstitial edema, cardiomegaly, and a standard 3-lead CRT device, with leads pacing the right atrium, right ventricle, and left ventricle. The LV lead is located in the coronary sinus, and the lead tip is position in the LV apex.

FOLLOW-UP AND MONITORING RESPONSE TO THERAPY

The relation between echocardiographic response and improved clinical outcomes has led clinicians to assess routinely response to CRT with an echocardiogram at approximately 6 months after implant, as a supplement to history, physical, and NYHA class assessment. By 6 months, approximately two-thirds of patients experience an improvement in EF, a decrease in LV end systolic volume, and/or class improvement in NYHA symptom class. Those who do not demonstrate improvement based on one or more of these metrics are referred to as nonresponders. Of note, although the term "nonresponder" is a frequently used classification in clinical practice and research, there is not a single agreed upon definition. The patient described in the clinical vignette would be considered a nonresponder based on lack of symptomatic improvement and decrement in EF. Though heterogeneity in the definitions of responder and nonresponder exist, it remains a clinically useful concept as changes in EF, LV end systolic volume, and symptom class provide important prognostic information regarding the success of CRT. Based on this, all patients should undergo complete assessment including echocardiogram and NYHA symptom class assessment at baseline and 6 months after implantation to assess responder status. It should be noted that more frequent clinical and echocardiographic assessment might be warranted for early detection of patients who are at risk of nonresponse.

The identification of CRT nonresponse should prompt a comprehensive evaluation for reversible causes. CRT nonresponse may be due to one or more of a number of factors, including suboptimal AV and/or VV optimization, anemia, arrhythmia, insufficient biventricular pacing, suboptimal lead positioning, suboptimal medical therapy, narrow QRS, and patient noncompliance. A comprehensive examination should include device interrogation, ECG, basic laboratory tests, PA and lateral chest x-ray, and echocardiogram with a trial of different AV and VV device settings. Multidisciplinary evaluation from electrophysiology, heart failure, and cardiac imaging perspectives should strongly be considered for all nonresponders.[7, 8] Therapy for nonresponders may include medication adjustment, device optimization, lead revision, catheter ablation, antiarrhythmic drugs, and cardioversion.

DETERMINANTS OF RESPONSE

Despite ongoing advances in CRT, nearly one-third of patients are nonresponders due to patient selection and/or device related issues. Characteristics commonly associated with increased risk of nonresponse include male sex, ischemic cardiomyopathy, non-LBBB morphology, narrow QRS, atrial fibrillation, low percentage of biventricular pacing, and suboptimal lead position.

QRS Duration

Although advanced conduction disease is typically associated with worsened cardiovascular disease and worsened outcomes in many populations, a prolonged QRS interval is associated with improved outcomes among those undergoing CRT.[9] This seemingly paradoxical finding is related to the fact that those with heart failure and a prolonged QRS frequently have heart failure at least in part due to conduction disease and resultant electrical dyssynchrony. Thus, a prolonged QRS represents an "electrical problem" that has the capacity to be treated by an electrical therapy (eg, CRT). Conversely, patients with severe heart failure and a narrower QRS are less likely to have an "electrical problem" underpinning pump dysfunction, and thus are less likely to respond to this pacing therapy.[10, 11]

Bundle Branch Morphology

Though QRS duration has emerged as an important determinant of response, a number of recent studies have strongly suggested that QRS morphology is at least as important.[12-14] Studies have demonstrated that patients with underlying LBBB prior to CRT are much more likely to respond to CRT than those with an RBBB or IVCD. This association is related to the fact that CRT predominantly resynchronizes the left ventricle, and those with RBBB and IVCD often have a substantial burden of right-sided conduction disease underlying clinical heart failure. Patients with an underlying paced rhythm have generally been excluded from major CRT trials and thus less thoroughly studied; however, outcomes after CRT appear to be nearly commensurate with LBBB patients. The findings regarding the impact of QRS duration and morphology have strongly informed the current CRT appropriate use guidelines (Table 70-1).

Cardiomyopathy Etiology

Ischemic cardiomyopathy has been associated with worsened outcomes in CRT.[12] This relation is likely related to the way scar is distributed across the myocardium in ischemic versus nonischemic cardiomyopathy. Ischemia-mediated cardiomopathy is often associated with dense transmural scar in areas corresponding to prior infarction. Areas of dense infarct often lead to poor lead capture and slowed conduction, precluding optimal ventricular resynchronization. This notion has been supported by research demonstrating that posterolateral scar (eg, scar in the preferred LV lead location) is associated with particularly poor outcomes.[15] Though the nonischemic cardiomyopathies represent a heterogeneous group of diseases, they are typically characterized by scar that is comparatively more diffuse and less likely to be transmural.

Atrial Fibrillation

Atrial fibrillation has been associated with decreased benefit from CRT. This finding is related to the fact that atrial fibrillation (particularly with rapid rates) can favor a higher incidence of native conduction compared to paced complexes and that being in atrial fibrillation also precludes the optimal use of AV optimization. Given the improved outcomes associated with normal sinus rhythm, physicians often opt for a rhythm control strategy when possible. Initial reports suggested that the presence of atrial fibrillation may preclude benefit from CRT. However, patients with atrial fibrillation appear to derive similar benefit from CRT as long as there is a high percentage of biventricular pacing.[16, 17] Of note, CRT response has been associated with decreased atrial fibrillation burden,[18] decrease in new onset atrial fibrillation,[19] and reversion to sinus rhythm in certain individuals.[20]

Percent Biventricular Pacing

Optimal resynchronization of the left ventricular requires a high percentage of biventricular pacing. While it is generally thought that 90% biventricular pacing is sufficient to derive benefit from CRT, it has been suggested that optimal response may require as much as 98.5% biventricular pacing.[21] Decreased biventricular pacing may be related to intrinsic AV conduction, premature ventricular beats, suboptimal device programming, and pacemaker dysfunction. Shortening of the

TABLE 70-1 Summary of Appropriate Use Criteria for Heart Failure Patients with an Ejection Fraction of Less Than 35%.

QRS duration, ms	QRS morphology	NYHA symptom class	Appropriate or may be appropriate?
>120	Any	III/IV	Yes
>120	LBBB	I/II	Yes
>150	Non-LBBB	I/II	Yes
120-149	Non-LBBB	I/II	No
<120	Any	Any	No
<120 with substantial RV pacing		Any	Yes

The source document[5] contains further information regarding the level of evidence for each patient subset. Abbreviations: LBBB, left bundle branch block; RV, right ventricle.

programmed AV interval to less than the intrinsic AV conduction is essential to ensure a high percent of biventricular pacing. Intrinsic AV conduction may occur despite optimal device programming in the context of atrial fibrillation and other atrial arrhythmias; for this reason, adequate nodal blockade is essential. AV nodal ablation is being used with increasing frequency in CRT patients to improve biventricular pacing. Pacemaker dysfunction, including lead dislodgement and oversensing, represents an important consideration when evaluating a patient with a reduced percentage of biventricular pacing. It should be noted that contemporary CRT devices tend to overestimate the percentage of true biventricular pacing because of difficulty in discriminating among true biventricular pacing, fusions beats, and pseudofusion.[22] Fusion complexes result when intrinsic and pacemaker induced wavefronts both contribute to a ventricular depolarization; these beats typically register as biventricular pacing on device counters, though they can be substantially more dyssynchronous than true biventricular pacing. Pseudofusion results when a pacemaker spike falls on an intrinsic QRS, giving the appearance of a fusion complex (Figure 70-3). As a result, Holter monitoring may be required for a full evaluation of nonresponders in whom fusion and pseudofusion is possible. A newer pacing strategy, termed "trigger pacing," has been used to increase biventricular synchrony in instances of intrinsic ventricular depolarizations (either via AV conduction or ventricular ectopy). In trigger pacing, an intrinsic ventricular deplorization is recognized by one of the ventricular leads, prompting a simultaneous pacemaker-induced depolarization by the other ventricular lead. This results in a fusion of the wavefronts from the intrinsic depolarization and the paced depolarization, improving ventricular synchrony.

Lead Position

Anatomic left ventricular lead location has emerged as a key determinant of outcomes in CRT.[23] Anatomic lead position is best defined using a validated 15-segment approach where the LV long axis is divided in the apical, midventricular, and basal segments, and the short axis is divided into anterior, anterolateral, lateral, posterolateral, and posterior segments[24, 25] (Figure 70-4). LV leads located in the basal or midventricular position along the long axis and the posterolateral segment along the short axis are generally associated with superior outcomes compared to other segments.[24, 25] While LV lead implantation should target an optimal anatomic location, options are sometimes limited by constraints of coronary venous anatomy, phrenic nerve stimulation, and the presence of focal scar precluding adequate capture.[23]

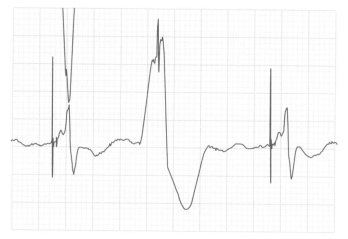

FIGURE 70-3 Pseudofusion with a premature ventricular beat between two biventricular paced complexes in lead V$_1$.

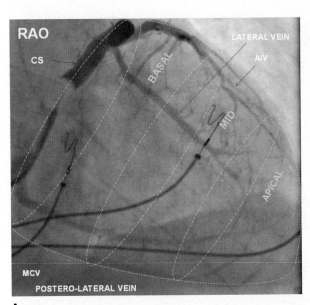
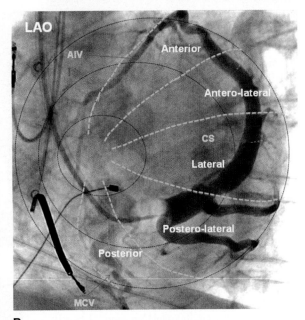

FIGURE 70-4 Angiographic classification of left ventricular lead position observed during intraprocedural coronary sinus venography demonstrating the validated 15-segment approach for defining LV lead position. (A) A right anterior oblique (RAO) view enables segmentation of the heart along the long axis into basal, midventricular (MID), and apical segments. (B) The left anterior oblique (LAO) view enables segmentation of the heart along the short axis into anterior, anterolateral, lateral, posterolateral, and posterior segments. Abbreviations: AIV, anterior interventricular vein; CS, coronary sinus; MCV, middle cardiac vein. (Reproduced with permission from Singh JP, Klein HU, Huang DT, Reek S, Kuniss M, Quesada A, Barsheshet A, Cannom D, Goldenberg I, McNitt S, Daubert JP, Zareba W, Moss AJ. Left ventricular lead position and clinical outcome in the multicenter automatic defibrillator implantation trial-cardiac resynchronization therapy (madit-crt) trial. Circulation. 2011;Mar 22;123(11):1159-1166.)

Lead position can additionally be defined by its electrical location by measuring the time between onset of the native QRS on the surface electrocardiogram and the sensed signal on the LV lead during intrinsic conduction. When this value is indexed for (eg, divided by) the native QRS duration, it is termed left ventricular lead electrical delay (LVLED); when this value is not indexed, it is termed "QLV." Longer delays are associated with enhanced CRT response and superior clinical outcomes, suggesting that intraprocedural assessment of electrical location may be useful during coronary sinus branch selection.[26, 27] Finally, it should be noted that electrical lead location assessment provides prognostic information that is complementary to traditional anatomic assessment, and as such, both can be considered during implantation.[27, 28]

Case Vignette

The patient in the case described at the beginning of the case possesses many risk factors for nonresponse. These factors include ischemic cardiomyopathy etiology, atrial fibrillation, non-LBBB morphology, decreased biventricular pacing, and suboptimal lead positioning. While many risk factors for nonresponse are not modifiable, it is prudent to attempt to correct all options that can be performed noninvasively. This would include attempts at rhythm control and device reprogramming with consideration for lead revision if noninvasive strategies fail.

MULTIDISCIPLINARY APPROACH TO THE CARE OF THE CRT PATIENT

The patients undergoing CRT represent some of the most complex cardiovascular patients and demand a deliberate and coordinated approach for ongoing care. Multidisciplinary care involving structured follow-up integrating heart failure, echocardiography, and electrophysiology care (Figure 70-5) may have the potential to improve outcomes in CRT. This approach incorporates frequent assessment of changes in symptom and functional status and in changes in cardiac

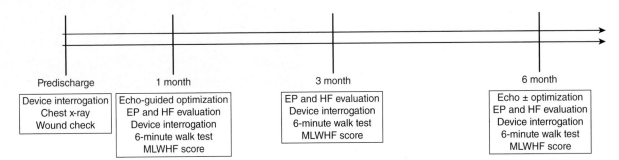

FIGURE 70-5 A diagram depicting a structured multidisciplinary care delivery strategy, integrating heart failure (HF), echocardiography (echo), and electrophysiology care during the first 6 months after device implantation. MLWHFQ indicates Minnesota Living with Heart Failure Questionnaire. (Reproduced with permission from Altman RK, Parks KA, Schlett CL, Orencole M, Park MY, Truong QA, Deeprasertkul P, Moore SA, Barrett CD, Lewis GD, Das S, Upadhyay GA, Heist EK, Picard MH, Singh JP. Multidisciplinary care of patients receiving cardiac resynchronization therapy is associated with improved clinical outcomes. Eur Heart J. 2012;Sep;33(17):2181-2188.)

structure and function as assessed by echocardiography. It allows for early identification of nonresponders and frequent device optimization (often with echocardiogram guidance), medication titration, and arrhythmia management when needed.

An important component of multidisciplinary care of the CRT patient involves optimization of the AV interval. Optimal AV duration is important to maximize coordination of the atria and ventricles, maximize left ventricular filling time, increase cardiac output, and facilitate ventricular synchrony. AV optimization can occur via proprietary device-based algorithms or via echocardiogram guidance utilizing one of many different approaches. One of the more popular methods for echocardiogram-based optimization involves optimization of the mitral inflow pattern using an iterative approach. With this approach, AV delay is initially increased until biventricular capture is lost. The AV delay is then decreased in 10 to 30 ms intervals until an optimal mitral inflow pattern (eg, optimal diastolic filling) is achieved (Figure 70-6).

Altman and colleagues[7] demonstrated that multidisciplinary care was associated with a 30% reduction in event-free survival at 2 years, compared to conventional care. A multidisciplinary approach has also been associated with a high rate of success in the evaluation and management of CRT nonresponders.[8] Despite intensive management, a certain proportion of patients will demonstrate progressive worsening despite CRT. In these cases, a multidisciplinary approach will afford a more seamless transition to consideration for advanced therapies including mechanical support (eg, left ventricular assist device) and cardiac transplantation.

SUMMARY

CRT is an advanced pacing therapy associated with a reduction in mortality and heart failure hospitalizations and improvements in functional status, quality of life, and cardiac function. Although CRT has been associated with improvement in most patients, a significant minority (approximately one-third) does not respond to this therapy. New implantation and optimization strategies, coupled with improved care coordination are needed to improve response rates and outcomes.

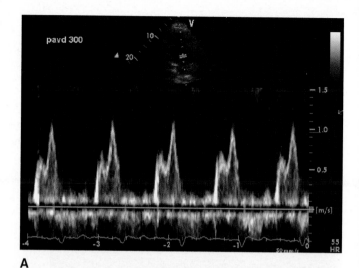

A

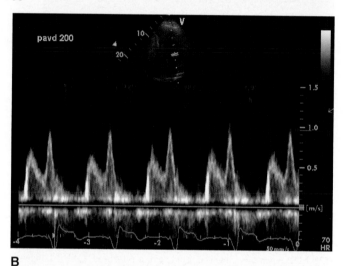

B

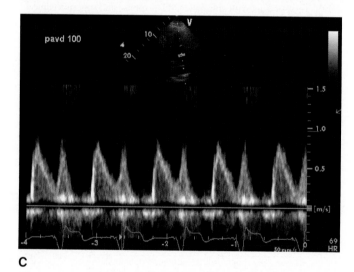

C

FIGURE 70-6 Mitral inflow pattern changes after successive decrements in programmed AV interval. The AV interval was progressively shortened from 300 ms to 80 ms until the E/A wave demonstrated an optimized mitral inflow profile at an AV interval of 80 ms. Representative inflow patterns using Doppler echocardiography with programmed AV intervals of (A) 300 ms, (B) 200 ms, (C) 100 ms, and (D) 80 ms.

REFERENCES

1. Tang AS, Wells GA, Talajic M, et al. Cardiac-resynchronization therapy for mild-to-moderate heart failure. *N Engl J Med.* 2010;363(25):2385-2395.

2. Moss AJ, Hall WJ, Cannom DS, et al. Cardiac-resynchronization therapy for the prevention of heart-failure events. *N Engl J Med.* 2009;361:1329-1338.

3. Bristow MR, Saxon LA, Boehmer J, et al. Cardiac-resynchronization therapy with or without an implantable defibrillator in advanced chronic heart failure. *N Engl J Med.* 2004;350:2140-2150.

4. Cleland JG, Daubert JC, Erdmann E, et al. Cardiac Resynchronization-Heart Failure Study I. The effect of cardiac resynchronization on morbidity and mortality in heart failure. *N Engl J Med.* 2005;352:1539-1549.

5. Russo AM, Stainback RF, Bailey SR, et al. ACCF/HRS/AHA/ASE/HFSA/SCAI/SCCT/SCMR 2013 appropriate use criteria for implantable cardioverter-defibrillators and cardiac resynchronization therapy: a report of the American College Of Cardiology Foundation Appropriate Use Criteria Task Force, Heart Rhythm Society, American Heart Association, American Society of Echocardiography, Heart Failure Society of America, Society for Cardiovascular Angiography and Interventions, Society of Cardiovascular Computed Tomography, and Society for Cardiovascular Magnetic Resonance. *Heart Rhythm.* 2013;10:e11-58.

6. Solomon SD, Foster E, Bourgoun M, et al. Effect of cardiac resynchronization therapy on reverse remodeling and relation to outcome: multicenter automatic defibrillator implantation trial: cardiac resynchronization therapy. *Circulation.* 2010;122:985-992.

7. Altman RK, Parks KA, Schlett CL, et al. Multidisciplinary care of patients receiving cardiac resynchronization therapy is associated with improved clinical outcomes. *Eur Heart J.* 2012.

8. Mullens W, Grimm RA, Verga T, et al. Insights from a cardiac resynchronization optimization clinic as part of a heart failure disease management program. *J Am Coll Cardiol.* 2009;53:765-773.

9. Bryant AR, Wilton SB, Lai MP, Exner DV. Association between QRS duration and outcome with cardiac resynchronization therapy: a systematic review and meta-analysis. *J Electrocardiol.* 2013;46:147-155.

10. Thibault B, Harel F, Ducharme A, et al; Lesser Earth Investigators. Cardiac resynchronization therapy in patients with heart failure and a QRS complex <120 milliseconds: the Evaluation of Resynchronization Therapy for Heart Failure (LESSER-EARTH) trial. *Circulation.* 2013;127:873-881.

11. Beshai JF, Grimm RA, Nagueh SF, et al. Cardiac-resynchronization therapy in heart failure with narrow QRS complexes. *N Engl J Med.* 2007;357:2461-2471.

12. Dupont M, Rickard J, Baranowski B, et al. Differential response to cardiac resynchronization therapy and clinical outcomes according to QRS morphology and QRS duration. *J Am Coll Cardiol.* 2012;60:592-598.

13. Gold MR, Thebault C, Linde C, et al. Effect of QRS duration and morphology on cardiac resynchronization therapy outcomes in mild heart failure: results from the resynchronization reverses remodeling in systolic left ventricular dysfunction (reverse) study. *Circulation.* 2012;126:822-829.

14. Zareba W, Klein H, Cygankiewicz I, et al; MADIT-CRT Investigators. Effectiveness of cardiac resynchronization therapy by QRS morphology in the multicenter automatic defibrillator implantation trial-cardiac resynchronization therapy (MADIT-CRT). *Circulation.* 2011;123:1061-1072.

15. Bleeker GB, Kaandorp TA, Lamb HJ, et al. Effect of posterolateral scar tissue on clinical and echocardiographic improvement after cardiac resynchronization therapy. *Circulation.* 2006;113:969-976.

16. Heist EK, Mansour M, Ruskin JN. Rate control in atrial fibrillation: targets, methods, resynchronization considerations. *Circulation.* 2011;124:2746-2755.

17. Upadhyay GA, Steinberg JS. Managing atrial fibrillation in the CRT patient: controversy or consensus? *Heart Rhythm.* 2012;9:S51-59.

18. Lellouche N, De Diego C, Vaseghi M, et al. Cardiac resynchronization therapy response is associated with shorter duration of atrial fibrillation. *Pacing Clin Electrophysiol.* 2007;30:1363-1368.

19. Brenyo A, Link MS, Barsheshet A, et al. Cardiac resynchronization therapy reduces left atrial volume and the risk of atrial tachyarrhythmias in MADIT-CRT (Multicenter Automatic Defibrillator Implantation Trial with Cardiac Resynchronization Therapy). *J Am Coll Cardiol.* 2011;58:1682-1689.

20. Gasparini M, Steinberg JS, Arshad A, et al. Resumption of sinus rhythm in patients with heart failure and permanent atrial fibrillation undergoing cardiac resynchronization therapy: a longitudinal observational study. *Eur Heart J.* 2010;31:976-983.

21. Hayes DL, Boehmer JP, Day JD, et al. Cardiac resynchronization therapy and the relationship of percent biventricular pacing to symptoms and survival. *Heart Rhythm.* 2011;8:1469-1475.

22. Kamath GS, Cotiga D, Koneru JN, et al. The utility of 12-lead holter monitoring in patients with permanent atrial fibrillation for the identification of nonresponders after cardiac resynchronization therapy. *J Am Coll Cardiol.* 2009;53:1050-1055.

23. Blendea D, Singh JP. Lead positioning strategies to enhance response to cardiac resynchronization therapy. *Heart Failure Rev.* 2011;16:291-303.

24. Merchant FM, Heist EK, McCarty D, et al. Impact of segmental left ventricle lead position on cardiac resynchronization therapy outcomes. *Heart Rhythm.* 2010;7:639-644.

25. Singh JP, Klein HU, Huang DT, et al. Left ventricular lead position and clinical outcome in the Multicenter Automatic Defibrillator Implantation Trial-Cardiac Resynchronization Therapy (MADIT-CRT) trial. *Circulation.* 2011;123:1159-1166.

26. Gold MR, Birgersdotter-Green U, Singh JP, et al. The relationship between ventricular electrical delay and left ventricular remodelling with cardiac resynchronization therapy. *Eur Heart J.* 2011;32:2516-2524.

27. Singh JP, Fan D, Heist EK, et al. Left ventricular lead electrical delay predicts response to cardiac resynchronization therapy. *Heart Rhythm.* 2006;3:1285-1292.

28. Friedman DJ, Upadhyay GA, Altman RK, et al. The anatomic and electrical location of the left ventricular lead predicts ventricular arrhythmia in cardiac resynchronization therapy. *Heart Rhythm.* 2012.

71 SUBCUTANEOUS DEFIBRILLATOR: PATIENT SELECTION AND IMPLANTATION TECHNIQUE

Christopher P. Rowley, MD, Peter H. Belott, MD, Michael R. Gold, MD, PHD

CASE PRSENTATION

A 35-year-old woman with hypertrophic cardiomyopathy, a family history of sudden cardiac death (SCD), and a 3.2-cm interventricular septal diameter presents for consideration of a primary prevention implantable cardioverter defibrillator (ICD). She has no other relevant past medical history. She has no history of atrial or ventricular dysrhythmias. A 12-lead electrocardiogram demonstrates sinus rhythm and LVH with normal PR interval and QRS duration of 121 ms.

EXPERT OPINION

This patient has a history of hypertrophic cardiomyopathy (HCM) with high-risk features for SCD and therefore has an indication for an ICD.[1] Until recently, traditional ICDs required either transvenous access to place leads endocardially, or less commonly, patches could be surgically placed on the epicardium. Whereas ICDs provide excellent protection from sudden death, long-term lead durability is imperfect, and lead failure often requires extraction of a chronic lead or placement of a new lead. Such procedures can be complicated by cardiac perforation, tamponade, or systemic infection due to the requirement for venous access. This is of particular importance in young patients whose life expectancy is anticipated to be far greater than battery longevity or lead durability. As such, a subcutaneous approach that does not require leads to be placed on or within the heart may be especially advantageous in younger populations that do not require pacing. In this regard, the subcutaneous defibrillator is not capable of sustained pacing for bradyarrhythmias or cardiac resynchronization therapy. This patient is young and has no current or anticipated indication for pacing and therefore may be offered a subcutaneous ICD (S-ICD) for SCD prevention.

SUBCUTANEOUS ICD

The S-ICD (Cameron Health/Boston Scientific) comprises a pulse generator and a single coil defibrillator lead placed to the left of and parallel with the sternum (Figure 71-1). The lead has a distal sensing electrode placed next to the manubriosternal junction and a proximal sensing electrode placed next to the xiphoid process. These electrodes flank an 8-cm shocking coil. The two sensing electrodes and pulse generator provide three sensing vectors for rhythm detection.

The S-ICD provides the following features:[2]

• The optimal sensing vector is automatically selected by the device and applies three algorithms to prevent double counting and T-wave oversensing.

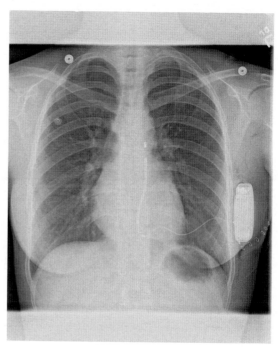

FIGURE 71-1 Posteroanterior (PA) chest X-ray demonstrating the left lateral position of the pulse generator as well as the parasternal lead location.

SUBCUTANEOUS DEFIBRILLATOR: PATIENT
SELECTION AND IMPLANTATION TECHNIQUE

SECTION IX
IMPLANTABLE CARDIAC DEVICES FOR
MANAGEMENT OF MALIGNANT

473

- One- or two-zone configurations are available for arrhythmia detection with a minimal rate of 170 bpm. Typically, a 2-zone configuration is programmed, and in a young patient with HCM, the l conditional zone, which utilizes discrimination criteria, would typically be programmed about 200 bpm with the shock zone (ie, no discrimination algorithm active) at about 230 bpm. The number of intervals to detect an episode is nonprogrammable, and the algorithm is designed as a rhythm rather than beat detector, which tends to prolong detection.

- Arrhythmia discrimination analysis is performed either to deliver therapy appropriately for lethal ventricular arrhythmias or withhold therapy for supraventricular arrhythmias, myopotentials, or noise.

- The S-ICD has excellent arrhythmia detection and discrimination when compared to transvenous systems using either single- or dual-lead devices.[3]

- Defibrillation is performed with 80 J shocks. If initially unsuccessful, the S-ICD automatically reverses shock polarity. Due to the higher energy requirement for subcutaneous defibrillation, the current generation pulse generator is larger at 69.9 cc compared to transvenous pulse generators which are typically 40% to 50% smaller (Figure 71-2). Though larger, the laterally placed pulse generator is well tolerated and has been successfully implanted without regard to body habitus.

- Up to 30 seconds of transcutaneous pacing is available for postshock bradycardia.

- In addition to an established safety profile, the S-ICD has been demonstrated to identify and terminate invoked as well as spontaneous ventricular arrhythmias effectively.[4]

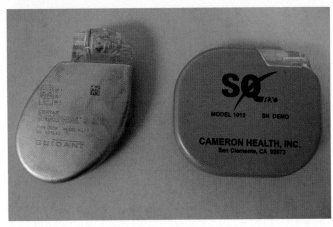

FIGURE 71-2 The S-ICD pulse generator (right) is larger than a typical transvenous pulse generator (left).

PATIENT SELECTION[5]

Good Candidates

- Young patients at risk for SCD may be particularly well suited for an S-ICD given the likely need for multiple pulse generator replacements and concerns regarding lead durability. This device is ideal for patients with channelopathies such as long QT syndrome and Brugada syndrome.

- Patients with congenital heart disease (CHD) may have anatomy that limits transvenous lead placement. The S-ICD can be placed without being limited by such anatomy.

- Immunocompromised patients may be at higher risk for systemic infection when transvenous access is required.

- The presence of indwelling catheters as well as active fistulas or grafts for hemodialysis may preclude standard transvenous approaches. Additionally, venous obstruction, as often found in this population, requires additional procedures such as venoplasty to place transvenous leads.

- Patients with previous transvenous device infections requiring lead extraction and pulse generator removal may have a lower risk of systemic infection by implanting an S-ICD. This can potentially avoid more costly options such as providing a wearable defibrillator vest while reimplantation is postponed for prolonged antibiotic treatment.

Poor Candidates

- Other than 30 seconds of pacing for postshock asystole, the S-ICD is not able to provide sustained bradyarrhythmia therapies. Therefore, patients with any pacing indication, including cardiac resynchronization therapy, are not candidates for the S-ICD.

- Monomorphic VT can frequently be terminated by using nonshock therapy such as antitachycardia pacing (ATP), thereby avoiding high-energy shocks. Since the S-ICD is not capable of nonshock therapy, it should be avoided in patients for whom ATP is likely to be needed.

IMPLANT TECHNIQUE

The S-ICD can be implanted in any standard sterile procedure or operating room without requiring fluoroscopy. Though fluoroscopy is not required, our practice has used a single fluoroscopic image to mark the ideal location of the pulse generator on the mid axillary line at the level of the apex. The S-ICD is then implanted in the following manner[6]:

- The left lateral wall and left chest are cleaned and draped in sterile fashion. Perioperative antibiotics are administered according to institutional policy. After the patient is sedated and local analgesic applied to the skin, an approximate 4-inch incision is made along the left mid axillary line and a subcutaneous pocket fashioned by standard technique utilizing electrocautery for hemostasis.

- Two incisions, inferior and superior, are made 1 to 2 cm to the left of the sternal border at the xiphoid process and manubriosternal junction (Figure 71-3). Of note, some implanters are avoiding the superior incision at the manubrium for cosmetic reasons.

- A tunneling tool is then used to guide the defibrillator lead in the subcutaneous space from the device pocket to the inferior incision and then from the inferior to superior incision. Suture sleeves are applied to the lead and anchored to the fascia to stabilize the lead (Figure 71-4).

- The pulse generator is then connected to the lead and placed within the pocket. The pocket and parasternal incisions are closed with suture in standard fashion (Figure 71-5).

- Defibrillation testing is typically performed at 65 J to establish an adequate safety margin, though the device is programmed to only deliver 80 J biphasic shocks.

TROUBLESHOOTING

An initially unsuccessful attempt at defibrillation warrants reevaluation of the pulse generator and lead location. Minor adjustment of these elements can significantly alter the shock vector and improve defibrillation success. For this reason our practice has been to place the pulse generator laterally with a preference for slight posterior rather than anterior placement.

FOLLOW-UP

Management of patients after S-ICD implantation is similar to management for transvenous ICDs. Device interrogation is typically performed within 24 hours of implant to ensure adequate sensing. Postoperative evaluation of incisions is performed in accord with

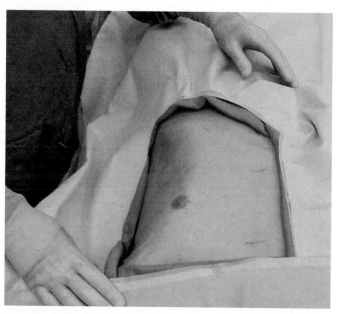

FIGURE 71-3 Two incisions are made 1 to 2 cm to the left of the sternum.

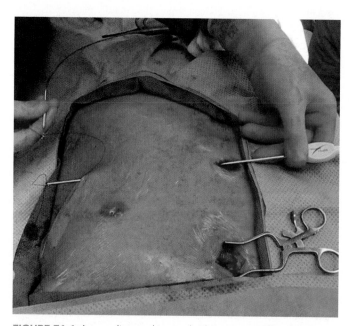

FIGURE 71-4 A tunneling tool is attached via suture to the distal end of the defibrillator lead and tunneled from the pocket to the inferior parasternal incision and then to the superior incision. The lead is secured by suture sleeves at both parasternal incision sites.

SUBCUTANEOUS DEFIBRILLATOR: PATIENT
SELECTION AND IMPLANTATION TECHNIQUE

SECTION IX
IMPLANTABLE CARDIAC DEVICES FOR
MANAGEMENT OF MALIGNANT

475

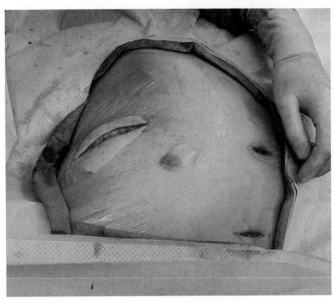

FIGURE 71-5 After the lead is secured, it is connected to the pulse generator, which is placed within the pocket. The pocket and parasternal incisions are closed in standard fashion.

institutional practice for transvenous systems. In contrast to transvenous ICDs, which are typically capable of remote monitoring, the S-ICD is not currently equipped with this feature and therefore requires in-person visits for follow-up interrogations. However, there are minimal parameters to measure, so it only takes 1 to 2 minutes to perform device interrogations and assessment of function.

REFERENCES

1. Epstein AE, Dimarco JP, Ellenbogen KA, et al. ACC/AHA/HRS 2008 guidelines for device-based therapy of cardiac rhythm abnormalities. *Heart Rhythm*. 2008;5(6):e1-62.

2. Bardy GH, Smith WM, Hood MA, et al. An entirely subcutaneous implantable cardioverter-defibrillator. *N Engl J Med*. 2010;363(1):36-44.

3. Gold MR, Theuns DA, Knight BP, et al. Head-to-head comparison of arrhythmia discrimination performance of subcutaneous and transvenous ICD arrhythmia detection algorithms: The START study. *J Cardiovasc Electrophysiol*. 2012;23(4): 359-366.

4. Weiss R, Knight BP, Gold MR, et al. The safety and efficacy of a totally subcutaneous implantable-defibrillator. *Circulation*. 2013;128(9):944-953.

5. Rowley CP, Gold MR. Subcutaneous implantable cardioverter defibrillator. *Circ Arrhythm Electrophysiol*. 2012;5(3):587-593.

6. Lobodzinski SS. Subcutaneous implantable cardioverter-defibrillator (S-ICD). *Cardiol J*. 2011;18(3):326-331.

72 SUBCUTANEOUS DEFIBRILLATOR: APPROPRIATE AND INAPPROPRIATE THERAPIES

Essa Essa, MD, Jose Tores, MD, Raul Weiss, MD

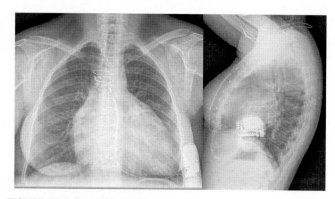

FIGURE 72-1 PA and lateral view of a chest X-ray of a 32-year-old patient with complex CHD and multiple corrective surgeries.

CASE PRESENTATION

The patient is a 32-year-old white woman, 125 pounds, with a body mass index of 23. She has complex congenital heart disease, has undergone multiple surgical repairs as a child, including repair of the atrial and ventricular septal defects, valvular replacement of the aortic, pulmonic, and tricuspid valves, as well as correction of subvalvular aortic stenosis. Originally she had a transvenous (TV) internal cardioverter defibrillator (ICD) that was implanted for a primary prevention indication. Her TV-ICD became infected after a routine generator replacement, requiring an extraction and replacement of the entire system. Unfortunately, a second infection in the newly implanted system occurred, but at this time it was complicated with prosthetic valve endocarditis. After 6 months of intensive care unit hospitalization and surgical interventions to remove the TV-ICD and replace the prosthetic valves, it was decided not to reimplant her with a TV-ICD. Approximately 1 year after discharged, she had an aborted sudden death episode, and she was referred for a secondary prevention ICD implantation. Given her past medical history a subcutaneous (S-ICD) was implanted (Figure 72-1). Baseline sensing was confirmed, ventricular fibrillation (VF) was induced, and her S-ICD converted VF at 65 J standard polarity two consecutive times.

During follow-up she received appropriate therapy for ventricular tachycardia, but she also experienced inappropriate therapies that were managed by reprogramming the sensing vector of the S-ICD.

FUNCTION OF S-ICD

Subcutaneous ICDs are commercially available for management of sudden cardiac death. Patients that potentially can benefit from this therapy are those who have accepted indications for ICD implantation,[1] who do not require antibradycardia pacing, or who have pace-terminable ventricular tachycardia.

Not every patient that has an ICD indication is suitable to be implanted with an S-ICD. Patients have to pass a prescreening 3-lead ECG in the supine and upright position. This prescreening ECG consists of three cutaneous electrodes placed in the proximity where the subcutaneous lead electrodes will be later implanted. This step has to be fulfilled in order to have the device implanted.

The advantage of the S-ICD is that there is no intravascular lead (Figure 72-2). Consequently, the implantation risks related to an intravascular procedure are eliminated, and the long-term risk of endocarditis due to lead infection and the risk associated with lead extraction are also minimal.

The ability of the S-ICD to sense and defibrillate ventricular arrhythmias has been originally questioned, but the safety and efficacy

SUBCUTANEOUS DEFIBRILLATOR: APPROPRIATE AND
INAPPROPRIATE THERAPIES

SECTION IX
IMPLANTABLE CARDIAC DEVICES FOR
MANAGEMENT OF MALIGNANT

477

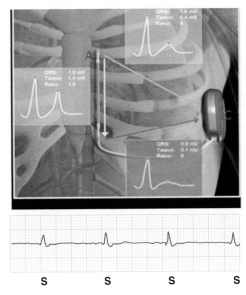
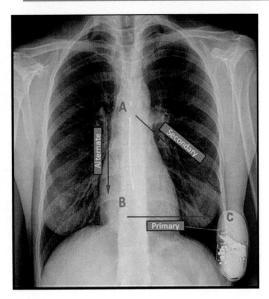

FIGURE 72-2 (A) Schematic representation of SICD pulse generator and subcutaneous electrode and sensing vectors. The electrogram obtained by the SICD is similar to an ECG tracing. (B) Chest x-ray of a patient with an SICD and a schematic representation of the vector.

of the system has recently been confirmed in a landmark study of 330 patients worldwide.[2]

The system consists of a subcutaneous electrode (SE) and a pulse generator (PG). The SE is a multistrand cable-core design, which is unlike a hollow core-design like TV leads. A multistrand design confers a stronger electrode. The polyurethane insulation was designed to withstand cardiopulmonary resuscitation forces, and the subcutaneous placement avoids intracardiac biomechanical stresses. This SE does not need to be as flexible as a TV lead. The PG is a 69-cc device capable of delivering 80 J, postshock, on-demand pacing at 50 beats per minute for up to 30 seconds and storing electrograms for approximately 48 episodes. The S-ICD can be programmed as a single zone in which the rate cut-off is the only determinant for providing therapy, or as a two-zone in which the second zone offers additional discriminators beyond just rate.

S-ICD SENSING AND INAPPROPRIATE SHOCKS

The sensing algorithm used by the S-ICD is a crucial component for appropriate detection and to minimize inappropriate therapies. It differs significantly from the TV ICD in two main ways.

The first difference between the S-ICD and TV-ICD systems is that there is no endocardial sensing lead with an S-ICD. Sensing, therefore, is accomplished via three electrodes. Two of the electrodes are located along the subcutaneous lead (electrode A is at the tip of the lead and electrode B is 15 cm from the tip), and the third electrode is the PG (C electrode) (Figure 72-2). From these three electrodes, three different vectors are generated. The S-ICD automatically chooses the vector with the largest QRS to T-wave ratio, but that vector can be overridden by reprogramming. The QRS to T-wave ratio may vary under different conditions. It can change with body position (patient in the supine versus upright position) or during exercise (Figures 72-3 to 72-5). We have learned that testing sensing during an exercise treadmill test, particularly in young patients, is quite useful in preventing T-wave oversensing (Figure 72-6). In the

patient presented in the case story, there were no further inappropriate therapies with reprogramming of the S-ICD sensing vector from secondary to primary vector configuration.

The second difference between S-ICD and TV-ICD sensing is that S-ICD utilizes a sophisticated sensing algorithm to help minimize inappropriate shocks. This algorithm evaluates the rhythm, but does not use a beat-to-beat assessment, which is the current methodology for a TV-ICD (Figure 72-7).

The S-ICD sensing algorithm has been thoroughly evaluated in the START study[2] and in a large clinical trial.[3] In the START study, the TV-ICD and the S-ICD sensitivity and specificity were compared. This study was performed by inducing VF (shockable rhythm) and atrial fibrillation (nonshockable rhythm) and then recording the rhythms simultaneously from a TV-ICD lead and from three cutaneous electrodes, which were then evaluated offline. The offline analysis passed the recordings through the TV-ICD sensing algorithms (Boston Scientific, Medtronic, and St Jude Medical) and through the sensing algorithm of the S-ICD (Cameron Health/Boston Scientific) in order to compare the sensitivity of the S-ICD to TV-ICDs. All devices, including the S-ICD, demonstrated 100% sensitivity, meaning that all VF episodes were appropriately detected as shockable rhythm. The specificity (the ability of a system to withhold therapy for nonshockable rhythms) was significantly superior for the S-ICD, 98%. The specificity for a single-chamber TV device was 77%, and for a dual-chamber device it was 68%.

In the largest published study,[3] appropriate detection and treatment occurred in 119 spontaneous VT/VF episodes in 21 patients who were treated by the S-ICD (appropriate shocks). In patients with single episodes of VT/VF, the S-ICD appropriately sensed and terminated all episodes (5% of patients required a second shock, and one patient converted while the device was charging to deliver a second shock). Patients with VT/VF storm were also successfully detected and treated by the S-ICD. One of the patients with VF storm is the patient presented in the case story. The ventricular arrhythmias were successfully detected and defibrillated four consecutive times

Sensing configuration: Secondary, gain 1X (initial programming)

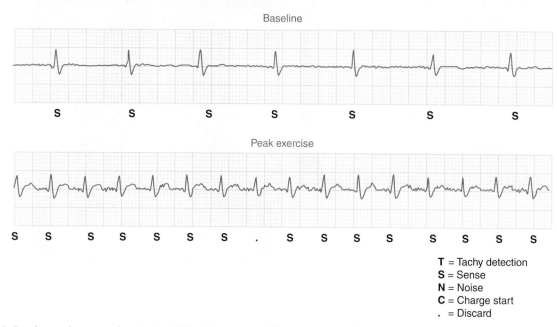

FIGURE 72-3 Baseline and exercise showing the QRS to T-wave ratio. This tracing discarded a single beat because that could not be classified (.).

Sensing configuration: Alternate, gain 1X

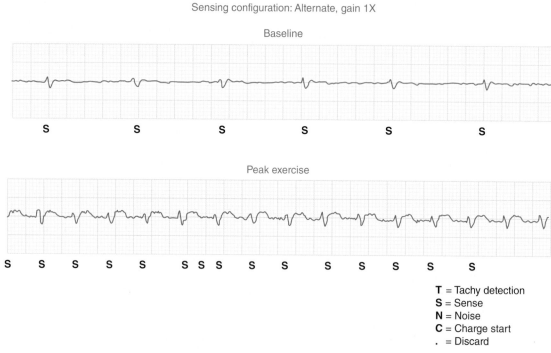

FIGURE 72-4 Shown is the change in the QRS to T-wave ratio in the alternate vector. At baseline sensing is appropriate, but during exercise the QRS to T ratio decreases, and there is occasional oversensing of the T wave.

SUBCUTANEOUS DEFIBRILLATOR: APPROPRIATE AND
INAPPROPRIATE THERAPIES

SECTION IX
IMPLANTABLE CARDIAC DEVICES FOR
MANAGEMENT OF MALIGNANT

479

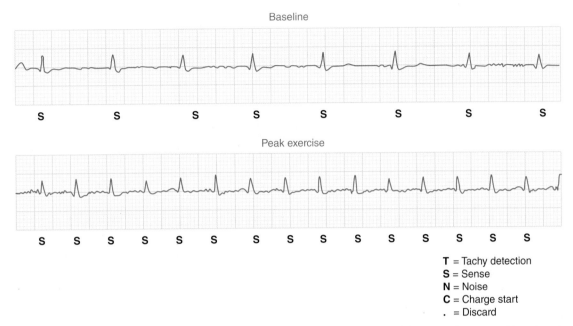

Sensing configuration: Primary, gain 1X (final programming)

Baseline

S   S   S   S   S   S   S   S

Peak exercise

S S S S S S S S S S S S S

T = Tachy detection
S = Sense
N = Noise
C = Charge start
. = Discard

FIGURE 72-5 In the primary vector configuration the QRS to T ratio is appropriate at baseline and during peak exercise. Note there is no increase in the amplitude of the T wave as occurred in the other configuration. There is no under- or oversensing of electrical signal.

(Figures 72-8 to 72-11). In the study, there was no SCD or death related to the S-ICD.

Due to the nature of the charge (nonprogrammable 80 J), the mean charge time is 14 seconds. This charge time allowed 63% of ventricular episodes to self-terminate and did not result in syncope (Figure 72-12). Similar observations were made in the MADIT-RIT trial.[4]

The incidence of inappropriate shocks over a follow-up of approximately 1 year was 13.1%. Supraventricular tachycardia in the high-rate zone (no discriminators), in which rate alone determines whether a shock is delivered, was the cause in 5.1% of patients (Figure 72-13). These inappropriate shocks were representative of normal sensing behavior by the S-ICD system at rates above the high-rate zone. No patient experienced an inappropriate shock in the lower, conditional zone. The most common cause of inappropriate shocks in this study was T-wave oversensing (see Figure 72-7). For our patient, T-wave oversensing was managed by changing vectors and programming a conditional zone. Programming the device and adding a conditional zone, which offers a detection criteria of rate cut off and discriminators, significantly decreased oversensing by 56% and inappropriate therapies for SVT by 70%. Inappropriate shocks

due to T-wave oversensing most often occurs during sinus tachycardia and can be screened by performing exercise treadmill testing and selecting a sensing vector with no T-wave oversensing.

CLINICAL HIGHLIGHTS

- S-ICD is a new device that is safe and effective in preventing sudden cardiac death.

- The sensing algorithm utilized by this device appropriately detects ventricular arrhythmias utilizing electrodes positioned subcutaneously and does not require a TV lead.

- The rate of inappropriate shocks with S-ICD is most often due to T-wave oversensing and is not higher than inappropriate shocks with TV-ICDs.

- Programming a second zone (conditional zone) significantly reduces the risk of inappropriate shocks.

- There is no discrimination error reported for atrial fibrillation in the conditional zone.

- Exercise stress testing is clinically helpful to select the best sensing vector to help reduce T-wave oversensing.

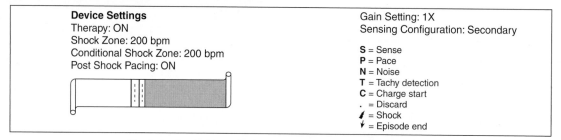

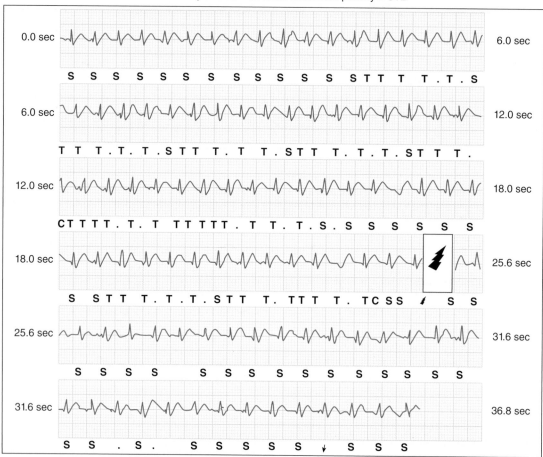

FIGURE 72-6 Sinus tachycardia during exercise with oversensing of the T wave that led to inappropriate shock due to overcounting. It is important to notice that the algorithm shown in Figure 72-2 does not apply because the device does not have any discrimination. Device is programmed as a single zone, cut off rate 200 in the secondary vector configuration.

SUBCUTANEOUS DEFIBRILLATOR: APPROPRIATE AND
INAPPROPRIATE THERAPIES

SECTION IX
IMPLANTABLE CARDIAC DEVICES FOR
MANAGEMENT OF MALIGNANT

481

The SICD system algorithm rhythm detection

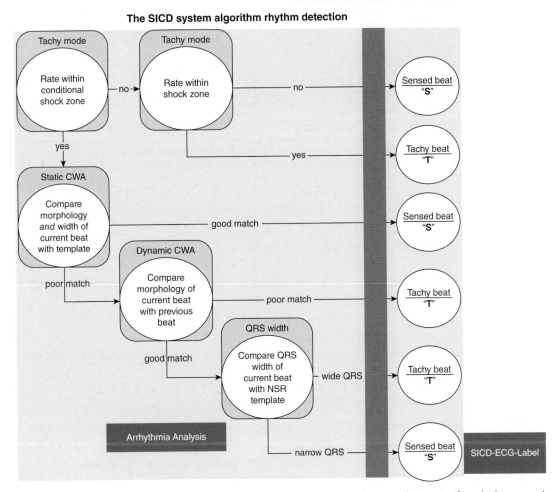

FIGURE 72-7 SICD algorithm for detection of ventricular arrhythmias. The programming of a second zone significantly decreases the number of inappropriate shocks.

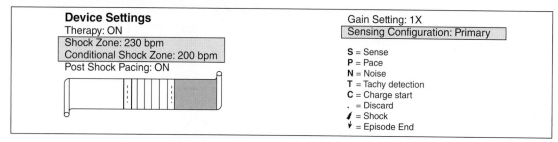

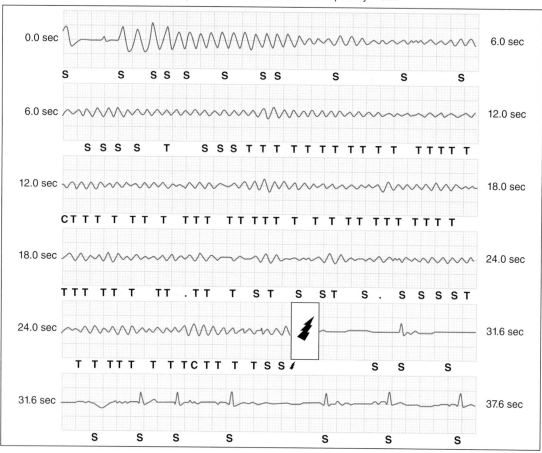

FIGURE 72-8 Approriate detection with occasional undersensing of Ventricular Fibrillation.

SUBCUTANEOUS DEFIBRILLATOR: APPROPRIATE AND
INAPPROPRIATE THERAPIES

SECTION IX
IMPLANTABLE CARDIAC DEVICES FOR
MANAGEMENT OF MALIGNANT

483

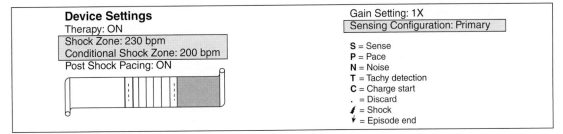

Device Settings
Therapy: ON
Shock Zone: 230 bpm
Conditional Shock Zone: 200 bpm
Post Shock Pacing: ON

Gain Setting: 1X
Sensing Configuration: Primary

S = Sense
P = Pace
N = Noise
T = Tachy detection
C = Charge start
. = Discard
⚡ = Shock
↓ = Episode end

Treated episode 003: 11/17/2010 01:03:44 AM 25 mm/sec 2.5 mm/mV
Shock impedance = 74 ohms Final shock polarity = STD

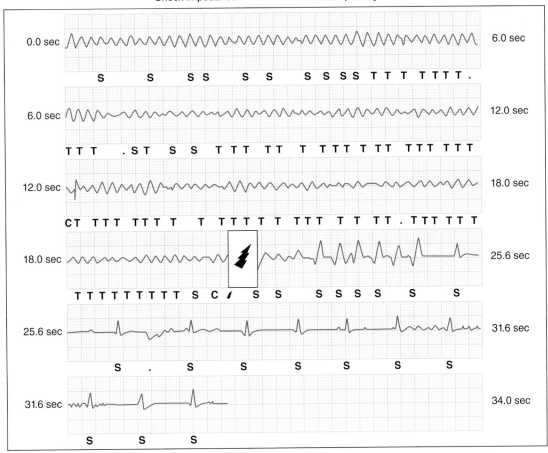

FIGURE 72-9 Appropriate detection and treatment of Ventricular Fibrillation.

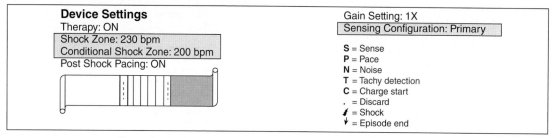

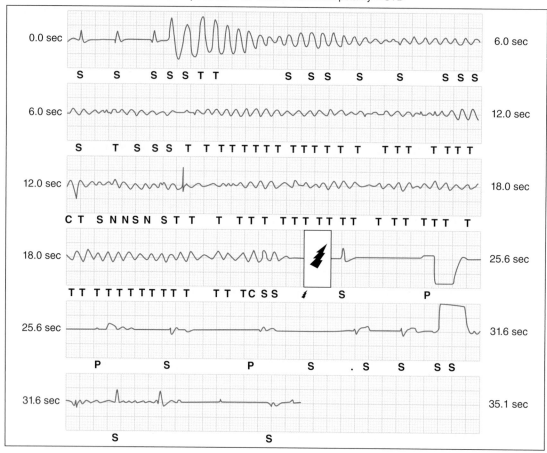

FIGURE 72-10 Appropriate detection and treatment of Ventricular Fibrillation. Also this figure shows post shock pacing (P).

SUBCUTANEOUS DEFIBRILLATOR: APPROPRIATE AND
INAPPROPRIATE THERAPIES

SECTION IX
IMPLANTABLE CARDIAC DEVICES FOR
MANAGEMENT OF MALIGNANT

485

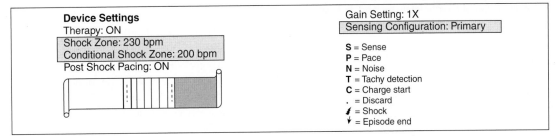

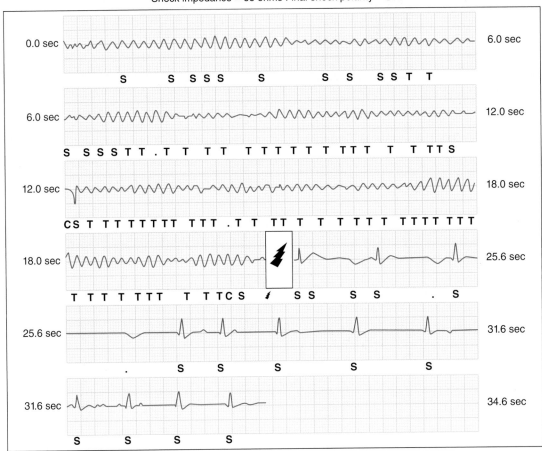

FIGURE 72-11 Initial undersensing of Ventricular Fibrillation with successful detection and appropriate the therapy and restoration of normal sinus rhythm.

Time to therapy:
Unnecesary therapy avoided

- The mean time to therapy for all inductions was 14.6±2.9 seconds, with a range of 9.6 to 29.7 seconds
- Therapy avoided in 63% of patients with VT//VF rhythms meeting criteria to charge without any reports of syncope

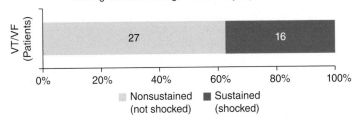

FIGURE 72-12 The charge time to 80 Joules in the SICD, although longer than the transvenous system, allows for spontaneous termination of ventricular rhythms. (Data from Weiss et al. Safety and efficacy of a totally subcutaneous implantable-cardioverter defibrillator. *Circulation.* 2013;Aug 27; 128(9):944-953.)

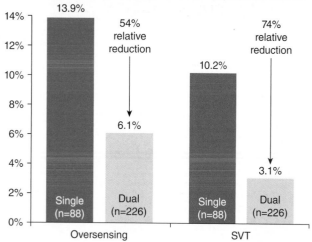

FIGURE 72-13 Reduction of inappropriate shocks by programing a conditional zone with all the rhythm discriminators shown in Figure 72-2. (Modified with permission from Weiss et al. Safety and efficacy of a totally subcutaneous implantable-cardioverter defibrillator. *Circulation.* 2013;Aug 27;128(9):944-953.)

CHAPTER 72

REFERENCES

1. Epstein AE, DiMarco JP, Ellenbogen KA, et al. 2012 ACCF/ AHA/HRS focused update incorporated into the ACCF/AHA/ HRS 2008 guidelines for device-based therapy of cardiac rhythm abnormalities: a report of the American College of Cardiology Foundation/American Heart Association Task Force on Practice Guidelines and the Heart Rhythm Society. *J Am Coll Cardiol.* 2013;61(3):e6-75.

2. Gold, MR, Theuns DA, Knight BP, et al. Head-to-head comparison of arrhythmia discrimination performance of subcutaneous and transvenous ICD arrhythmia detection algorithms: the START Study. *J Cardiovasc Electrophysiol.* 2012;23:359-366.

3. Weiss R, Knight BP, Gold MR, et al. Safety and efficacy of a totally subcutaneous implantable-cardioverter defibrillator. *Circulation.* 2013;128:944-953.

4. Moss AJ, Schuger C, Beck CA, et al; MADIT-RIT Trial Investigators. Reduction in inappropriate therapy and mortality through ICD programming *N Engl J Med.* 2012;367:2275-2283.

DEVICE TROUBLESHOOTING:
CASE I—DIAGNOSIS OF SVT VERSUS VT

SECTION IX
IMPLANTABLE CARDIAC DEVICES FOR
MANAGEMENT OF MALIGNANT

487

73 DEVICE TROUBLESHOOTING: CASE I—DIAGNOSIS OF SVT VERSUS VT

Kelly M.W. McDonnell, DO, Shawn Campbell, MEM,
Kenneth A. Ellenbogen, MD, FHRS

CASE PRESENTATION

A 60-year-old man is seen in evaluation for an ICD shock. He has a history of sick sinus syndrome, nonischemic cardiomyopathy, ejection fraction of 30%, and New York Heart Association class II heart failure symptoms with a dual chamber, single coil ICD for primary prevention of sudden cardiac death. The patient has no history of device therapy but has reported intermittent palpitations prior to this event that he describes as "fast and regular" with sudden onset. Baseline laboratory studies and ECG were normal. The patient denied changes in his medications or baseline health status. The stored event is depicted in Figure 73-1 and demonstrates a tachycardia with 1:1 atrial to ventricular activity.

CASE EXPLANATION

- This is a case of 1:1 tachycardia resulting in ICD therapy. Evaluation of an arrhythmia resulting in a shock requires careful evaluation of the stored electrograms, interval plots, tachycardia initiation, response to antitachycardia pacing (ATP), and arrhythmia termination to determine if the therapy was appropriate or inappropriate.

- Inappropriate shocks are shocks that occur for rhythms other than ventricular tachycardia or ventricular fibrillation and occur in up to 30% of patients with ICD shocks.[1] They are most common due to supraventricular tachycardia (SVT), which gets classified by the device as ventricular tachycardia (VT). It is essential to determine the appropriateness of the shock to guide programming and medical therapy.

- The differential diagnosis of this event with 1:1 AV relationship includes ventricular tachycardia with retrograde atrial activation versus supraventricular tachycardia.

PATHOPHYSIOLOGY

The quintessential reason for implanting an ICD is to provide therapy for a life-threatening rhythm that if left untreated would result in sudden death. Differentiating VT from SVT is a key component of device algorithms to appropriately classify tachycardia events. Enhancements to tachycardia detection include rhythm stability, tachycardia onset, electrogram morphology, atrial to ventricular ratios, and atrial to ventricular timing. No algorithm is perfect in differentiating ventricular tachycardia from supraventricular tachycardia, but each detection enhancement aids in correctly identifying the rhythm.

- Rhythm stability helps differentiate atrial fibrillation with rapid ventricular response from ventricular tachycardia due to the variable R-R intervals seen in atrial fibrillation.

- Onset: Sinus tachycardia tends to gradually increase in rate; whereas other types of supraventricular tachycardia and ventricular tachycardia occur abruptly with a premature complex.

- Morphology templates: Newer algorithms store a baseline morphology of the intrinsic QRS. This is used during rhythm discrimination; SVT usually results in preserved QRS morphology, and VT results in a change in morphology due to the activation sequence. This algorithm is less reliable in patients with a baseline bundle

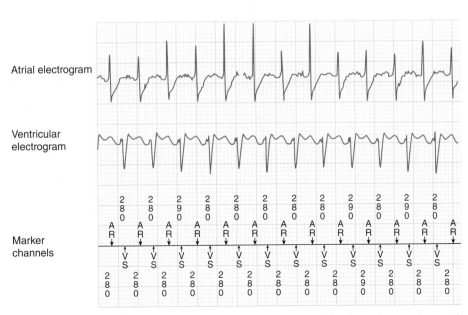

FIGURE 73-1 Documented tachycardia with atrial and ventricular electrograms and marker channel annotations with measured intervals in milliseconds.

branch block or when aberrancy develops during supraventricular tachycardia. Limitations to morphology algorithm, even when the template is regularly updated, include changes in the baseline QRS morphology, problems with alignment in the baseline and tachycardia morphology, and clipping of the signal.

- Atrial to ventricular ratios also assist. In general, A > V suggests SVT or atrial tachycardia, A = V suggest SVT or VT, and V > A suggests ventricular tachycardia.

DIAGNOSIS

The approach to evaluating an episode should be performed in a stepwise fashion.

- The episode text will outline the event, including the classification, duration, and therapy received as seen in Figure 73-2. The device has classified this rhythm as VT and provided therapy.

- The interval plot shows the A-V relationship throughout the event and illustrates the rate in relationship to the programmed VT and VF zones (Figure 73-3). Initially there are slight variations between the atrial and ventricular rhythm followed by an abrupt onset of tachycardia. The interval plot shows that the tachycardia initiated with a V marker and then has a consistent ventricular to atrial relationship. The rate of the rhythm falls into the programmed ventricular tachycardia zone, which triggers the device to detect the event. After detection of the tachycardia, ATP is delivered, which

Episode Summary

Type:	VT
A. Median Cycle:	290 ms
V. Median Cycle:	290 ms
V. Average Cycle:	290 ms
V. Interval Stability:	0 ms - 10 ms
Last Therapy:	VF Rx 1 - Defib. Successful
VT/VF Duration:	20 sec

SVT Criteria Triggered Prior to VT/VF Detection

None

Therapy Sequence

VT Rx 1 Burst	Seq 1	
VF Rx 1 Defib	Energy	0.0 - 28.0 J
	Charge Time	8.13 sec
	Waveform	Biphasic
	Pathway	AX>B
	Delivered Energy	28.1 J
	Impedance	45 ohms

Episode Termination

Parameter Settings

VF	On	290 ms (207 bpm)
FVT	Off	
VT	On	330 ms (182 bpm)

	NID Initial	NID Redetect
VF	12/16	9/12
VT	16	12

Dual Chamber SVT Criteria

AFib/AFlutter	On
Sinus Tach	On
Other 1:1 SVTs	On
SVT Limit	290 ms

Ventricular SVT Criteria

VT Stability	Off

Sensitivity

A. Sensitivity	0.3 mV
V. Sensitivity	0.3 mV

	EGM 1	EGM 2
EGM Source	Atip to Aring	Vtip to Vring
EGM Range	+/– 8 mV	+/– 16 mV

FIGURE 73-2 Event text summary with documentation of the programmed VT and VF zones and detection intervals.

DEVICE TROUBLESHOOTING:
CASE I—DIAGNOSIS OF SVT VERSUS VT

SECTION IX
IMPLANTABLE CARDIAC DEVICES FOR
MANAGEMENT OF MALIGNANT

489

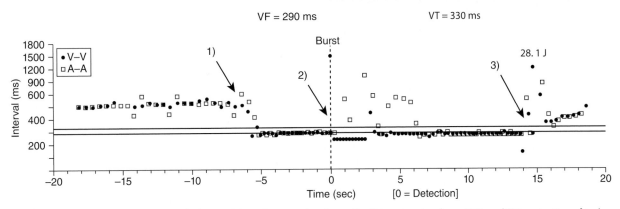

FIGURE 73-3 Interval plot showing baseline rhythm and then 1) onset of tachycardia, 2) burst pacing from ATP, and 3) termination of tachycardia with a 26.1-J shock.

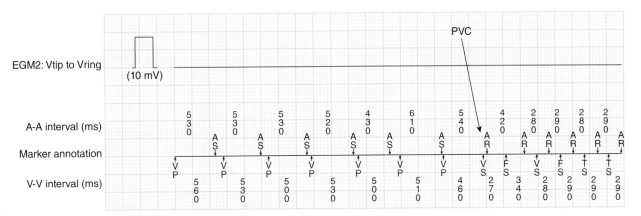

FIGURE 73-4 Initiation of tachycardia with PVC (arrow).

results in AV dissociation and then acceleration of the ventricular rate into the ventricular fibrillation zone. Then a shock is delivered.

- Initiation of tachycardia is seen in Figure 73-4. This event initiates with a PVC, which increases the likelihood of VT but does not exclude SVT (Figure 73-4).
  - The PVC is labeled as VS and occurs at a coupling interval shorter than the previously paced rhythm. The presence of VA conduction is demonstrated with the PVC. Evaluating the marker channels, there is an AR (atrial refractory) immediately after the PVC, consistent with retrograde conduction to the atrium due to the PVC.
  - At onset does the V-V interval predict the cycle length of the next A-A interval (the ventricle is driving the rhythm) or does the A-A predict the V-V (the atrium is driving the rhythm)? In this case it appears that the atrial cycle length predicts the next ventricular rate but then becomes constant at 290 ms. This demonstrates that the ventricle and atrium are linked.
- Evaluate the response to ATP. The change in atrial activity during ventricular pacing makes atrial tachycardia less likely and increases the likelihood of ventricular tachycardia (Figure 73-5).
  - Atrial tachycardia occurs independent of the ventricle and therefore will not be affected by ventricular pacing, although it can terminate if retrograde conduction exists and the atrial rate is increased to the pacing rate during ATP.

  - ATP is also seen to accelerate the ventricular rate and slow the atrial rate (Figure 73-6), more consistent with ventricular tachycardia. This also suggests that there is a rate sensitive relationship between the VA conduction during VT. If this were SVT, the ventricular rate would have slowed in conjunction with the atrial rate.
- Termination: Rhythm stability and duration has been met, and the rhythm is terminated with a 26-J shock (Figure 73-7).

  This patient has ventricular tachycardia with 1:1 retrograde conduction.

MANAGEMENT AND PATIENT EDUCATION

This patient had appropriate detection of his ventricular tachycardia and received appropriate therapy. His programming should reflect changes for secondary prevention of ventricular tachycardia with a detection zone at least 40 ms slower than his slowest VT. The current programming provides this, so he does not require programming changes. The patient had no evidence of reversible causes of his ventricular tachycardia and no change in his baseline status. At this time he does not need further medical intervention. If he has recurrent events then he may be considered for antiarrhythmic therapy or ablation.

The patient must be advised that he is not to drive for a minimum of 6 months due to rapid, hemodynamically significant ventricular tachycardia.

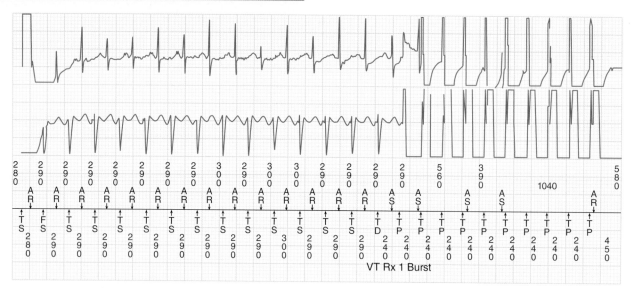

FIGURE 73-5 Initiation of ATP as indicated by TP (tachy pacing) on the marker channel. There is AV dissociation during ATP.

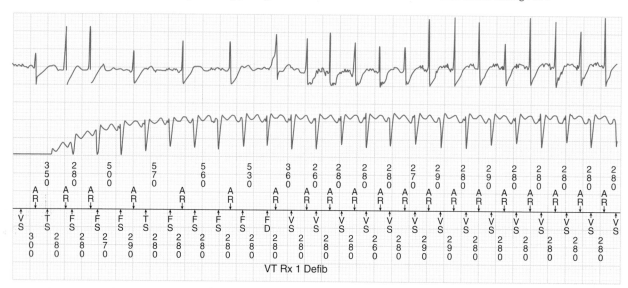

FIGURE 73-6 Termination of ATP with acceleration of the ventricular rate and initial slowing of the atrial rate.

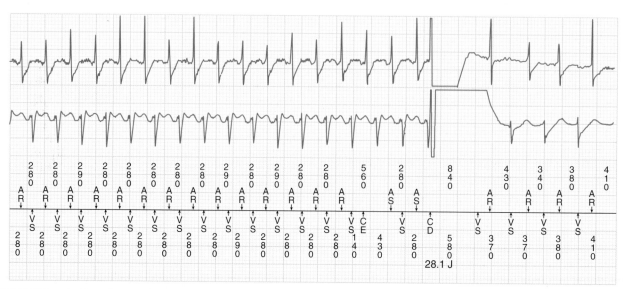

FIGURE 73-7 Termination of ventricular tachycardia with ICD shock.

DEVICE TROUBLESHOOTING:
CASE I—DIAGNOSIS OF SVT VERSUS VT

SECTION IX
IMPLANTABLE CARDIAC DEVICES FOR
MANAGEMENT OF MALIGNANT

491

FOLLOW-UP

The patient should continue to have routine scheduled office or remote follow-up with device checks every 3 months. This will allow for early identification in changes in the patient's rhythm burden.

REFERENCES

1. Ellenbogen KA, Kay GN, Lau CP, Wilkoff BL. *Clinical Cardiac Pacing, Defibrillation and Resynchronization Therapy*. 4th ed. Philadelphia, PA: Elsevier; 2011.

2. Al-Ahmad A, Ellenbogen KA, Natale A, Wang PJ. *Pacemakers and Implantable Cardioverter Defibrillators*. Minneapolis, MN: Cardiotext; 2010.

3. Ellenbogen KE, Wood MA. *Cardiac Pacing and ICDs*. 5th ed. Hoboken, NJ: Blackwell; 2009.

4. Koneru JN, Swerdlow CD, Wood MA, Ellenbogen KA. Minimizing inappropriate or "unnecessary" implantable cardioverter-defibrillator shocks: appropriate programming. *Circ Arrhythm Electrophysiol*. 2011;4(5):778-790.

74 DEVICE TROUBLESHOOTING: CASE II—LEAD/DEVICE NOISE

Kelly M.W. McDonnell, DO, Shawn Campbell, MEM, Kenneth A. Ellenbogen, MD, FHRS

CASE PRESENTATION

A 75-year-old man is seen in the emergency department after receiving multiple shocks from his ICD. He has a history of symptomatic bradycardia, coronary artery disease, ischemic cardiomyopathy, ejection fraction of 20%, and New York Heart Association class II heart failure. A dual chamber ICD was implanted 5 years earlier for primary prevention. The patient has a history of nonsustained ventricular tachycardia with no history of previous ICD therapy delivery. He denies change in medications or clinical status. He has had consistent follow-up with normal device function and lead parameters since implant. Evaluation of the clinical event is demonstrated with the interval plot in Figure 74-1 and the electrograms in Figure 74-2. This demonstrates the appearance of multiple ventricular-sensed events accelerating into the ventricular fibrillation zone and the delivery of multiple shocks during a single event prior to termination.

CASE EXPLANATION

- This is a case of nonphysiologic ventricular-sensed events on the ventricular lead resulting in the classification of ventricular fibrillation and delivery of therapy. Careful evaluation of all telemetered information is required to fully evaluate and classify therapy as appropriate or inappropriate.

- A complete evaluation includes assessment of lead integrity (sensing, impedance, and threshold values), lead parameter trends, device implant history, and imaging studies.

- The differential diagnosis of these events includes both physiologic and nonphysiologic events, such as ventricular fibrillation, lead noise, and electromagnetic interference (EMI).

ETIOLOGY/PATHOPHYSIOLOGY

The delivery of appropriate therapies is the *pièce de résistance* of ICDs. The delivery of multiple shocks can lead to great psychological distress; including depression for patients. When this occurs secondary to oversensing of nonphysiologic events, patients can develop fear and distrust of the reliability of the device designed to save their lives. Rapid intervention to prevent further shocks is essential. If therapy is found to be inappropriate secondary to noise, immediately inactivate all therapies while the patient and the device are evaluated.

The etiology of lead noise can be differentiated based on the number of leads demonstrating noise.

- Noise that is sensed on multiple leads suggests EMI.

- Noise sensed on a single lead can occur secondary to loose set screw, lead fracture, conduction failure, lead dislodgement, or air in the header.

Lead noise can represent lead integrity failure. In 2011, 150 386 new right ventricular ICD leads were implanted in the United States.[1] Lead failure is estimated to occur in 0.58% per year of modern ICD lead implants.[2]

DIAGNOSIS

The approach to determining the etiology of noise artifact in this case includes assessing multiple aspects of the device.

- Clinical history: The patient's history may provide key insight into the etiology of the noise artifact. Inquiry into possible sources of EMI should be made; including magnetic sources, TENS units, or operation of high voltage equipment.

- Implant information: Evaluate the device indication, implant techniques, leads used, or need for device revisions. Timing of noise from device implant or generator change should also be identified.

- Electrocardiogram (ECG): A 12-lead ECG should be performed on all patients with implantable devices. This allows for evaluation of the paced morphology. In particular, it is essential in patients with

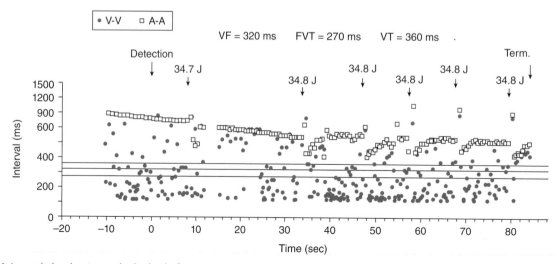

FIGURE 74-1 Interval plot showing multiple shocks for a patient with a lead fracture. The v-v intervals are less than 200 ms and are non-physiologic.

DEVICE TROUBLESHOOTING:
CASE II—LEAD/DEVICE NOISE

SECTION IX
IMPLANTABLE CARDIAC DEVICES FOR
MANAGEMENT OF MALIGNANT

493

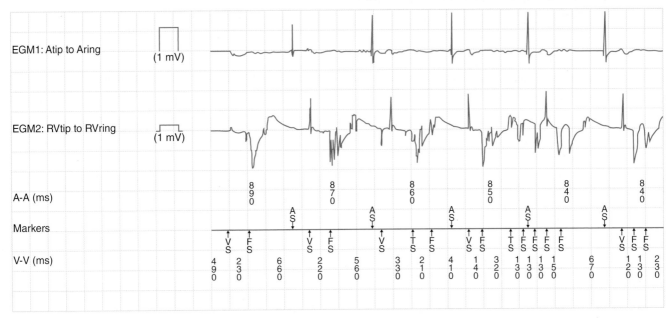

FIGURE 74-2 Intracardiac electrograms from patient with prior dot plot (74-1) showing noise. The tracing shows the typical sporadic, intermittent, high frequency non physiologic signals recorded from the sensed bipolar electrogram.

biventricular devices to assess pacing morphology. It is also useful to compare the implant ECG to the presenting ECG. Sudden change of a right ventricular-paced morphology from a left to right bundle branch block pattern may suggest lead migration or septal perforation.

- Chest X-ray (CXR): Ideally the implant CXR should be compared to a current CXR to assess the device system. The CXR should be used to assess the device location, course of the lead near the clavicle and first rib junction, evaluation of the header with visualization of the lead pin across the set screw, lead integrity with breach of the insulation, and the position of the leads in the cardiac chambers. Comparison with the original CXR will assist with identification of lead position changes or dislodgement. The CXR may also identify defects in the lead or positioning of the lead in the header of the pulse generator.

- Interrogation: A complete device interrogation should be performed on all patients who are identified with lead integrity issues. Lead parameters, programming, trends, histograms, and mode switches should all be clearly assessed. The diagnostic evaluation should also include further maneuvers to exclude myopotential sensing.
  - Sensing counters: Attention should be paid to sensing counters, which will rapidly identify nonphysiologic-sensed signals, which are termed "short V-V intervals" in Medtronic devices. These counters identify ventricular-sensed events that occur at very short cycle lengths and are suggestive of lead damage (Figure 74-3).
  - Lead diagnostics and trends: Sudden changes in a lead parameter typically indicate acute fracture or dislodgement of the lead, versus slow, chronic changes that may indicate changes at the electrode myocardial interface or lead failure. It is important to know that data trends are developed by daily measurements on the leads and represent only a single point in time and do not collect continuous information about lead function. Therefore, lead

integrity problems may not be highlighted if there is intermittent noise or artifact (Figure 74-4).

- Lead recalls: It is prudent to have knowledge of all lead recalls or leads with a higher failure rate. Although all leads carry a risk of lead failure, leads with particular problems should be assessed regularly and have active alerts in place to rapidly identify problems with the lead function.

This patient has lead noise secondary to a lead fracture. His intrinsic rhythm can be seen through the noise artifact (Figure 74-5). He has a Sprint Fidelis RV defibrillation lead with a previously recognized increased risk of lead failure.

MANAGEMENT

The initial management of this patient includes disabling therapy for VT/VF to prevent further unnecessary shocks. He will then need replacement of the ICD lead. The options are replacement of the ICD lead with a new ICD lead if the vein is patent, placement of a new pace-sense lead (again assuming the vein is patent), or lead extraction of the failed ICD lead and placement of a new ICD lead.

Device algorithms have been designed to deal with lead noise. These algorithms include noise reversion algorithms, lead noise algorithms, and lead integrity alerts (LIA).

- Noise reversion algorithms protect against pacing inhibition from artifact sensing. The response to sensed-rapid signals suggestive of nonphysiologic artifact is transient reversion to asynchronous pacing. These algorithms are more difficult to implement in ICDs due to the need to recognize ventricular fibrillation and the risk of undersensing ventricular fibrillation and withholding appropriate therapy.

- Lead noise algorithms (RV lead noise) compares near field electrograms to far field electrograms to determine the presence of noise when short V-V events occur. Noise should be isolated to the near field electrogram (RV tip to RV ring sensed channel in a dedicated

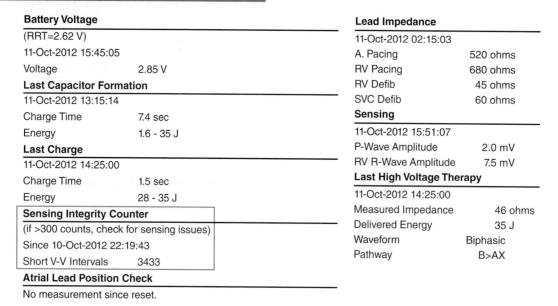

Battery Voltage

(RRT=2.62 V)	
11-Oct-2012 15:45:05	
Voltage	2.85 V

Last Capacitor Formation

11-Oct-2012 13:15:14	
Charge Time	7.4 sec
Energy	1.6 - 35 J

Last Charge

11-Oct-2012 14:25:00	
Charge Time	1.5 sec
Energy	28 - 35 J

Sensing Integrity Counter

(if >300 counts, check for sensing issues)	
Since 10-Oct-2012 22:19:43	
Short V-V Intervals	3433

Atrial Lead Position Check

No measurement since reset.

Lead Impedance

11-Oct-2012 02:15:03	
A. Pacing	520 ohms
RV Pacing	680 ohms
RV Defib	45 ohms
SVC Defib	60 ohms

Sensing

11-Oct-2012 15:51:07	
P-Wave Amplitude	2.0 mV
RV R-Wave Amplitude	7.5 mV

Last High Voltage Therapy

11-Oct-2012 14:25:00	
Measured Impedance	46 ohms
Delivered Energy	35 J
Waveform	Biphasic
Pathway	B>AX

FIGURE 74-3 Interrogated data for patient with the lead fracture showing an elevated sensing integrity counter.

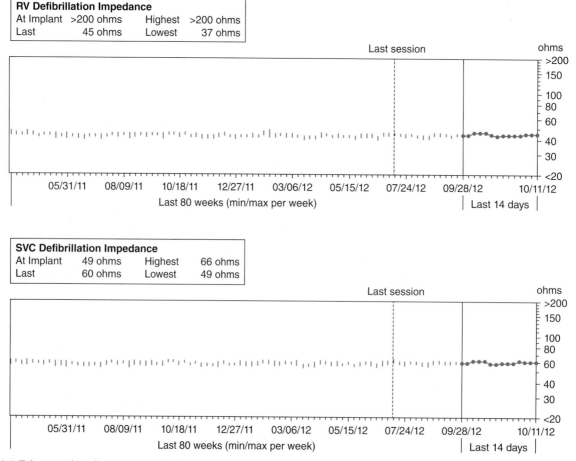

FIGURE 74-4 Telemetry data showing normal right ventricular (RV) and superior vena cava (SVC) defibrillation impedance.

DEVICE TROUBLESHOOTING:
CASE II—LEAD/DEVICE NOISE

SECTION IX
IMPLANTABLE CARDIAC DEVICES FOR
MANAGEMENT OF MALIGNANT

495

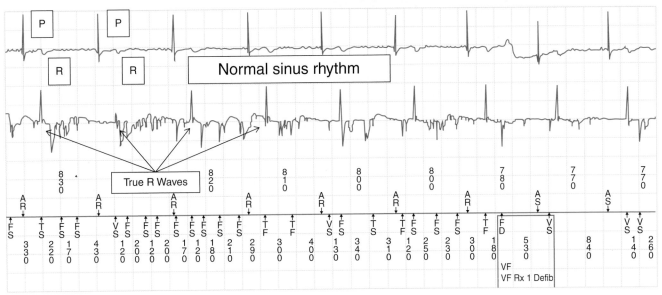

FIGURE 74-5 Intracardiac tracing (atrial electrogram on top, RV pace/sense electrogram in the middle and marker channel on bottom showing noise and non physiologic signals on the right ventricular electrogram.

bipolar ICD lead). If short V-V intervals are noted on both near field and far-field electrograms, then one must be concerned about EMI, noise not limited to the ICD rate sense component, or a true ventricular arrhythmia. If the event is classified as noise, a timeout window is initiated for a nominal 45 seconds, during which detection and therapy is withheld. After the timeout period is completed, redetection is initiated.

- Lead integrity alerts (LIA) are in place to identify possible lead failures and were created for the Sprint Fidelis lead. When two of the three components have fallen outside of the normal parameters, an audible alert sounds for the patient and a transmitted report will be sent to the physician if remote monitoring is being utilized. The components are:

  ○ Greater than 30 short V-V intervals (≤130 ms) in 3 days.
  ○ Abnormal RV lead impedance, defined as a significantly higher or lower value then the calculated baseline. Specifically, a 75% increase or 50% decrease from baseline.
  ○ Nonsustained ventricular episodes (>2 events) with >5 intervals that are shorter then 220 ms.

If noise has been identified and is determined to not be due to lead failure, programming changes can be made. Sensitivity can be increased, but testing to make certain that ventricular fibrillation can still be sensed is mandatory. The VT/VF detection intervals or durations can also be extended. If there is significant concern or proof of lead failure, then ICD lead replacement is necessary.

FOLLOW-UP

Patients with lead concerns should be followed very closely and have remote monitoring for early identification of a problem. Efforts should be made for early intervention and lead revision. After lead revision, the patients will require regular follow-up per standard guidelines for device implants.

REFERENCES

1. Kremers MS, Hammill SC, Berul CL, et al. The National ICD Registry Report: version 2.1 including leads and pediatrics for years 2010 and 2011. *Heart Rhythm*. 2013;10(4):e59-e65.

2. Kalahasty G, Ellenbogen KA. Management of the patient with implantable cardioverter-defibrillator lead failure. *Circulation*. 2011;123:1352-1354.

3. Al-Ahmad A, Ellenbogen KA, Natale A, Wang PJ. *Pacemakers and Implantable Cardioverter Defibrillators*. Minneapolis, MN: Cardiotext; 2010.

4. Ellenbogen KA, Kay GN, Lau CP, Wilkoff BL. *Clinical Cardiac Pacing, Defibrillation and Resynchronization Therapy*. 4th ed. Philadelphia, PA: Elsevier; 2011.

5. Swerdlow CD, Gunderson BD, Ousdigian KT, et al. Downloadable algorithm to reduce inappropriate shocks caused by fractures of implantable cardioverter-defibrillator leads. *Circulation*. 2008;118:2122-2129.

Page numbers followed by f and t refer to figures and tables, respectively.